Food Carotenoids

IFT Press

The *IFT Press* series reflects the mission of the Institute of Food Technologists—to advance the science of food, contributing to healthier people everywhere. Developed in partnership with Wiley, *IFT Press* books serve as leading-edge handbooks for industrial application and reference and as essential texts for academic programs. Crafted through rigorous peer review and meticulous research, *IFT Press* publications represent the latest, most significant resources available to food scientists and related agriculture professionals worldwide. Founded in 1939, the Institute of Food Technologists is a nonprofit scientific society with 18,000 individual members working in food science, food technology, and related professions in industry, academia, and government. IFT serves as a conduit for multidisciplinary science thought leadership, championing the use of sound science across the food value chain through knowledge sharing, education, and advocacy.

WILEY Blackwell

Food Carotenoids

Chemistry, Biology, and Technology

Delia B. Rodriguez-Amaya

University of Campinas, Universidade Federal da Fronteira Sul, Brazil

IFT Press

WILEY Blackwell

Registered Office
John Wiley & Sons, Ltd, The Atrium, Southern Gate, Chichester, West Sussex, PO19 8SQ, UK

Editorial Offices
9600 Garsington Road, Oxford, OX4 2DQ, UK
The Atrium, Southern Gate, Chichester, West Sussex, PO19 8SQ, UK
111 River Street, Hoboken, NJ 07030-5774, USA

For details of our global editorial offices, for customer services, and for information about how to apply for permission to reuse the copyright material in this book, please see our website at www.wiley.com/wiley-blackwell.

Library of Congress Cataloging-in-Publication Data

Rodriguez-Amaya, Delia B., author.
Food carotenoids : chemistry, biology and technology / Delia B. Rodriguez-Amaya.
p. ; cm. – (IFT Press series)
Includes bibliographical references and index.
ISBN 978-1-118-73330-1 (cloth)
I. Title. II. Series: IFT Press series.
[DNLM: 1. Carotenoids. QU 110]
QP671.C35
612′.01528–dc23

2015018743

A catalogue record for this book is available from the British Library.

Wiley also publishes its books in a variety of electronic formats. Some content that appears in print may not be available in electronic books.

Cover image: © Laguna Design/Science Source

Set in 10.5/12.5pt Times by SPi Global, Pondicherry, India
Printed and bound in Singapore by Markono Print Media Pte Ltd

1 2016

Titles in the IFT Press series

- *Accelerating New Food Product Design and Development* (Jacqueline H. Beckley, Elizabeth J. Topp, M. Michele Foley, J.C. Huang, and Witoon Prinyawiwatkul)
- *Advances in Dairy Ingredients* (Geoffrey W. Smithers and Mary Ann Augustin)
- *Anti-Ageing Nutrients: Evidence-Based Prevention of Age-Related Diseases* (Deliminda Neves)
- *Bioactive Compounds from Marine Foods: Plant and Animal Sources* (Blanca Hernandez-Ledesma and Miguel Herrero)
- *Bioactive Proteins and Peptides as Functional Foods and Nutraceuticals* (Yoshinori Mine, Eunice Li-Chan, and Bo Jiang)
- *Biofilms in the Food Environment* (Hans P. Blaschek, Hua H. Wang, and Meredith E. Agle)
- *Calorimetry in Food Processing: Analysis and Design of Food Systems* (Gönül Kaletunç)
- *Coffee: Emerging Health Effects and Disease Prevention* (YiFang Chu)
- *Food Carbohydrate Chemistry* (Ronald E. Wrolstad)
- *Food Industry Design, Technology and Innovation* (Helmut Traitler, Birgit Coleman, and Karen Hofmann)
- *Food Ingredients for the Global Market* (Yao-Wen Huang and Claire L. Kruger)
- *Food Irradiation Research and Technology, second edition* (Christoper H. Sommers and Xuetong Fan)
- *Foodborne Pathogens in the Food Processing Environment: Sources, Detection and Control* (Sadhana Ravishankar, Vijay K. Juneja, and Divya Jaroni)
- *Food Oligosaccharides: Production, Analysis and Bioactivity* (F. Javier Moreno and Maria Luz Sanz
- *Food Texture Design and Optimization* (Yadunandan Lal Dar and Joseph M. Light)
- *High Pressure Processing of Foods* (Christopher J. Doona and Florence E. Feeherry)
- *Hydrocolloids in Food Processing* (Thomas R. Laaman)
- *Improving Import Food Safety* (Wayne C. Ellefson, Lorna Zach, and Darryl Sullivan)
- *Innovative Food Processing Technologies: Advances in Multiphysics Simulation* (Kai Knoerzer, Pablo Juliano, Peter Roupas, and Cornelis Versteeg)
- *Mathematical and Statistical Methods in Food Science and Technology* (Daniel Granato and Gastón Ares)
- *Membrane Processes for Dairy Ingredient Separation* (Kang Hu and James M. Dickson)
- *Microbial Safety of Fresh Produce* (Xuetong Fan, Brendan A. Niemira, Christopher J. Doona, Florence E. Feeherry, and Robert B. Gravani)
- *Microbiology and Technology of Fermented Foods* (Robert W. Hutkins)
- *Multiphysics Simulation of Emerging Food Processing Technologies* (Kai Knoerzer, Pablo Juliano, Peter Roupas, and Cornelis Versteeg)
- *Multivariate and Probabilistic Analyses of Sensory Science Problems* (Jean-François Meullenet, Rui Xiong, and Christopher J. Findlay)
- *Nanoscience and Nanotechnology in Food Systems* (Hongda Chen)
- *Nanotechnology and Functional Foods: Effective Delivery of Bioactive Ingredients* (Cristina Sabliov, Hongda Chen, and Rickey Yada)
- *Natural Food Flavors and Colorants* (Mathew Attokaran)
- *Nondestructive Testing of Food Quality* (Joseph Irudayaraj and Christoph Reh)
- *Nondigestible Carbohydrates and Digestive Health* (Teresa M. Paeschke and William R. Aimutis)
- *Nonthermal Processing Technologies for Food* (Howard Q. Zhang, Gustavo V. Barbosa-Cánovas, V.M. Balasubramaniam, C. Patrick Dunne, Daniel F. Farkas, and James T.C. Yuan)

- *Nutraceuticals, Glycemic Health and Type 2 Diabetes* (Vijai K. Pasupuleti and James W. Anderson)
- *Organic Meat Production and Processing* (Steven C. Ricke, Ellen J. Van Loo, Michael G. Johnson, and Corliss A. O'Bryan)
- *Packaging for Nonthermal Processing of Food* (Jung H. Han)
- *Practical Ethics for the Food Professional: Ethics in Research, Education and the Workplace* (J. Peter Clark and Christopher Ritson)
- *Preharvest and Postharvest Food Safety: Contemporary Issues and Future Directions* (Ross C. Beier, Suresh D. Pillai, and Timothy D. Phillips, Editors; Richard L. Ziprin, Associate Editor)
- *Processing and Nutrition of Fats and Oils* (Ernesto M. Hernandez and Afaf Kamal-Eldin)
- *Processing Organic Foods for the Global Market* (Gwendolyn V. Wyard, Anne Plotto, Jessica Walden, and Kathryn Schuett)
- *Regulation of Functional Foods and Nutraceuticals: A Global Perspective* (Clare M. Hasler)
- *Resistant Starch: Sources, Applications and Health Benefits* (Yong-Cheng Shi and Clodualdo Maningat)
- *Sensory and Consumer Research in Food Product Design and Development* (Howard R. Moskowitz, Jacqueline H. Beckley, and Anna V.A. Resurreccion)
- *Sustainability in the Food Industry* (Cheryl J. Baldwin)
- *Thermal Processing of Foods: Control and Automation* (K.P. Sandeep)
- *Trait-Modified Oils in Foods* (Frank T. Orthoefer and Gary R. List)
- *Water Activity in Foods: Fundamentals and Applications* (Gustavo V. Barbosa-Cánovas, Anthony J. Fontana Jr., Shelly J. Schmidt, and Theodore P. Labuza)
- *Whey Processing, Functionality and Health Benefits* (Charles I. Onwulata and Peter J. Huth)

WILEY Blackwell

Contents

Preface

Foods are man's major sources of carotenoids, and numerous papers on food carotenoids are published every year. Yet published books on carotenoids rarely focus on food carotenoids. The present book aims to fill a long-standing need for a comprehensive treatise dedicated specifically to the multiple facets of food carotenoids. Because of the vast literature on the different aspects of this topic, the task of putting together all pertinent information in one volume has been challenging, often daunting. Nevertheless, it is hoped that the objective has been fulfilled.

The book commences with basic information on food carotenoids, covering nomenclature and structures of carotenes, xanthophylls, *E-Z* isomers, and apocarotenoids (Chapter 1). Also included are physicochemical properties (size, shape, solubility, light absorption, color), antioxidant activity (quenching of singlet oxygen, free radical scavenging), prooxidant effects, and interactions with other antioxidants.

With the successful cloning of the genes for carotenogenic enzymes, the carotenoid biosynthetic pathway is now well established (Chapter 2). It is also now amply documented that the formation of isopentenyl diphosphate in plants occurs primarily through the 2-C-methyl-D-erythritol-4-phosphate (MEP) pathway rather than the mevalonic pathway, as previously thought. Regulation of carotenogenesis and its enhancemernt during fruit ripening are better understood.

Qualitative and quantitative analyses are discussed in Chapter 3, with emphasis on how best to carry out each step and the various errors that can be introduced. Chromatographic separation has been carried out for over two decades by HPLC, but UHPLC is increasingly employed. The importance and applications of UV-visible spectrometry and MS, NMR, NIRS, and Raman spectroscopy are discussed, as well as chemical reactions used in identification. Method validation and quality assurance to guarantee the reliability of analytical data are addressed. The merits and limitations of in vitro assays to assess bioaccessibility and antioxidant capacity are dealt with in Chapter 4.

The enormous efforts directed toward the determination of the carotenoid compositions of foods, along with investigations of the factors that affect the composition, have yielded a wealth of information invaluable to agriculture, food science and technology, nutrition, chemistry, biology, public health, and the medical sciences (Chapter 5). The results obtained attest to the biodiversity of carotenoid sources worldwide. In addition, genetic engineering of the carotenoid biosynthetic pathway in crop plants is being harnessed to obtain higher content or better composition of carotenoids.

Fruits and vegetables, the principal sources of dietary carotenoids, are perishable and mostly seasonal; thus, processing is necessary. Losses of carotenoids, especially during thermal processing, have been a major concern, as shown by the numerous papers on processing effects (Chapter 6). In recent years, nonthermal processing technologies have been introduced to avoid detrimental effects of heating on sensory attributes (color, taste, and texture) and to minimize losses of carotenoids and other bioactive compounds.

Recent studies on microencapsulation and nanoencapsulation to protect carotenoids during processing and storage, and possibly to increase bioavailability, are also presented. Surprisingly, knowledge of the chemistry behind carotenoid losses during processing remains limited and fragmentary, although the general degradation scheme, involving geometric isomerization and oxidation, is known (Chapter 7).

In terms of food quality, the importance of carotenoids lies in their role as food colorants and precursors of aroma compounds (Chapter 8). Carotenoids as food colorants have been extensively studied in earlier years. Presently, research on this topic has centered on biotechnological (microbial) production of potential food colorants. A more recent interest is the investigation of carotenoids as precursors of aroma compound, with enzymatic oxidation being better studied than nonenzymatic oxidation.

Carotenoid bioavailability and the many dietary factors affecting it, including food processing, are discussed in Chapter 9. As background information, current knowledge of absorption, metabolism, and transport of carotenoids in the human body is presented.

The best established function of carotenoids in human health is the provitamin A activity. Chapter 10 discusses bioconversion and the difficulty in establishing vitamin A equivalency of provitamin A carotenoids. Vitamin A deficiency continues to be a serious public health problem in many developing countries. It is evident that there is no single solution for this persisting problem. Countries should choose the strategy that best fits their particular needs and conditions, and simultaneous implementation of interventions is likely to be needed. Periodic supplementation with high-dose vitamin A capsules, food fortification, and dietary diversification have long been proposed. More recently, biofortification and conservation of biodiversity for food and nutrition have been advocated.

The final chapter deals with the other health benefit attributed to carotenoids—their association with reduced risk of several chronic health disorders, including some forms of cancer, cardiovascular diseases, cataract, and macular degeneration. This is a widely discussed topic, addressed in detail in numerous review articles, book chapters, and books, so the reader is referred to these publications for a more detailed discussion. An overview is given in Chapter 11, including a discussion of inherent difficulties in obtaining proof of efficacy.

This book came into being with the support and assistance of many people. I am indebted to my husband Jaime Amaya Farfan, daughters Katherine Grace Amaya Barros and Melisa Ann Amaya, and son-in-law Eduardo Barros for the family atmosphere so conducive to the writing of the book. Knowing that I am not computer savvy, Jaime made sure that my computer was working properly throughout the writing process. I acknowledge with gratitude the efforts of David McDade, who invited me to write the book, project editor Audrie Tan, editorial assistant Lea Abot, and Sandeep Kumar at SPi-Global. Special thanks are due to the dedicated, competent copy editor Skye Loyd and my former secretary Débora de Assis Subirá, who helped me with the figures.

Finally, I wish to thank all carotenoid researchers around the world for the wealth of knowledge that they have provided about these fascinating, multifaceted, multifunctional, but complicated and difficult to investigate natural pigments. I tried to include all relevant papers in the book, but with the enormous literature on this topic, it is likely that I may have missed some important papers. To the authors of papers I may have overlooked, I apologize.

Delia B. Rodriguez-Amaya

1 Nomenclature, structures, and physical and chemical properties

1.1 INTRODUCTION

Carotenoids are naturally occurring yellow, orange, or red pigments, notable for their wide distribution, structural diversity, and multiple functions and actions. It is estimated that about 100 million tons of these compounds are produced annually in nature (Isler et al., 1967). According to the last compilation, approximately 750 naturally occurring carotenoids have been reported, of which about 500 have been properly characterized (Britton et al., 2004). Currently, the total number of reported carotenoids is probably about 800, of which between 520 and 550 have been fully characterized (Britton, personal communication). This number includes the enormous variety of carotenoids in algae, bacteria, and fungi. In foods, they are not as numerous, but the composition can still be complex and variable.

1.2 NOMENCLATURE

A semisystematic nomenclature for carotenoids (Table 1.1) that conveys structural information, including the stereochemistry (three-dimensional structure), was devised by the International Union of Pure and Applied Chemistry and the International Union of Biochemistry (IUPAC/IUB, 1975; Weedon and Moss, 1995). The names are based on the stem name "carotene," preceded by Greek-letter prefixes (β, ε, ψ, κ), that denotes the two end groups, together with the numbering system for the carbon atoms. The numbering of the carotenoid skeleton is shown for lycopene and β-carotene in Figure 1.1. Changes in hydrogenation and the presence of oxygen-containing substituents are indicated by standard prefixes and suffixes used in organic chemistry. The absolute stereochemistry of chiral, optically active carotenoids is indicated by the R/S designation.

Carotenoids have trivial names, usually derived from the biological sources from which they were first isolated. For the sake of simplicity, these short and familiar trivial names will be used throughout this book. The *E/Z* designation is now preferred to indicate the configuration of the double bonds and will be used in this book instead of the still widely used *trans/cis* terminology.

Food Carotenoids: Chemistry, Biology, and Technology, First Edition. Delia B. Rodriguez-Amaya.

Table 1.1 Trivial and semisystematic names of food carotenoids.

Trivial Name	Semisystematic Name
Antheraxanthin	(3S,5R,6S,3′R)-5,6-epoxy-5,6-dihydro-β,β-carotene-3,3′-diol
β-Apo-8′-carotenal	8′-apo-β-caroten-8′-al
β-Apo-10′-carotenal	10′-apo-β-caroten-10′-al
Astaxanthin	(3S,3′S)-3,3′-dihydroxy-β,β-carotene-4,4′-dione
	(3R,3′R)-3,3′-dihydroxy-β,β-carotene-4,4′-dione
	(3R,3′S)-3,3′-dihydroxy-β,β-carotene-4,4′-dione
Aurochrome	5,8,5′,8′-diepoxy-5,8,5′,8′-tetrahydro-β,β-carotene
Auroxanthin	(3S,5R,8RS,3′S,5′R,8′RS)-5,8,5′,8′-diepoxy-5,8,5′,8′-tetrahydro-β,β- carotene-3,3′-diol
Bixin	methyl hydrogen (9′Z)-6,6′-diapocarotene-6,6′-dioate
Canthaxanthin	β,β-carotene-4,4′-dione
Capsanthin	(3R,3′S,5′R)-3,3′-dihydroxy-β,κ-caroten-6′-one
Capsorubin	(3R,5R,3′S,5′R)-3,3′-dihydroxy-κ,κ-carotene-6,6′-dione
α-Carotene	(6′R)-β,ε-carotene
β-Carotene	β,β-carotene
β-Carotene-5,6-epoxide	(5R,6S)-5,6-epoxy-5,6-dihydro-β,β-carotene
β-Carotene-5,6,5′,6′-diepoxide	5,6,5′,6′-diepoxy-5,6,5′,6′-tetrahydro-β,β-carotene
δ-Carotene	(6R)-ε,ψ-carotene
ε-Carotene	(6R,6′R)-ε,ε-carotene
γ-Carotene	β,ψ-carotene
ζ-Carotene	7,8,7′,8′-tetrahydro-ψ,ψ-carotene
Citranaxanthin	5′,6′-dihydro-5′-apo-18′-nor-β-caroten-6′-one
Crocetin	8,8′-diapocarotene-8,8′-dioic acid
β-Citraurin	(3R)-3-hydroxy-8′-apo-β-caroten-8′-al
Cryptoflavin	5,8-epoxy-5,8-dihydro-β,β-caroten-3-ol
α-Cryptoxanthin	(3′R,6′R)-β,ε-caroten-3′-ol
β-Cryptoxanthin	(3R)-β,β-caroten-3-ol
β-Cryptoxanthin-5,6-epoxide	5,6-epoxy-5,6-dihydro-β,β-caroten-3-ol
Echinenone	β,β-caroten-4-one
Fucoxanthin	(3S,5R,6S,3′S,5′R,6′R)-5,6-epoxy-3′-ethanoyloxy-3,5′-dihydroxy-6′,7′-didehydro-5,6,7,8, 5′,6′-hexahydro-β,β-caroten-8-one
Isocryptoxanthin	β,β-caroten-4-ol
Isozeaxanthin	β,β-carotene-4,4′-diol
Lactucaxanthin	(3R,6R,3′R,6′R)-ε,ε-carotene-3,3′-diol
Lutein	(3R,3′R,6′R)-β,ε-carotene-3,3′-diol
Lutein-5,6-epoxide	(3S,5R,6S,3′R,6′R)-5,6-epoxy-5,6-dihydro-β,ε-carotene-3,3′-diol
Luteochrome	5,6,5′,8′-diepoxy-5,6,5′,8′-tetrahydro-β,β-carotene
Luteoxanthin	5,6,5′,8′-diepoxy-5,6,5′,8′-tetrahydro-β,β-carotene-3,3′-diol
Lycopene	ψ,ψ-carotene
Lycophyll	ψ,ψ-carotene-16,16′-diol
Lycoxanthin	ψ,ψ-caroten-16-diol
Mutatochrome	5,8-epoxy-5,8-dihydro-β,β-carotene
Mutatoxanthin	(3S,5R,8RS,3′R)-5,8-epoxy-5,8-dihydro-β,β-carotene-3,3′-diol
Neochrome	5′,8′-epoxy-6,7-didehydro-5,6,5′,8′-tetrahydro-β,β-carotene-3,5,3′-triol
Neoxanthin	(3S,5R,6R,3′S,5′R,6′S)-5′,6′-epoxy-6,7-didehydro-5,6,5′,6′-tetrahydro-β,β-carotene-3,5,3′-triol
Neurosporene	7,8-dihydro-ψ,ψ-carotene
Phytoene	7,8,11,12,7′,8′,11′12′-octahydro-ψ,ψ-carotene
Phytofluene	7,8,11,12,7′,8′-hexahydro-ψ,ψ-carotene
Rubixanthin	(3R)-β,ψ-caroten-3-ol
Violaxanthin	(3S,5R,6S,3′S,5′R,6′S)-5,6,5′,6′-diepoxy-5,6,5′,6′-tetrahydro-β,β-carotene-3,3′-diol
α-Zeacarotene	(6R)-7′,8′-dihydro-ε,ψ-carotene
β-Zeacarotene	7′,8′-dihydro-β,ψ-carotene
Zeaxanthin	(3R,3′R)-β,β-carotene-3,3′-diol
Zeinoxanthin	(3R,6′R)-β,ε-carotene-3-ol

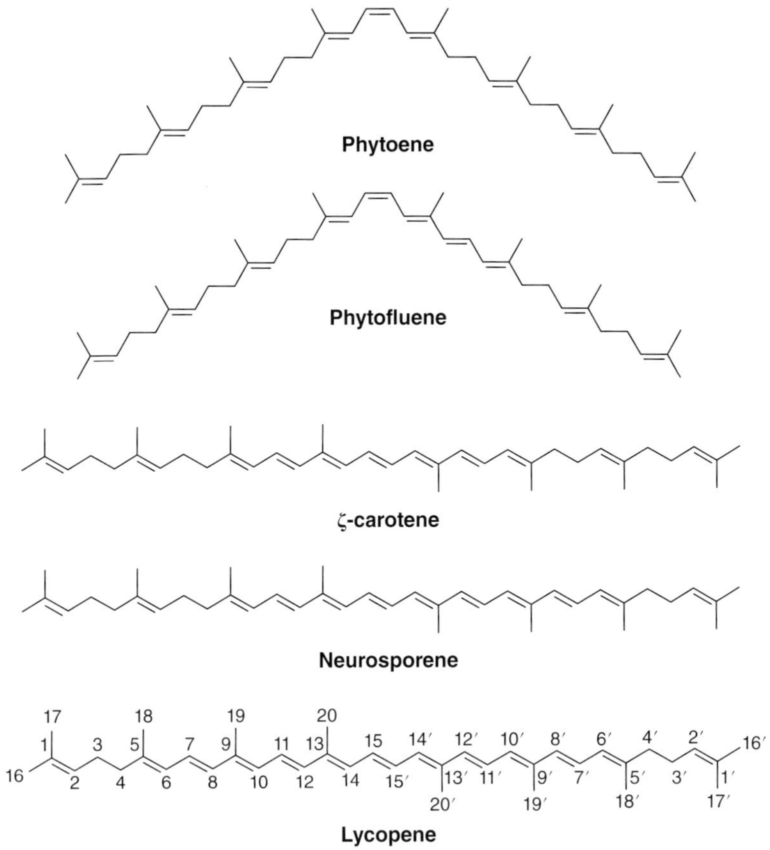

Figure 1.1 Structures of food carotenes.

1.3 NATURE OF CAROTENOIDS IN FOODS

Carotenoids in foods are generally C_{40} tetraterpenes/tetraterpenoids formed from eight C_5 isoprenoid units joined head to tail, except at the center where a tail-to-tail linkage reverses the order, resulting in a symmetrical molecule (Figure 1.1). The most distinctive structural feature is a centrally located, long system of alternating double and single bonds, in which the π-electrons are effectively delocalized throughout the entire polyene chain. This conjugated double-bond system constitutes the light-absorbing chromophore that gives carotenoids their attractive color and is mainly responsible for their special properties and many functions. However, it also renders the molecule susceptible to geometric isomerization and oxidative degradation.

The basic linear and symmetrical skeleton has lateral methyl groups separated by six C-atoms at the center and the others by five C-atoms. Modification occurs in many ways, including cyclization, hydrogenation, dehydrogenation, introduction of oxygen-containing groups, migration of the double bonds, rearrangement, chain shortening or extension, or combinations thereof, resulting in a wide array of structures.

Carotenoids may be acyclic (e.g., lycopene, ζ-carotene) or may have a six-membered ring at one (e.g., γ-carotene, δ-carotene) or both ends (e.g., β-carotene, α-carotene) of the molecule. Exceptionally, capsanthin and capsorubin have five-membered rings.

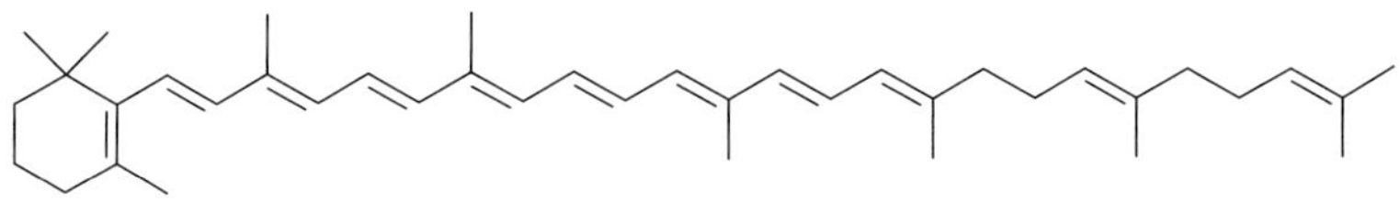

β-zeacarotene

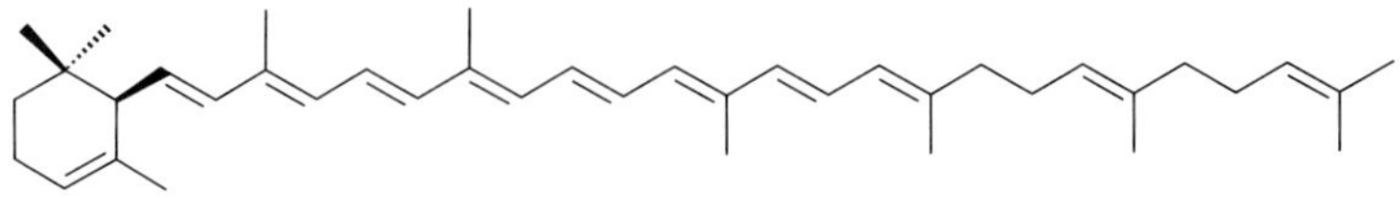

α-zeacarotene

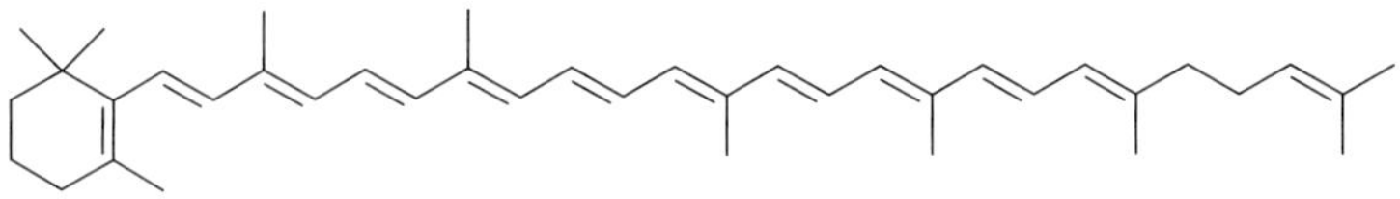

γ-carotene

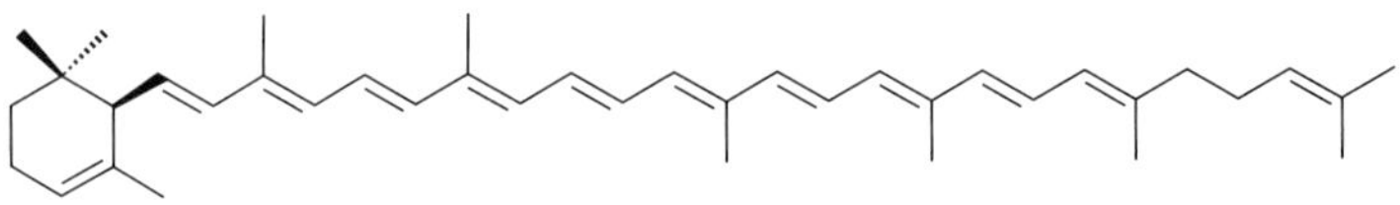

δ-carotene

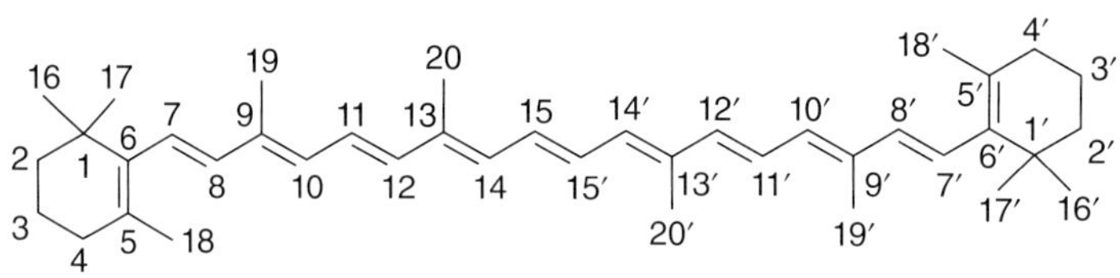

β-carotene

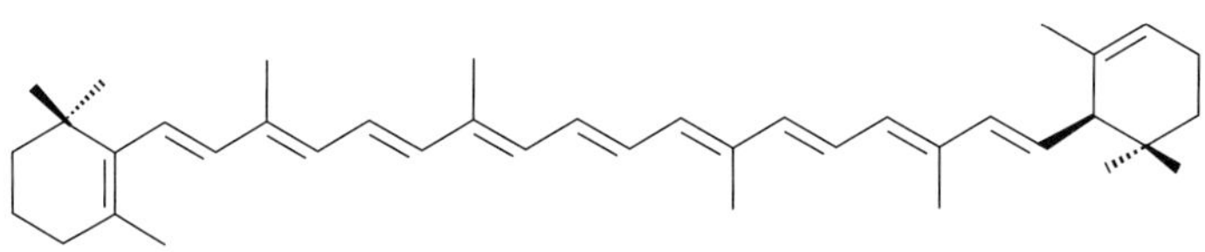

α-carotene

Figure 1.1 (*Continued*)

Hydrocarbon carotenoids (e.g., β-carotene, lycopene) are known as carotenes, and the oxygenated derivatives are called xanthophylls. Common oxygen-containing groups are hydroxyl (as in β-cryptoxanthin), keto (as in canthaxanthin), epoxy (as in violaxanthin), and aldehyde (as in β-citraurin) substituents. These functional groups are mainly responsible for the degree of polarity, solubility, and chemical behavior of the xanthophylls.

In foods, about a hundred carotenoids have been found. Typically a plant food would have one to five major carotenoids with a series of carotenoids in trace or very small amounts (Rodriguez-Amaya, 1999). Because plants are able to synthesize carotenoids de novo, along with the principal carotenoids, low levels of their biosynthetic precursors and derivatives are also found. The carotenoid composition is variable and usually complex. These carotenoids are located in subcellular organelles (plastids), mainly associated with proteins in the chloroplasts and deposited in crystalline form or as oily droplets in chromoplasts (Bartley and Scolnik, 1995).

Unable to biosynthesize carotenoids, animals are limited to absorbing dietary carotenoids, which are accumulated unchanged or slightly altered to form carotenoids typical of animal species. Consequently, carotenoids are not as widely distributed in foods of animal origin and the composition is simpler.

1.3.1 Carotenes

Of the acyclic carotenes (Figure 1.1), lycopene and ζ-carotene are the most common. Lycopene is not as widely encountered as ζ-carotene, but when found in fruits and fruit vegetables, it is usually the predominating pigment. Examples of lycopene food sources are red- or pink-fleshed tomato, watermelon, papaya, guava, grapefruit, and the Brazilian fruit pitanga (Rodriguez-Amaya et al., 2008).

ζ-carotene is ubiquitous, but it is usually present at low levels except in Brazilian passion fruit and in carambola, in which it occurs as a major pigment. Phytoene and phytofluene are probably more widely distributed than reported; because they are both colorless, their presence may often be overlooked. Neurosporene, when found in foods, is usually in small amounts.

The bicyclic β-carotene (Figure 1.1) is the most widespread of all food carotenoids, found in virtually all foods analyzed, as a minor or as the major pigment (Rodriguez-Amaya et al., 2008). Examples of foods where β-carotene is the main carotenoid are acerola, apricot, carrot, loquat, melons, orange-fleshed sweet potato, and palm fruits. The bicyclic α-carotene and the monocyclic γ-carotene sometimes accompany β-carotene, generally at much lower concentrations. Appreciable amounts of α-carotene are found in carrot, red palm oil, and some varieties of squash and pumpkin. High levels of γ-carotene are found in rose hips and pitanga. Less frequently encountered is δ-carotene, although it is the principal carotenoid of the high delta strain of tomato and the Brazilian peach palm fruit.

1.3.2 Xanthophylls

A wide variety of xanthophylls are found in foods (Figure 1.2). The hydroxylated lycopenes, lycoxanthin and lycophyll, are rarely encountered; they are sometimes found in trace amounts in tomato. Rubixanthin, a derivative of γ-carotene, is the main pigment of rose hips (Hornero-Méndez and Mínguez-Mosquera, 2000) and also occurs in appreciable amount in pitanga. β-Cryptoxanthin is the main pigment of many orange-fleshed fruits, such as peach, nectarine, orange-fleshed papaya, persimmon, fruit of the tree tomato, and the Brazilian fruit *Spondias lutea* (Rodriguez-Amaya et al., 2008). It often appears as a secondary pigment.

Interestingly, in contrast to the relative abundance of the parent carotenes, with β-carotene predominating over α-carotene, lutein (dihydroxy derivative of α-carotene) is normally present in plant tissues at considerably higher levels than zeaxanthin (dihydroxy derivative of β-carotene). Lutein is the predominant carotenoid in yellow edible flowers,

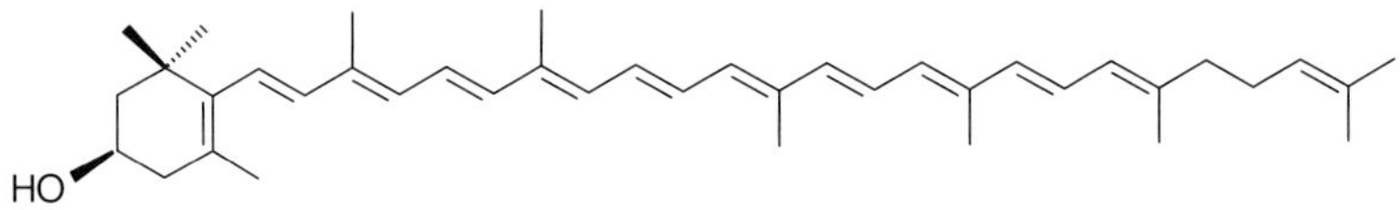

Rubixanthin

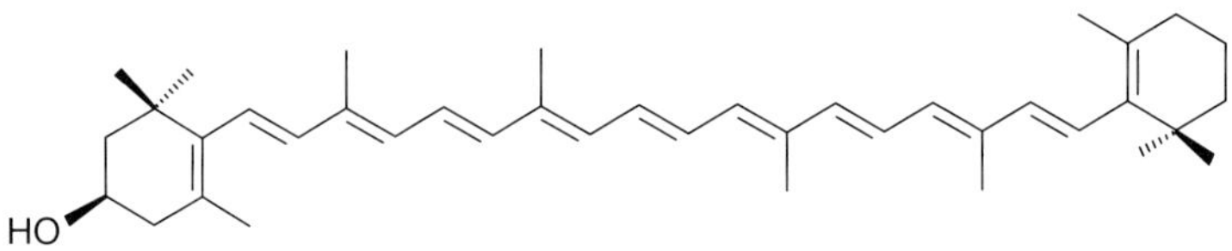

β-cryptoxanthin

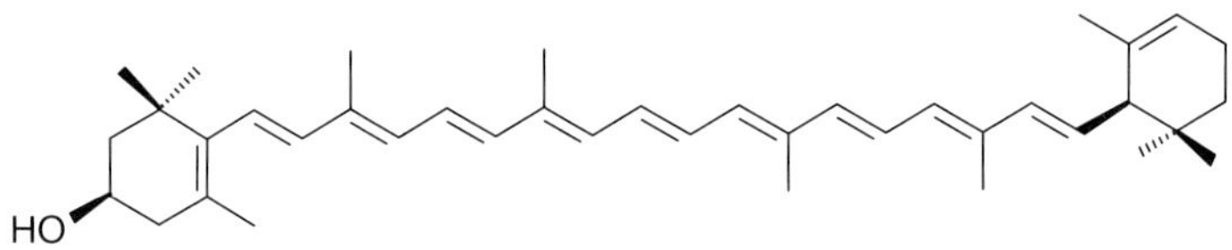

Zeinoxanthin

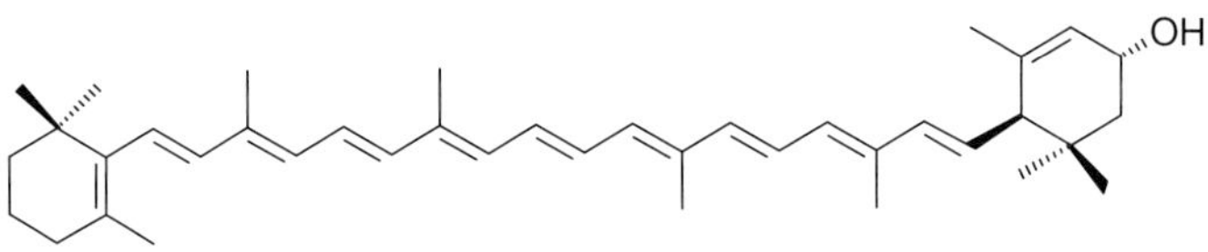

α-cryptoxanthin

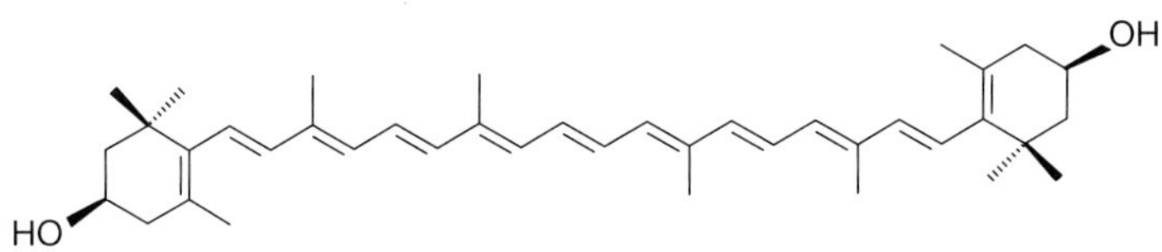

Zeaxanthin

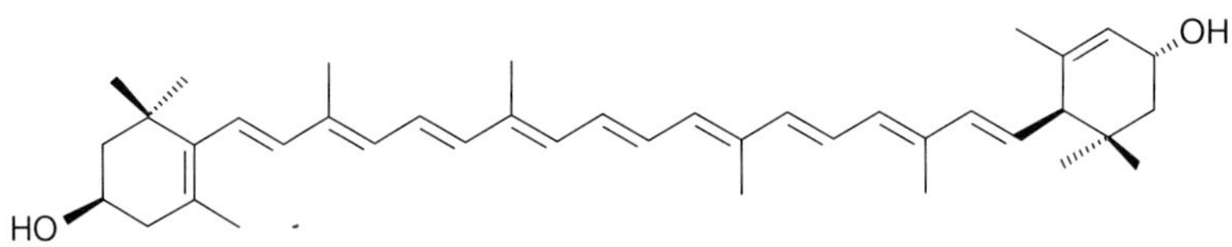

Lutein

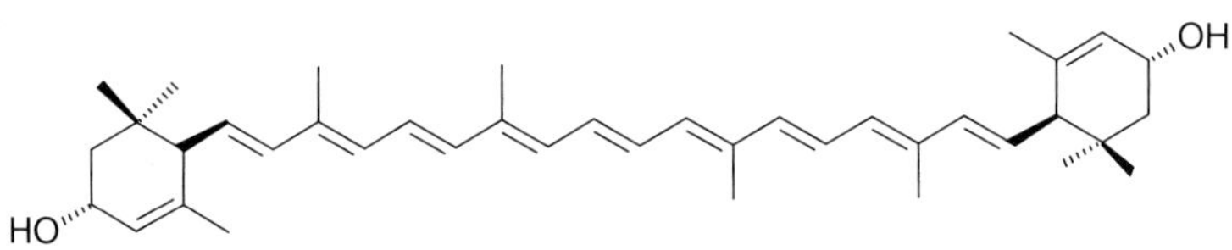

Lactucaxanthin

Figure 1.2 Structures of food xanthophylls.

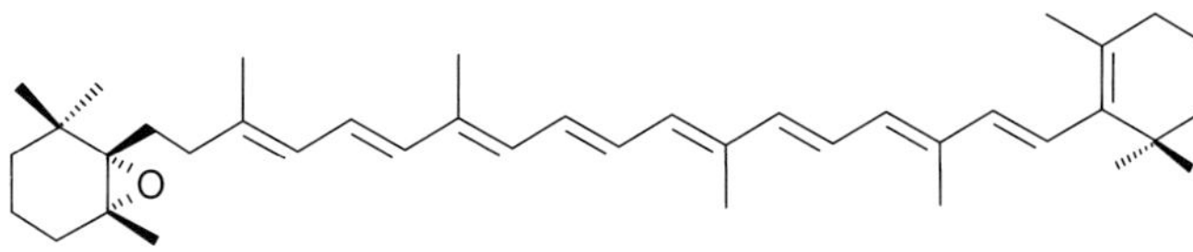

β-carotene-5,6-epoxide

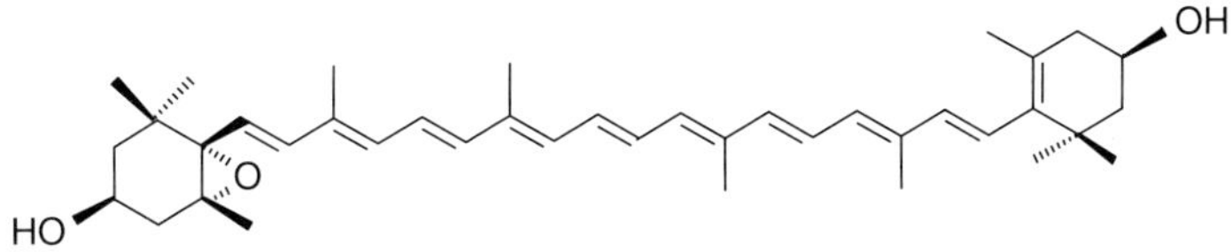

Antheraxanthin

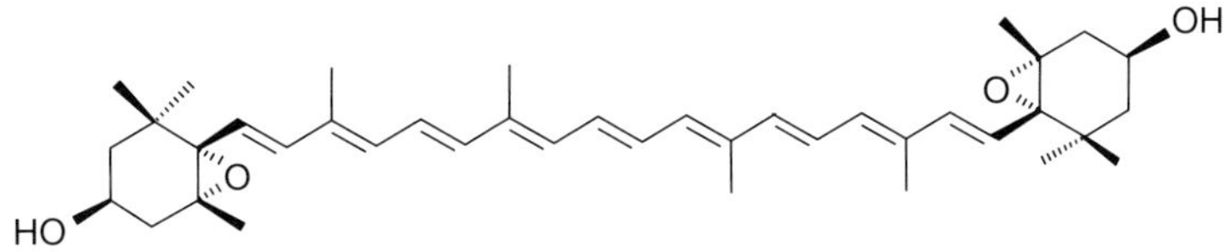

Violaxanthin

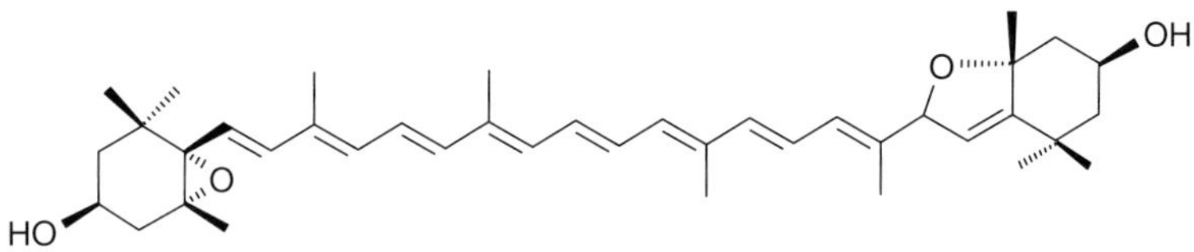

Luteoxanthin

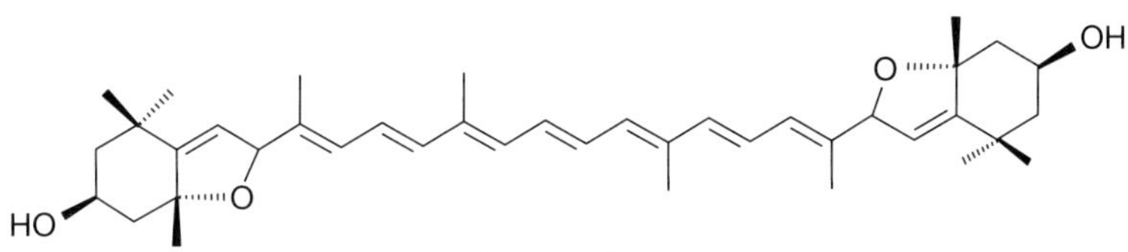

Auroxanthin

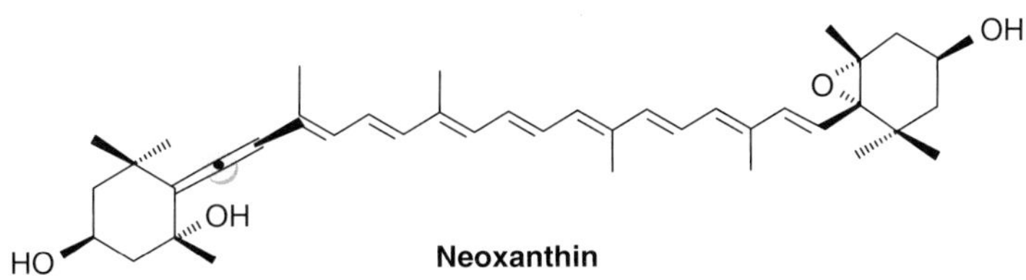

Neoxanthin

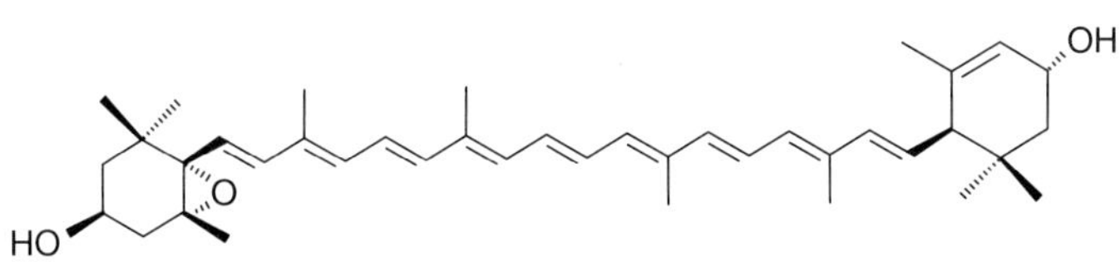

Lutein-5,6-epoxide

Figure 1.2 *(Continued)*

green leaves and other green vegetables, and some varieties of *Cucurbita maxima* (Rodriguez-Amaya et al., 2008). Except for yellow corn, the Brazilian fruit *Cariocar villosium*, and the East Asian fruit goji (*Lycium barbarium*) (Peng et al., 2005), in which it is the major pigment, zeaxanthin is a minor food carotenoid. It does not usually reach high levels because biosynthesis often stops at the precursor β-carotene, which is the preponderant pigment of many foods. Moreover, when formed, zeaxanthin is easily transformed to violaxanthin. Lutein appears to undergo limited epoxidation. The monohydroxy derivatives of α-carotene, α-cryptoxanthin, and zeinoxanthin, are minor carotenoids of some foods.

Carotenols in green leaves (Kobori and Rodriguez-Amaya, 2008) are unesterified, and those of corn (Rodriguez-Amaya and Kimura, 2004; Oliveira and Rodriguez-Amaya, 2007) are mostly unesterified. Carotenols in ripe fruits are generally esterified with fatty acids. However, the carotenols of a few fruits, particularly those that remain green when ripe, such as kiwi (Gross, 1987), undergo limited or no esterification. The principal carotenoid, lutein, occurs free or esterified in one (monoester) or both hydroxyl groups (diester) in the edible nasturtium (Niizu and Rodriguez-Amaya, 2005) and marigold (Breithaupt et al., 2002) flowers, with the esters predominating. Esterification, which occurs progressively during maturation, appears to be important physiologically. Acylation increases the lipophilic character of the xanthophylls, facilitating their accumulation in the chromoplasts (Gross, 1987).

Epoxy carotenoids comprise a large group of xanthophylls in foods. The zeaxanthin epoxide derivatives, antheraxanthin, mutatoxanthin, violaxanthin, luteoxanthin, auroxanthin, and neoxanthin, are widely encountered. The 5,8-epoxide of neoxanthin, neochrome, is occasionally detected.

The epoxides derived from β-carotene, β-carotene-5,6-epoxide, β-carotene-5,8-epoxide (mutatochrome), β-carotene-5,6,5′,6′-diepoxide, β-carotene-5,6,5′,8′-diepoxide (luteochrome), and β-carotene-5,8,5′,8′-diepoxide (aurochrome), and those of β-cryptoxanthin, especially β-cryptoxanthin-5,6-epoxide and β-cryptoxanthin-5,8-epoxide (cryptoflavin), are also frequently found.

Except for violaxanthin and neoxanthin, carotenoid epoxides are usually detected in trace levels. Because they can be generated during analysis, in spite of their wide distribution, their natural occurrence is often questioned. Easily degraded, violaxanthin may be underestimated in foods, as was shown in mango (Mercadante and Rodriguez-Amaya, 1998). In commercially processed mango juice, violaxanthin, the main carotenoid of the unprocessed fruit, was not detected. Instead the 5,8,5′,8′-diepoxy derivative, auroxanthin, appeared in appreciable amounts.

The existence of species-specific carotenoids (Figure 1.3) has also been demonstrated. The most prominent examples are capsanthin and capsorubin, the predominant pigments of red pepper. Carotenoids with two ε-rings are rare, and of the many leafy vegetables and fruits already analyzed, lactucaxanthin (Figure 1.2) has been found only in lettuce.

Although not as widely distributed and not as structurally diverse as in plants, carotenoids also occur in animal products. Astaxanthin (Figure 1.4) is the main carotenoid of some fish, such as salmon and trout, as well as crustaceans (e.g., shrimp, lobster, and crab). In salmon, it occurs in three optical forms: 75%–85% (3S,3′S), 12%–17%

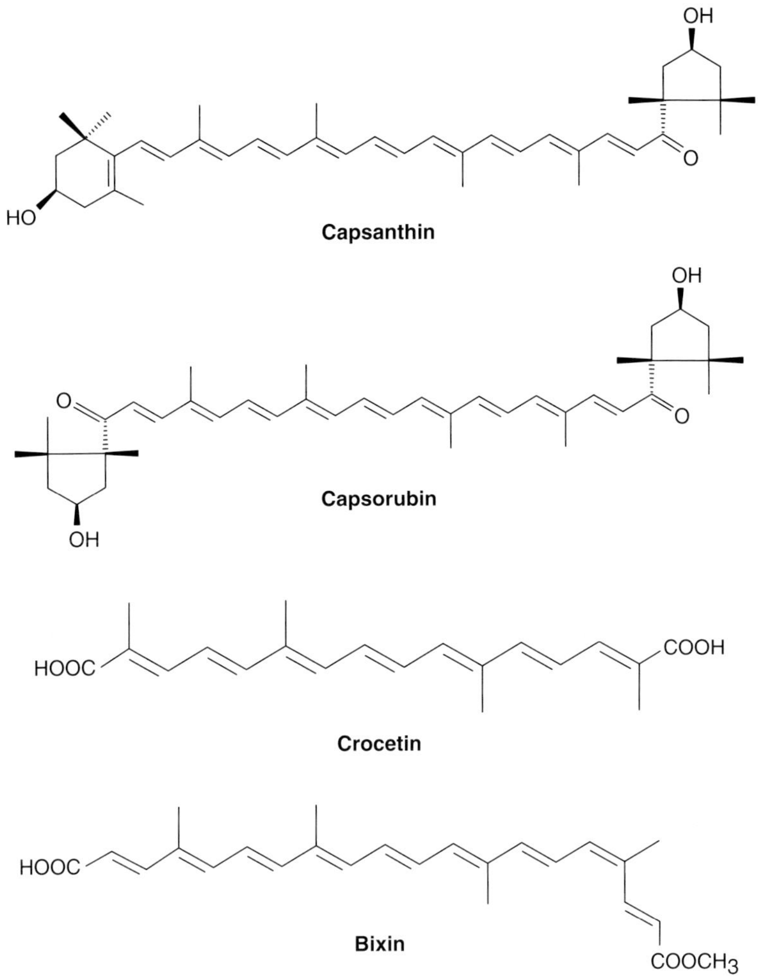

Figure 1.3 Structures of major carotenoids in food colorants.

(3R,3′R), and 2%–6% (3R,3′S, *meso*) (Schiedt, 1998). The three isomers are also found in shrimp as a 1:2 (meso form):1 mixture. In lobster all three isomers are equally well bound in the blue crustacyanin astaxanthin complex (Renstrom et al., 1982). The marketed synthetic astaxanthin is also a 1:2 (meso form):1 mixture, whereas that produced by the alga *Haematococcus* sp. is the optically pure (3S,3′S) isomer. The intermediates in the transformation of dietary carotenoids to astaxanthin, such as canthaxanthin, echinenone, isocryptoxanthin, and isozeaxanthin, are often detected as accompanying minor carotenoids. Tunaxanthin in its various stereoisomeric forms is also a major carotenoid of fish.

Astaxanthin may be found free, esterified in one or both hydroxyl groups with fatty acids, or as a complex with proteins (carotenoproteins) or lipoproteins (carotenolipoproteins) (Shahidi and Brown, 1998). Crustacean astaxanthin is a mixture of the three

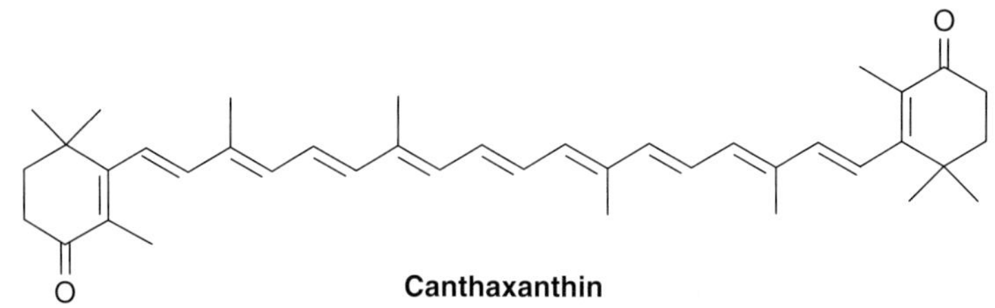

Canthaxanthin

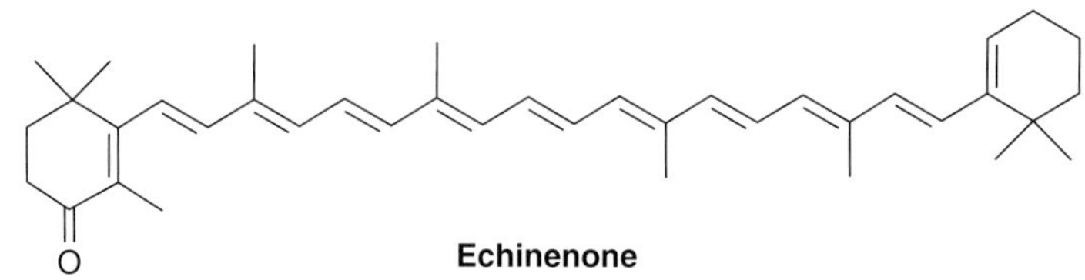

Echinenone

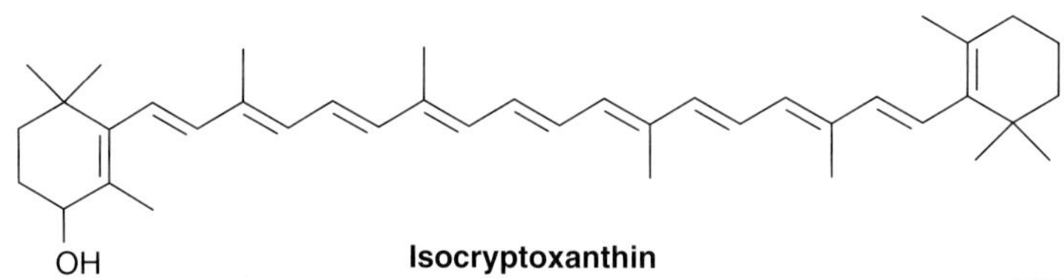

Isocryptoxanthin

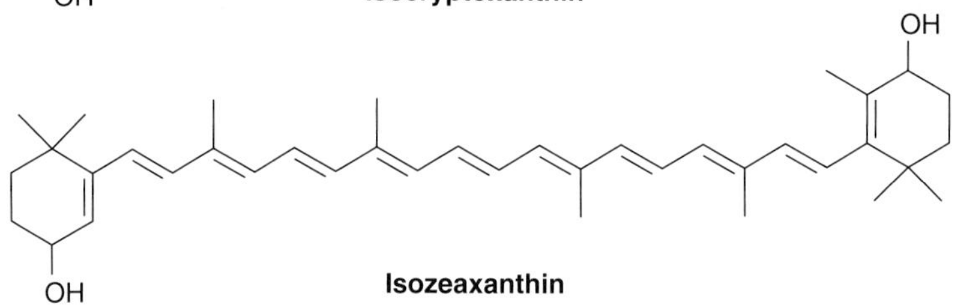

Isozeaxanthin

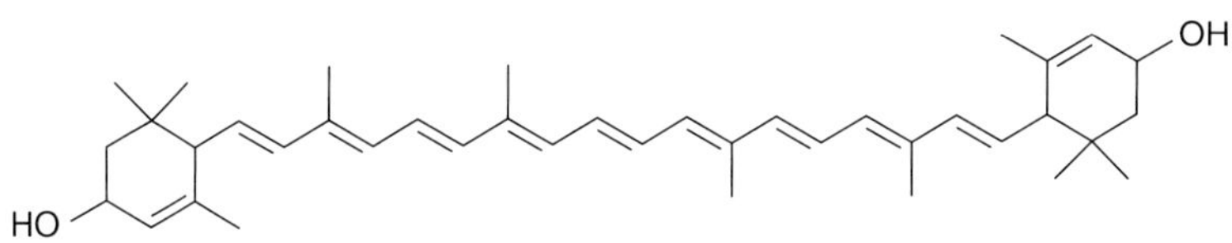

Tunaxanthin

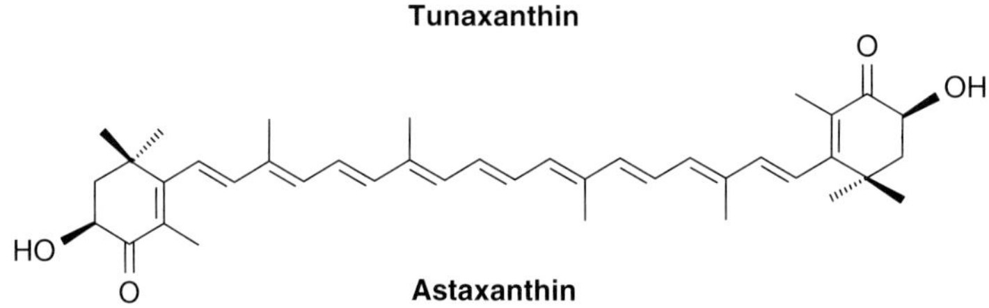

Astaxanthin

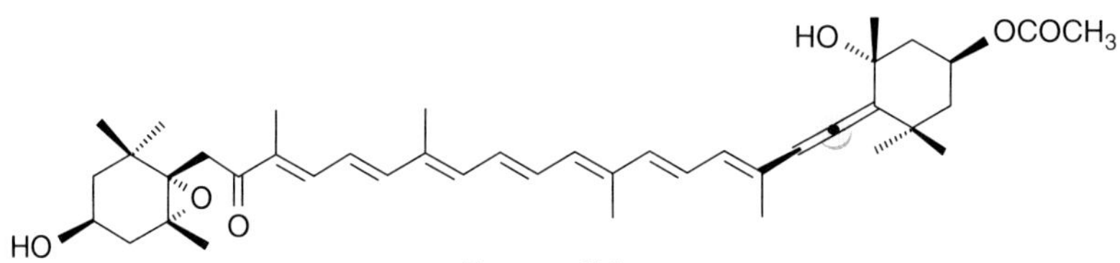

Fucoxanthin

Figure 1.4 Structures of typical animal and algal carotenoids.

forms. Found in algae, it is always esterified; synthetic astaxanthin is not esterified (Johnson and An, 1991). In the red crab langostilla (*Pleuroncodes planipes*), astaxanthin diesters comprised approximately 70%, monoesterified astaxanthin approximately 12%, and unesterified astaxanthin approximately 8% of the total carotenoids (Coral-Hinostroza and Bjerkeng, 2002).

Although of limited occurrence in foods, fucoxanthin (Figure 1.4) is among the most abundant carotenoids in nature. It is found in edible brown algae (Yan et al., 1999; Miyashita et al., 2011; Christaki et al., 2012), largely consumed in Asian countries. It has a more complicated structure than most food carotenoids, having an allenic bond, several functional substituents, including secondary and tertiary hydroxyl, epoxy, and keto, and is a natural acetate.

1.3.3 *Z*-isomers

In nature, carotenoids exist primarily in the generally more thermodynamically stable all-*E* configuration. The structures in Figures 1.1 to 1.4 are generally in this form. The first two carotenoids formed biosynthetically, phytoene and phytoflene, have the 15-*Z* configuration in most natural sources. Another exception is bixin, which occurs naturally in the *Z*-form. As the improved efficiency of chromatographic methods permitted their separation, small amounts of *Z*-isomers have been increasingly reported in raw foods. On the other hand, it is well known that thermal processing enhances geometric isomerization, increasing the levels of *Z*-isomers in processed foods.

Theoretically, each carbon-carbon double bond in the polyene chain of carotenoids may exhibit *E*-*Z* isomerization. However, some double bonds are prevented from undergoing this isomerization because the *Z*-configuration is sterically hindered (Figure 1.5) (Zechmeister et al., 1941). This is the case with C-7,8, C-11,12, C-7′,8′ and C-11′,12′ double bonds, in which steric hindrance between a hydrogen atom and a methyl group prevents a *Z*-configuration (Weedon and Moss, 1995). Thus, the *Z*-isomers of symmetrical β-carotene (Figure 1.6) (Lessin et al., 1997; Marx et al., 2000; Dachtler et al., 2001) and zeaxanthin (Dachtler et al., 2001; Humphries and Khachik, 2003; Updike and Schwartz, 2003; Aman et al., 2005) commonly found in foods are the 9-*Z*-, 13-*Z*-, and the 15-*Z*-isomers, the formation of which has relatively little hindrance as it comes from two hydrogen atoms.

Carbon-carbon double bonds located in the cyclic part of the carotenoid structure, as the C-5,6 double bond in β-carotene, are also sterically hindered and are not isomerized. However, this double bond in the acyclic lycopene is unhindered and 5-*Z*-lycopene is

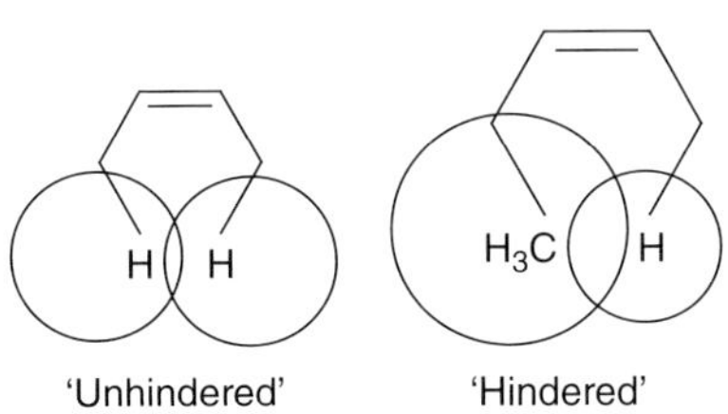

Figure 1.5 Sterically unhindered and hindered *Z*-configurations.

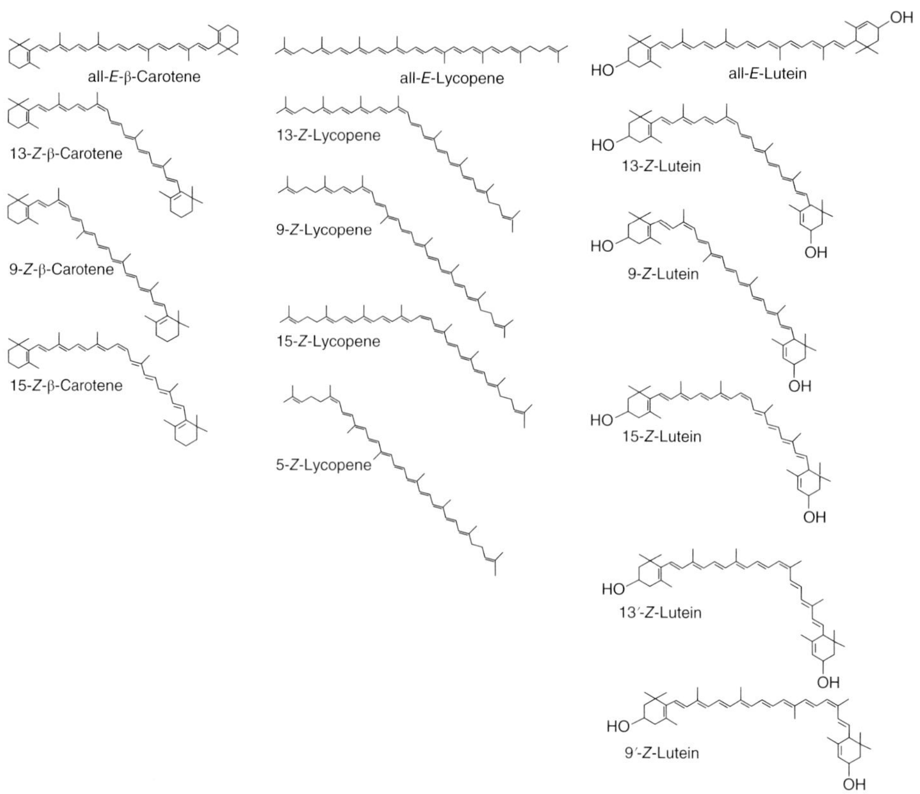

Figure 1.6 Geometric isomers of β-carotene, lycopene, and lutein commonly found in foods.

increasingly detected in tomato and tomato products, along with the 9-*Z*-, 13-*Z*-, and the 15-*Z*-isomers (Figure 1.6) (Tiziani et al., 2006; Li et al., 2012; Stinco et al., 2013).

Being unsymmetrical, all-*E*-α-carotene (Lessin et al., 1997), all-*E*-β-cryptoxanthin (Lessin et al., 1997), and all-*E*-lutein (Figure 1.6) (Dachtler et al., 2001; Humphries and Khachik, 2003; Updike and Schwartz, 2003; Aman et al., 2005; Achir et al., 2010) give rise to 13′-Z- and 9′-Z-isomers in addition to 13-Z-, 9-Z-, 15-Z-isomers in foods.

1.3.4 Apocarotenoids

Carotenoids in which the carbon skeleton has been shortened by removal of fragments from one or both ends of the usual C_{40} structure are called apocarotenoids. Natural examples are bixin, the major pigment of the food colorant annatto, and crocetin, the main coloring component of saffron (Figure 1.3). They are believed to be produced by Glover-Redfearn degradation of C_{40} carotenoids.

As with the epoxy carotenoids, apocarotenoids are initial products of the oxidative degradation of carotenoids. Thus, traces of these compounds are often found in foods.

β-Apo-8′-carotenal, β-Apo-10′-carotenal, and β-citraurin (Table 1.1), for example, are common minor pigments of citrus fruits.

1.4 PHYSICOCHEMICAL PROPERTIES

The major structural features that account for variations in properties and biological activities of carotenoids are length and rigidity of the molecule, length of the conjugated double-bond system, cyclized or acyclic end groups, and presence of polar substituents in the predominantly hydrocarbon molecule.

The physical and chemical properties of carotenoids in vitro provide valuable insights, but these properties in vivo are affected by a wide range of factors other than their basic chemical characteristics, including interactions with other molecules in their microenvironment, and may be significantly different from those of free carotenoids in organic solvent solution. Thus, extrapolations of in vitro results to in vivo situations should be done with caution.

1.4.1 Size and shape

The overall molecular geometry (size, shape, presence of functional groups) is essential in ensuring that carotenoids fit into cellular and subcellular structures in the correct location and orientation, so that they can function efficiently (Britton, 1995).

Acyclic carotenoids such as lycopene are long, linear molecules. Cyclization shortens the overall length of the molecule and increases the effective bulk of the end groups and the space they occupy.

The size and shape of *Z*- and all-*E* isomers are substantially different, with marked influence on their properties and biological actions and functions. The all-*E* isomers are linear and rigid molecules, whereas the Z-isomers are bent—thus their ability to assemble in supramolecular structure, fit into subcellular structures, and interact with enzymes differs. The tendency of Z-isomers to crystallize or aggregate is usually much less; thus, *Z*-isomers have lower melting point and may be more readily solubilized, absorbed, and transported than their all-*E* counterparts (Britton, 1995; Schieber and Carle, 2005).

1.4.2 Solubility

Carotenoids are highly lipophilic. They are insoluble in water and soluble in varying degrees in organic solvents such as acetone, alcohol, ethyl ether, chloroform, and ethyl acetate. Carotenes are readily soluble in petroleum ether, hexane, and toluene; xanthophylls dissolve better in methanol and ethanol. Crystalline carotenoids may be difficult to dissolve in the above solvents but do dissolve in benzene and dichloromethane (Schiedt and Liaaen-Jensen, 1995). Both β-carotene and the xanthophyll lutein have excellent solubility in tetrahydrofuran (Craft and Soares, 1992).

In the cell, carotenoids are expected to be restricted to hydrophobic areas, such as the inner core of membranes, but association with protein allows them access to aqueous environments (Britton, 1995).

1.4.3 Light absorption and color

Because the π electrons of the extended conjugated double bond system are highly delocalized and the excited state is of comparatively low energy, the excitation energy required is relatively small, corresponding to light in the visible region in the wavelength range of 400–500 nm. Carotenoids are therefore brightly colored. The transition involved is $\pi \rightarrow \pi^*$, in which one of the bonding π electrons of the conjugated double bond system is raised to a previously unoccupied π^* antibonding orbital.

The conjugated double bond system is the chromophore that gives carotenoids their color and provides the visible absorption spectra that serve as basis for their identification and quantification. At least 7 conjugated double bonds are needed for a carotenoid to have perceptible color, as in ζ-carotene, which is light yellow. Phytoene (3 conjugated double bonds) and phytofluene (5 conjugated double bonds) are colorless. Lycopene, with 11 conjugated double bonds in an acyclic structure, is red. Cyclization takes the π electrons of the ring double bond out of plane with those of the chain because of steric hindrance between the ring methyl group at C-5 and the hydrogen at C-8 of the polyene chain. Consequently, the monocyclic γ-carotene and the bicyclic β-carotene, although possessing the same number of conjugated double bonds as lycopene, are red-orange and yellow-orange, respectively. Hydroxy substituents do not affect the chromophore; thus, both α-carotene and its dihydroxy derivative, lutein, are pale yellow. Similarly, the monohydroxy and dihydroxy derivatives of β-carotene, β-cryptoxanthin and zeaxanthin, have the same color as β-carotene.

Capsanthin, with its conjugated double bond system consisting of nine double bonds in the polyene chain, one in the β-ring, and the carbonyl group double bond, and capsorubin, with its nine conjugated double bonds in the polyene chain extended by the double bonds of two carbonyl groups, give the intense color of red pepper. Astaxanthin, having nine conjugated double bond in the polyene chain extended by two double bonds in β-rings and two carbonyl group double bonds, is responsible for the vivid red color of cooked shrimp, lobster, and crabs. In the raw crustaceans, astaxanthin is complexed with protein, transforming the color to blue, black, or grey. Heating denatures the protein and the red color of free astaxanthin appears. The reddish color of salmon and trout flesh also comes from astaxanthin.

1.5 ANTIOXIDANT PROPERTIES

An antioxidant is defined as any substance that when present at low concentrations compared to those of an oxidizable substrate, significantly delays or prevents oxidation. Carotenoids are natural antioxidants of importance in foods and in humans. They may enhance the stability and extend the shelf life of foods. On the other hand, the antioxidant activity is the most cited mode of action of carotenoids in the reduction of the risk of chronic degenerative diseases. Most researchers in the last two to three decades have focused attention on the antioxidant role of food carotenoids in human health rather than in the food itself.

The antioxidant properties of carotenoids are due to their exceptional singlet oxygen ($^1O_2$) quenching ability and their free-radical scavenging activity.

1.5.1 Quenching of singlet oxygen

Photosensitizers in biological systems (e.g., chlorophyll, riboflavin, myoglobin) can absorb energy from light and, in its excited triplet state, transfer energy to atmospheric triplet-state oxygen ($^3O_2$), forming the highly reactive and destructive singlet oxygen ($^1O_2$).

Carotenoids can interfere in this process in two ways: (1) by deactivating the triplet state phosensitizer, thus preventing the formation of singlet oxygen, and (2) converting singlet-state oxygen back to its ground triplet state. In both cases, transferred energy is released as heat.

It is well documented that carotenoids quench $^1O_2$ (Krinsky, 1989, 2001; Edge et al., 1997). This occurs through physical or chemical quenching, the efficacy of the former greatly exceeding that of the latter. Physical quenching involves the transfer of excitation energy from $^1O_2$ to the carotenoid; oxygen then returns to its ground state and the carotenoid is elevated to its excited triplet state. The energy is dissipated through rotational and vibrational interactions between the excited carotenoid and the surrounding solvent, yielding ground state carotenoid and thermal energy. The carotenoid remains intact and can undergo further cycles of singlet oxygen quenching.

$$^1O_2 + CAR \rightarrow {}^3O_2 + {}^3CAR^*$$

$$^3CAR^* \rightarrow CAR + heat$$

In chemical quenching, the carotenoid combines with oxygen or is oxidized, leading to its destruction (bleaching) and yielding a variety of oxidized products.

Carotenoids can also quench the excited triplet-state chlorophyll or other excited sensitizers, thereby preventing the formation of $^1O_{2.}$

$$^3CHL^* + CAR \rightarrow CHL + {}^3CAR^*$$

The quenching ability of carotenoids increases with increasing number of conjugated double bonds, maximum protection being given by those having nine or more double bonds (Foote et al., 1970). To a lesser extent, it is also affected by the carotenoid end groups (cyclic or acyclic) and the nature of the substituents in cyclic end groups.

Oxygen quenching depends on the environment. Efficient $^1O_2$ quenchers in solvents may be inefficient in the cell membrane (Edge and Truscott, 2009). The aggregation and the orientation of a carotenoid in the lipid bilayer may be major factors in determining the $^1O_2$ quenching efficiency.

Singlet oxygen is involved in the photooxidation of vegetable oils and oil-containing foods. Addition of various carotenoids to foods containing unsaturated fatty acids improves the shelf life, mainly because of $^1O_2$ quenching (Kiokias and Gordon, 2004).

1.5.2 Free radical scavenging

Although not as efficient as in quenching $^1O_{2,}$ carotenoids can also scavenge free radicals, thereby breaking chain propagation. Interaction with free radicals can occur in three main ways (Young and Lowe, 2001; El-Agamey et al., 2004; Skibsted, 2012):

$$CAR + ROO^{\bullet} \rightarrow CAR^{\bullet+} + ROO^{-}\left(\text{electron transfer}\right)$$

$$CAR + ROO^{\bullet} \rightarrow CAR^{\bullet} + ROOH\left(\text{hydrogen abstraction}\right)$$

$$CAR + ROO^{\bullet} \rightarrow \left(ROO - CAR\right)^{\bullet}\left(\text{addition}\right)$$

The factors that can affect the rates and mechanisms of free-radical reactions include the nature of the free radical and its environment (aqueous or lipid regions) and structural features of the carotenoid (number of conjugated double bonds, cyclic or acyclic, polar or apolar end groups, redox properties) (Everett et al., 1996; Mortensen and Skibsted, 1997; Rice-Evans et al., 1997; El-Agamey et al., 2004). The nature of the radical species appears to have greater effect than the carotenoid structure (Mortensen et al., 1997; Martinez et al., 2009).

Carotenoids react with a wide range of radicals, such as $CCl_3O_2^{\bullet}$, $RSO_2^{\bullet}$, $NO_2^{\bullet}$, and various arylperoxyl radicals through electron transfer, producing the radical cation $CAR^{\bullet+}$ (Everett et al., 1996; Mortensen and Skibsted, 1997; Mortensen et al., 2001). Glutathione and 2-mercaptoethanol thiyl radicals react via radical addition to generate carotenoid-thiyl radical adducts $(RS\text{-}CAR)^{\bullet}$ (Everett et al., 1996; Mortensen and Skibsted, 1997). The $RSO^{\bullet}_2$ radical (generated by conjugation of the $RS^{\bullet}$ radical with molecular oxygen) undergoes both radical addition, producing $(RSO_2\text{-}CAR)^{\bullet}$, and electron abstraction, forming $CAR^{\bullet+}$ (Everett et al., 1996; Mortensen and Skibsted, 1997). With less strongly oxidizing radicals, such as akylperoxyl radicals, hydrogen atom transfer can occur, leading to the neutral carotenoid radical (Mortensen et al., 2001). Hydrogen abstraction, characteristic of lipid oxidation, has often been suggested as a mechanism of carotenoid antioxidant activity (Woodall et al., 1997a; El-Agamey and McGarvey, 2003).

Steady-state photolysis experiments showed that alkyl, alkoxyl, and alkylperoxyl radicals all reacted with β-carotene (Mortensen and Skibsted, 1998). However, laser flash photolysis experiments indicated that the reaction with peroxyl radicals was slower than with alkyl and alkoxyl radicals, indicating that β-carotene was a poor direct scavenger of peroxyl radicals. The authors suggested that scavenging of peroxyl radicals by this carotenoid proceeded not by electron transfer but by adduct formation and/or hydrogen abstraction.

El-Algamey and McGarvey (2003) observed that the carotenoid radical formed depends on the polarity of the solvent medium. Only addition radicals are formed in apolar solvents, whereas these adducts decay to carotenoid radical cations in polar solvents.

The β-carotene radical cation and adduct radicals are highly resonance stabilized and undergo slow bimolecular decay to nonradical products (Everett et al., 1996). In the scavenging of lipid-derived peroxyl radicals ($LOO^{\bullet}$), the carotenoid radicals are less reactive than the $LOO^{\bullet}$; carotenoids thus act as chain-breaking antioxidants in lipid peroxidation.

Carotenoids may also be reduced, forming radical anions:

$$CAR + ROO^{\bullet} \rightarrow CAR^{\bullet-} + ROO^{+}$$

The balance between electron donation and electron acceptance forming radical cations and radical anions, respectively, varies among carotenoids and is important in their role in antioxidant networks (Skibsted, 2012).

Structural features of the carotenoid govern not only their reactivity but also their location and orientation within the lipid bilayer (Britton, 1995) and even their tendency to self-aggregate under polar conditions (Ruban et al., 1993). β-Carotene and other carotenes lie parallel with the membrane surface, deep within the hydrophobic core

(Johansson et al., 1981; van de Ven et al., 1984). The dihydroxy zeaxanthin spans the membrane entirely.

1.5.3 Relative efficacy of individual carotenoids

Comparison of the effectiveness of carotenoids as antioxidant has been carried out in homogenous solution and liposomes (cell membrane models). The results are somewhat inconsistent but can be better understood when the different influencing factors are considered. Noting that the efficiency of carotenoids as antioxidants did not follow their capability as radical scavengers or the order of their oxidation potential, J. Liang et al. (2009) suggested that the long-standing controversy about the function of carotenoids as antioxidant might be related to the extrapolation of properties determined in solution to more complex biological systems, where other factors (e.g., spatial organization and interaction between antioxidants) become important.

Having an extended conjugated double bond system in an acyclic structure, lycopene has been shown in different systems to be one of the most potent antioxidants (Mascio et al., 1989; Mortensen et al., 1997; Woodall et al., 1997b; Cantrell et al., 2003; Stahl and Sies, 2003). In a mixed solvent system, its singlet oxygen quenching ability was twice as high as β-carotene and 10 times higher than that of α-tocopherol (Mascio et al., 1989). It was twice as efficient as β-carotene in scavenging nitrogen dioxide radical (Tinkler et al., 1994; Böhm et al., 1995). According to real-time kinetic studies, it was also more efficient than zeaxanthin, lutein, echinenone, canthaxantin, and astaxanthin as reductive scavengers of radicals (Mortensen and Skibsted, 1997).

Astaxanthin quenched $^1O_2$ in a mixed solvent system (Mascio et al., 1989), model membrane (Cantrell et al, 2003), and chlorophyll-sensitized and photooxidized soybean oil (Lee and Min, 1990). Its quenching capacity in a mixed solvent system was lower than lycopene, almost equivalent to γ-carotene, slightly higher than canthaxanthin, and greater than α- and β-carotene (Mascio et al., 1989).

As with other carotenoids, astaxanthin's free radical scavenging efficiency depends on the nature of the free radical, the scavenging mechanism, and the environment. In a free radical–initiated system, Terão (1989) found canthaxanthin and astaxanthin better antioxidants than β-carotene and zeaxanthin. Astaxanthin and canthaxanthin and other carotenoids containing keto-groups in the 4 position of the β-ionone ring were found more effective than β-carotene and zeaxanthin in preventing free-radical oxidation of methyl linoleate in solution (Jorgensen and Skibsted, 1993). In organic solvent and liposomal media, astaxanthin showed higher activity toward peroxyl radical generated by the lipophilic generator AMVN (2,2′-azobis-2,4-dimethylvaleronitrile) than lutein, lycopene, α- and β-carotene, and α-tocopherol (Naguib, 2000). Goto et al. (2001) reported that astaxanthin is twice as effective as β-carotene in inhibiting the production of peroxides induced by ADP and Fe^{2+} in liposomes. This potent antiperoxidative activity of astaxanthin was attributed to efficient radical trapping at the surface and inside the phospholipid membrane.

On the other hand, astaxanthin and canthaxanthin ranked among the least efficient reductive scavengers of radicals according to both theoretical calculations and real-time kinetic studies (Skibsted, 2012). Real-time detection following laser flash photolysis of transient carotenoid radical cations formed in chloroform with phenoxyl radicals established the antioxidant hierarchy as follows: lycopene > β-carotene > zeaxanthin > lutein > echinenone > canthaxanthin ~ β-apo-8′-carotenal > astaxanthin (Mortensen and Skibsted, 1997).

Differences in the reactivity of carotenoids had been related to differences in their electron density. For example, the presence at C-4 and C-4′ of hydroxy (as in isozeaxanthin) and especially keto groups (as in astaxanthin and canthaxanthin) decreased reactivity by preventing hydrogen abstraction from these positions (Britton, 1995; Woodall et al., 1997a, b).

β-cryptoxanthin and zeaxanthin were found to be more protective than β-carotene against peroxyl radicals in liposomal membranes (Woodall et al., 1997a). Since all three carotenoids have 11 conjugated double bonds, and β-carotene and zeaxanthin behaved similarly when tested against peroxyl radicals in solution, the presence of one and two hydroxyl groups in β-cryptoxanthin and zeaxanthin, respectively, accounts only partially for the difference. Chemical reactivity of the carotenoid toward peroxyl radicals, as demonstrated in homogenous solution, is not the only factor that determines its ability to protect membranes against oxidation; the position and orientation of the carotenoid in the lipid bilayer are additional important factors (Woodall et al., 1997a; Young and Lowe, 2001). The hydrocarbons lycopene and β-carotene are located in the hydrophobic inner core of the bilayer and are not in a position to readily intercept free radicals entering the membrane from the aqueous phase. Carotenoids with polar end groups span the bilayer with their end groups located near the hydrophobic-hydrophilic interface where free radicals attack first.

Sujak et al. (1999) investigated the effect of lutein and zeaxanthin on oxidative damage of egg yolk lecithin liposomal membranes induced by exposure to UV radiation and incubation with the water-soluble peroxyl radicals generator AAPH (2,2′-azobis (2-methylpropionamidine)dihydrochloride). Lutein and zeaxanthin protected lipid membranes against free radical attack with almost the same efficacy. Both carotenoids also slowed down UV-induced lipid oxidation at a very similar rate at the initial stage of the experiments, but zeaxanthin appeared to be a better photoprotector during prolonged UV exposure. The difference in protective efficacy was attributed to a different organization of zeaxanthin-lipid and lutein-lipid membranes.

1.6 PROOXIDANT EFFECT

A possible prooxidant property of carotenoids came into focus as an aftermath of intervention studies that showed an increase rather than a decrease in the incidence of lung cancer with β-carotene supplementation. According to Palozza (1998), there is evidence for a prooxidant activity of carotenoids in vitro and in vivo. The carotenoids shift from being antioxidants to prooxidants, depending on their redox potential and the biological environment. Both Krinsky (2001) and Young and Lowe (2001), however, considered it unlikely that carotenoids would act as prooxidants in biological systems, although they may lose their effectiveness as antioxidants at high concentrations or at high partial pressures of oxygen.

The concept that carotenoids can be prooxidants arose from the findings of Burton and Ingold (1984) that at high, nonphysiologic, oxygen tensions (760 torr, 100%

oxygen) and high carotenoid concentrations (>500 μM), β-carotene behaves as a prooxidant. A close look at the data, however, strongly suggested that it was actually a decrease in antioxidant activity under those conditions and not necessarily a prooxidant effect (Krinsky, 2001). Moreover, the oxygen tension in the lung would only be 150 torr for inspired air, dropping rapidly to 15 torr or less in the tissues; at this level there was no indication of a decrease in antioxidant capacity. Evidence of prooxidant action has also been obtained at high, nonphysiologic concentrations (50 μM). Even in the major intervention trials where individuals received between 20 and 25 mg/d of β-carotene for extended periods, the plasma β-carotene concentration ranged from 0.4 to 5 μM, well below the levels where it had been reported to act as prooxidant.

It is also important to consider that studies on the antioxidant-prooxidant potential are carried out with the carotenoids dissolved in organic solvents. In biological systems, these compounds are predominantly found associated with protein or lipoprotein structures and, in this condition, behave differently from those in solution (Young and Lowe, 2001).

The factors that may influence the antioxidant or prooxidant activities of carotenoids in biological systems are: (1) the structure (i.e., size, shape, and the nature, position, and number of substituent groups) and physical form (aggregated or monomeric, *Z* or *E* configuration, etc.) of the carotenoid molecule, (2) the location or site of action of the carotenoid molecule within the cell, (3) the potential for interaction with other carotenoids or antioxidants (especially vitamins C and E), (4) the concentration of the carotenoid, and (5) the partial pressure of oxygen (Britton, 1995; Young and Lowe, 2001).

1.7 INTERACTION WITH OTHER ANTIOXIDANTS

In the human organism, carotenoids are part of the antioxidant defense system, interacting synergistically with other antioxidants (Stahl and Sies, 2003). Combinations of carotenoids or carotenoids with other antioxidants are more effective than single compounds.

Truscott (1996) proposed a mechanism for the interaction of vitamins C and E with β-carotene whereby the carotenoid molecule repairs the vitamin E radical and the resulting carotenoid cation radical is, in turn, repaired by vitamin C. An additive response was observed with β-carotene and vitamin E; a synergistic response was seen only in the presence of vitamin C.

$$\mathrm{CAR} + \mathrm{TOH}^{\bullet+} \rightarrow \mathrm{CAR}^{\bullet+} + \mathrm{TOH}$$

$$\mathrm{CAR}^{\bullet+} + \mathrm{ASCH}_2 \rightarrow \mathrm{CAR} + \mathrm{ASCH}^{\bullet} + \mathrm{H}^+$$

$$\mathrm{CAR}^{\bullet+} + \mathrm{ASCH}^- \rightarrow \mathrm{CAR} + \mathrm{ASCH}^{\bullet-} + \mathrm{H}^+$$

Synergistic protection of human cells both in vivo and in vitro by β-carotene with vitamins E and C against lethal damage by both $NO_2\cdot$ and $OONO^-/HOONO$ (formed from NO· and the superoxide radical $O_2^{\cdot-}$) was reported by Böhm et al. (1998).

On the other hand, in red palm oil, the carotenes appeared to be the primary substrate for lipid-derived radicals and tocopherols/tocotrienols regenerated the carotenes

(Schroeder et al., 2006). Regeneration of the carotenes by tocopherols or tocotrienols also seemed to explain the antioxidant synergism observed for liposomes.

The synergistic effect was shown to be dependent on the type of antioxidant and its concentration (Shi et al., 2007). In a homogenous solution of linoleic acid methyl ester and in linoleic acid methyl ester oxidation induced by an azo-initiator, lycopene appeared to interact synergistically with vitamin E at a specific concentration and ratio, but β-carotene showed no synergistic effect with vitamin E at the levels used in the study.

A synergistic response among carotenoids had been also reported (Stahl et al., 1998). A combination of lutein and lycopene was found to be most effective against AMVN-induced oxidation in multilamellar liposomes. In a phosphatidyl choline liposome, a combination of astaxanthin with β-carotene or astaxanthin with lycopene showed significant antioxidant synergism (J. Liang et al., 2009). It was suggested that astaxanthin, anchored in the water/lipid interface, acted as a radical transfer bridge, scavenging radicals at the interface and transferring an electron from a nonpolar and more reducing carotenoid in the membrane interior.

Skibsted (2012) envisioned carotenoids forming antioxidant networks based on one-electron transfer with other carotenoids, depending on the balance between ionization energy and electron affinity of the individual carotenoids, as demonstrated by real-time kinetic studies and quantum mechanical calculations. The more hydrophilic xanthophylls serve as molecular wiring across membranes in these networks, anchoring in water/lipid interfaces, resulting in synergism with more lipophilic carotenoids.

Synergism had also been observed between isoflavonoids and β-carotene (Han et al., 2007, 2010; R. Liang et al., 2010). This seems to involve the regeneration of the carotenoid radical cation formed in the lipid phase by the isoflavonoid in the lipid/water interfaces. The monoanionic and dianionic forms of the isoflavonoids, not the neutral forms, regenerated the oxidized carotenoid, and electron transfer from the isoflavonoids was faster for astaxanthin than for the other carotenoids, in agreement with its highest electron accepting index (Han et al., 2010).

The coexistence of carotenoids and polyphenols in foods is advantageous because carotenoids are efficient in $^1O_2$ quenching but not as effective in free radical scavenging, whereas polyphenols are very good free radical quenchers but not as efficient in $^1O_2$ quenching. Together, they have at least an additive effect.

References

Achir N, Randrianatoandro VA, Bohuon P, Laffargue A, Avallone S. 2010. Kinetic study of β-carotene and lutein degradation in oils during heat treatment. *Eur J Lipid Sci Technol* 112:349–61.

Aman R, Biehl J, Carle R, Conrad J, Beifuss U, Schieber A. 2005. Application of HPLC coupled with DAD, APcI-MS and NMR to the analysis of lutein and zeaxanthin stereoisomers in thermally processed vegetables. *Food Chem* 92:753–63.

Bartley GE, Scolnik PA. 1995. Plant carotenoids: Pigments for photoprotection, visual attraction, and human health. *Plant Cell* 7:1027–38.

Böhm F, Edge R, McGarvey D J, Truscott TG. 1998. Beta-carotene with vitamins E and C offers synergistic cell protection against NO_x. *FEBS Lett* 436:387–9.

Böhm F, Tinkler JH, Truscott TG. 1995. Carotenoids protect against cell membrane damage by nitrogen dioxide radical. *Nature Med* 1:98–9.

Breithaupt D, Wirt U, Bamedi A. 2002. Differentiation between lutein monester regioisomers and detection of lutein diesters from marigold flowers (*Tagetes erecta* L.) and several fruits by liquid chromatography-mass spectrometry. *J Agric Food Chem* 50:66–70.

Britton G. 1995. Structure and properties of carotenoids in relation to functions. *FASEB J* 9:1551–8.

Britton G, Liaaen-Jensen S, Pfander H. 2004. *Carotenoid handbook*. Basel: Birkhaüser Verlag.

Burton GW, Ingold KU. 1984. β-Carotene: An unusual type of lipid antioxidant. *Science* 224:569–73.

Cantrell A, McGarvey DJ, Truscott TG, Rancan F, Bohn F. 2003. Singlet oxygen quenching of dietary carotenoids in a model membrane. *Arch Biochem Biophys* 412:47–54.

Christaki E, Bonos E, Giannenas I, Florou-Paneri P. 2012. Functional properties of carotenoids originating from algae. *J Sci Food Agric* 93:5–11.

Coral-Hinostroza GN, Bjerkeng B. 2002. Astaxanthin from the red crab langostilla (*Pleuroncodes planipes*): Optical *R/S* isomers and fatty acid moieties of astaxanthin esters. *Comp Biochem Physiol Part B* 133:437–44.

Craft NE, Soares JH Jr. 1992. Relative solubility, stability, and absorptivity of lutein and β-carotene in organic solvents. *J Agric Food Chem* 40:431–4.

Dachtler M, Glaser T, Kohler K, Albert K. 2001. Combined HPLC-MS and HPLC-NMR on-line coupling for the separation and determination of lutein and zeaxanthin stereoisomers in spinach and in retina. *Anal Chem* 73:667–74.

Edge R, McGarvey DJ, Truscott TG. 1997. The carotenoids as anti-oxidants—a review. *J Photochem Photobiol* 41:189–200.

Edge R, Truscott G. 2009. Properties of carotenoid radicals and excited states and their potential role in biological systems. In: Landrum JT. editor. *Carotenoids: Physical, chemical and biological functions and properties*. Boca Raton: CRC Press, p 283–307.

El-Agamey A, Lowe GM, McGarvey DJ, Mortensen A, Phillip DM, Truscott TG, Young AJ. 2004. Carotenoid radical chemistry and antioxidant/pro-oxidant properties. *Arch Biochem Biophys* 430:37–48.

El-Agamey A, McGarvey DJ. 2003. Evidence for a lack of reactivity of carotenoid addition radicals towards oxygen: A laser flash photolysis study of the reactions of carotenoids with acylperoxyl radicals in polar and non-polar solvents. *J Am Chem Soc* 125:3330–40.

Everett SA, Dennis MF, Patel KB, Maddix S, Kundu SC, Willson RL. 1996. Scavenging of nitrogen dioxide, thiyl, and sulfonyl free radicals by the nutritional anti-oxidant β-carotene. *J Biol Chem* 271:3988–94.

Foote CS, Chang YC, Denny RW. 1970. Chemistry of singlet oxygen. X. Carotenoid quenching parallels biological protection. *J Am Chem Soc* 92:5216–8.

Goto S, Kogure K, Abe K, Kimata Y, Kitahama K, Yamashita E, Terada H. 2001. Efficient radical trapping at the surface and inside the phospholipid membrane is responsible for highly potent antiperoxidative activity of the carotenoid astaxanthin. *Biochim Biophys Acta* 1512:251–8.

Gross J. 1987. *Pigments in fruits*. London: Academic Press.

Han R-M, Chen C-H, Tian Y-X, Zhang J-P, Skibsted LH. 2010. Fast regeneration of carotenoids from radical cations by isoflavonoid dianions: Importance of the carotenoid keto group for electron transfer. *J Phys Chem A* 114:126–32.

Han R-M, Tian Y-X, Becker EM, Andersen ML, Zhang J-P, Skibsted LH. 2007. Puerarin and conjugate bases as radical scavengers and antioxidants: Molecular mechanism and synergism with β-carotene. *J Agric Food Chem* 55:2384–91.

Hornero-Mendéz D, Mínguez-Mosquera MI. 2000. Carotenoid pigments in *Rosa mosqueta* hips, an alternative carotenoid source for foods. *J Agric Food Chem* 48:825–8.

Humphries JM, Khachick F. 2003. Distribution of lutein, zeaxanthin, and related geometrical isomers in fruit, vegetables, wheat and pasta products. *J Agric Food Chem* 51:1322–7.

Isler O, Rüegg R, Schweiter U. 1967. Carotenoids as food colorants. *Pure Appl Chem*14:245–63.

IUPAC Commission of Nomenclature of Organic Chemistry, IUPAC-IUB Commission on Biochemical Nomenclature. 1975. Nomenclature of carotenoids. *Pure Appl Chem* 41:405–31.

Johansson LB-A, Lindblom G, Wieslander A, Arvidson G. 1981. Orientation of β-carotene and retinal in lipid bilayers. *FEBS Lett* 128:97–9.

Johnson EA, An G-H. 1991. Astaxanthin from microbial sources. *Crit Rev Biotechnol* 11:297–326.

Jorgensen K, Skibsted LH. 1993. Carotenoid scavenging of radicals. Effect of carotenoid structure and oxygen partial pressure on antioxidant activity. *Z Lebensm Unters Forsch* 196:423–9.

Kiokias S, Gordon MH. 2004. Antioxidant properties of carotenoids in vitro and in vivo. *Food Rev Int* 20:99–121.

Kobori CN, Rodriguez-Amaya DB. 2008. Uncultivated Brazilian green leaves are richer sources of carotenoids than commercially produced leafy vegetables. *Food Nutr Bull* 29:333–41.
Krinsky NI. 1989. Antioxidant functions of carotenoids. *Free Radic Biol Med* 7:617–35.
Krinsky NI. 2001. Carotenoids as antioxidants. *Nutr* 17:815–7.
Lee SH, Min DB. 1990. Effects, quenching mechanisms, and kinetics of carotenoids in chlorophyll sensitized photoxidation of soybean oil. *J Agric Food Chem* 38:1630–4.
Lessin WJ, Catigani GL, Schwartz SJ. 1997. Quantification of *cis-trans* isomers of provitamin A carotenoids in fresh and processed fruits and vegetables. *J Agric Food Chem* 45:3728–32.
Li H, Deng Z, Liu R, Loewen S, Tsao R. 2012. Ultra-performance liquid chromatographic separation of geometric isomers of carotenoids and antioxidant activities of 20 tomato cultivars and breeding lines. *Food Chem* 132:508–17.
Liang J, Tian Y-X, Yang F, Zhang J-P, Skibsted LH. 2009. Antioxidant synergism between carotenoids in membranes: Astaxanthin as a radical transfer bridge. *Food Chem* 115:1437–42.
Liang R, Chen C-H, Han R-M, Zhang J-P, Skibsted LH. 2010. Thermodynamic versus kinetic control of antioxidant synergism between β-carotene and (iso)flavonoids and their glycosides in liposomes. *J Agric Food Chem* 58:9221–7.
Martinez A, Vergas R, Galano A. 2009. What is important to prevent oxidative stress? A theoretical study on electron-transfer reactions between carotenoids and free radicals. *J Phys Chem B* 113:12113–20.
Marx M, Schieber A, Carle R. 2000. Quantitative determination of carotene stereoisomer in carrot juices and vitamin supplemented (ATBC) drinks. *Food Chem* 70:403–8.
Mascio P di, Kaiser S, Sies H. 1989. Lycopene as the most efficient biological carotenoid singlet oxygen quencher. *Arch Biochem Biophys* 274:532–8.
Mercadante AZ, Rodriguez-Amaya DB. 1998. Influence of ripening, cultivar differences, and processing on the carotenoid composition of mango. *J Agric Food Chem* 46:128–30.
Miyashita K, Nishikawa S, Beppu F, Tsukui T, Abe M, Hosokawa M. 2011. The allenic carotenoid fucoxanthin, a novel marine nutraceutical from brown seaweeds. *J Sci Food Agric* 91:1166–74.
Mortensen A, Skibsted LH. 1997. Relative stability of carotenoid radical cations and homoloque tocopheroxyl radicals. A real time kinetic study of antioxidant hierarchy. *FEBS Lett* 417:261–6.
Mortensen A, Skibsted LH. 1998. Reactivity of β-carotene towards peroxyl radicals studied by laser flash and steady-state photolysis. *FEBS Lett* 426:392–6.
Mortensen A, Skibsted LH, Sampson J, Rice-Evans C, Everett SA. 1997. Comparative mechanisms and rates of free radical scavenging by carotenoid antioxidants. *FEBS Lett* 418:91–7.
Mortensen A, Skibsted LH, Truscott TG. 2001. The interaction of dietary carotenoids with radical species. *Arch Biochem Biophys* 385:13–9.
Naguib YMA. 2000. Antioxidant activities of astaxanthin and related carotenoids. *J Agric Food Chem* 48:1150–4.
Niizu PY, Rodriguez-Amaya DB. 2005. The flowers and leaves of *Tropaeolum majus* as rich sources of lutein. *J. Food Sci* 70:S605–9.
Oliveira GPR de, Rodriguez-Amaya DB. 2007. Processed and prepared products of corn as sources of lutein and zeaxanthin. Compositional variation in the food chain. *J Food Sci* 72:S79–S85.
Palozza P. 1998. Prooxidant actions of carotenoids in biologic systems. *Nutr Rev* 56: 257–65.
Peng Y, Ma C, Li Y, Leung KS-Y, Jiang Z-H, Zhao Z. 2005. Quantification of zeaxanthin dipalmitate and total carotenoids in *Lycium* fruits (Fructus lycii). *Plant Foods Hum Nutr* 60:161–4.
Renstrom B, Ronneberg H, Borch G, Liaaen-Jensen S. 1982. Animal carotenoids 28. Further studies on the carotenoproteins crustacyanin and ovoverdin. *Comp Biochem Physiol* 71B:249–52.
Rice-Evans CA, Sampson J, Bramley PM, Holloway DE. 1997. Why do we expect carotenoids to be antioxidants in vivo? *Free Radical Res* 26:381–98.
Rodriguez-Amaya DB. 1999. *A guide to carotenoid analysis in foods*. Washington DC: International Life Sciences Institute (ILSI) Press.
Rodriguez-Amaya DB, Kimura M. 2004. *HarvestPlus handbook for carotenoid analysis*. Washington: International Food Policy Research Institute.
Rodriguez-Amaya DB, Kimura M, Godoy HT, Amaya-Farfan J. 2008. Updated Brazilian database on food carotenoids: factors affecting carotenoid composition. *J Food Comp Anal* 21:445–63.
Ruban AV, Horton P, Young AJ. 1993. Aggregation of higher plant xanthophylls: Differences in absorption spectra and in dependency on solvent polarity. *J Photobiol Photobiochem B* 21:229–34.
Schieber A, Carle R. 2005. Occurrence of carotenoid cis-isomers in food: Technological, analytical, and nutritional implications. *Trends Food Sci Technol* 16:416–22.

Schiedt K. 1998. Absorption and metabolism of carotenoids in birds, fish and crustaceans. In: Britton G, Liaaen-Jensen S, Pfander H. editors. *Carotenoids, vol. 3, Biosynthesis and metabolism*. Basel: Birkhäuser Verlag, p 285–358.

Schiedt K, Liaaen-Jensen S. 1995. Isolation and analysis. In: Britton G, Liaaen-Jensen S, Pfander H. editors. *Carotenoids, vol. 1A, Isolation and analysis*. Basel: Birkhaüser Verlag, p 81–108.

Schroeder MT, EM, Skibsted LH. 2006. Molecular mechanism of antioxidant synergism of tocotrienols and carotenoids in palm oil. *J Agric Food Chem* 54:3445–53.

Shahidi F, Brown JA. 1998. Carotenoid pigments in seafoods and aquaculture. *Crit Rev Food Sci Nutr* 38:1–67.

Shi J, Qu Q, Kakuda Y, Xue SJ, Jiang Y, Koide S, Shim Y-Y. 2007. Investigation of the antioxidant and synergistic activity of lycopene and other natural antioxidants using LAME and AMVN model systems. *J Food Comp Anal* 20:603–8.

Skibsted LH. 2012. Carotenoids in antioxidant networks. Colorants or radical scavengers. *J Agric Food Chem* 60:2409–17.

Stahl W, Junghans A, de Boer B, Driomina ES, Briviba K, Sies H. 1998. Carotenoid mixtures protect multilamellar liposomes against oxidative damage: Synergistic effects of lycopene and lutein. *FEBS Lett* 427:305–8.

Stahl W, Sies H. 2003. Antioxidant activity of carotenoids. *Mol Aspects Med* 24:345–51.

Stinco CM, Rodríguez-Pulido FJ, Escudero-Gilete ML, Gordillo B, Vicario IM, Meléndez-Martínez AJ. 2013. Lycopene isomers in fresh and processed tomato products: Correlations with instrumental color measurements by digital image analysis and spectroradiometry. *Food Res Int* 50:111–20.

Sujak A, Gabrielska J, Grudzinski W, Borc R, Mazurek P, Gruszecki WI. 1999. Lutein and zeaxanthin as protectors of lipid membranes against oxidative damage: The structural aspects. *Arch Biochem Biophys* 371:301–7.

Terão J. 1989. Antioxidant activity of beta-carotene related carotenoids in solution. *Lipids* 24:659–62.

Tinkler JH, Boehm F, Schalch W, Truscott TG. 1994. Dietary carotenoids protect human cells from damage. *J Photochem Photobiol* 26:283–5.

Tiziani S, Schwartz SJ, Vodovotz Y. 2006. Profiling of carotenoids in tomato juice by one- and two-dimensional NMR. *J Agric Food Chem* 54:6094–100.

Truscott TG. 1996. β-Carotene and disease: A suggested pro-oxidant and anti-oxidant mechanism and speculations concerning its role in cigarette smoking. *J Photochem Photobiol B* 35:233–5.

Updike AA, Schwartz SJ. 2003. Thermal processing of vegetables increases *cis* isomers of lutein and zeaxanthin. *J Agric Food Chem* 51:6184–90.

van de Ven M, Kattenberg M, van Ginkel G, Levine YK. 1984. Study of the orientational ordering of carotenoids in lipid bilayers by resonance-Raman spectroscopy. *Biophys J* 45:1203–9.

Weedon BCL, Moss GP. 1995. Structure and nomenclature. In: Britton G, Liaaen-Jensen S, Pfander H. editors. *Carotenoids, vol. 1A, Isolation and analysis*. Basel: Birkhaüser Verlag, p 27–70.

Woodall AA, Britton G, Jackson MJ. 1997a. Carotenoids and protection of phospholipids in solution or in liposomes against oxidation by peroxyl radicals: Relationship between carotenoid structure and protective ability. *Biochim Biophys Acta* 1336:575–86.

Woodall AA, Lee SW-M, Weesie RJ, Jackson MJ, Britton G. 1997b. Oxidation of carotenoids by free radicals: Relationship between structure and reactivity. *Biochem Biophys Acta* 1336:33–42.

Yan X, Chuda Y, Suzuki M, Nagata T. 1999. Fucoxanthin as the major antioxidant in *Hijikia fusiformis*, a common edible seaweed. *Biosci Biotechnol Biochem* 63:605–7.

Young AJ, Lowe GM. 2001. Antioxidant and prooxidant properties of carotenoids. *Arch Biochem Biophys* 385:20–7.

Zechmeister L, LeRosen AL, Went FW, Pauling L. 1941. Prolycopene, a naturally occurring stereoisomer of lycopene. *Proc. Natl Acad Sci USA*. 27:468–74.

2 Biosynthesis and metabolism

2.1 INTRODUCTION

The sequence of reactions that make up the carotenoid biosynthetic pathway was mostly established by the 1960s, based on classical biochemical procedures that employed specific inhibitors, labeled precursors, and naturally occurring mutants. However, attempts to purify and characterize individual enzymes were largely unsuccessful. These membrane-associated enzymes are typically present in low amounts, are sensitive to detergents used for solubilization, and may require additional plastid components for activity (Hirschberg et al., 1997; Cunningham and Gantt, 1998; Sandmann, 2001). In the 1990s, the successful cloning of genes for carotenogenic enzymes, from the early steps to the predominant xanthophylls, allowed their characterization and greatly advanced knowledge and understanding of carotenogenesis at the molecular level (Hirschberg et al., 1997; Cunningham and Gantt, 1998).

2.2 BIOSYNTHESIS IN PLANTS

The biosynthesis of carotenoids is now well established, including the enzymes responsible for the different steps, and has been comprehensively reviewed (Cunningham and Gantt, 1998; Fraser and Bramley, 2004; Bouvier et al., 2005b; Domonkos et al., 2013).

In higher plants, carotenoids are biosynthesized in plastids by nuclear-coded enzymes. Carotenoid biosynthesis can be divided into five main stages. The early stages consist of (1) formation of isopentenyl diphosphate (IPP) (Figure 2.1) and (2) chain elongation to geranylgeranyl diphosphate (GGPP) and formation of phytoene (Figure 2.2). The later stages consist of (1) desaturation from phytoene to lycopene, (2) cyclization of neurosporene or lycopene, and (3) formation of the xanthophylls (Figure 2.3). The early stages up to the formation of GGPP are common to the biosynthesis of all isoprenoid compounds. The first step that is specific to carotenoids is the condensation of two molecules of GGDP to form phytoene, the first C_{40} carotenoid in the biosynthetic pathway.

Food Carotenoids: Chemistry, Biology, and Technology, First Edition. Delia B. Rodriguez-Amaya.

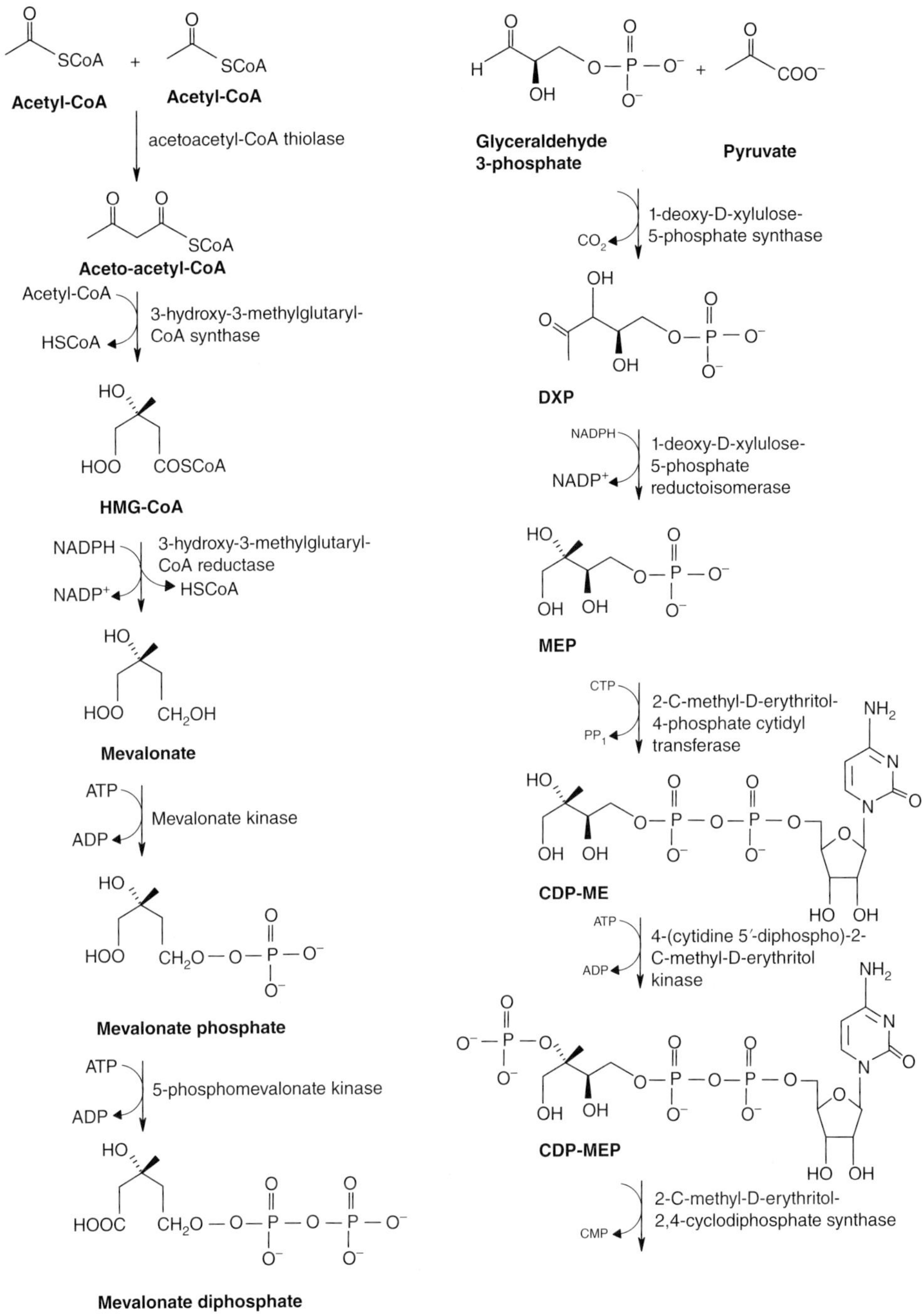

Figure 2.1 Two routes for the formation of isopentenyl diphosphate. Bouvier et al. (2005b). Reproduced with permission from Elsevier.

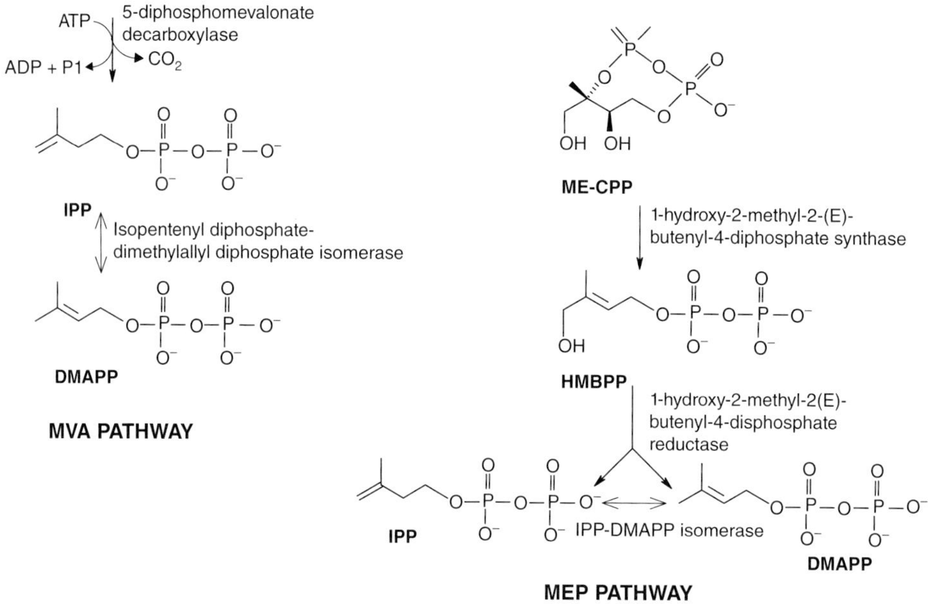

Figure 2.1 (*Continued*)

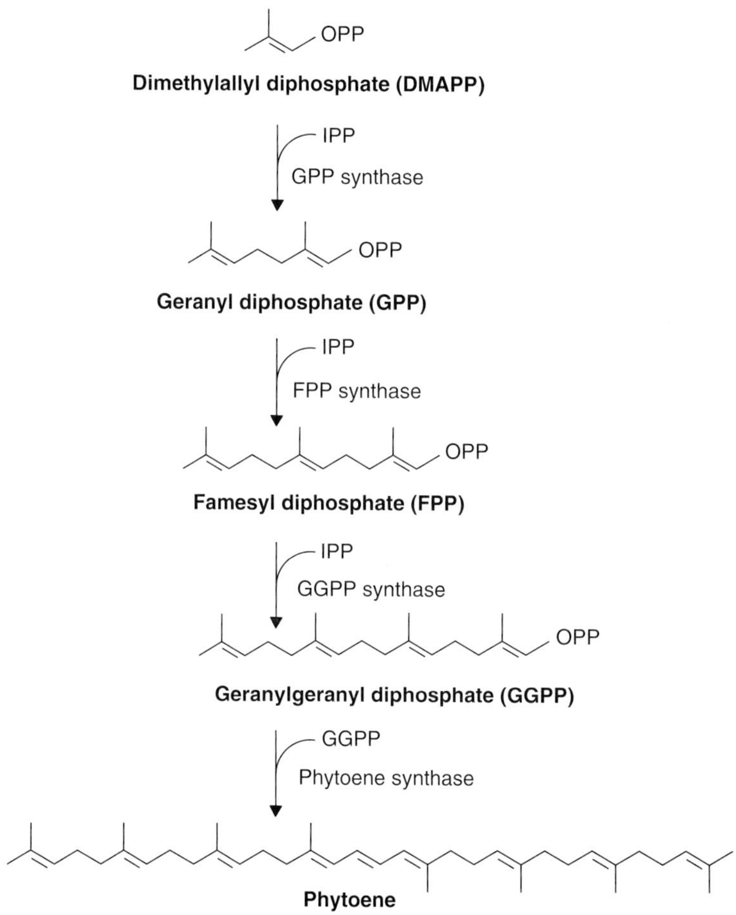

Figure 2.2 Chain elongation and formation of phytoene. Adapted from Cunningham and Gantt (1998).

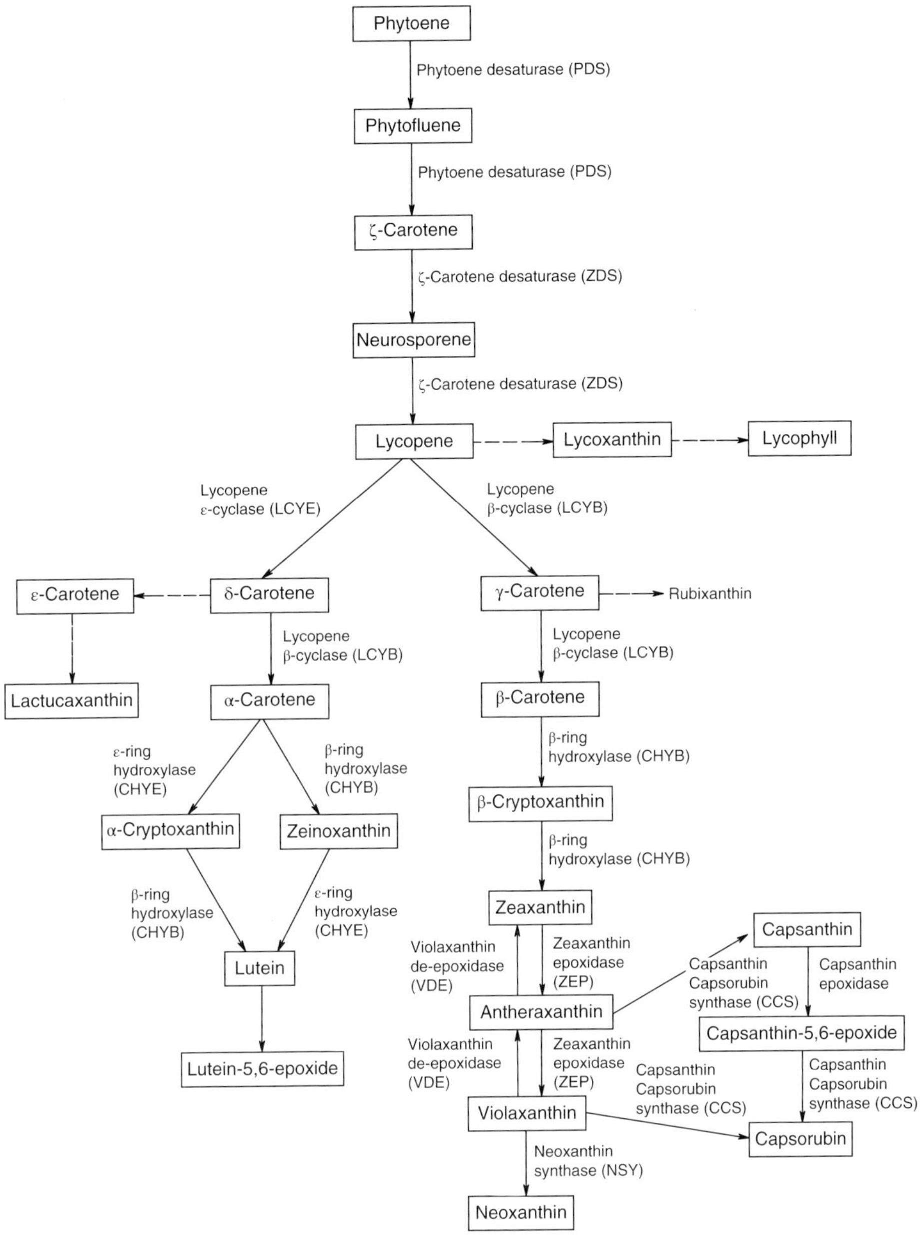

Figure 2.3 Later stages of carotenoid biosynthesis.

2.2.1 Formation of isopentenyl diphosphate

There are two routes for the synthesis of isopentenyl diphosphate (IPP), the universal precursor of isoprenoids, and its isomer dimethylallyl diphosphate (DMAPP) (Figure 2.1). For a long time it was thought that all isoprenoids, including carotenoids, were produced through the well-known mevalonic acid (MVA) pathway (Chappell, 1995; McGarvey and Croteau, 1995). A MVA-independent pathway was later discovered (Rohmer et al., 1993, 1996; Lichtenthaler et al., 1997; Rohmer, 1999; Lichtenthaler, 2000) and is now well documented in plants, the 1-deoxy-D-xylulose-5-phosphate (DXP) pathway, currently better known as the 2-C-methyl-D-erythritol-4-phosphate (MEP) pathway (Eisenreich et al., 2001, 2004; Rodríguez-Concepción and Boronat, 2002). It is now believed that plants synthesize carotenoids mainly by the MEP pathway rather than the MVA pathway as previously assumed (Bramley, 2002). The MVA pathway is responsible for the formation of sterols, sesquiterpenoids, and triterpenoids in the cytosol, while the MEP pathway leads to the formation of plastidic isoprenoids, such as carotenoids, phytol, plastoquinone-9, and diterpenes (Lichtenthaler, 1999; Bouvier et al., 2005b), although the formation of plastid isoprenoids at some developmental stages can arise partly from the MVA pathway. Cross-talk between the two pathways occur, with exchange of intermediates (IPP, GPP, FPP) between the cytoplasm and the plastids (Arigoni et al., 1997; Rohmer, 1999; Taylor and Ramsey, 2005). All genes encoding enzymes of the MEP and MVA pathways have been cloned and functionally analyzed (Bouvier et al., 2005a).

In the MVA pathway, condensation of two molecules of acetyl-CoA mediated by the enzyme acetoacetyl-CoA thiolase (AACT) produces acetoacetyl-CoA (Rodríguez-Concepción and Boronat, 2002; Lombard and Moreira, 2011). Acetoacetyl-CoA condenses with a third molecule of acetyl-CoA, forming 3-hydroxy-3-methylglutaryl-CoA (HMG-CoA), in the presence of HMG-CoA synthase (HMGS). HMG-CoA is reduced to MVA by HMG-CoA reductase (HMGR), phosphorylated by mevalonate kinase (MVK) and further phosphorylated by phosphomevalonate kinase (PMK) to mevalonate diphosphate (MVPP). In an ATP-dependent reaction, decarboxylation by MVPP decarboxylase (DPMDC or PMD) finally generates IPP. A molecule of IPP is isomerized to its isomer dimethylallyl diphosphate (DMAPP), catalyzed by IPP isomerase (IPPI).

The MEP pathway commences with the condensation of pyruvate with D-glyceraldehyde-3-phosphate (G3P), producing 1-deoxy-D-xylulose 5-phosphate (DXP), in the presence of DXP synthase (DXS). The carboxyl group of pyruvate is lost as CO_2. DXS uses thiamine diphosphate as cofactor and requires a divalent cation, such as Mg^{2+} or Mn^{2+}. Intramolecular skeletal rearrangement and subsequent reduction of DXP forms MEP, considered the first committed precursor of the pathway (Rohmer et al., 1996; Arigoni et al., 1997). The enzyme that catalyzes this reaction, DXP reductoisomerase (DXR), requires NADPH and Mn^{2+} as cofactors. MEP cytidyl transferase (MCT), also designated as CMS (CDP-ME synthase), transfers a cytidyl phosphate moiety to MEP transforming it to 4-(cytidine 5'-diphospho)-2-C-methyl-D-erythritol (CDP-ME), and phosphorylation of the tertiary hydroxyl group of CDP-ME is catalyzed by CDP-ME kinase (CMK). Formation of 2-C-methyl-D-erythritol-2,4-cyclodiphosphate (MECPP) is mediated by MECPP synthase (MCS) (Rodríguez-Concepción and Boronat, 2002), via intramolecular transphosphorylation releasing CMP. With the enzyme hydroxymethylbutenyl synthase (HDS), MECPP is converted to 1-hydroxy-2-methyl-2-(*E*)-butenyl-4-diphosphate (HMBPP), which is finally transformed by the enzyme HMBPP reductase (HDR) into a 5:1 mixture of IPP and DMAPP.

Most of the enzymes of the MEP pathway have been characterized structurally (Hunter, 2007). *DXS* genes have been isolated from a variety of plants, such as pepper (Bouvier et al., 1998b), tomato (Lois et al., 2000), peppermint (Lange et al., 1998), marigold (Moehs et al., 2001), soybean (Zhang et al., 2009), and corn (Cordoba et al., 2011), and functionality has been demonstrated.

Plastidic forms of IPP isomerase has been purified from pepper (Dogbo and Camara, 1987). For optimum activity, a divalent ion, typically Mg^{2+} or Mn^{2+}, is required. The gene encoding this enzyme has been identified in marigold (Moehs et al., 2001).

2.2.2 Chain elongation to GGPP and formation of phytoene

For both MEP and MVA pathways, DMAPP serves as the primer for the sequential and linear chain elongation, catalyzed by the respective synthases (also called prenyl transferases) (Figure 2.2). Successive additions of IPP in a head to tail fashion yield in sequence C_{10} geranyl diphosphate (GPP), C_{15} farnesyl diphosphate (FPP), and C_{20} GGPP, catalyzed by GPP synthase (GPPS), FPP synthase (FPPS) and GGPP synthase (GGPPS), respectively. These reactions involve the attack of a carbonium ion to the electron-rich C-3,4 double bond of the IPP molecule with the concurrent loss of inorganic phosphate.

GGPPS has been purified from the chromoplast of pepper (Dogbo and Camara, 1987). The pepper cDNA has been cloned, sequenced, and expressed (Kuntz et al., 1992), and that of tomato has been isolated (Römer et al., 1993).

The tail-to-tail condensation of two molecules of GGPP, catalyzed by phytoene synthase (PSY), produces phytoene, passing through prephytoene diphosphate as an intermediate (Dogbo and Camara, 1987; Hirschberg, 2001). This is considered the rate-limiting and most important step in carotenoid biosynthesis. The colorless phytoene (three conjugated double bonds), the first C_{40} carotenoid in the pathway, is formed by elimination of the diphosphate group and stereospecific proton abstraction (Sandmann, 2001).

Genes encoding PSY have been identified and isolated from pepper (Dogbo et al., 1988), tomato (Römer et al., 1993); melon (Karvouni et al., 1995), maize (Buckner et al., 1996), marigold (Moehs et al., 2001) and Satsuma mandarin (Ikona et al., 2001). Two *PSY* genes have been found in tomato (Bartley and Scolnik, 1993; Fray and Grierson, 1993; Misawa et al., 1994; Giorio et al., 2008). *PSY1* is expressed in ripening fruit, whereas *PSY2* is expressed in green tissues and has no role in ripening fruit (Fraser et al., 1999). Detailed characterization of this enzyme has been carried out with pepper (Dogbo et al., 1988) and tomato chromoplasts and chloroplasts (Fraser et al., 2000). The pepper PSY requires only Mn^{2+} while that of tomato requires ATP as well as the divalent ion.

2.2.3 Desaturations from phytoene to lycopene

Starting with phytoene, a series of desaturation reactions sequentially remove two hydrogens from adjoining positions each time, introducing double bonds at alternate sides of the conjugated double bond system (Figure 2.3). This extends the chromophore, giving rise first to colorless phytofluene (5 conjugated double bonds), then to yellow ζ-carotene (7 conjugated double bonds), the orange neurosporene (9 conjugated double bonds), and finally the red lycopene (11 conjugated double bonds). These four sequential desaturations proceed in two steps, catalyzed by two enzymes, phytoene desaturase (PDS) (phytoene to ζ-carotene with phytofluene as intermediate) and ζ-carotene desaturase (ZDS) (ζ-carotene to lycopene with neurosporene as intermediate) (Sandmann, 1994; Cunningham and Gantt, 1998). Phytoene is found in carotenogenic plants as the 15-*Z* geometric isomer, whereas lycopene is in the all-*E* form; thus, geometric isomerization occurs at some stage during desaturation (Fraser and Bramley, 2004), particularly in the ZDS-mediated desaturation (Isaacson et al., 2004).

PDS genes have been identified and isolated from soybean (Bartley et al., 1991), pepper (Hugueney et al., 1992), tomato (Pecker et al., 1992), and maize (Z.H. Li et al., 1996). Encoding genes of *ZDS* have been identified and characterized in pepper (Albrecht et al., 1995; Breitenbach et al., 1999), tomato (Bartley and Ishida, 1999), and maize endosperm (Matthews et al., 2003).

Two carotenoid isomerases have been isolated from plants. *Z*-carotene isomerase (Z-ISO), which converts 9,15,9′-*Z*-ζ-carotene to 9, 9′-*Z*-ζ-carotene via the isomerization of the 15-*Z*-double bond, was isolated from a corn mutant (Chen and Wurtzel, 2010). The gene for the second isomerase (*CRTISO*) was cloned from tomato (Isaacson et al., 2002), expressed in *Escherichia coli*, and the biochemical properties of the enzyme were investigated (Isaacson et al., 2004). It was concluded that CRTISO functions in parallel with ζ-carotene desaturation by converting 7,9,9′-tri-*Z*-neurosporene to 9′-*Z*-neurosporene and 7′,9′-di-*Z*-lycopene to all-*E*-lycopene.

When *CRTISO* is not functional, the unique bright orange pigment pro-lycopene (7Z,9Z,7′Z,9′Z-lycopene) is accumulated because the α- and β-cyclase enzymes are specific to all-*E*-lycopene. Mutants accumulating pro-lycopene instead of all-*E*-lycopene as their major carotenoid have been reported in tomato (Zechmeister et al., 1941), watermelon (Tadmor et al., 2005) and melon (Galpaz et al., 2013). It is hypothesized that the function of carotene isomerase in plants is to enable carotenoid biosynthesis to occur in the dark and in nonphotosynthetic tissues (Isaacson et al., 2002). In photosynthetic tissues, ζ-carotene and lycopene can undergo both enzymatic isomerization and photoisomerization (Isaacson et al., 2004).

2.2.4 Cyclization to β-carotene and α-carotene

Cyclization occurs at one or both ends of the acyclic molecule (Figure 2.3), initiated by proton attack at the C-2 carbon of the terminal, isolated C-1,2 double bond, forming a six-membered ring. Cyclization creates a branching point. Lycopene, the usual acyclic precursor, is cyclized at one end of the molecule by lycopene ε-ring cyclase (LCYE), producing the monocyclic δ-carotene, or by lycopene β-cyclase (LCYB), yielding γ-carotene, which is also monocyclic. Cyclization at the other end of the molecule by β-ring cyclase results, respectively, in the dicyclic carotenes α-carotene and β-carotene. α-Carotene may also be produced through γ-carotene, the β-ring being formed before the ε-ring. Since β- and α-zeacarotenes are sometimes found in plant foods, it is possible that neurosporene is also cyclized.

LCYB gene has been cloned from pepper (Hugueney et al., 1995) and papaya (Skelton et al., 2006). Two lycopene-β-cyclases have been isolated and characterized from tomato, one of which is chromoplast-specific (Pecker et al., 1996; Ronen et al., 2000). *LCYE* gene has been isolated from romaine lettuce, one of the few plant species known to contain substantial amounts of lactucaxanthin, a carotenoid with two ε-rings (Cunningham and Gantt, 2001).

Lycopene cyclases proceed via a carbocationic mechanism (Bouvier et al., 1997), a mechanism shared by capsanthin-capsorubin synthase (Bouvier et al., 1994). In lettuce, a single lycopene bicyclase catalyzes the formation of ε-carotene, the precursor of lactucaxanthin (Cunningham and Gantt, 2001).

2.2.5 Formation of xanthophylls

Oxygen functions are normally introduced as the final steps in carotenoid biosynthesis, forming xanthophylls (Figure 2.3). Catalyzed by hydroxylases (Fraser and Bramley, 2004; Botella-Pavía and Rodríguez-Concepción, 2006), hydroxylation can give rise to rubixanthin (monohydroxy) from γ-carotene, and to lycoxanthin (monohydroxy) and lycophyll (dihydroxy) from lycopene. These hydroxylations are based on structural considerations of carotenoids found in foods but have not been demonstrated with the enzymes concerned, so the reaction is shown with broken lines in Figure 2.3.

Hydroxylases introduce hydroxy groups at the C-3 and C-3' positions of either the β- or ε-ring. Introduction of a hydroxyl group in β-carotene, catalyzed by carotenoid β-ring hydroxylase (CHYB), results in β-cryptoxanthin and of a second hydroxyl group, in zeaxanthin. Similar modifications of α-carotene produces the monohydroxy α-cryptoxanthin or zeinoxanthin and the dihydroxy lutein, mediated by β- and ε- hydroxylase (CHYE).

Two genes encoding β-carotene hydroxylases that convert β-carotene to β-cryptoxanthin and zeaxanthin were cloned from pepper (Bouvier et al., 1998c). As with PSY and LCYB, there are two β-carotene hydroxylases in tomato (Hirschberg, 1998).

Epoxidation of β-carotene, β-cryptoxanthin, zeaxanthin, and lutein yields a large number of epoxy carotenoids. Zeaxanthin epoxidase (ZEP) introduces a 5,6-epoxy group into the 3-hydroxy-β-ring of zeaxanthin, forming antheraxanthin. Epoxidation of the other ring yields violaxanthin, which can be converted to neoxanthin by neoxanthin synthase (NSY). Neoxanthin has a single allenic group, assumed to originate from proton abstraction from C-7, which is adjacent to the 5,6-epoxy-5,6-dihydro-β-ring of violaxanthin. The epoxy group then rearranges to 5-hydroxy. In the chloroplast, neoxanthin is in the 9-*Z* form (Domonkos et al., 2013).

Pepper β-cyclohexenyl xanthophyll epoxidase cDNA was cloned and the corresponding enzyme overexpressed and purified from *Escherichia coli* (Bouvier et al., 1996). The epoxidase acted specifically on the β-ring of xanthophylls such as β-cryptoxanthin, zeaxanthin, and antheraxanthin, the proposed reaction mechanism for epoxidation involving the formation of a transient carbocation. It was also shown that the epoxidase gene was up-regulated during oxidative stress and when chloroplasts undergo differentiation into chromoplasts in pepper fruit.

A cDNA for neoxanthin synthase was isolated from tomato (Bouvier et al., 2000). The enzyme was found to be mechanistically and structurally similar to lycopene cyclase and capsanthin-capsorubin synthase (CCS).

De-epoxidation of violaxanthin to regenerate zeaxanthin comprises what is known as the xanthophyll, violaxanthin, or epoxide cycle (Yamamoto, 1979; Demmig-Adams et al., 1996; Young et al., 1997). A violaxanthin de-epoxidase (VDE) cDNA was obtained from romaine lettuce (Bugos and Yamamoto, 1996).

The enzyme capsanthin-capsorubin synthase transforms antheraxanthin and violaxanthin into the unique carotenoids capsanthin and capsorubin, respectively. These ketohydroxycarotenoids of ripe fruits of red pepper are characterized by an unusual five-membered cyclopentane κ-ring, formed from the 3-hydroxy-5,6-epoxy β-ring of violaxanthin and antheraxanthin. The pepper capsanthin/capsorubin synthase has been purified and characterized (Bouvier et al., 1994).

2.3 CLEAVAGE TO APOCAROTENOIDS

The apocarotenoids, such as the β-apocarotenals, bixin, and crocetin, are believed to be generated by cleavage of fragments from the ends of the C_{40} molecule. Carotenoid dioxygenases that catalyze the initial steps in the formation of bixin in *Bixa orellana* seeds and crocin in *Crocus sativus* stigma have been identified and functionally characterized.

Three genes from *Bixa orellana* govern bixin formation (Bouvier et al., 2003a). These genes code for lycopene cleavage dioxygenase, bixin aldehyde dehydrogenase, and norbixin carboxyl methyltransferease. Lycopene 5,6,5′,6′-cleavage initiates bixin formation (Figure 2.4). The bixin dialdehyde produced is converted first to norbixin, then to bixin (Bouvier et al., 2003a).

In *C. sativus*, a chromoplast zeaxanthin 7,8,7′,8′-cleavage dioxygenase initially generates crocetin dialdehyde (Bouvier et al., 2003b; Camara and Bouvier, 2004),

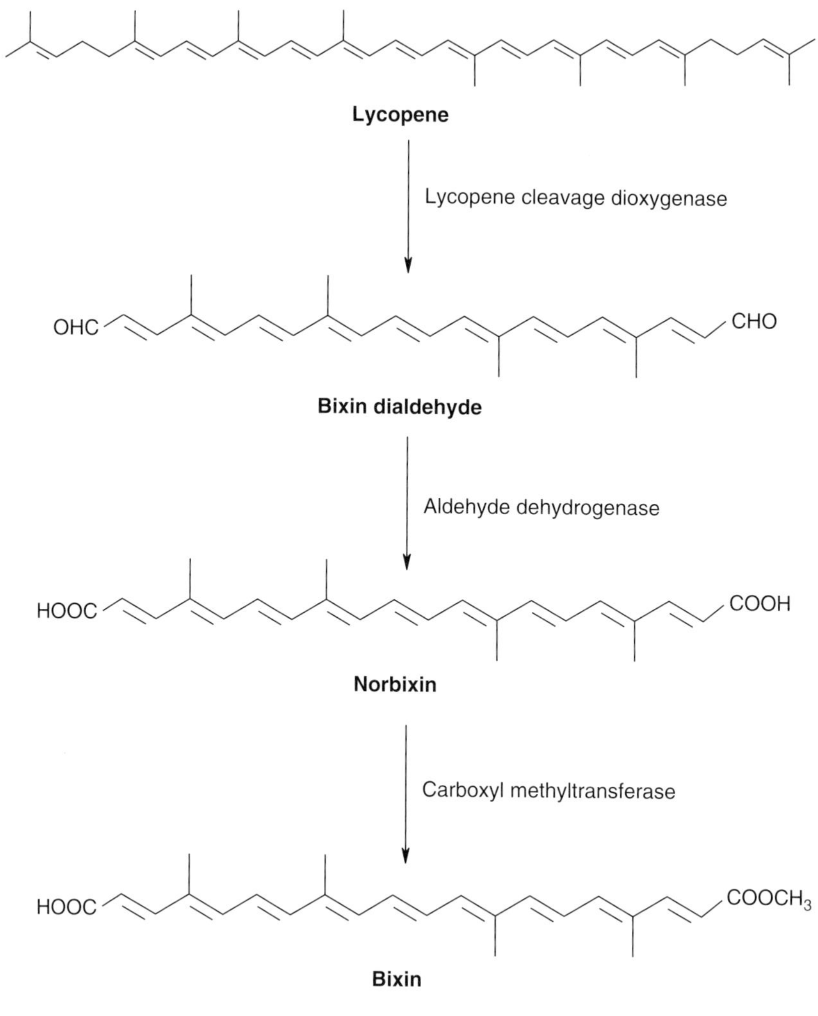

Figure 2.4 Formation of bixin. Adapted from Bouvier et al. (2003a) and Camara and Bouvier (2004).

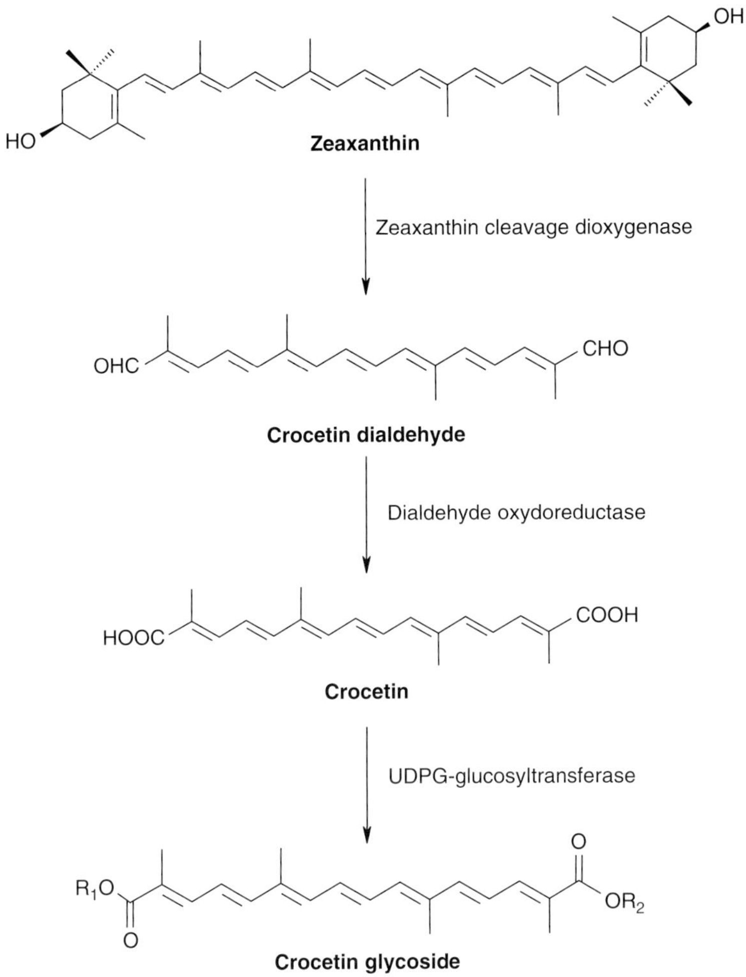

Figure 2.5 Formation of crocin. Adapted from Bouvier et al. (2003b) and Camara Bouvier (2004).

which is subsequently converted to crocetin by an aldehyde oxido-reductase (Figure 2.5). Crocetin is transformed into crocin through the action of UDP-glycosyltransferase.

Neoxanthin and violaxanthin in the light-harvesting complex are believed to be in the *Z*-form (Liu et al., 2004), and it is in this configuration that they serve as precursors of abscisic acid (Parry et al., 1990; Schwartz et al., 1997; Qin and Zeevaart, 1999). VP14 (also called PvNCED1 or 9-*Z*-epoxycarotenoid dioxygenase) catalyzes the first step for the formation of abscisic acid by cleaving the 11,12 (11′,12′) double bond of 9-*Z*-violaxanthin or 9-*Z*-neoxanthin, forming C_{25} apocarotenoids and C_{15} xanthoxin, which is then converted to abscisic acid. Abscisic acid is a phytohormone involved in various physiological processes of plants, such as seed development and dormancy, and in plant responses to environmental stresses (Seo and Koshiba, 2002).

Enzymatic cleavage of carotenoids yields volatile compounds that become part of the typical aroma/flavor of ripe fruits. This topic is discussed in Chapter 8.

2.4 REGULATION OF CAROTENOID BIOSYNTHESIS

Carotenoid biosynthesis in fruits (and flowers) is controlled by regulatory mechanisms that are different from those in photosynthetic tissues. Carotenogenesis in developing chloroplasts proceeds together with the assembly of the light-harvesting antennae and reaction centers with which these pigments are associated. The amounts and identities of carotenoids in the photosynthetic membranes of green plants are relatively constant. In contrast, the carotenoids in nongreen tissues vary considerably both in quantity and composition. The genes coding for components of pathways at photosynthetically active tissues may be under greater selection constraints, and therefore less able to tolerate genotypic diversity, than gene members active only in flowers or fruits (Taylor and Ramsay, 2005). Robust feedback mechanisms also exert control over carotenoid synthesis and accumulation in plant chloroplasts (Cunningham, 2002). The regulation of chromoplast biogenesis plays a crucial role in controlling carotenoid content in plants (L. Li and Yuan, 2013).

Considering that the pathway consists of many steps and the early stages are shared with a large range of noncarotenoid compounds, carotenoid regulation is likely to occur at several levels, involving both transcriptional and post-transcriptional events (Namitha and Negi, 2010).

DXP serves as precursor, not only of IPP, but also of thiamin and pyridoxyl, which are necessary for the functions of plastids. Thus, the formation of MEP from DXP has been considered the first regulatory step in the formation of IPP (Takahashi et al., 1998). The DXS mRNA accumulates when the fruit color changes from mature green to orange or red, indicating that DXS is induced at the onset of ripening. Up-regulation of DXS during chloroplast to chromoplast differentiation was observed in pepper (Bouvier et al., 1998b) and tomato (Lois et al., 2000). FPPS is also considered an important and regulatory enzyme because of its role in directing the carbon flow away from the central portion of the isoprenoid biosynthetic pathways to various important metabolites such as carotenoids, sterols, and ubiquinones (Dhar et al., 2013).

There is ample evidence to indicate that the reaction catalyzed by PSY is an important control point for the regulation of flux into and through the carotenoid pathway (Fraser et al., 2002). Calculation of flux control coefficients allowed the assessment of the control exerted by each step in the pathway (Fraser et al., 2002). Based on these data, PSY1 exerts the greatest control over pathway flux. Large quantities of lycopene accumulate in ripe tomato by increasing the acyclic carotenes of the pathway and blocking the cyclization step. Expression of PSY1 and PDS in tomato is controlled by both environmental and developmental signals (Pecker et al., 1992; Giuliano et al., 1993; Bartley and Scolnik, 1995).

Although the control of gene expression is believed to be the main regulatory mechanism for carotenoids, post-transcriptional regulation has also been cited, including feedback inhibition (Bramley, 2002). Direct inhibition of enzyme activity by carotenoid end products has been demonstrated to a certain extent (Fraser et al., 2000). Expression of a bacterial carotenoid gene (*crtI*) encoding the enzyme PDS in transgenic tomatoes did not elevate total carotenoid levels although β-carotene content increased about threefold, suggesting a feedback inhibition in the pathway (Römer et al., 2000). End-product regulation of the carotenoid biosynthetic pathway is likely to exist in photosynthetic tissues, as noted with PDS gene transcription (Corona et al., 1996).

Transcriptional regulation resulting in increased enzymatic activities had also been observed in ripening of pepper fruit (Römer et al., 1993). Oxidative stress, which enhances carotenoid biosynthesis during chromoplast differentiation, has also been shown to up-regulate expression of carotenoid genes (Bouvier et al., 1998a). Up-regulation of carotenoid gene expression during flower development of marigold (Moehs et al., 2001), as well as melon and citrus fruit (Ikoma et al., 2001) development and ripening, has been reported.

Light and its intensity have been reported to be an important factor in the regulation of carotenoid biosynthesis in plants (Römer and Fraser, 2005), appearing to alter carotenogenesis by increasing the expression of some genes (Fraser and Bramley, 2004). Observing that red light/far red light regulation of PSY activity in tomato was not reflected in PSY1 transcript levels, Schofield and Paliyath (2005) suggested that PSY may be subject to phytochrome post-translational regulation.

Two other likely control points of the carotenoid pathway in plants are the availability of the substrate and the branching of the pathway (Cunningham, 2002).

Substrate specificity of the LCY enzymes is suggested as a mechanism for regulating the partitioning of β- and ε-ring carotenoids (Cunningham and Gantt, 2001).

2.5 CAROTENOGENESIS AND FRUIT RIPENING

With the fundamental roles of carotenoids in plant development and adaptation, their biosynthesis appears to be coordinated with other developmental processes such as plastid formation, flowering, and fruit development (Fraser and Bramley, 2004). Differential transcriptional regulation of carotenoid biosynthesis genes appears to determine the type and amount of carotenoids that accumulate during fruit ripening.

The main regulation mechanisms described to date can be grouped into three categories: (a) control of expression of genes encoding enzymes involved in carotenoid biosynthesis, (b) regulation of enzyme activities, and (c) availability of storage structures (Rodríguez-Concepción and Stange, 2013).

Carotenogenesis during the ripening of tomato fruit has been studied extensively. It is a complex process that occurs along with the differentiation of chloroplast into chromoplast and changes in the sensory properties (Bramley 2002). Developmentally regulated transcription is the major mechanism that governs lycopene accumulation in the ripening fruit (Ronen et al., 2000).

At the breaker stage, the red color of lycopene begins to appear as the chlorophyll content decreases. Carotenoid concentration increases 10- to 14-fold, mainly due to accumulation of lycopene (Fraser et al., 1994), arising from the up-regulation of the early part of the pathway, leading to the synthesis of lycopene, and a down-regulation of the later part of the pathway, preventing lycopene cyclization. Higher expression of isoprenoid genes in the central pathway occurs, notably *DXS* (Lois et al., 2000) and also *HDR* (Botella-Pavía et al., 2004), suggesting that the MEP pathway may be crucial in the overall regulation of lycopene formation in tomato. Additionally, the mRNA levels of both *PSY-1* and *PDS* increase significantly (Pecker et al., 1992, Giuliano et al., 1993; Fraser et al., 1994; Corona et al., 1996), although *PSY* expression increases more than 20-fold while *PDS* expression is raised less than 3-fold (Giuliano et al., 1993). At the same time the mRNAs of both *LCYB* and *LCYE* decrease (Pecker et al., 1996; Ronen et al., 1999). The levels of upstream genes encoding *DXR, HDR, PSY, PDS,* and *ZDS* increase by 2–4 fold at the breaker stage as compared to the leaf (Bramley, 2002; Namitha et al., 2011). Although the control of gene expression is considered to be the main regulatory mechanism, post-transcriptional regulation has also been reported, including feedback inhibition.

DXS is also up-regulated during chloroplast to chromoplast differentiation in pepper (Bouvier et al., 1998b). Expression of the *GGPPS* gene is strongly induced during chloroplast to chromoplast transistion in ripening pepper, correlated with an increase in enzyme activity (Kuntz et al., 1992), and expression of *PSY*, *CHYB*, *ZEP,* and *CCS* (capsanthin-capsorubin synthase) is induced. CCS catalyzes the synthesis of the ketocarotenoids characteristic of pepper fruit (Bartley and Scolnik, 1995). The expression of this gene is under genetic control of the y gene.

In five red pepper cultivars, lutein and neoxanthin, both characteristic of chloroplast pigments, decreased with ripening and eventually disappeared (Hornero-Méndez et al., 2000a). β-Carotene, antheraxanthin, and violaxanthin increased and other pigments were biosynthesized de novo: zeaxanthin, β-cryptoxanthin, capsanthin, capsorubin, capsanthin-5,6-epoxide, and cucurbitaxanthin A. Esterification appeared to be part of the ripening process, the changes in the fractions of free and partially and totally esterified carotenoids being similar among five pepper cultivars (Hornero-Méndez and Mínguez-Mosquera, 2000b). From the first stages of ripening, the fraction of totally esterified pigments (zeaxanthin, β-cryptoxanthin, capsanthin, and capsorubin diesters) made up almost 50% of the total carotenoid content. The proportion of the partially esterified pigment fraction (zeaxanthin, capsanthin, and capsorubin monoesters) increased, with a gradual decrease in the fraction of free pigments (β-cryptoxanthin, β-carotene, zeaxanthin, capsanthin, capsorubin).

In orange (Kato et al., 2004; Rodrigo et al., 2004) and mandarin (Kato et al., 2004, 2007), as the color changes from green to orange, the biosynthesis shifts from β,ε-carotenoids to β,β-carotenoids. The results of Rodrigo et al. (2004) collectively indicated that *PDS* gene expression correlated with carotenoid content in the developing fruit, and up-regulation of *PSY* and *ZDS* genes at the onset of fruit coloration would enhance the production of linear carotenes and the flux into the pathway. The shift from the β,ε-branch to the β,β-branch of the pathway during fruit coloration could be explained by the down-regulation of LCYE and by the increase in LCYB. Expression of genes that produce β,β-xanthophylls (*PSY, PDS, ZDS, LCYB, CHYB,* and *ZEP*) increased dramatically during the pronounced accumulation of β-cryptoxanthin, all-*E*-violaxanthin, and 9′-*Z*-violaxanthin (Kato et al., 2004, 2007). During the β,β-xanthophyll accumulation, the gene expression of carotenoid cleavage dioxygenases (*CCD1, NCED2,* and *NCED3*) increased in the mandarin varieties.

Three *DXS* and three *PSY* were identified in citrus, but *PSY1* and *DXS1* were identified as the main gene members controlling the carotenoid biosynthesis in this fruit

(Peng et al., 2013). Similar results were obtained in 16 citrus cultivars regarding the expression of *DXS1* and *PSY1* and carotenoid accumulation in peel and flesh.

In watermelon, Bang et al. (2007) found that the *LCYB* gene might be the genetic determinant for canary yellow or red flesh color. In five varieties, Kang et al. (2010) investigated the relation between carotenoid profiles and expression of carotenoid-related genes, including *PSY*, *PDS*, *ZDS*, *CRTISO*, *LCYB*, *CHYB*, *NCED1*, *NCED2*, and *NCED3*, during fruit development. In red and pink color varieties, the decrease of gene expression for *LCYB* and *CHYB* at 30 days after pollination might be consistent with the high accumulation of lycopene and β-carotene. In the yellow variety, expression of the genes increased markedly with the onset of maturation, but little carotenoid accumulation was detected, which might be due to a high level of carotenoid cleavage dioxygenases.

Carotenoid accumulation and the expression of the carotenogenic genes, *PSY1, PDS, ZDS, LCYB, LCYE, HYB,* and *ZEP*, were analyzed in two cultivars of Japanese apricot (Kita et al., 2007). In "Orihime" fruits, large increases in carotenoids occurred with the induction of *PSY1* and the downstream genes *LCYB, HYB* and *ZEP*. In "Nanko" fruits, carotenoid accumulation happened mainly after harvest, correlating with appreciable induction of *PSY1* expression, but the downstream genes were not induced, which could explain the lower carotenoid content of this cultivar. In both cultivars, a decrease in *LCYE* expression and increased or constant *LCYB* expression could cause the metabolic shift from the β,ε-synthesis to β,β-carotenoid synthesis that occurs as ripening approaches.

Transcriptional expression patterns of carotenogenic genes were investigated in relation to different carotenoid composition during fruit development in *Cucurbita* species (Nakkanong et al., 2012).The carotenoid (mainly α-carotene and β-carotene) content and the expression of all the genes detected, especially the *PSY1* gene, were low in the pale orange *C. moschata* flesh compared to those in other squashes. The proportion of *CHYB* and *ZEP* activity could account for the almost equal concentrations of violaxanthin and lutein, the predominant carotenoids, in the yellow-fleshed *C. maxima*. In two interspecific inbred lines, the expression of *ZEP* was lower compared to the *CHYB* gene throughout ripening, correlating with the higher concentration of lutein than of violaxanthin and neoxanthin. Gene expression in this study, however, could not explain the observed β-carotene accumulation in the hybrids.

In kiwi fruit, accumulation of β-carotene, the major carotenoid, appeared to be controlled by the level of expression of the *LCYB* gene (Ampomah-Dwamena et al., 2009). *PDS* expression was the least variable among the different genotypes, while *ZDS, CHYB,* and *CHYE* showed some variation in gene expression.

The mRNA levels of 15 carotenogenesis-related genes were analyzed during fruit development and ripening of loquat (Fu et al., 2012). After the breaker stage, the mRNA levels of *PSY1* and *LYCB* were higher in the peel, and *LYCB* and *CHYB* mRNAs were higher in the flesh of red-fleshed, compared with white-fleshed, loquat. The lower carotenoid content in white-fleshed fruit was associated with the lower mRNA levels of *PSY1*, *LYCB*, and *CHYB*, but the failure to develop normal chromoplasts was considered the most convincing explanation for the lack of carotenoid accumulation.

2.6 CAROTENOGENESIS AND SEED AND ROOT DEVELOPMENT

Carotenoids accumulate in corn seed in starch-bearing amyloplasts, principally in the endosperm and, to a lesser extent, in the embryo. During corn endosperm development, carotenoid accumulation is accompanied by increased levels of *PSY* transcripts, whereas *PDS* transcripts are constant (Z.H. Li et al., 1996).

The expression patterns of the major genes encoding the enzymes of the carotenoid biosynthetic pathway were compared in high carotenoid and low carotenoid potato tubers during development and storage (Morris et al., 2004). Significant differences in the profiles were observed, indicating that transcriptional control or mRNA stability was responsible for the large differences in tuber carotenoid content. In particular, there was an inverse relation between the *ZEP* transcript level and the tuber carotenoid content.

Eight genes encoding carotenoid biosynthetic enzymes (*PSY1, PSY2, PDS, ZDS1, ZDS2, LCYE, LCYB1* and *ZEP*) were investigated during the development of white, yellow, orange, and red carrots (Clotault et al., 2008). All eight genes were expressed in the white cultivar although it did not contain carotenoids. In the colored carrots, the expression of the carotenogenic genes began during the early stages of development, increasing progressively for most of the genes during root development as the carotenoid level increased. The high expression of genes encoding ZDS and LCYE in red and yellow cultivars appeared consistent with the accumulation of lycopene and lutein, respectively. Illuminated carrot root sections do not enlarge as much as the dark-grown roots and they contain chloroplasts with high levels of lutein, instead of the β-carotene-rich chromoplasts found in underground roots (Rodríguez-Concepción and Stange, 2013).

2.7 FUNCTIONS IN PLANTS

As vital components of the photosynthetic apparatus, carotenoids are universally found in green tissues, located in the chloroplast thylakoid membranes, associated with the reaction centers and antenna complexes of photosystems I and II. They are in pigment-protein complexes to ensure the right positioning and orientation essential for efficient energy transfer. Photosystem I is enriched in β-carotene and photosystem II in lutein (Demmig-Adams et al., 1996).

Carotenoids play diverse roles in photosynthesis: (1) light harvesting, (2) photoprotection, (3) dissipation of excess energy, (4) structure stabilization and assembly, and (5) regulation of membrane fluidity (Britton, 1995; Demmig-Adams et al., 1996; Frank and Cogdell, 1996). The two principal functions of carotenoids in photosynthesis involve interaction with chlorophyll in different directions (Demmig-Adams et al., 1996). While light collection for photosynthesis requires passing energy to chlorophyll, photoprotection involves channeling energy away from chlorophyll. Photoprotective processes prevent or minimize generation of oxidizing molecules, scavenge reactive oxygen species efficiently, and repair damage that inevitably occurs (Niyogi, 1999).

Carotenoids (mainly the xanthophylls) act as accessory light-harvesting pigments, absorbing light at wavelengths where chlorophylls do not absorb, and passing their excitation energy to chlorophyll.

Carotenoids in the reaction centers and antenna complexes react with and efficiently quench triplet chlorophyll, singlet oxygen, and superoxide anion radicals (Demmig-Adams and Adams, 1994; Britton, 1995; Frank and Cogdell, 1996). Carotenoids are especially important in providing protection against photooxidation by singlet oxygen ($^1O_2$) (Niyogi, 1999). When the light-harvesting chlorophylls absorb more light than needed for photosynthesis, some chlorophyll molecules will undergo intersystem crossing to form the excited state, ^{3}CHL. The energy of ^{3}CHL can be transferred to ground state triplet oxygen ($^3O_2$) to yield $^1O_2$, a highly reactive species that can rapidly damage lipids, proteins, membranes, and tissues. Carotenoids, particularly β-carotene, can efficiently quench ^{3}CHL, thus preventing the formation of $^1O_2$. They can also quench $^1O_2$ if formed.

There is a clear correlation between the dissipation of excess excitation energy and the formation of zeaxanthin from violaxanthin in the light-harvesting complexes of plants (Young et al., 1997). When photosynthetic tissues are exposed to excess light, not all the absorbed light can be utilized for photosynthesis and should be removed to avoid damage. *VDE* catalyzes the two-step deepoxidation that transforms violaxanthin to zeaxanthin via antheraxanthin (Figure 2.3) (Yamamoto, 1979; Demmig-Adams et al., 1996). This is a reversible reaction, and under low-light conditions transformation of zeaxanthin into violaxanthin can occur, mediated by *ZEP*. *VDE* has been purified and its gene cloned from romaine lettuce (Bugos and Yamamoto, 1996).

This interconversion of zeaxanthin and violaxanthin is called the xanthophyll cycle, the participating components of which were first fully identified by Yamamoto (1979). It is a key for plant adaptation to changing environmental conditions. The acclimation of the carotenoid composition of leaves to a shade environment, with a high demand for efficient light collection, versus a fully sun-exposed site, with a high demand for photoprotection, has been described in many species of higher plants (Thayer and Björkman,1990; Demmig-Adams and Adams, 1994; Demmig-Adams et al., 1996). The deepoxidized xanthophylls zeaxanthin and antheraxanthin, along with a low pH within the photosynthetic membrane, facilitate the harmless dissipation of excess excitation energy directly within the light-harvesting chlorophyll antennae (Demmig-Adams et al., 1996).

Aside from their well-established function as collectors of light energy for photosynthesis and as quenchers of triplet chlorophyll and singlet oxygen, carotenoids of higher plant chloroplasts might also play an important structural role (Havaux, 1998).

Xanthophylls that contain polar groups at the two ends of the molecule, particularly those having all-*E* configuration, are positioned in the membrane in a way that permits anchoring of their terminal groups in the two opposite polar zones of the bilayer, forming hydrogen bonds with the hydrophilic groups of the lipids (Gruszecki and Strzalka, 2005). Such localization and orientation favors van der Waals interaction with the alkyl chains of membrane lipids. These interactions between xanthophyll molecules and membrane lipids result in a decrease in membrane fluidity, an increase in membrane thermostability, and a lowered susceptibility to lipid peroxidation (Havaux, 1998).

Carotenoids can also protect nonphotosynthetic tissues against $^1O_2$, which can be generated in the presence of photosensitizers other than chlorophyll. Moreover, they serve as precursors for the plant growth regulator abscisic acid (Zeevart and Creelman, 1988; Parry et al., 1990) and act as coloring agents in flowers and fruits to attract

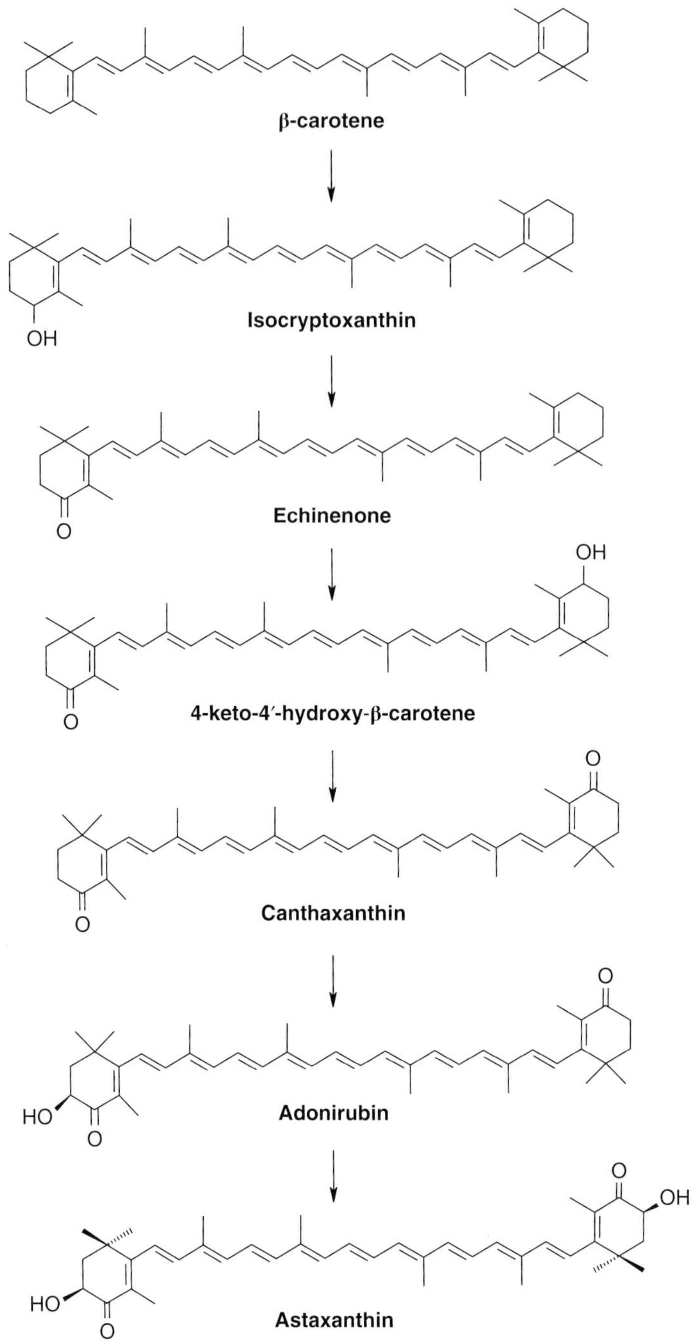

Figure 2.6 Formation of astaxanthin from β-carotene. Adapted from Simpson et al. (1981) and Shahidi and Brown (1998).

pollinators and agents of seed dispersal. Cleavage of carotenoids to apocarotenoids has attracted attention in recent years. Apocarotenoids act as visual or volatile signals to attract pollinating and dispersal agents and may also play a role in plant defense (Bouvier et al., 2005a). They may also convey signals that regulate plant architecture.

2.8 METABOLISM IN ANIMALS

Animals are unable to synthesize carotenoids de novo so they are obtained from the diet. Ingested carotenoids are either accumulated unchanged or are slightly modified into typical animal carotenoids.

Avian species preferentially deposit their ingested carotenoids in the liver, eggs, body fat, skin, feathers, beak, and shanks (Marusich and Bauernfeind, 1981). β-Carotene is not an effective pigmenter because it is efficiently converted to vitamin A. In dairy cow, however, β-carotene is both a pigmenter and a provitamin source. Ingested β-carotene that is not converted to vitamin A is stored in the fatty tissues of the body and the butterfat of milk.

Pigmentation of poultry involves primarily the skin coloration of meat chickens and the degree and shade of egg yolk color (Marusich and Bauernfeind, 1981). Consumers generally prefer broilers with uniformly well pigmented skin and shanks, a yellow coloration being often associated with quality and health. With eggs, a uniformly light to deep yellow yolk color is generally preferred by consumers. The xanthophylls lutein and zeaxanthin are preferentially deposited in eggs.

Wild fish obtain astaxanthin from marine bacteria and microalgae. For fish (e.g., salmon) grown in aquaculture, astaxanthin must be provided through the feed to give the typical reddish pink color to their flesh. In Arctic char (*Salvelinus alpinus* L.) fed with diets containing astaxanthin, canthaxanthin, and a mixture of both, carotenoids were absorbed without chemical change in the flesh or the skin (Shahidi et al., 1994).

When astaxanthin is not provided, the most common modification is the introduction of a carbonyl function at C-4 and C-4′, producing echinenone and canthaxanthin when β-carotene is the substrate (Figure 2.6) in fish (Simpson et al., 1981) and crustaceans (Shahidi and Brown, 1998). Hydroxylation at C-3 and C-3′ following the introduction of the keto groups forms astaxanthin.

References

Albrecht M, Klein A, Hugueney P, Sandmann G, Kuntz M. 1995. Molecular cloning and functional expression in *E. coli* of a novel plant enzyme mediating ζ-carotene desaturation. *FEBS Lett* 372:199–202.

Ampomah-Dwamena C, McGhie T, Wibisono R, Montefiori M, Hellens RP, Allan AC. 2009. The kiwi lycopene beta-cyclase plays a significant role in carotenoid accumulation in fruit. *J Exp Bot* 60:3765–79.

Arigoni D, Sagner S, Latzel C, Eisenreich, W, Bacher A, Zenk MH. 1997. Terpenoid biosynthesis from 1-deoxy-D-xylulose in higher plants by intramolecular skeletal rearrangement. *Proc Natl Acad Sci USA* 94:10600–5.

Bang H, Kim S, Leskovar D, King S. 2007. Development of a codominant CAPS marker for allelic selection between canary yellow and red watermelon based on SNP in lycopene β-cyclase *(LCYB)* gene. *Mol Breed* 20:63–72.

Bartley GE, Ishida BK. 1999. ζ-Carotene desaturase (Accession No. AF195507) from tomato. *Plant Physiol* 121:1383.
Bartley GE, Scolnik PA. 1993. cDNA cloning, expression during development, and genome mapping of PSY2, a second tomato gene encoding phytoene synthase. *J Biol Chem* 268:25718–21.
Bartley GE, Scolnik PA. 1995. Plant carotenoids: Pigments for photoprotection, visual attraction and human health. *Plant Cell* 7:1027–38.
Bartley GE, Viitanen PV, Pecker I, Chamovitz D, Hirschberg J, Scolnik PA. 1991. Molecular cloning and expression in photosynthetic bacteria of a soybean cDNA coding for phytoene desaturase, an enzyme of the carotenoid biosynthesis pathway. *Proc Natl Acad Sci* 88:6532–6.
Botella-Pavía P, Besumbes O, Phillips MA, Carretero-Paulet L, Boronat A, Rodríguez-Concepción M. 2004. Regulation of carotenoid biosynthesis in plants: Evidence for a key role of hydroxymethylbutenyl diphosphate reductase in controlling the supply of plastidial isoprenoid precursors. *Plant J* 40:188–99.
Botella-Pavía P, Rodríguez-Concepción M. 2006. Carotenoid biotechnology in plants for nutritionally improved foods. *Physiol Plant* 126:369–81.
Bouvier F, Backhaus RA, Camara B. 1998a. Induction and control of chromoplast-specific carotenoid genes by oxidative stress. *J Biol Chem* 273:30651–9.
Bouvier F, d'Harlingue A, Backhaus RA, Kumagai MH, Camara B. 2000. Identification of neoxanthin synthase as a carotenoid cyclase paralog. *Eur J Biochem* 267:6346–52.
Bouvier F, d'Harlingue A, Camara B. 1997. Molecular analysis of carotenoid cyclase inhibition. *Arch Biochem Biophys* 346:53–64.
Bouvier F, d'Harlingue A, Hugueney P, Marin E, Marion-Poll A, Camara B. 1996. Xanthophyll biosynthesis: Cloning, expression, functional reconstitution, and regulation of β-cyclohexenyl carotenoid epoxide from pepper (*Capsicum annuum*). *J Biol Chem* 271:28861–7.
Bouvier F, d'Harlingue A, Suire C, Backhaus RA, Camara B. 1998b. Dedicated roles of plastid transketolases during the early onset of isoprenoid biogenesis in pepper fruits. *Plant Physiol* 117:1423–31.
Bouvier F, Dogbo O, Camara B. 2003a. Biosynthesis of the food and cosmetic plant pigment bixin (annatto). *Science* 300:2089–91.
Bouvier F, Hugueney P, d'Harlingue A, Kuntz M, Camara B. 1994. Xanthophyll biosynthesis in chromoplasts: Isolation and molecular cloning of an enzyme catalyzing the conversion of 5,6-epoxycarotenoids into ketocarotenoids. *Plant J* 6:45–54.
Bouvier F, Keller Y, d'Harlingue A, Camara B. 1998c. Xanthophyll biosynthesis: Molecular and functional characterization of carotenoid hydroxylases from pepper fruits (*Capsicum annuum* L.). *Biochem Biophys Acta* 1391:320–8.
Bouvier F, Isner J-C, Dogbo O, Camara B. 2005a. Oxidative tailoring of carotenoids: A prospect towards novel functions in plants. *Trends Plant Sci* 10:187–94.
Bouvier F, Rahier A, Camara B. 2005b. Biogenesis, molecular regulation and function of plant isoprenoid. *Prog Lipid Res* 44:357–429.
Bouvier F, Suire C, Mutterer J, Camara B. 2003b. Oxidative remodeling of chromoplast carotenoids: Identification of the carotenoid dioxygenase CsCCD and CsZCD genes involved in Crocus secondary metabolite biogenesis. *Plant Cell* 15:47–62.
Bramley PM. 2002. Regulation of carotenoid formation during tomato fruit ripening and development. *J Exp Bot* 53:2107–13.
Breitenbach J, Kuntz M, Takaichi S, Sandmann G. 1999. Catalytic properties of an expressed and purified higher plant type ζ-carotene desaturase from *Capsicum annuum*. *Eur J Biochem* 265:376–83.
Britton G. 1995. Structure and properties of carotenoids in relation to functions. *FASEB J* 9:1551–8.
Buckner B, San Miguel P, Janick-Buckner D, Bennetzen JL. 1996. The yl gene of maize codes for phytoene synthase. *Genetics* 143:479–88.
Bugos RC, Yamamoto HY. 1996. Molecular cloning of violaxanthin de-epoxidase from romaine lettuce and expression in *Escherichia coli*. *Proc Natl Acad Sci* 93:6320–5.
Camara B, Bouvier F. 2004. Oxidative remodeling of plastid carotenoids. *Arch Biochem Biophys* 430:16–21.
Chappell J. 1995. Biochemistry and molecular biology of the isoprenoid biosynthetic pathway in plants. *Annu Rev Plant Physiol Mol Biol* 46:521–47.
Chen Y, Li F, Wurtzel ET. 2010. Isolation and characterization of the *Z-ISO* gene encoding a missing component of the carotenoid biosynthesis in plants. *Plant Physiol* 153:66–79.
Clotault J, Peltier D, Berruyer R, Thomas M, Briard M, Geoffriau E. 2008. Expression of carotenoid biosynthesis genes during carrot root development. *J Exp Bot* 59:3563–73.

Cordoba E, Porta H, Arroyo A, San-Roman C, Medina, L, Rodriguez-Concepcion M, Leon P. 2011. Functional characterization of three genes encoding 1-deoxy-D-xylulose 5-phosphate synthase in maize. *J Exp Bot* 62:2023–38.

Corona V, Aracri B, Kosturkova G, Bartley GE, Pitto L, Giorgetti L, Scolnik PA, Giuliano G. 1996. Regulation of a carotenoid biosynthesis gene promoter during plant development. *Plant J* 9:505–12.

Cunningham FX Jr. 2002. Regulation of carotenoid synthesis and accumulation in plants. *Pure Appl Chem* 74:1409–17.

Cunningham FX Jr, Gantt E. 1998. Genes and enzymes of carotenoid biosynthesis in plants. *Annu Rev Plant Physiol Plant Mol Biol* 49:557–83.

Cunningham FX Jr, Gantt E. 2001. One ring or two? Determination of ring number in carotenoids by lycopene ε-cyclases. *Proc Natl Acad Sci* 98:2905–10.

Demmig-Adams B, Adams WW III. 1994. Capacity for energy dissipation in the pigment bed in leaves with different xanthophyll cycle pools. *Aust J Plant Physiol* 22:575–88.

Demmig-Adams B, Gilmore AM, Adams WW III. 1996. Carotenoids 3: *In vivo* function of carotenoids in higher plants. *FASEB J* 10:403–12.

Dhar MK, Koul A, Kaul S. 2013. Farnesyl pyrophosphate synthase: A key enzyme in isoprenoid biosynthetic pathway and potential molecular target for drug development. *New Biotechnol* 30:114–23.

Dogbo O, Camara B. 1987. Purification of isopentenyl isomerase and geranylgeranyl pyrophosphate synthase from *Capsicum* chromoplasts by affinity chromatography. *Biochem Biophys Acta* 920:140–8.

Dogbo O, Laferriere A, d'Harlingue A, Camara B. 1988. Carotenoid biosynthesis: Isolation of bifunctional enzyme catalyzing the synthesis of phytoene. *Proc. Natl Acad Sci* 85:7054–8.

Domonkos I, Kis M, Gombos Z, Ughy B. 2013. Carotenoids, versatile components of oxygenic photosynthesis. *Prog Lipid Res* 52:539–61.

Eisenreich W, Bacher A, Arigoni D, Rohdich F. 2004. Biosynthesis of isoprenoids via the non-mevalonate pathway. *Cell Mol Life Sci* 61:1401–26.

Eisenreich W, Rohdich F, Bacher A. 2001. Deoxyxylulose phosphate pathway to terpenoids. *Trends Plant Sci* 6:78–84.

Frank HA, Cogdell RJ. 1996. Carotenoids in photosynthesis. *Photochem Photobiol* 63:257–64.

Fraser PD, Bramley PM. 2004. The biosynthesis and nutritional uses of carotenoids. *Prog Lipid Res* 43:228–65.

Fraser PD, Kiano JW, Truesdale MR, Schuch W, Bramley PM. 1999. Phytoene synthase-2 enzyme activity in tomato does not contribute to carotenoid synthesis in ripening fruit. *Plant Mol Biol* 40:687–98.

Fraser PD, Römer S, Shipton CA, Mills PB, Kiano JW, Misawa N, Drake RG, Schuch W, Bramley PM. 2002. Evaluation of transgenic tomato plants expressing an additional phytoene synthase in a fruit-specific manner. *Proc Natl Acad Sci USA* 99:1092–7.

Fraser PD, Schuch W, Bramley PM. 2000. Phytoene synthase from tomato (*Lycopersicon esculentum*) chloroplasts: Partial purification and biochemical properties. *Planta* 211:361–9.

Fraser PD, Truesdale MR, Bird CR, Schuch W, Bramley PM. 1994. Carotenoid biosynthesis during tomato fruit development: Evidence for tissue-specific gene expression. *Plant Physiol* 105:405–13.

Fray RG, Grierson D. 1993. Identification and genetic analysis of normal and mutant phytoene synthase genes of tomato by sequencing, complementation and co-suppression. *Plant Mol Biol* 22:589–602.

Fu XM, Kong WB, Peng G, Zhou J, Azam M, Xu C, Grierson D, Chen K. 2012. Plastid structure and carotenogenic gene expression in red- and white-fleshed loquat (*Eriobotrya japonica*) fruits. *J Exp Bot* 63:341–54.

Galpaz N, Burger Y, Lavee T, Tzuri G, Sherman A, Melamed T, Eshed R, Meir A, Portnoy V, Bar E, Shimoni-Shor E, Feder A, Saar Y, Saar U, Baumkolder F, Lewinsohn E, Schaffer AA, Katzir N, Tadmor Y. 2013. Genetic and chemical characterization of an EMS induced mutation in *Cucumis melo* CRTISO gene. *Arch Biochem Biophys* 539:117–25.

Giorio G, Stigliani AL, D'Ambrosio C. 2008. Phytoene synthase genes in tomato (*Solanum lycopersicum* L.): New data on the structures, the deduced amino acid sequences and the expression patterns. *FEBS J* 275:527–35.

Giuliano G, Bartley GE, Scolnik PA. 1993. Regulation of carotenoid biosynthesis during tomato fruit development. *Plant Cell* 5:379–87.

Gruszecki WI, Strzalka K. 2005. Carotenoids as modulators of lipid membrane physical properties. *Biochim Biophys Acta Mol B Dis* 1740:108–15.

Havaux M. 1998. Carotenoids as membrane stabilizers in chloroplasts. *Trends Plant Sci* 3:147–51.

Hirschberg J. 1998. Molecular biology of carotenoid biosynthesis. In: Britton G, Liaaen-Jensen S, Pfander H. editors. *Carotenoids, vol. 3. Biosynthesis and metabolism.* Basel: Birkhäuser Verlag, p 149–94.

Hirschberg J. 2001. Carotenoid biosynthesis in flowering plants. *Curr Opin Plant Biol* 4:210–8.

Hirschberg J, Cohen M, Harker M, Lotan T, Mann V, Pecker I. 1997. Molecular genetics of the carotenoid biosynthesis pathway in plants and algae. *Pure Appl Chem* 69:2151–8.

Hornero-Méndez D, Guevara RG-L de, Mínguez-Mosquera MI. 2000a. Carotenoid biosynthesis changes in five red pepper (*Capsicum annuum* L.) cultivars during ripening. Cultivar selection for breeding. *J Agric Food Chem* 48:3857–64.

Hornero-Méndez D, Mínguez-Mosquera MI. 2000b. Xanthophyll esterification accompanying carotenoid overaccumulation in chromoplast of *Capsicum annuum* ripening fruits is constitutive process and useful for ripeness index. *J Agric Food Chem* 48:1617–22.

Hugueney P, Badillo A, Chen H-C, Klien A, Hirschberg J, Camara B, Kuntz M. 1995. Metabolism of cyclic carotenoids: A model for the alteration of this biosynthetic pathway in *Capsicum annuum* chromoplasts. *Plant J* 8:417–24.

Hugueney P, Römer S, Kuntz M, Camara B. 1992. Characterization and molecular cloning of a flavoprotein catalyzing the synthesis of phytofluene and ζ-carotene in *Capsicum* chromoplasts. *Eur J Biochem* 209:399–407.

Hunter WN. 2007. The non-mevalonate pathway of isoprenoid precursor biosynthesis. *J Biol Chem* 282:21573–7.

Ikoma Y, Komatsu A, Kita M, Ogawa K, Omura M, Yano M, Moriguchi T. 2001. Expression of a phytoene synthase gene and characteristic accumulation during citrus fruit development. *Physiol Plant* 111:232–8.

Isaacson T, Ohad I, Beyer P, Hirschberg J. 2004. Analysis in vitro of the enzyme CRTISO establishes a poly-cis-carotenoid biosynthesis pathway in plants. *Plant Physiol* 136:4246–55.

Isaacson T, Ronen G, Zamir D, Hirschberg J. 2002. Cloning of *tangerine* from tomato reveals a carotenoid isomerase essential for the production of β-carotene and xanthophylls in plants. *Plant Cell* 14:333–42.

Kang B, Zhao W-E, Hou Y, Tian P. 2010. Expression of carotenogenic genes during development and ripening of watermelon fruit. *Sci Hort* 124:368–75.

Karvouni Z, John I, Taylor JE, Watson CF, Turner AJ, Grierson D. 1995. Isolation and characterisation of a melon cDNA clone encoding phytoene synthase. *Plant Mol Biol* 27:1153–62.

Kato M, Ikoma Y, Matsumoto H, Sugiura M, Hyodo H, Yano M. 2004. Accumulation of carotenoids and expression of carotenoid biosynthetic genes during maturation in citrus fruit. *Plant Physiol* 134:824–37.

Kato M, Matsumoto H, Ikoma Y, Kuniga T, Nakajima N, Yoshida T, Yano M. 2007. Accumulation of carotenoids and expression of carotenoid biosynthetic genes and carotenoid cleavage dioxygenase genes during fruit maturation in the juice sacs of 'Tamami,' 'Kiyomi' tangor, and 'Wilking' mandarin. *J Japan Soc Hort Sci* 76:103–11.

Kita M, Kato M, Ban Y, Honda C, Yaegaki H, Ikoma Y, Moriguchi T. 2007. Carotenoid accumulation in Japanese apricot (*Prunus mume* Siebold & Zucc.): Molecular analysis of carotenogenic gene expression and ethylene regulation. *J Agric Food Chem* 55:3414–20.

Kuntz M, Römer S, Suire C, Hugueney P, Weil JH, Schantz R, Camara B. 1992. Identification of a cDNA for the plastid-located geranylgeranyl pyrophosphate synthase from *Capsicum annuum*: Correlative increase in enzyme activity and transcript level during fruit ripening. *Plant J* 2:25–34.

Lange BM, Wildung MR, McCaskill D, Croteau R. 1998. A family of transketolases that directs isoprenoid biosynthesis via mevalonate-independent pathway. *Proc Natl Acad Sci* 95:2100–4.

Li ZH, Matthews PD, Burr B, Wurtzel ET. 1996. Cloning and characterization of maize cDNA encoding phytoene desaturase, an enzyme of the carotenoid biosynthetic pathway. *Plant Mol Biol* 30:269–79.

Li L, Yuan H. 2013. Chromoplast biogenesis and carotenoid accumulation. *Arch Biochem Biophys* 539:102–9.

Lichtenthaler HK. 1999. The 1-deoxy-D-xylulose-5-phosphate pathway of isoprenoid biosynthesis in plants. *Annu Rev Plant Physiol Plant Mol Biol* 50:47–65.

Lichtenthaler HK. 2000. Non-mevalonate isoprenoid biosynthesis: enzymes, genes and inhibitors. *Biochem Soc Trans* 28:785–9.

Lichtenthaler HK, Schwender J, Disch A, Rohmer M. 1997. Biosynthesis of isoprenoids in higher plant chloroplasts proceeds via a mevalonate-independent pathway. *FEBS Lett* 400:271–4.

Liu Z, Yan H, Wang K, Kuang T, Zhang J, Gui L, An X, Chang W. 2004. Crystal structure of spinach major light-harvesting complex at 2.72 A resolution. *Nature* 428:287–92.

Lois LM, Rodríguez-Concepción M, Gallego F, Campos N, Boronat A. 2000. Carotenoid biosynthesis during tomato fruit development: Regulatory role of 1-deoxy-D-xylulose 5-phosphate synthase. *Plant J* 22:503–13.

Lombard J, Moreira D. 2011. Origins and early evolution of the mevalonate pathway of isoprenoid biosynthesis in the three domains of life. *Mol Biol Evol* 28:87–99.

Marusich WL, Bauernfeind JC. 1981. Oxycarotenoids in poultry feeds. In: Bauernfeind JC. editor. *Carotenoids as colorants and vitamin A precursors. Technological and nutritional applications.* New York: Academic Press, p 319–462.

Matthews PD, Luo RB, Wurtzel ET. 2003. Maize phytoene desaturase and ζ-carotene desaturase catalyse a poly-*Z* desaturation pathway: Implications for genetic engineering of carotenoid content among cereal crops. *J Exp Bot* 54:2215–30.

McGarvey DJ, Croteau R. 1995. Terpenoid metabolism. *Plant Cell* 7, 1015–26.

Misawa N, Truesdale MR, Sandmann G, Fraser PD, Bird C, Schuch W, Bramley PM. 1994. Expression of a tomato cDNA coding for phytoene synthase in *Escherichia coli*, phytoene formation *in vivo* and *in vitro*, and functional analysis of the various truncated gene products. *J Biochem* 116:980–5.

Moehs CP, Tian L, Osteryoung KW, DellaPenna D. 2001. Analysis of carotenoid biosynthetic gene expression during marigold petal development. *Plant Mol Biol* 45:281–93.

Morris WL, Ducreux L, Griffiths DW, Stewart D, Davies HV, Taylor MA. 2004. Carotenogenesis during tuber development and storage in potato. *J Exp Bot* 55:975–82.

Nakkanong K, Yang JH, Zhang MF. 2012. Carotenoid accumulation and carotenogenic gene expression during fruit development in novel interspecific inbred squash lines and their parents. *J Agric Food Chem* 60:5936–44.

Namitha KK, Archana SN, Negi PS. 2011. Expression of carotenoid biosynthetic pathway genes and changes in carotenoids during ripening in tomato (*Lycopersicon esculentum*). *Food Funct* 2:168–73.

Namitha KK, Negi PS. 2010. Chemistry and biotechnology of carotenoids. *Crit Rev Food Sci Nutr* 50:728–60.

Niyogi KK. 1999. Photoprotection revisited: Genetic and molecular approaches. *Annu Rev Plant Physiol Plant Mol Biol* 50:333–59.

Parry AD, Babiano MJ, Horgan R. 1990. The role of *cis*-carotenoids in abscisic acid biosynthesis. *Planta* 182:118–28.

Pecker I, Chamovitz D, Linden H, Sandmann G, Hirschberg J. 1992. A single polypeptide catalyzing the conversion of phytoene to ζ-carotene is transcriptionally regulated during tomato fruit ripening. *Proc Natl Acad Sci* 89:4962–6.

Pecker I, Gabbay R, Cunningham FX Jr, Hirschberg J. 1996. Cloning and characterisation of the cDNA for lycopene β-cyclase from tomato reveals a decrease in its expression during tomato ripening. *Plant Mol Biol* 30:807–19.

Peng G, Wang C, Song S, Fu X, Azam M, Grierson D, Xu C. 2013. The role of 1-deoxy-D-xylulose-5-phosphate synthase and phytoene synthase gene family in citrus carotenoid accumulation. *Plant Physiol Biochem* 71:67–76.

Qin X, Zeevaart JAD. 1999. The 9-*cis*-epoxycarotenoid cleavage reaction is the key regulatory step of abscisic acid biosynthesis in water-stressed bean. *Proc Natl Acad Sci USA* 96:15354–61.

Rodrigo M-J, Marcos JF, Zacarias L. 2004. Biochemical and molecular analysis of carotenoid biosynthesis in flavedo of orange (*Citrus sinensis* L.) during fruit development and maturation. *J Agric Food Chem* 52:6724–31.

Rodríguez-Concepción M, Boronat A. 2002. Elucidation of the methylerythritol phosphate pathway for isoprenoid biosynthesis in bacteria and plastids. A metabolic milestone achieved through genomics. *Plant Physiol* 130:1079–89.

Rodríguez-Concepción, Stange C. 2013. Biosynthesis of carotenoids in carrot: An underground story comes to light. *Arch Biochem Biophys* 539:110–6.

Rohmer M. 1999. The mevalonate-independent methylerythritol 4-phosphate (MEP) pathway for isoprenoid biosynthesis, including carotenoids. *Pure Appl Chem* 71:2279–84.

Rohmer M, Knani M, Simonin P, Sutter B, Sahm H. 1993. Isoprenoid biosynthesis in bacteria: A novel pathway for early steps leading to isopentenyl diphosphate. *Biochem J* 295:517–24.

Rohmer M, Seemann M, Horbach S, Bringer-Meyer S, Sahm H. 1996. Glyceraldehyde 3-phosphate and pyruvate as precursors of isoprenic units in an alternative non-mevalonate pathway for terpenoid biosynthesis. *J Am Chem Soc* 118:2564–6.

Römer S, Fraser PD. 2005. Recent advances in carotenoid biosynthesis, regulation and manipulation. *Planta* 221:305–8.

Römer S, Fraser PD, Kiano JW, Shipton CA, Misawa N, Schuch W, Bramley PM. 2000. Elevation of the provitamin A content of transgenic tomato plants. *Nat Biotechnol* 18:666–9.

Römer S, Hugueney P, Bouvier F, Camara B, Kuntz M. 1993. Expression of the genes encoding the early carotenoid biosynthetic enzymes in *Capsicum annuum*. *Biochem Biophys Res Commun* 196:1414–21.

Ronen G, Carmel-Goren L, Zamir D, Hirschberg J. 2000. An alternative pathway to β-carotene formation in plant chromoplasts discovered by map-based cloning of *Beta and old-gold* color mutations in tomato. *Proc Natl Acad Sci* 97:11102–7.

Ronen G, Cohen M, Zamir D, Hirschberg J. 1999. Regulation of carotenoid biosynthesis during tomato fruit development: Expression of the gene for lycopene epsilon cyclase is down-regulated during ripening and is elevated in the mutant delta. *Plant J* 17:341–51.

Sandmann G. 1994. Carotenoid biosynthesis in microorganisms and plants. *Eur J Biochem* 223:7–24.

Sandmann G. 2001. Carotenoid biosynthesis and biotechnological application. *Arch Biochem Biophys* 385:4–12.

Schofield A, Paliyath G. 2005. Modulation of carotenoid biosynthesis during tomato fruit ripening through phytochrome regulation of phytoene synthase activity. *Plant Physiol Biochem* 43:1052–60.

Schwartz SH, Tan BC, Gage DA, Zeevart JAD, McCarty DR. 1997. Specific oxidative cleavage of carotenoids by VP14 of maize. *Science* 276:1872–4.

Seo M, Koshiba T. 2002. Complex regulation of ABA biosynthesis in plants. *Trends Plant Sci* 7, 41–65.

Shahidi F, Brown JA. 1998. Carotenoid pigments in seafoods and aquaculture. *Crit Rev Food Sci Nutr* 38:1–67.

Shahidi F, Synowiecki J, Penney RW. 1994. Chemical nature of xanthophylls in flesh and skin of cultured Arctic char (*Salvelinus alpinus* L.). *Food Chem* 51:1–4.

Simpson KL, Katayama T, Chichester CO. 1981. Carotenoids in fish feeds. In: Bauernfeind JC. editor. *Carotenoids as colorants and vitamin A precursors. Technological and nutritional applications.* New York: Academic Press, p 463–538.

Skelton RL, Yu Q, Srinivasan R, Manshardt R, Moore PH, Ming R. 2006. Tissue differential expression of lycopene β-cyclase gene in papaya. *Cell Res* 16:731–9.

Tadmor Y, King S, Levi A, Davis A, Meir A, Wasserman B, Hirschberg J, Lewinsohn E. 2005. Comparative fruit colouration in watermelon and tomato. *Food Res Int* 38:832–41.

Takahashi S, Kuzuyama T, Watanabe H, Seto H. 1998. A 1-deoxy-D-xylulose 5-phosphate reductoisomerase catalyzing the formation of 2-C-methyl-D-erythritol 4-phosphate in an alternative nonmevalonate pathway for terpenoid biosynthesis. *Proc Natl Acad Sci USA* 95:9879–84.

Taylor M, Ramsay G. 2005. Carotenoid biosynthesis in plant storage organs: Recent advances and prospects for improving plant food quality. *Physiol Plant* 124:143–51.

Thayer SS, Björkman O. 1990. Leaf xanthophyll content and composition in sun and shade determined by HPLC. *Photosynth Res* 23:331–43.

Yamamoto HY. 1979. Biochemistry of the violaxanthin cycle in higher plants. *Pure Appl Chem* 51:639–48.

Young AJ, Phillip D, Ruban AV, Horton P, Frank HA. 1997. The xanthophyll cycle and carotenoid-mediated dissipation of excess excitation energy in photosynthesis. *Pure Appl Chem* 69:2125–30.

Zechmeister L, LeRosen AL, Went FW, Pauling L. 1941. Prolycopene, a naturally occurring stereoisomer of lycopene. *Proc Natl Acad Sci USA* 27:468–74.

Zeevart JA, Creelman RAD. 1988. Metabolism and physiology of abscisic acid. *Annu Rev Plant Physiol Plant Mol Biol* 39:439–73.

Zhang M, Li K, Zhang CH, Gai JY, Yu DY. 2009. Identification and characterization of class 1 DXS gene encoding 1-deoxy-D-xylulose-5-phosphate synthase, the first committed enzyme of the MEP pathway from soybean. *Mol Biol Rep* 36:879–87.

3 Qualitative and quantitative analyses

3.1 INTRODUCTION

Analytical methods are basic tools in appraising the quality, safety, and health effects of foods. Because of their importance as natural pigments and as health-promoting compounds, the need for accurate analytical data on food carotenoids has been widely recognized. Unreliable data will lead to erroneous conclusions and recommendations, with potentially grave consequences.

Selection or development of methods is guided not only by the methods' performance but also by the intended use of the analytical data. Indeed, trends in carotenoid analysis reflect not only refinements in analytical methodology or instrumentation but also current knowledge of their functions or action.

3.2 STRUCTURE ELUCIDATION AND QUALITATIVE ANALYSIS

The intensive, meticulous work on structure elucidation undertaken in the 1970s, mostly by organic chemists, led to the tremendous number of natural carotenoids with established structure. Mass spectrometry (MS) and nuclear magnetic resonance (NMR) spectroscopy aided by UV-visible absorption spectrometry, specific group chemical reactions, and synthesis were employed. Through optical rotary dispersion and circular dichroism, the absolute configuration of many of these carotenoids was also established.

Among other purposes, qualitative analysis is currently carried out to: (a) obtain a rapid overview of the carotenoids in a sample, (b) study carotenoid compositions in the natural environment, (c) verify the conformational changes of carotenoids, and (d) classify samples (Rivera and Canela-Garayoa, 2012). Spectroscopic methods, principally MS, NMR, and Raman spectroscopy, have been used for this purpose.

Several ionization methods have been used for the MS analysis of carotenoids: electron impact (EI), fast atom bombardment (FAB), matrix-assisted laser desorption/ionization (MALDI), electrospray (ESI), atmospheric pressure chemical ionization (APCI),

Food Carotenoids: Chemistry, Biology, and Technology, First Edition. Delia B. Rodriguez-Amaya.

atmospheric pressure photoionization (APPI), and atmospheric pressure solids analysis probe (ASAP) (Enzell and Back, 1995; van Breemen, 1995, 1997; Dachtler et al., 2001; Aman et al., 2005).

EI used to be the most common ionization method. Carotenoids generally give good molecular ions, and many fragmentations diagnostic of particular structural features had been identified (Enzell and Back, 1995). EI requires sample vaporization prior to ionization, which is a disadvantage in the analysis of the thermally labile and nonvolatile carotenoids.

APCI has rapidly become the most widely used ionization technique. APCI produces molecular ions and/or protonated or deprotonated molecules, depending upon the mobile phase conditions, and abundant fragment ions, especially for xanthophylls (van Breeman, 1997). The main advantage of APCI is its high linearity of detector response over a carotenoid concentration range of at least three orders of magnitude, suggesting that APCI LC/MS might be the preferred mass spectrometric technique for carotenoid quantification. Disadvantages of APCI include the multiplicity of molecular ion species, which might lead to ambiguous molecular weight determinations because it tends to reduce the abundance of the molecular ions.

APCI and electrospray provide high sensitivity for carotenoids (low pmol level), are among the easiest interfaces to operate, and may be operated unattended by use of an autosampler (van Breeman, 1997). The soft ionization of electrospray, which produces molecular ions without fragmentation, greatly facilitates molecular weight confirmation and might be preferable to APCI for identification of carotenoids in mixtures and biological extracts, since APCI can produce abundant fragment ions.

The sensitivity of the ESI-MS detection is two orders of magnitude higher than that of UV-visible absorption spectrometry detection (e.g., a detection limit of 0.7 pmol for β-carotene). APCI in positive or negative modes gives detection limits of 1–13 pmol (Feltl et al., 2005).

Fruits and flowers have a complicated mixture of esterified carotenoids, which are difficult to identify in the ester form. HPLC (high-performance liquid chromatography)-APCI/MS was used for the identification of carotenoid esters in mango (Pott et al., 2003), red-orange essential oils (Dugo et al., 2008), marigold flowers, several fruits (Breithaupt et al., 2002), and tritordeum grains (Mellado-Ortega and Hornero-Méndez, 2012).

Tandem mass spectrometry (MS/MS) offers many advantages for the analysis of carotenoids. Analyzing zeaxanthin and its oxidation products in biological samples, Prasain et al. (2005) affirmed that tandem mass spectrometric analysis offers added selectivity and specificity and requires minimal sample cleanup, leading to high sample throughput. It reduces interference by impurities in the extract and allows the following: (a) minimal sample cleanup, (b) distinguishing between carotenoids that coelute, (c) information about structural isomers, and (d) a decrease in overall analysis time (Rivera and Canela-Garayoa, 2012).

MALDI/TOF-MS, ASAP-MS, and Raman spectroscopy are used to profile rapidly and analyze qualitatively carotenoids in different crude extracts. Such detection can be used directly for the analysis of samples without the need for sample preparation or chromatographic separation. Consequently, they allow for the fast screen of multiple analytes. McEwen et al. (2005) reported the qualitative detection of carotenoids in spinach leaves by ASAP-MS, which can offer a direct (without sample pretreatment or chromatographic separation) analysis within minutes.

MALDI/TOF-MS was used to distinguish tomato genotypes and mutants, rapidly profiling and displaying alterations in carotenoid content (Fraser at al., 2007). NMR was used for rapid fingerprinting in metabolome analysis (Hollywood et al., 2006). Raman and ASAP-MS have also been employed for direct analysis of carotenoids (Schulz et al., 2005; McEwen et al., 2005).

HPLC-NMR (Aman et al., 2005; Dachtler et al., 2001; Glaser et al., 2003) and off-line NMR (Tiziani et al., 2006) have also been utilized, particularly to identify the geometric isomers, which are not distinguished by MS. One- and two-dimensional NMR successfully determined the carotenoid profile of typical tomato juice, including the *Z*-isomers, with minimal purification procedures (Tiziani et al., 2006).

A prerequisite for reliable results in direct coupling of HPLC-NMR is a complete separation of all the isomers (Feltl et al., 2005). Measurement of NMR spectra requires pure components in higher amounts than UV-visible and MS detection modes (Feltl et al., 2005). LC-NMR has been utilized to obtain unambiguous identification of carotenoids (Dachtler et al., 2001). However, this method is not applicable to small sample size from a complex matrix.

Carotenoid molecules are among the most efficient Raman scatterers (Feltl et al., 2005). Raman spectra of carotenoids show strong bands within the 1500–1550 cm^{-1} and 1150–1170 cm^{-1} ranges due to in-phase c=c (v_1) and c-c stretching (v_2) vibrations of the polyene chain.

Raman spectroscopy can be used for sensitive detection of carotenoids in living tissues, and Raman mapping provides further information about their spatial distribution in the plant sample. Near-infrared Fourier transform (NIR-FT) Raman spectroscopy measured β-carotene, lycopene, and α-carotene/lutein (with strong bands at 1520, 1510, and 1527 cm^{-1}, respectively) in situ in carrot roots of different color without preliminary sample preparation (Baranska et al., 2006a). The Raman mapping technique revealed that β-carotene in the secondary phloem increased gradually from the periderm toward the core but declined in cells close to the vascular cambium. α-Carotene was deposited in younger cells at a higher rate than β-carotene, while lycopene in red carrots accumulated throughout the whole secondary phloem at the same level. FT-Raman spectroscopy was also utilized in in situ analysis of carotenoids in red pepper, nectarine, yellow carrot root, pumpkin, and corn seed (Schulz et al., 2005).

3.3 QUANTITATIVE ANALYSIS

A detailed description of the procedure for quantitative analysis is beyond the scope of this book. Instead, the underlying principles and precautions to avoid errors in each step in the quantification of carotenoids will be presented. The readers are referred to Rodriguez-Amaya (1999) and Rodriguez-Amaya and Kimura (2004) for detailed procedures (including weights, volumes, and calculations).

3.3.1 Storage of samples

Ideally, laboratory work should be planned so that the samples are analyzed as soon as they are collected because it is difficult to avoid changes in the carotenoid composition during storage, even at very low temperature. Additionally, because carotenoid concentration is expressed per unit weight of sample, changes in the food's weight (e.g., due to loss or gain of water during storage) also affect the final result.

When storage is unavoidable, raw food samples are better stored intact. Tissue disintegration should be postponed until after storage and then carried out immediately before or simultaneously with extraction to avoid enzymatic oxidation of the carotenoids (Rodriguez-Amaya, 1999). Moreover, loss of moisture and volatile compounds is greater with disintegrated tissues, concentrating the carotenoids and leading to overestimation of the concentrations, if corrections are not made. Storage of extracts should also be avoided or limited to a very short period. Once extracted, carotenoids lose the natural protection of the plant's cellular structure and degrade rapidly even at low temperature. In carotenoid extracts from banana, for example, a breakdown rate of around 5% per day was observed even in the dark at –20°C and in the presence of antioxidants (Davey et al., 2009a).

Lyophilization (freeze-drying) is considered the appropriate means of preserving samples that have to be stored before analysis. Davey et al. (2006, 2009a) reported no significant difference in the recoveries of total provitamin A carotenoids from lyophilized and fresh banana, and no further significant loss during storage of lyophilized tissue in the dark at –20°C, whereas variable losses occurred in frozen pulp tissues. However, degradation of carotenoids, especially of lycopene, does occur during lyophilization (Craft et al., 1993); further, it increases sample porosity and, consequently, exposure to oxygen during storage. Moreover, to transform the carotenoid concentrations obtained with lyophilized samples to those of the foods as purchased or as consumed, the preferred form in databases, the moisture content is used. Determination of moisture is simple, but it is proximate analysis; the error from this macrocomponent analysis can be carried over and appreciably affect the microcomponent concentration.

3.3.2 Total carotenoid content

Determination of the total carotenoid content, through the visible absorption at the λ_{max} of the principal carotenoid, although still done and attractive for its simplicity, yields insufficient information. It is not adequate for human health purposes but can still be employed for the quick appraisal of color loss and for initial screening of a large number of samples as in breeding projects (Kimura et al., 2007).

Carotenoids in solution obey the Beer-Lambert law: their absorbance is directly proportional to the concentration. Thus, carotenoids are quantified spectrometrically.

The carotenoids of the food sample are extracted with acetone, transferred to petroleum ether, and the visible absorption spectrum is taken. The total concentration is calculated according to the following formulas:

$$x(\mu g) = \frac{A \times y(\text{mL}) \times 10^6}{A_{1\text{cm}}^{1\%} \times 100}$$

$$x(\mu g / g) = \frac{x(\mu g)}{(g)}$$

where x is the weight or concentration of the principal carotenoid, y is the volume of the solution that gives an absorbance of A at a specified wavelength, $A^{1\%}_{1cm}$ is the absorption coefficient of the major carotenoid in the solvent used, and (g) is the weight of the sample. For example, for petroleum ether extracts with β-carotene as the main carotenoid, the absorbance (A) at 450 nm and an $A^{1\%}_{1cm}$ of 2592 should be used. $A^{1\%}_{1cm}$ is the absorbance at a given wavelength of a 1% solution in a cuvette with a 1-cm light path and can be found tabulated in several publications (e.g., Britton, 1995; Rodriguez-Amaya, 1999).

The formula presented above is also used for the spectrometric quantification of standards in HPLC quantification, using the respective $A^{1\%}_{1cm}$ of the carotenoid standards.

3.3.3 Quantification of individual carotenoids

To appraise food quality and understand better the health benefits of carotenoids, including their mechanisms of action, comprehensive and reliable quantitative information on these compounds in foods is needed. Since carotenoids differ in their properties (e.g., polarity, stability, bioavailability, antioxidant activity) and efficacy and health-promoting actions (e.g., the highest provitamin A activity is attributed to β-carotene, action against prostate cancer to lycopene, and against cataract and macular degeneration to lutein and zeaxanthin), the total carotenoid content is of limited use. Analytical methods for the accurate identification and quantification of individual carotenoids are essential.

The adoption of an analytical method or strategy depends on the purpose of analysis, and the nature of both the food sample and the analyte. Because of the varied nature of food matrices and the qualitative and quantitative variation in the carotenoid composition of foods, a single analytical method/procedure is not likely to be appropriate for different foods (Rodriguez-Amaya, 1999; Rodriguez-Amaya and Kimura, 2004; Kimura et al., 2007). Method optimization (e.g., Sá and Rodriguez-Amaya, 2004), development/validation (e.g., Hart and Scott, 1995; Kimura and Rodriguez-Amaya, 2002; Kimura et al., 2007; Akhtar and Bryan, 2008), and evaluation of performance in the analyst's laboratory even when using a validated method (e.g., Dias et al., 2008) should precede data generation. The method should be optimized for each food matrix, particularly in terms of the preparation of the analytical sample and extraction and chromatographic conditions.

Quantitative carotenoid analysis generally consists of (1) sampling, (2) preparation of the analytical sample, (3) extraction, (4) partition to a solvent compatible with the subsequent chromatographic step, (5) saponification and washing (optional), (6) concentration or evaporation of solvent, (7) chromatographic separation, (7) identification, (8) quantification, and (9) data processing and interpretation (Figure 3.1).

3.3.3.1 Sampling

Carotenoids are among the food constituents most affected by genetic and environmental factors. Aside from the remarkable variation between foods, in a given food, compositional variation also occurs due to factors such as cultivar/variety, maturity at harvest, climate/season/geographic site of production, part of the plant utilized, farming practices, harvesting and postharvest handling, and processing and storage conditions

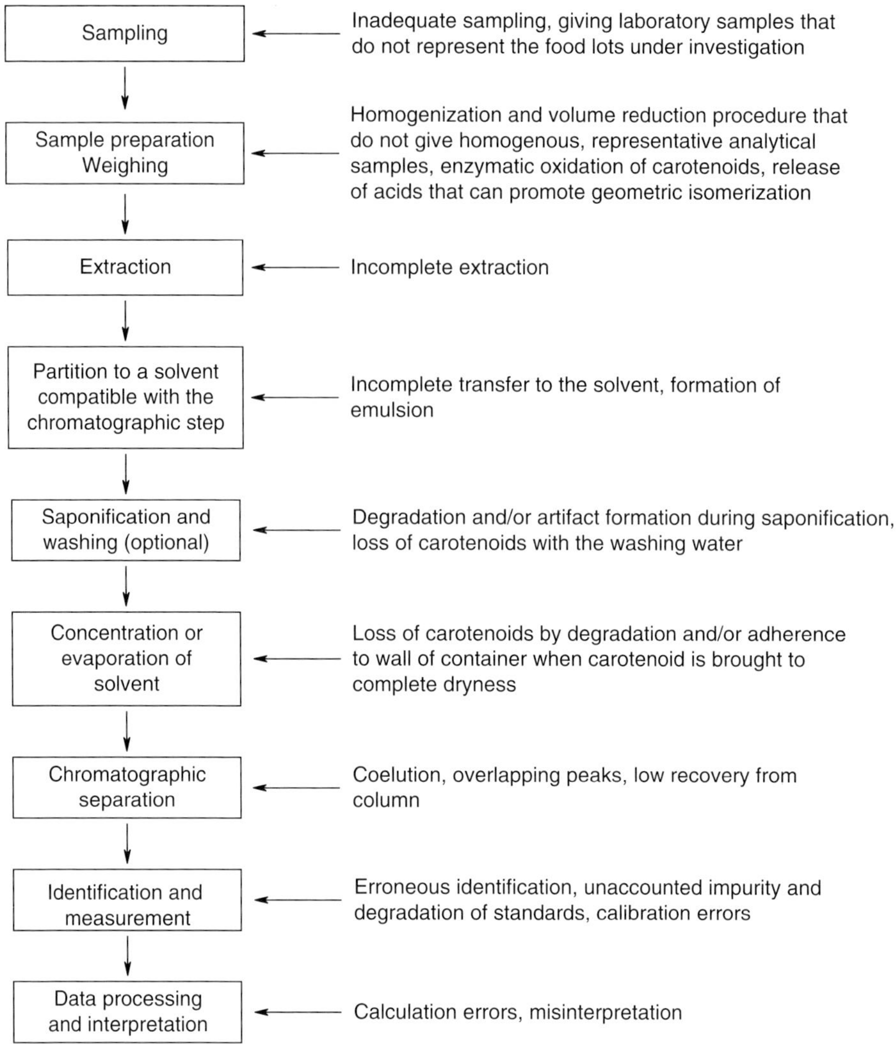

Figure 3.1 General procedure for carotenoid analysis and sources of errors in each step. Exposure to light will promote photoisomerization and photodegradation at any step from extraction. Rodriguez-Amaya (2015). Reproduced with permission of Elsevier.

(Rodriguez-Amaya et al., 2006, 2008). The analytical data can only be reliable and truly useful if the sample taken for analysis is representative of the lot under investigation and is adequately prepared for analysis. Errors introduced in these initial steps cannot be compensated for in the subsequent steps. Natural variation should be clearly distinguished from analytical errors and compositional data should be accompanied by pertinent information such as the variety, stage of maturity, geographical origin, season, and part of the plant analyzed.

Obtaining a portion that is representative of the whole is not an easy task. The following factors should be considered: purpose of the analysis, nature of the food and the analyte, distribution of the analyte within the population, the analysis to be performed, and the desired accuracy and precision of the analytical results (Rodriguez-Amaya, 1999, 2008).

Evidently, the more heterogeneous the food is, the greater the difficulty and effort needed to obtain a representative sample. Representativity can be enhanced by increasing the sample size, weight of the subsample submitted to analysis (analytical sample), degree of comminuting, and number of analytical runs. The more sensitive modern methods become, the smaller the portions of the original lots submitted to actual analysis become, making it more challenging to minimize sampling errors. Because of the heterogeneity of food samples, a large number of samples should ideally be analyzed. In practice, however, the sampling and sample preparation procedures adopted are usually a compromise between heterogeneity considerations and operational costs.

In data generation for food composition tables and databases, for which representative mean compositional values are desired, all factors that can potentially influence the composition should be accounted for in the sampling plan. Several increments randomly taken from across the sample lot are combined and blended to obtain a homogeneous composite, subsamples of which are analyzed. Several different sample lots are individually submitted to analysis and mean values are reported, accompanied by a statement of uncertainty, usually expressed in terms of the standard deviation.

The number of analytical runs needed per food depends on the compositional variability. In tomato fruit, Darrigues et al. (2008) observed that between-plot field variation accounted for 50% and 52% of the total variation for lycopene and β-carotene, respectively. The corresponding contributions of within-plot variation were 7% and 3%, and of uncontrolled error 43% and 45%. There was no significant variance due to replicated extraction or replicated HPLC injection for either carotenoid. Also working with tomato, Dias et al. (2008) concluded, from the results of 12 samples harvested in the same region, that analyzing 5 primary samples would be sufficient to estimate the population mean value with a level of confidence of 95%.

The heterogeneous distribution of carotenoids in food is well illustrated in African bananas and plantains (Davey et al., 2007). Analysis of the between-plant, within-plant, within-hand, and within-fruit variations of *Musa* varieties cultivated under standardized field conditions demonstrated that the provitamin A carotenoid content varied significantly across all sample groups. Since the extent of these variations appeared to be genotype dependent, in spite of the large overall variations in the mean provitamin A contents, once the within-bunch variability had been accounted for, the between-plant variations of a variety were found to generally fall within acceptable levels. It was necessary to collect fruits from hands at the proximal end, the middle, and the distal end of the bunch to obtain representative values. The samples in this case came from plants grown under the same environmental conditions and harvested at the same time. It is not known whether the same conclusion could be drawn with actual samples (of the same variety) that would come from plants cultivated under different conditions, harvested at different times.

3.3.3.2 Preparation of the analytical sample

The sample that is collected and brought to the laboratory is usually too large, both in bulk and particle size, for direct analysis. It must be transformed into a homogeneous, small sample for analysis while maintaining its representativeness. The procedure for the preparation of the analytical sample should be adapted to the nature of the food, the analyte, the analytical method, and the distribution of the analyte in the food. Sample preparation and extraction remain the most time-consuming and error-prone steps in the food analysis process.

Variation in the carotenoid concentration along the longitudinal and across the transversal axes of the cassava root was shown by Chávez et al. (2008). The carotenoid content was higher in the part of the root closest to its attachment to the stem (proximal section), gradually decreasing toward the opposite end (distal section). Across the root, carotenoid content was higher in the core and lower toward the periphery. Quartering roots and fruits longitudinally is therefore the appropriate manner of reducing the sample's volume to obtain the analytical sample.

Subsampling and homogenization may be done simultaneously. Physical operations, such as chopping, cutting into pieces, mixing, milling, blending, and sieving, are carried out, along with bulk reduction, for example, by quartering and riffling. The process can be done manually or through commercially available mills, blenders, grinders, riffle cutters, etc. Because the food product is usually analyzed in the form in which it is commonly consumed, inedible portions (i.e., peel, seed, shell, etc.) are initially removed.

Once homogenization is done, the analytical sample should be weighed and extraction should immediately follow because tissue disruption releases enzymes (e.g., lipoxygenase) that catalyze carotenoid oxidation and acids that promote *E-Z* isomerization. In fact, sample maceration, homogenization, and extraction with an organic solvent are usually carried out simultaneously.

3.3.3.3 Extraction

Using a Placket-Burman experimental design, Periago et al. (2007) examined 15 factors that affect the extraction and quantification of lycopene from tomato and tomato products: sample weight; volume of extraction solution; antioxidant (BHT) concentration; neutralizing agent ($MgCO_3$) concentration; light presence during extraction; homogenization velocity and time; agitation time; temperature during the extraction process; water volume for separation of polar/nonpolar phases; presence of inert atmosphere throughout the process; time, temperature, and light presence during separation of phases; and time delay for reading. The sample weight, neutralizing agent concentration, and water volume for separation of polar/nonpolar phases could be considered the key factors for raw and processed tomato. For tomato sauce, sample weight and volume of extraction solution had the greatest impact on the results.

A good extraction procedure should effectively release all the carotenoids from the food matrix without causing structural and concentration changes. Because carotenoids are found in a variety of foods, the extraction procedure should be adapted to suit the food being analyzed. The solvent chosen should efficiently extract the range of carotenoids present in the sample. Foods generally contain large amounts of water; thus, water-miscible organic solvent, such as acetone, methanol, ethanol, or mixtures thereof are used as extracting solvents to allow better solvent penetration. Dried materials can be extracted with water-immiscible solvents, but extraction is usually more efficient if the samples are rehydrated prior to extraction with water-miscible solvents.

Acetone has been the traditional solvent for carotenoid extraction. It has three advantages: (a) it dissolves both carotenes and xanthophylls efficiently, (b) it penetrates the food matrix well, and (c) subsequent partitioning to an apolar solvent occurs more easily. Our HPLC method (Figure 3.2) makes use of acetone as extracting solvent; this method has been validated in our laboratory using a certified reference material (Kimura et al., 2007) and in an international interlaboratory study (Rodriguez-Amaya et al., 2012).

With the advent of HPLC, tetrahydrofuran (THF) has become a popular extracting solvent. Solubility of both β-carotene and lutein in this solvent was shown to be excellent (Craft and Soares, 1992). Other solvents, such as hexane, petroleum ether, methanol, and ethanol have also been used. The first two solvents readily dissolve carotenes but not xanthophylls; on the other hand, methanol and ethanol dissolve the xanthophylls efficiently but not the carotenes. Thus, mixtures of solvents such as hexane:ethanol (Taungbodhitham et al., 1998; Lin and Chen, 2003; Cortés et al., 2004), hexane:acetone:ethanol (Periago et al., 2004: Barba et al., 2006), and

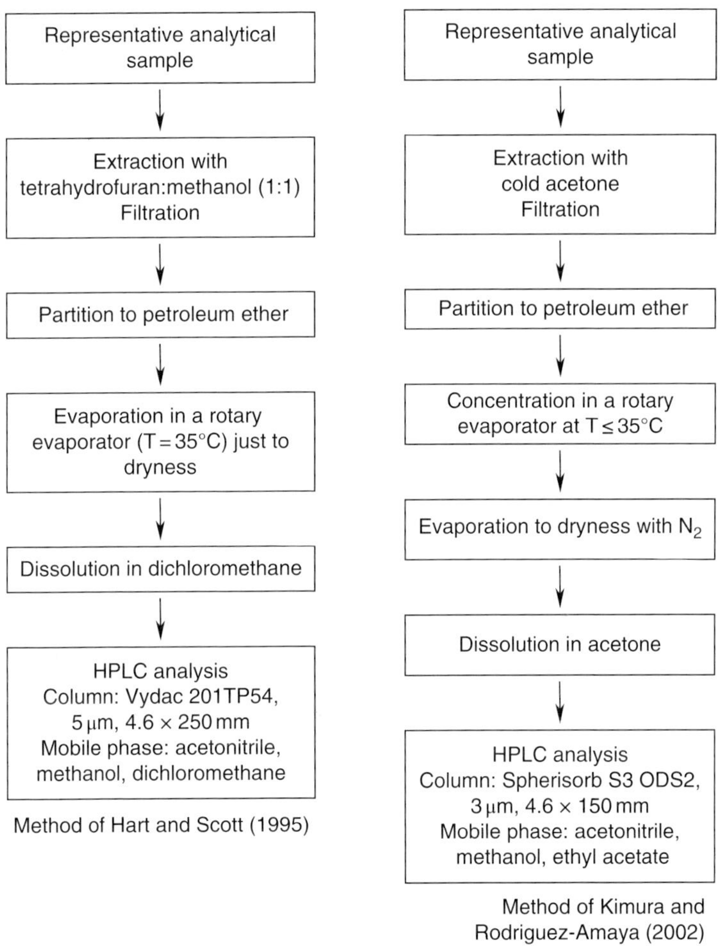

Figure 3.2 Schematic diagrams of two widely used, validated HPLC methods for the quantitative analysis of carotenoids.

hexane:ethanol:acetone:toluene (J.P. Chen et al., 2004) are utilized. The widely used method of Hart and Scott (1995) employs THF:methanol (Figure 3.2). This method was validated in the European interlaboratory study of Scott et al. (1996).

Extraction should be carried out under a fume hood to protect the analyst from inhaling solvent vapor. The sample is generally homogenized with celite (or Hyflosupercel) and the solvent in a suitable mechanical blender for 1–2 minutes or with a mortar and pestle. Celite facilitates both tissue disintegration and the subsequent filtration. A Waring blender is fast and efficient for mechanical disruption and homogenization of soft fruits and juice. Increasingly, the Polytron homogenizer is used because it provides rapid and uniform homogenization. Vortexing has also been employed, but it should only be used for finely ground and easy to extract samples. For samples such as fresh leaves, the simple mortar and pestle is better because small pieces of leaves, which can escape the blender blades, can be well ground. Leaves and other difficult-to-extract matrices may also need previous soaking in the extracting solvent (about 15 minutes for leaves) to soften the cell wall. Prolonged soaking should be avoided to prevent isomerization and degradation of the carotenoids.

To prevent isomerization, $MgCO_3$ or other neutralizing agent is often added to neutralize the acids liberated by tissue disintegration. Oxidation can be reduced by directing nitrogen into the blending vessel or by adding dry ice before homogenization. In our experience, using cold acetone (left in the refrigerator for a short time before use) and doing the extraction immediately or simultaneously with sample maceration not only prevents enzymatic oxidation but also makes the addition of neutralizing agents unnecessary.

Filtration can be done with a sintered glass funnel (porosity 3; pore size 20–30 μm) or with a Buchner funnel. The solid residue is returned to the blender and re-extracted with fresh solvent; extraction and filtration are repeated until the residue is colorless (three extractions are usually sufficient).

3.3.3.4 Partition

The extract usually contains a substantial amount of water, which can be removed by partition to hexane, petroleum ether, diethyl ether, dichloromethane, or mixtures of these solvents. This partition also serves as a cleanup step. Diethyl ether or a mixture of ether with hexane or petroleum ether is preferred for extracts with large amounts of xanthophylls, part of which is lost with the washing water during partition with pure hexane or petroleum ether (Kobori and Rodriguez-Amaya, 2013).

Partition can be carried out by adding small portions of the extract to petroleum ether or another appropriate solvent in a separatory funnel (Rodriguez-Amaya, 1999). After each addition, water is added gently to avoid formation of an emulsion, preferably by allowing the water to flow along the walls of the funnel. The two layers are allowed to separate, without agitation, and the lower aqueous phase (with the water miscible extracting solvent) is discarded. When the entire extract has been added, the petroleum ether phase is washed four or five times with water to remove residual extracting solvent. In our experience, this procedure is efficient and emulsions are less likely to form.

Alternatively, the acetone extract can be added to petroleum ether in the separatory funnel all at once, followed by addition of water. Some workers then agitate the mixture, but this practice leads to the formation of an emulsion, which is difficult to break and results in loss of carotenoids to the aqueous phase. After separation of phases, the lower layer is drawn off and re-extracted with fresh petroleum ether. The combined petroleum ether solution is then washed five times with water.

The solvents used in extraction or partition are subsequently removed or at least reduced by evaporation; thus, solvents with low boiling points are chosen to avoid prolonged heating. The lower-boiling fractions of petroleum ether (b.p. 30–60 or 40°C–60°C) are used instead of the higher-boiling fractions. Dichloromethane (b.p. 42°C) is preferred instead of chloroform (b.p. 61°C).

3.3.3.5 *Saponification*

Saponification is effective in removing chlorophylls and unwanted lipids, which may interfere with the chromatographic separation and shorten the column's life in HPLC. With saponified extracts of green vegetables, chlorophyllide (with phytol removed from chlorophyll) goes to the washing water. In samples such as fruits, it also hydrolyzes the carotenol esters, thereby simplifying the chromatographic separation, identification, and quantification because the free carotenols are analyzed instead of the carotenol esters, which usually occur as a difficult-to-separate mixture of esters with a variety of fatty acids.

Saponification, however, extends the analysis time and is error prone; it should therefore be included in the analytical procedure only when indispensable. It is unnecessary, for example, in the analysis of leafy vegetables, tomato, and carrot, all of which are low-lipid materials and essentially free of carotenol esters. The chlorophylls coextracted with carotenoids from leaves can be separated during chromatography. For the high-lipid dry corn, saponification is dispensable when gradient elution is used, removing the lipids from the column (Rodriguez-Amaya and Kimura, 2004).

For food samples requiring saponification, this step should be thoroughly evaluated and optimized and the subsequent washing carefully done to avoid losing carotenoids with the aqueous phase (e.g., de Sá and Rodriguez-Amaya, 2004). It is best done after transferring the carotenoids to petroleum ether or hexane, by adding an equal volume of 10% methanolic potassium hydroxide. The mixture is left overnight at room temperature in the dark, after which the carotenoid solution is washed about five times with water to remove the alkali. To avoid losing carotenoids into the washing water, especially the more polar xanthophylls, this step should be done in the same manner as in partition, described above. When apocarotenals (e.g., β-citraurin in citrus) are present in the sample, all traces of acetone must be removed before saponification to avoid aldol condensation between the apocarotenals and acetone.

3.3.3.6 *Concentration or evaporation of the solvent*

The carotenoid solution, after partitioning of unsaponified samples or after washing of saponified samples, is dried with anhydrous sodium sulfate and concentrated in a rotary evaporator at reduced pressure and a temperature ≤35°C. If complete removal of the solvent is desired, concentration in the rotary evaporator is done first, and evaporation to dryness is accomplished with a stream of nitrogen or argon. Bringing the carotenoid solution to complete dryness in the rotary evaporator increases the possibility of degradation, especially of lycopene (Tonucci et al., 1995), and may leave the carotenoids tightly adhered to the glass walls, making quantitative removal from the flask difficult.

3.3.3.7 Chromatographic separation

For over two decades, reversed-phase high performance liquid chromatography (HPLC) has been the chromatographic technique most widely used for quantitative carotenoid analysis. Compilation of HPLC methods for carotenoids can be found in review articles (Oliver and Palou, 2000; Schoefs, 2002; Su et al., 2002; Quirós and Costa, 2006; Rivera and Canela-Garayoa, 2012; Amorim-Carrilho et al., 2014). Two examples of widely used, validated HPLC methods are shown in Figure 3.2.

Two important developments in HPLC have advanced carotenoid analysis considerably: (a) columns that provide baseline separation of the range of carotenoids in a given food, now up to the separation of geometric isomers, and (b) the photodiode array detector that provides the visible absorption spectra of the separated carotenoids online.

For some time, the most widely used column for carotenoid separation was the polymeric C_{18} Vydac 201TP54 (250 × 4.6 mm, 5 μm) column. It has been surpassed by the polymeric C_{30} YMC (250 × 4.6 mm, 5 μm) column in recent years. Especially designed for the separation of carotenoid isomers (Sander et al., 1994), the C_{30} stationary phases have gained wide application in food analysis (Sander et al., 2000).

Carotenoid separation has been carried out with 5 μm spherical particles packed in a 250 × 4.6 mm column. The C18 column with 5 μm particles have often been found not to provide adequate separation of food carotenoids, especially the geometric isomers. Shorter columns with smaller particles have demonstrated greater separation efficiency and require much less mobile phase. The C18 Spherisorb ODS 2 (150 × 4.6 mm, 3 μm) column used in our laboratory, for example, has provided excellent chromatograms for the carotenoids of different foods, including those with complex carotenoid composition, such as leafy vegetables (Kimura and Rodriguez-Amaya, 2002; Kobori and Rodriguez-Amaya, 2008), squashes and pumpkins (Azevedo-Meleiro and Rodriguez-Amaya, 2007), pepper (Azevedo-Meleiro and Rodriguez-Amaya, 2009), and the tropical fruit *Eugenia uniflora* L. (Azevedo-Meleiro and Rodriguez-Amaya, 2004).

As mobile phases for carotenoids, the primary solvents have been acetonitrile and methanol. In all our work using the 3 μm C_{18} column and in most of those employing the Vydac column, the mobile phase has these two solvents. On the other hand, a combination of methanol and methyl-*tert*-butyl ether has been used by the majority of those who utilize the C_{30} column.

Aside from the primary solvents, small amounts of other solvents are added to obtain the desired retention, increase solubility, and improve resolution. Often used for this purpose are chlorinated solvents (e.g., chloroform and dichloromethane) because of their good solvent properties and effects on selectivity, although these solvents can be contaminated with traces of hydrochloric acid. Other solvents used as modifiers are tetrahydrofuran, ethyl acetate, hexane, acetone, and water. Some methanol has also been added to acetonitrile-based mobile phase. Craft et al. (1992) investigated the effect of nine solvent modifiers on the separation of seven carotenoids, and found tetrahydrofuran to be the most beneficial modifier of methanol. They cautioned against the use of mixtures of three or more solvents because it can make the method more complicated, enhance demixing, and result in different evaporation rates, causing variation in the retention times during the course of the day.

Ammonium acetate improved the recovery of carotenoids from the column when added to acetonitrile-based solvents. Addition of triethylamine to the mobile phase containing ammonium acetate further increased recovery, from around 60% to over 90% (Hart and Scott 1995).

Since geometric isomers of carotenoids have different bioavailability, as discussed in Chapter 8, when measurable amounts of the *Z*-isomers are present, their separation and quantification should be carried out in health-oriented studies. Examples of foods in which quantification of the *Z*-isomers is important are thermally prepared or processed foods (Lessin et al., 1997), such as tomato and tomato products (Tavares and Rodriguez-Amaya, 1994), prepared/processed corn (Aman et al., 2005; de Oliveira and Rodriguez-Amaya, 2007), carrot juice (Marx et al., 2000), and cooked spinach (Glaser et al., 2003). Fresh foods generally have negligible amounts of *Z*-isomers (Godoy and Rodriguez-Amaya, 1994, 1998). An exception is cassava root, in which appreciable levels of 9-*Z*-β-carotene and 13-*Z*-β carotene accompany the principal carotenoid, all-*E*-β-carotene (Kimura et al., 2007). Two columns cited above can be used for this separation: the 3 μm C18 column and the C30 column developed for this purpose. Identification is easier in the former because the *Z*-isomers elute close to the corresponding all-*E*-carotenoid, but separation of the isomers is better in the latter. Equivalent results were obtained for all-*E*-, 9-*Z*- and 13-*Z*-β-carotene of cassava when these two columns were used (Kimura et al., 2007). For corn, which has a complex carotenoid composition, the concentrations of zeaxanthin, lutein, β-cryptoxanthin, and β-carotene in the all-*E*-configuration, obtained with the two columns, did not differ significantly, but the *Z*-isomers were difficult to locate in the chromatogram obtained with the C30 column. The chromatograms, together with the photodiode array spectra, of the carotenoids of corn obtained with the two columns are presented in Figure 3.3.

Gradient elution should be used only when the analysis cannot be done isocratically. Isocratic separation is rapid, can be performed with simple equipment (with a single high-pressure pump and premixed solvent), and results in stable baseline and more reproducible retention times. Gradient elution, on the other hand, has the advantages of greater resolving power, improved sensitivity, and elution of strongly retained compounds. It is more likely to resolve the whole range of carotenoids found in a given food. However, it has several disadvantages: (a) increased complexity, (b) requirement for more sophisticated and expensive equipment, (c) need for column reequilibration between runs, (d) greater differential detector's response (i.e., different detector's signals for the same concentration of different compounds), and (e) often poor reproducibility. Good solvent miscibility is required to prevent baseline disturbance resulting from outgassing and refractive index effects (Craft, 1992).

3.3.3.8 Identification

Since inconclusive or even erroneous identifications could be found in the literature, Schiedt and Liaaen-Jensen (1995) recommended the following minimum criteria for the identification of carotenoids: (1) the visible (or ultraviolet for shorter chromophores)

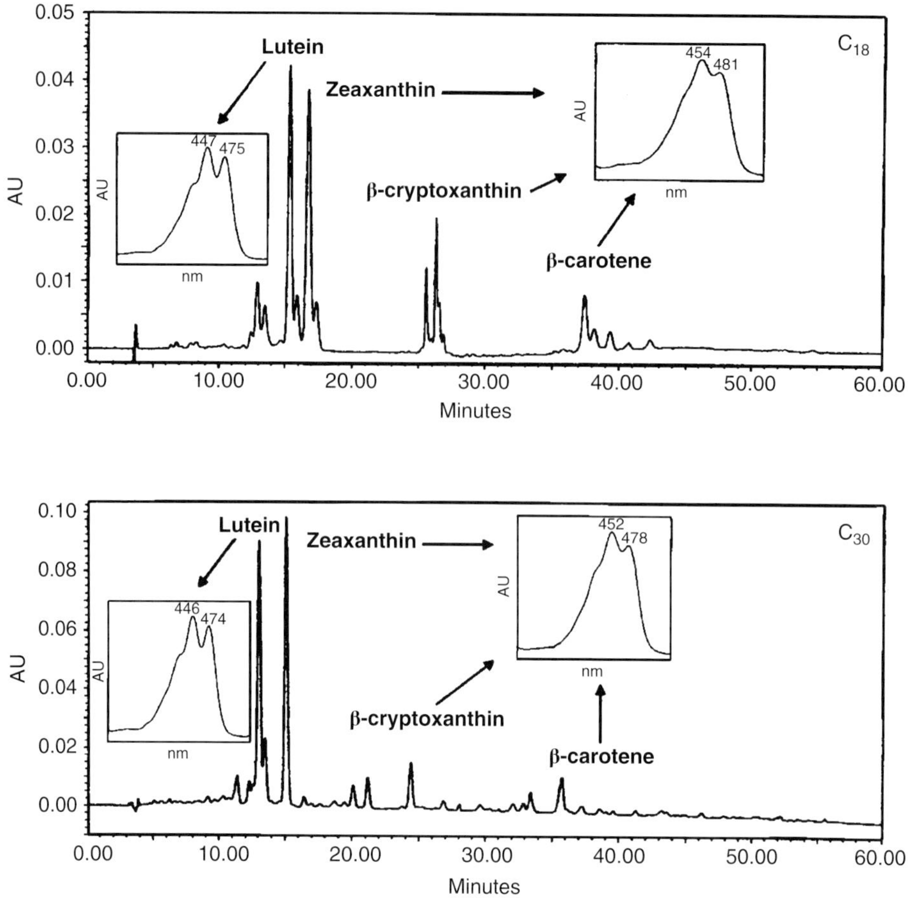

Figure 3.3 HPLC chromatograms and photodiode array spectra of the carotenoids of dry corn, variety Assum Preto. C_{18} column: monomeric Spherisorb ODS2, 3 μm, 4.6 × 150 mm. C_{30} column: YMC polymeric, 3 μm, 4.6 × 250 mm. Taken from Rodriguez-Amaya (1999).

absorption spectrum (λ_{max} and fine structure) in at least two different solvents must be in agreement with the chromophore suggested; (2) chromatographic properties must be identical in two systems, preferably thin-layer chromatography (TLC) (R_F) and HPLC (t_R), and co-chromatography with an authentic sample should be demonstrated; and (3) a mass spectrum should be obtained, which allows at least the confirmation of the molecular mass.

The chromatographic behavior and the ultraviolet and visible absorption spectrum provide the first clues for the identification of carotenoids. Both the position of the absorption maxima (λ_{max}) and the shape (fine structure) of the spectrum reflect the chromophore. However, identification of carotenoids based solely on the retention times/co-chromatography with standards or the absorption spectra may lead to erroneous conclusions. Different carotenoids can have the same retention time in a given chromatographic system, and different carotenoids may have the same chromophore, thus presenting the same absorption spectrum. However, carotenoids with well-known structure can be conclusively identified by the combined and judicious use of chromatographic behavior, UV-visible absorption spectra, and, for xanthophylls, specific group chemical reactions (Azevedo-Meleiro and Rodriguez-Amaya, 2004). In the absence of mass spectra, the chemical tests can confirm the type, location, and number of functional groups (Eugster, 1995; Rodriguez-Amaya, 1999). MS and NMR are indispensable in the elucidation of the structure of an unknown carotenoid.

3.3.3.8.1 UV-visible absorption spectrometry

The UV-visible absorption spectrum is still the first diagnostic tool for the identification of carotenoids. HPLC-DAD has allowed the acquisition of the spectra of individual carotenoids within a short time (Figure 3.3). Both the position of the absorption maxima (λ_{max}) and the shape (spectral fine structure) of the spectrum are characteristic of the polyene chromophore. Tables giving the λ_{max} values for carotenoids are available in many reviews and books published through the years (e.g., Britton, 1995; Rodriguez-Amaya, 1999).

The absorption spectra of most carotenoids have three peaks or two peaks with a shoulder (Figure 3.4). The characteristic λ_{max} values of common carotenoids in petroleum ether will be quoted here. In a given solvent, the greater the number of conjugated double bonds, the higher the λ_{max} values. This is best seen in the acyclic series. The most unsaturated acyclic carotenoid lycopene, with 11 conjugated double bonds, absorbs at the longest wavelengths (λ_{max} at 444, 470, and 502 nm) (Figure 3.4a). Being also acyclic, ζ- carotene has a spectrum with three well-defined peaks, but these are at wavelengths much lower than those of lycopene (λ_{max} at 378, 400, and 425 nm), commensurate with its conjugated system of 7 double bonds (Figure 3.4b). The two carotenoids that precede ζ-carotene in the desaturation biosynthetic pathway, phytoene (3 conjugated double bonds) and phytofluene (5 conjugated double bonds), are colorless and absorb maximally at 276, 286, and 297 nm and at 331, 348, and 367 nm, respectively. The degree of spectral fine structure is small for phytoene; it increases through phytofluene and ζ-carotene, then decreases again as the chromophore is extended. Neurosporene, which has a structure intermediate between ζ-carotene and lycopene (9 conjugated double bonds), exhibits maximum absorption at 414, 439, and 467 nm.

Cyclization results in steric hindrance between the ring methyl group at C-5 and the hydrogen at C-8 of the polyene chain, taking the π electrons of the double bond in the ring out of plane with those of the chain. Consequently, a hypsochromic shift (displacement of λ_{max} to lower wavelength), hypochromic effect (decrease in absorbance), and loss of fine structure (spectrum with less-defined peaks) are observed.

Thus, bicyclic β-carotene, which has the same number of conjugated double bonds as lycopene, has λ_{max} at 450 and 477 nm and a mere inflection (shoulder) at 425 nm (Figure 3.4a). Monocyclic γ-carotene has a structure with half of the molecule resembling lycopene and the other half resembling β-carotene. Thus, it exhibits a spectrum intermediate between those of lycopene and β-carotene in λ_{max} and shape (Figure 3.4a). The double bond in the ε-ring of α-carotene is out of conjugation, leaving 10 conjugated double bonds (9 in the polyene chain and 1 in the β-ring). Consequently, its absorption spectrum is more defined with λ_{max} at slightly shorter wavelengths (422, 445, and 473 nm) than those of β-carotene (Figure 3.4a).

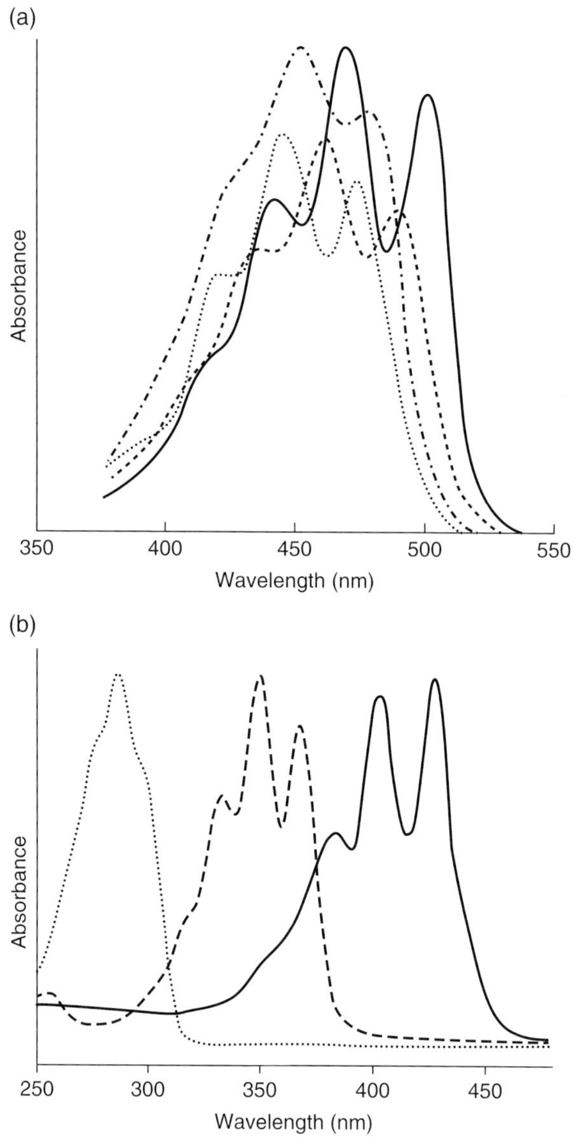

Figure 3.4 (a) Visible absorption spectra of lycopene (—), γ-carotene (- - -) β-carotene (-·-·-·), and α-carotene (.....) in petroleum ether. (b) Photodiode array spectra of ζ-carotene (–), phytofluene (- - -), and phytoene (......). Mobile phase: acetonitrile/ethyl acetate/methanol (85:10:5). Taken from Rodriguez-Amaya (1999).

The introduction of hydroxy and methoxy substituents in the carotenoid molecule does not affect the chromophore and therefore has virtually no effect on the absorption spectrum. Thus, the spectra of lutein, zeinoxanthin, and α-cryptoxanthin resemble that of α-carotene, and those of β-cryptoxanthin and zeaxanthin are identical to that of β-carotene (Figure 3.3).

The 5,6-monoepoxide and 5,6,5′,6′-diepoxides of cyclic carotenoids, having lost one and two ring double bonds, respectively, absorb maximally at wavelengths about

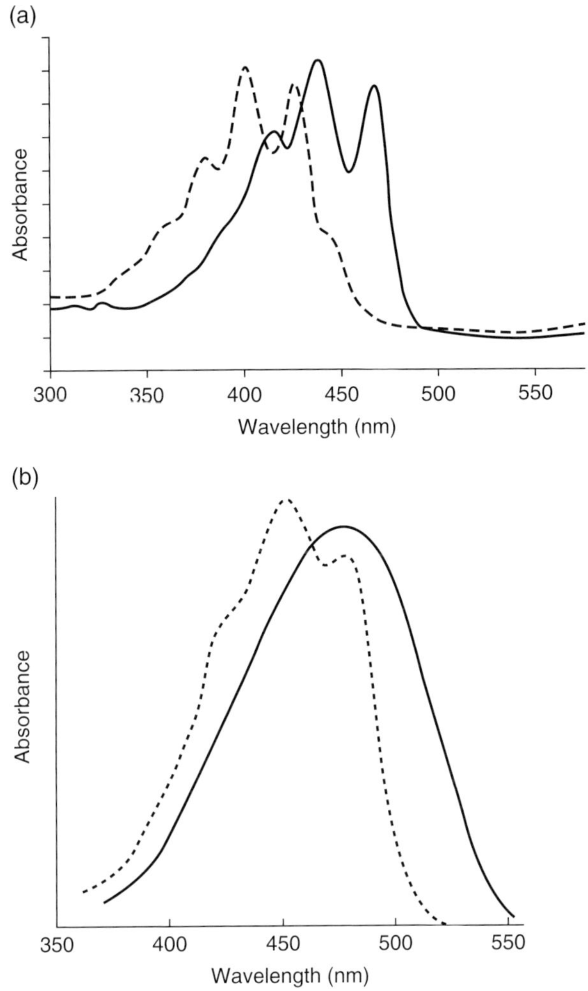

Figure 3.5 (a) Visible absorption spectra of violaxanthin (—) and its epoxide-furanoid rearrangement product (- - - -) in petroleum ether; (b) Visible absorption spectra of canthaxanthin (–) and its reduction product (- - - -) in petroleum ether. Taken from Rodriguez-Amaya (1999).

5 and 10 nm lower (Figure 3.5a). When a 5,6-epoxide is rearranged to the 5,8-epoxide (furanoid), an additional double bond, this time from the polyene chain, is lost. Thus, the λ_{max} of the 5,8-monoepoxide and 5,8,5′,8′-diepoxide are 20–25 and 50 nm lower, respectively, than those of the parent carotenoids (Figure 3.5a). Because only the polyene chain conjugated double bonds remain, the degree of spectral fine structure increases, resembling that of acyclic carotenoids.

An isolated carbonyl group (i.e., not in conjugation with the chromophore) does not affect the spectrum, but a carbonyl group in conjugation with the polyene chain double bonds extends the chromophore. The latter's effect is manifested in a bathochromic shift (displacement to higher wavelengths) and loss of spectral fine structure, to the extent that the spectrum consists of a single broad curve instead of the three-maxima spectrum.

The absorption spectrum of echinenone (orange) has an unsymmetrical peak with λ_{max} at 458 nm and a shoulder at 482 nm. The absorption peak of canthaxanthin (red-orange) is symmetrical with the λ_{max} at 466 (Figure 3.5b).

Z-isomerization of a chromophore's double bond causes a slight loss in color, a small hypsochromic shift (usually 2 to 6 nm for mono-*Z*), and a hypochromic effect. A *cis* peak may appear in or near the ultraviolet region (Figure 3.6), about 142 nm hypsochromically displaced from the longest wavelength maximum of the *E*-isomer. The intensity of the *cis* band is greater as the *cis* double bond is nearer the center of the molecule. Thus, the *cis* peak of the 15-*Z* isomer, which has a *cis* double bond at the center of the molecule, is intense; it decreases in intensity in 13-*Z* and practically disappears in the 9-*Z* isomer (Figure 3.5). 5-*Z*-lycopene had been overlooked until recently because of the difficulty in separating it from all-*E*-lycopene, and the all-*E*- and the 5-*Z*-isomers have identical visible absorption spectra (Liaaen-Jensen, 2004). Moreover, since the *cis* double is located at the terminal double bond, 5-*Z*-lycopene does not exhibit the characteristic *cis* peak.

Understandably, slightly different λ_{max} values are reported in the literature, considering that the reproducibility of recording spectrophotometer in the 400–500 nm region is about 1–2 nm. Instrumental errors should be kept at a minimum by calibrating the instruments (e.g., using a holmium oxide filter and recording the spectra of authentic carotenoid standards).

The absorption spectra of carotenoids are markedly solvent dependent. This has to be remembered when spectra are taken by the photodiode array detector in high-performance liquid chromatography (HPLC), in which the spectra are taken in mixed solvents in isocratic elution and in varying mixed solvents in gradient elution. The λ_{max}

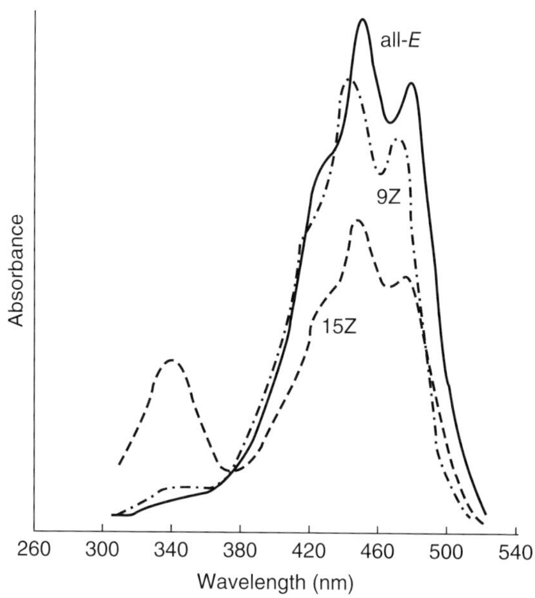

Figure 3.6 Absorption spectra of geometric isomers of β-carotene in hexane. Taken from Rodriguez-Amaya and Kimura (2004). Reproduced with permission of HarvestPlus.

values recorded in hexane, petroleum ether, diethyl ether, methanol, ethanol, and acetonitrile are practically the same, but they are higher by 2–6 nm in acetone, 10–20 nm in chloroform, 10–20 nm in dichloromethane, and 18–24 nm in toluene (Britton, 1995).

The absorption spectra are now rarely presented in published papers. To give an idea of the spectral fine structure, the %III/II can be presented, along with the λ_{max} values. The %III/II is the ratio of the height of the longest wavelength absorption peak, designated III, and that of the middle absorption peak, designated II, taking the minimum between the two peaks as baseline, multiplied by 100 (Britton, 1995). In a few cases, such as ζ-carotene, III is greater than II; thus, the %III/II value is slightly higher than 100. For conjugated ketocarotenoids, such as canthaxanthin and echinenone, the spectrum consists of a broad single maximum with no defined fine structure; thus, %III/II is 0.

3.3.3.8.2 Mass spectrometry

Many laboratories around the world now have access to HPLC-MS. Aside from the molecular formula, important characteristic fragment ions facilitate identification of the carotenoids. Enzell and Back (1995) tabulated data for 170 different carotenoid end groups. Only some examples of typical fragmentation patterns (Enzell and Back, 1995; Rivera and Canela-Garayoa, 2012) will be presented here.

Losses of 92 (toluene) and 106 (xylene) mass units, producing the ions $[M-92]^{+\cdot}$, $[M-92]^{+}$, $[M+H-92]^{+}$ and the ions $[M-106]^{+\cdot}$, $[M-106]^{+}$, and $[M+H-106]^{+}$ (obtained by means of EI, ESI, and APCI, respectively) are characteristics of carotenoids in general, indicating the extensive conjugation of the polyene chain.

Loss of 56 mass unit indicates carotenoids containing ε-ring, with the production of ions $[M-56]^{+\cdot}$, $[M-56]^{+}$, and $[M+H-56]^{+}$ by means of EI, ESI, and APCI, respectively. A ψ end group gives rise to ions $[M-69]^{+\cdot}$, $[M-69]^{\cdot}$, and $[M-69]^{+}$ by EI and APCI.

The removal of a molecule of water, generating ions $[M-17]^{+-}$ or $[M+H-18]^{+}$, is characteristic of the presence of a hydroxyl group, as in β-cryptoxanthin or lutein. Zeinoxanthin and α-cryptoxanthin have the same chemical formula but are distinguishable by the position of the hydroxyl group. For carotenoid epoxides, the fragments at *m/z* 221 and 181 indicate that the epoxy group is in a ring bearing a hydroxyl group.

A limitation of MS for carotenoids is its inability to distinguish between all-*E*- and *Z*-isomers and between 5,6- and 5,8-epoxy carotenoids.

HPLC-MS (APCI) was used to unequivocally identify and quantify zeaxanthin esters in wolfberries, Chinese lanterns, orange pepper, and sea buckthorn (Weller and Breithaupt, 2003).

3.3.3.8.3 Reactions of functional groups

Xanthophylls undergo functional group chemical reactions that can serve as simple and rapid tests for the identification of carotenoids (Eugster 1995; Rodriguez-Amaya 1999). Many of the chemical reactions in extensive use in the late 1960s and early 1970s have now been supplanted by MS and NMR. However, some reactions remain useful and can be performed quickly with only a small amount of the test carotenoid and are amenable to rapid monitoring by UV-visible spectrometry, TLC, or HPLC.

Primary and secondary hydroxyl groups are acetylated by acetic anhydride in pyridine. Allylic hydroxyls, isolated or allylic to the chromophore, are methylated with acidic methanol. In both reactions a positive response is shown by a marked increase in the silica TLC RF value or the retention time in reversed-phase HPLC, the extent of the increase depending on the number of hydroxyl substituents. Both the acetylated and methylated products have unchanged chromophore and thus unaltered ultraviolet and visible spectra, but they are less polar than the original carotenoids.

Epoxy groups in the 5,6 or 5,6,5′,6′ positions are easily detected by their facile conversion to the furanoid derivatives in the presence of an acid catalyst, reflected by a hypsochromic shift of 20–25 nm or 40–50 nm, respectively (Figure 3.5a).

Ketocarotenoids, such as echinenone and canthaxanthin, and apocarotenals undergo reduction with LiAlH4 or NaBH4, manifested by the appearance of the three-maxima spectra of the resulting hydroxycarotenoid, in lieu of the single broad band of the original ketocarotenoid or apocarotenal (Figure 3.6b).

Iodine-catalyzed *E-Z* isomerization, which can be done directly in the spectrometer cuvette, results in a 3–5 nm shift of the λ_{max}s of all-*E*-carotenoids to lower wavelengths, whereas those of *Z*-carotenoids (such as 15-*Z*- and 13-*Z*-β-carotene) will shift to longer wavelengths after 1–5 minute exposure to light.

3.3.3.9 Quantitation

HPLC quantitation is usually carried out by external calibration with the respective standards, although internal standardization has also been used. Because carotenoids absorb maximally at different wavelengths and have different coefficients of absorption, a carotenoid cannot be quantified accurately using another carotenoid as standard, as is sometimes seen in the literature. Carotenoid standards are costly, unstable, and often unavailable. Open-column chromatography can be used to separate and isolate standards with purity comparable or even better than that of commercial standards (Kimura and Rodriguez-Amaya, 2002; Rodriguez-Amaya and Kimura, 2004; Kimura et al., 2007). This procedure has been used in other laboratories (e.g., Morris et al., 2004; Gama and Sylos, 2007; Giuffrida et al., 2007; Griffiths et al., 2007).

The purity of the standards should be verified and the concentrations of the standard solutions should be corrected accordingly. In the calibration process, for each carotenoid being quantified, the analyst has to prepare standard solutions of varying concentrations (usually five concentrations), inject each solution usually in triplicate, and construct the standard curve. The standard curve should be linear, pass through the origin, and should bracket the expected concentrations of the food samples.

The concentration of the standard solution is determined by visible absorption spectrometry as in measuring the total carotenoid content (Section 3.3.2), using the absorption coefficient of the carotenoid being quantified. Absorption coefficients of the major all-*E*-carotenoids in foods in specific solvents are available (Britton, 1995; Rodriguez-Amaya, 1999). For *Z*-carotenoids, the absorption coefficients of the corresponding all-*E*-carotenoid is used. Since the coefficients for *cis* isomers are generally lower, this practice underestimates the *Z*-isomer contents (Liaaen-Jensen, 2004).

Even when HPLC-MS was used for identification, quantification had been carried out mostly with the DAD detector. As exceptions, Frenich et al. (2005), Matsumoto et al. (2007), and Slavin et al. (2009) quantified with HPLC-MS by selective ion monitoring (SIM). Weller and Breithaupt (2003) also quantified zeaxanthin esters by HPLC-MS. The HPLC-DAD-MS instrument is a powerful tool, allowing easier identification and quantification of the carotenoids (Figure 3.7).

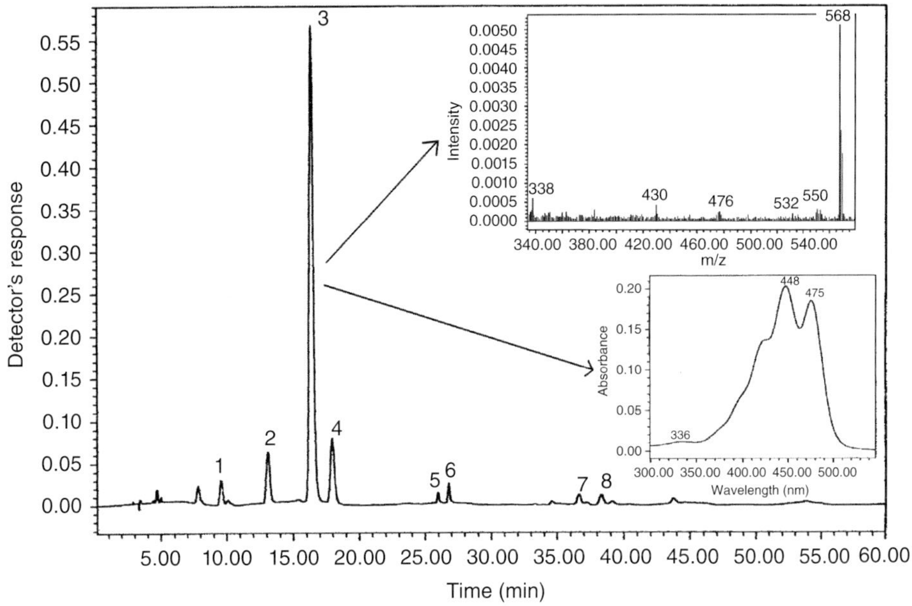

Figure 3.7 Typical HPLC chromatogram of the carotenoids of a saponified sample of *Tropaeolum majus* L. flowers. Peak identification: 1. violaxanthin, 2. antheraxanthin, 3. lutein, 4. zeaxanthin, 5. zeinoxanthin, 6. β-cryptoxanthin, 7. α-carotene, 8. β-carotene. Inset: mass and visible absorption spectra of lutein. Taken from Niizu and Rodriguez-Amaya (2005).

3.3.4 Sources of errors and precautionary measures

The overall error in an analytical data is the sum of the errors stemming from sampling, preparation of the analytical sample, the analysis per se, data processing, and interpretation. For any analyte, accurate quantitative analysis requires representative sampling, a validated method, a quality assurance system, and an adequately trained analyst. Critical points in the analytical process and sources of errors, as well as means to avoid them, must be known.

Carotenoid analysis in foods is particularly and inherently challenging because of the following:

- the large number of different carotenoids in foods
- the substantial qualitative and quantitative composition variation between foods and between samples of the same food
- the wide differences in the carotenoid levels in a given food
- the diversity and complexity of food matrices
- the distribution of carotenoids which is not uniform within a sample or between samples of a given food
- the susceptibility of the highly unsaturated carotenoid molecule to isomerization and oxidation during analysis and during storage of samples and standards
- the low levels (μg/g) of carotenoids in foods, together with other compounds at much higher concentrations that can interfere in the analysis or at least make complete extraction difficult.

Analysis at low levels usually means that analytical errors are magnified. A further confounding factor is the rapid pre- and postharvest physiological changes that occur in fruits and vegetables, the major dietary sources of carotenoids.

Especially in the 1990s, a lot of effort has been directed to obtaining reliable quantitative data for food carotenoids. Sources of errors and critical points have been identified, interlaboratory studies have been carried out, and certified reference materials are available. The carotenoid analyst should take advantage of these advances in ensuring data quality to avoid errors that can still be perceived in the literature. A summary of the errors at each step of the analytical procedure is presented in Figure 3.1.

Currently, the major errors in carotenoid analysis appear to arise from the sampling/sample preparation schemes. Obtaining representative and homogeneous samples for analysis is a difficult but essential task. Unfortunately, in many papers the sampling plan and reduction of the gross sample to the analytical sample are not described at all or if they are, only superficially; frequently, a single sample lot is analyzed per food. Errors from these initial steps are not observed in intralaboratory and interlaboratory evaluations in which the same homogenized samples are analyzed by the participating analysts/laboratories.

With the highly sensitive analytical instrumentation currently available, along with environmental and economic concerns, a possible emerging source of error is the use of extremely low sample masses (down to mg) with concomitant reduction of the amount of extracting solvent (down to μL). There is a limit to miniaturization as the smaller the sample submitted to analysis, the more difficult it is to guarantee representativity. Moreover, reduction in sample size makes sample manipulation more difficult and is likely to magnify the analytical errors of such trace analysis. As noted by Blake (2007), analytical samples of 2 to 10 g are specified in AOAC official methods and 5 to 10 g in European Committee for Standardization (CEN) procedures for the determination of β-carotene. A possible solution is to start with the smallest amount of analytical sample that guarantees representativity, and after extraction, take aliquots for the rest of the analytical process, as is done in mycotoxin analysis.

Susceptibility of carotenoids to isomerization and oxidation is a major cause of analytical errors. Irrespective of the analytical method chosen, precautionary measures to avoid formation of artifacts and quantitative losses should be routine practices in the laboratory. These include completion of the analysis within the shortest possible time, exclusion of oxygen, protection from light, avoiding high temperature and contact with acid, use of high-purity solvents free from harmful impurities (e.g., peroxides), addition of antioxidants (e.g., butylated hydroxytoluene, pyrogallol, and ascorbyl palmitate) and neutralizing agents (e.g., $MgCO_3$) (Schiedt and Liaaen-Jensen, 1995; Rodriguez-Amaya, 1999), and adequate storage conditions or execution of analysis immediately after sample collection (Rodriguez-Amaya, 1999). The analyst should take advantage of the carotenoids' color to monitor the different steps of carotenoid analysis. Loss or change of color at any time during the analysis is an indication of degradation or structural modification. A complicating factor is that the instability varies with different carotenoids. Adding an internal standard to correct for losses during the different steps will not be of much help since the stability will differ between the standard and the carotenoids and, in fact, between the carotenoids.

Oxygen, especially in combination with light and heat, is highly destructive. The presence of even traces of oxygen in stored samples (even at deep freeze temperatures) and of peroxides in solvents (e.g., diethyl ether and tetrahydrofuran), or of any oxidizing agent in extracts of carotenoids, can rapidly lead to bleaching and the formation of artifacts, such as epoxy carotenoids and apocarotenals (Britton, 1991). Oxygen can be excluded at several steps during analysis and during storage with the use of vacuum and a nitrogen or argon atmosphere. As stated above, antioxidants may also be used, especially when the analysis is prolonged. They can be added during sample disintegration or saponification or added to solvents (e.g., tetrahydrofuran), standard solutions, and isolates.

Carotenoid work must be done under subdued light. Speed of manipulation and protection from light, especially direct sunlight and ultraviolet light, are particularly important in extracts containing chlorophylls (e.g., extracts of green leafy or nonleafy vegetables) or other potential sensitizers. In the presence of these sensitizers, photodegradation and isomerization occur very rapidly, even with brief exposure to light. Gold lighting is used by some laboratories to filter out visible light. It was shown by O'Neil and Schwartz (1995), however, that this lighting does not prevent but only slows down sensitized photoisomerization.

Carotenoids may decompose, dehydrate, or isomerize in the presence of acids. 5,6-epoxycarotenoids, such as violaxanthin and neoxanthin, readily undergo rearrangement to the 5,8-epoxides. A neutralizing agent (e.g., calcium carbonate, magnesium carbonate, or sodium bicarbonate) may be added during extraction to neutralize acids liberated from the food sample itself. Strong acids and acidic reagents should not be used in rooms where carotenoids are handled. Most carotenoids are stable toward alkali.

Fractions or isolates should be kept dry under nitrogen or argon or dissolved in a hydrocarbon solvent, petroleum ether or hexane, and kept at −20°C or lower when not in use. Leaving carotenoids in solvents such as cyclohexane, dichloromethane, diethyl ether (Craft and Soares, 1992), and acetone can lead to substantial degradation. Carotenoids extracted with acetone should be immediately transferred to petroleum ether.

Currently the preferred technique, HPLC itself is subject to several sources of errors: (a) incompatibility of the injection solvent and the mobile phase which results in peak splitting; (b) inconclusive or erroneous identification; (c) impurity, instability, and unavailability of standards; (d) quantification of overlapped peaks; (e) variable and low recovery from the HPLC column; (f) inaccuracy in the preparation of standard solutions and in the calibration procedure; and (g) calculation errors (Craft, 1992; Epler et al., 1992; Scott, 1992; Hart and Scott, 1995; Kimura and Rodriguez-Amaya, 1999; Rodriguez-Amaya, 1999; Rodriguez-Amaya and Kimura, 2004).

Saponification continues to be a critical step in carotenoid analysis. Considerable losses during this step and the subsequent washing have been reported through the years, especially of lutein, zeaxanthin, violaxanthin, and other dihydroxy, trihydroxy, and epoxycarotenoids (Khachik et al., 1986; Rodriguez-Amaya et al., 1988; Kimura et al., 1990; Marsili and Callahan, 1993; Riso and Porrini, 1997; Yue et al., 2006), although provitamin A carotenoids (α-carotene, β-carotene, γ-carotene, β-cryptoxanthin) appeared stable (Rodriguez-Amaya et al., 1988; Kimura et al., 1990). The extent of carotenoid degradation depends on the conditions used, being greater with higher concentration of alkali and hot saponification (Kimura et al., 1990). If required, this step should be thoroughly evaluated and optimized, and the subsequent washing carefully done to avoid losing carotenoids with the discarded aqueous phase (de Sá and Rodriguez-Amaya, 2004). Complete hydrolysis of carotenol esters to the free carotenoids should also be verified.

Principally because of losses during saponification and the subsequent washing, lutein is frequently underestimated, as in leafy vegetables. Except in lettuce, if the lutein content is almost equal to or lower than that of β-carotene in a leafy vegetable, as is sometimes seen in the literature, lutein loss during analysis is strongly indicated.

Concern about the negative effects of saponification has led analysts to shorten the duration of ambient temperature saponification (e.g., to 1 or 2 hours). In our experience, however, longer saponification times are required for complete hydrolysis of carotenol esters.

In the 1990s, lycopene drew concern analytically because of reported low recoveries from the HPLC column (Konings and Roomans, 1997), high intralaboratory (Hart and Scott, 1995) and interlaboratory (Scott et al., 1996) coefficients of variation, and low range of linearity (Riso and Porrini, 1997). Each laboratory should verify if their analytical procedure and/or chromatographic system leads to loss of this carotenoid.

In HPLC, the concentrations of analytes are calculated by comparing the detector response with those of standard solutions of known concentration. Errors introduced in the preparation of the standard solutions, determination of the concentrations, and construction of the calibration curves will be reflected in the analytical results. The purity of the standards should be verified and the concentrations of the standard solutions corrected accordingly. If necessary (i.e., low purity), the standards should be repurified.

Instability of carotenoid standards is a serious problem. Standard carotenoid crystals should be sealed in ampoules under N_2 or argon and stored at −20°C or preferably at −70°C until use. Stock and working solutions, even when kept at low temperature, have limited validity; the analyst should know when degradation commences under the conditions of his/her laboratory.

3.3.5 Method validation and quality assurance

Methods should be validated before use. Validation can reveal weaknesses of the method that were not perceived during development. Periodic evaluation of the method and the analyst's performance (Kobori and Rodriguez-Amaya, 2013) should be part of the quality assurance system of any laboratory.

Method accuracy can be verified in the laboratory by recovery tests, method comparisons, and analyses of certified reference material. The widely employed recovery test (i.e., spiking of samples with standards) is of questionable validity for compounds such as carotenoids, which are well protected by membranes and cell walls and can be linked to other components in food samples. The added analytes do not behave in the same way as the endogenous compounds, and overestimated recoveries are reported. The efficiency of extraction, a critical step in carotenoid analysis, is not assessed. However, a low recovery percentage is a good indicator of losses, physical or degradative, during analysis.

Comparable results obtained with methods of differing principles/procedures indicate good reliability of the methods. However, analysis of a certified reference material is the preferred procedure for verifying method performance and the laboratory's capability for obtaining accurate results. Unlike the recovery test, the analytical process from extraction to instrumental measurement can be assessed. For carotenoids, two certified reference materials have been developed: Community Bureau of Reference BCR485 (freeze-dried mixed vegetables) and NIST SRM 2383 (baby food composite) (Sharpless et al., 2000; Phillips et al., 2007).

Because of the limited availability of certified reference materials, the development of in-house reference materials that resemble the food samples of interest in terms of matrix and carotenoid composition/concentrations is recommended. As with certified reference materials, processed foods are generally used for this purpose because of their longer shelf life and homogeneity. The food's perishability (aside from the carotenoids' instability) makes reference materials of raw foods, which are generally more difficult to analyze than processed foods, inviable.

Interlaboratory studies play an important role in quality assurance, in evaluating laboratory and method performance and certifying reference materials. These studies have been conducted for carotenoids, each reporting findings that greatly impact the quality of analytical data. Participation in interlaboratory trials is encouraged because it enables laboratories to assess and demonstrate objectively the reliability of the data that they are producing (Thompson et al., 2006). The results also demonstrate certain features of the analysis that are not so apparent in single laboratory evaluations. Opportunities to participate in these trials are, however, rare.

A European study with 17 participating laboratories investigated various possible problem areas, including the chromatographic systems, standardization of carotenoid stock solutions, extraction procedures, and data handling (Scott et al., 1996). A lyophilized vegetable mix, which became the certified reference material BCR CRM 485, was used. The effect of the chromatographic system did not appear to be the major variable. In the more experienced laboratory, variation in the standardization of the carotenoid solution was also not thought to be a significant problem. The results suggested that the preparation of the extract might account for about 13% of the overall variance of around 23%. Among the carotenoids analyzed (lutein, zeaxanthin, lycopene, α-carotene, and β-carotene), greater variations occurred for lycopene calibration and measurement.

In a second European study involving 14 laboratories, β-carotene and its *cis* isomers were determined in commercial processed foods (margarine, vitamin drink, pudding powder, and natural mixed vegetable), which were chosen according to type of matrix, range of concentration, and availability in food stores (Schüep and Schierle, 1997). The best repeatability and reproducibility were obtained with the supplemented drink and the worst results with the pudding powder. Considerable differences were observed in the reported values between total β-carotene and all-*E*-β-carotene, depending on the separation efficiency of the HPLC system used. The authors concluded that excluding *Z*-isomers from quantification of β-carotene would result in significant underestimation of this carotenoid.

In an interlaboratory study among 26 U.S. and European laboratories (Sharpless et al., 1999), a baby food composite was used, which is now known as certified reference material NIST SRM 2383. The relative expanded uncertainties were higher than those generally expected for certified values, attesting to the complexity of carotenoid analysis. Certified concentrations were provided for some carotenoids, but only reference values could be given for other carotenoids. For lycopene, for example, only reference values were provided because of greater variation in the values obtained, attributed to degradation of this analyte in some participating laboratories.

An international interlaboratory study was conducted in 2005 by our laboratory for the international project HarvestPlus, involving 19 Asian, African, European, Latin American, and U.S. laboratories with widely differing laboratory conditions and experience in carotenoid analysis. Using sweet potato, cassava, and corn flours as test materials, it was demonstrated that (1) incomplete extraction was a major problem; (2) HarvestPlus had several laboratories capable of determining the carotenoid concentrations in sweet potato and cassava, but more work was needed for corn, the test material with a more complex carotenoid composition; and (3) training of the analysts was very important. Since the test materials were dehydrated products, from which carotenoids were harder to extract than the fresh produce, those laboratories that rehydrated the products prior to extraction had better results. Analysts who were newcomers but had undergone the HarvestPlus hands-on training on carotenoid analysis did as well as those who had done this analysis for some time.

3.3.6 UHPLC-DAD methods

For over two decades, HPLC-DAD has been the method of choice and has provided a large body of reliable and detailed data on carotenoid composition of foods. However, environmental and economic concerns have encouraged the continued search for faster methods that use less organic solvents.

Efforts to improve HPLC further have led to ultra-high performance liquid chromatography (UHPLC). This technique, in comparison with HPLC, uses narrow bore, shorter columns (2.1 × 50 mm vs. 4.6 × 200 mm); less run time (10 min vs. 30 min); lower flow rate (0.3 mL/min vs. 1 mL/min); lower injection volume (1.4 μL vs. 20 μL) and solvent volume/sample (4.0 mL vs. 27 mL); smaller particle size (2 μm vs. 2-5 μm); and much higher back pressure (up to 103.5 MPa vs. 35–40 MPa) (Bohoyo-Gil et al., 2012; Rivera and Canela-Garayoa, 2012). High-strength silica (HSS) C18 and T3 and ethylene bridged hybrid (BEH) C18 stationary phases have been successfully used to separate carotenoids.

UHPLC has several advantages over conventional chromatography, including (a) faster analyses due to shorter retention times; (b) narrower peaks, giving increased signal-to-noise ratio; and (c) higher resolution and sensitivity (Rivera and Canela-Garayoa, 2012). Moreover, it is estimated that UHPLC typically saves at least 80% of mobile phase compared to HPLC (S. Chen and Kord, 2009); much lower solvent consumption is in line with current initiative to promote environmentally friendly green analytical chemistry. As with the HPLC methods, however, UHPLC methods have to undergo rigorous method standardization as well as intralaboratory and interlaboratory validation to guarantee data reliability. Special attention should be given to sampling and sample preparation because, as discussed above, the smaller the analytical sample, the more difficult it is to guarantee representativity. There is also a tendency to transform the sample into dried or lyophilized, ground fine powder (Li et al., 2012, 2013; Rivera and Canela, 2012; Kaulmann et al., 2014), considered to be more amenable to small-scale analysis. Both drying and grinding can lead to substantial losses of carotenoids (Rodriguez-Amaya, 2010).

UHPLC has been used for the quantification of carotenoids in corn (Rivera and Canela-Garayoa, 2012; Rivera et al., 2013), *Brassica* vegetables (Guzman et al., 2012), durum wheat (Hung and Hatcher, 2011), milk (Chauveau-Duriot et al., 2010), tomato (Li et al., 2012, 2013; van Meulebroek et al., 2012), honeybee pollen, pumpkin, nectarine (Bohoyo-Gil et al., 2012), buckthorn berries and leaves (Pop et al., 2014), *Brassica oleracea*, and plum varieties (Kaulmann et al., 2014). In milk, the UPLC method gave similar concentration of all-*E*-β-carotene (mean of 0.24 μg/mL of milk) to that obtained by an HPLC method (mean of 0.22 μg/mL of milk) (Chauveau-Duriot et al., 2010). Using seven carotenoid standards, UHPLC was compared to HPLC and the quantified concentrations were statistically indistinguishable (Bohoyo-Gil et al., 2012).

3.3.7 Other methods

Carotenoid extraction with organic solvents generates large amounts of waste, the disposal of which is an environmental problem. An environmentally friendly alternative is supercritical fluid extraction with CO_2, which also has the advantages of inertness and low toxicity and reactivity. This technique has been applied to the extraction of carotenoids from food samples without a modifier (Gómez-Prieto et al., 2003) or with ethanol or methanol as modifier (Barth et al., 1995; Mathiasson et al., 2002; López et al., 2004). β-carotene results obtained with a supercritical CO_2 procedure with ethanol as modifier, performed in approximately 30 min, averaged 23% higher than those of ethanol-pentane extraction, performed in 90 min (Marsili and Callahan, 1993).

Other environmentally friendly extraction methods have been introduced, such as microwave-assisted extraction (Xiao et al., 2012; Hiranvarachat 2013), accelerated solvent extraction (Breithaupt, 2004; H. Sun et al., 2012), and ultrasound-assisted extraction (T. Sun et al., 2006; Yue et al., 2006; Lianfu and Zelong, 2008; Li et al., 2013). Microwave-assisted extraction (Kiss et al., 2000), which shortens the extraction time and improves the yield of the extraction, is simple and is not limited by solvent selectivity. Ultrasound-assisted extraction was used in quantifying lutein from chicken liver by HPLC (T. Sun et al., 2006). With three samples, the concentrations of lutein in the ultrasound-assisted solvent-extracted samples had higher levels (6.0, 10.4, and 5.5 μg/g) than those of saponified solvent-extracted samples (2.9, 4.5, 2.5 μg/g).

Matrix solid-phase dispersion has been proposed for the rapid, mild (without artifact formation), complete, and reproducible extraction of carotenoid *Z*/*E*-isomers as shown with raw and cooked spinach samples (Glaser et al., 2003). It was also used for carotenoids in corn flour and kiwi (Gentili and Caretti, 2011). In comparison to liquid-liquid extraction and solid-phase extraction, matrix solid-phase dispersion (MSPD) is easy to handle because the solid or viscous biological tissue can be directly mixed with the sorbent material, and so MSPD combines the advantages of being time saving and requiring less solvent (Dachtler et al., 2001). As the carotenoids elute in a small fraction, the evaporation of large amounts of solvent, as is usual in liquid-liquid extraction, is not necessary. With MSPD, the carotenoids are protected against oxidation and isomerization during the quick and gentle extraction process, avoiding the formation of artifacts.

Isocratic separation and determination of carotenoids in vegetables by capillary electrochromatography was found to resolve β-carotene, lycopene, and lutein well (Herrero-Martínez et al., 2006). The concentrations of β-carotene and lutein in carrot and spinach, and of lycopene in tomato obtained with this technique were within the ranges reported in the literature. Recently, ultra-high-performance supercritical fluid chromatogaphy (UHPSFC) was applied to carotenoids in paprika oleoresin (Berger and Berger, 2013).

With the advantages of rapidity, simplicity, safety, and low operational costs, nondestructive techniques have been applied to carotenoid analysis, such as near infrared spectroscopy (NIRS) (Berardo et al., 2004; Brenna and Berardo, 2004; Pedro and Ferreira, 2005; Clément et al., 2008; Bonierbale et al., 2009; Davey et al., 2009b), attenuated total reflection Fourier transform infrared spectroscopy (ATR-IR) (Baranska et al., 2006b; Nardo et al., 2009), Fourier transform infrared spectroscopy (FTIR) (Rubio-Diaz et al., 2011), and Raman spectroscopy (Bhosale et al., 2004; Darwin et al., 2007). For these techniques, the results obtained were shown to have high correlation with those of HPLC. Application of reflectance colorimetry in carotenoid analysis has also been investigated (Pinho and Lima Reis, 2012).

For screening, high-correlation coefficients may be sufficient. However, for quantitative carotenoid composition, equivalency rather than correlation of the results obtained with those of validated HPLC methods should be demonstrated (Rodriguez-Amaya, 2010). In a recent paper comparing spectrophotometric and HPLC methods for carotenoid determination, Luterotti et al. (2013) concluded that reliable picture on the data compliance for carotenoid contents in food could not be always obtained through the R-values and t-tests.

Brenna and Berardo (2004) did show that the mean values obtained by NIRS and HPLC for six carotenoids in samples of maize flour were similar. However, in a comparison of Fourier transform-Raman (FT-Raman), ATR-IR, and NIRS for measuring lycopene and β-carotene, ATR-IR showed the best statistics. The prediction quality of Raman was poorer, and NIRS had the worst prediction potential (Baranska et al., 2006b).

Several analytical techniques and approaches relying on photothermal phenomena have been recently shown to be applicable for pretreatment-free and rapid screening of low quantities of carotenoids in foods (Bicanic et al., 2010; Bicanic, 2011). Laser photoacoustic spectroscopy was used for the determination of the total carotenoid content of corn and sweet potato flours, using UV-visible spectrometry as reference method (Luterotti et al., 2011).

It was also shown that X-ray photoelectron spectroscopy and time-of-flight secondary ion mass spectrometry could be used for direct measurement of the major carotenoid in the annatto seed (Felicissimo et al., 2004).

As with the HPLC methods, these alternative procedures or methodologies should undergo method standardization and validation, including interlaboratory studies, before they can be adopted for wider use.

3.4 CALCULATION OF RETENTION IN COOKED AND PROCESSED FOOD

Because of the instability of carotenoids, it is important to monitor losses during cooking and processing. Optimum conditions for the maximum retention of these important compounds in the foods served for consumption can then be ascertained.

Loss of carotenoids had been calculated in published papers simply by the difference of the carotenoid concentrations before (e.g., μg/g raw weight) and after cooking or processing (e.g., μg/g cooked weight). This calculation does not account for changes in the food weight during cooking (due to loss of water and soluble solids or gain of water or oil) and therefore does not indicate true losses of the carotenoids.

Calculations that account or compensate for loss or gain of food weight during cooking can be done by the formula of Murphy et al. (1975) and by calculation on a dry weight basis:

$$\%\ \text{retention} = \frac{\text{carotenoid content per g of cooked food} \times \text{g of food after cooking}}{\text{carotenoid content per g of raw food} \times \text{g of food before cooking}} \times 100$$

$$\%\ \text{retention} = \frac{\text{carotenoid content per g of raw food (dry basis)}}{\text{carotenoid content per g of cooked or processed food (dry basis)}} \times 100$$

Calculation on a dry weight basis overestimates retention, but it is not always feasible to obtain data on weights of foods before and after thermal processing, especially under industrial production conditions.

Carotenoid retentions of over 100% in cooked or processed foods are sometimes reported. Since it is not possible for carotenoids to be biosynthesized during heat treatment, these results are not true increases. Heating, in fact, inactivates the enzymes responsible for carotenogenesis and stimulates isomerization and oxidative degradation of carotenoids, as discussed in Chapter 7.

These alleged increases could be due simply to the greater ease with which carotenoids are extracted from cooked or processed samples compared with carotenoids in fresh foods, where they are physically protected or combined with other food components. Extraction efficiency of fresh samples must be enhanced to make it as equivalent as possible to that of cooked samples (such as soaking the sample in water or extracting solvent before extraction), and extraction must be exhaustive. Apparent increases may also be due to appreciable leaching of soluble solids, as in carrots, concentrating the carotenoids per unit weight of food. Calculating the retention on the insoluble solid basis has been proposed in this case. Moreover, enzymatic oxidation of carotenoids can substantially lower their concentrations in raw samples, especially when these samples are left standing for some time after being cut or grated.

In contrast to sampling for databases, to study the effects of industrial processing and home cooking, raw and processed/cooked samples are taken from the same sample lot. Replicate analyses of paired samples are carried out so that differences in the results obtained are due solely to processing/cooking, without the influence of raw material variability. In reporting the results, it is important to specify the processing and storage conditions (time, temperature, etc.).

Paired samples (i.e., equivalent raw and cooked samples) are used in these studies to offset between-sample natural variations (e.g., varietal differences, seasonal or climatic effects, degree of maturity, etc.) For example, in our study on the retention of β-carotene in carrot, the carrots were quartered longitudinally, two opposite sections were taken for analysis of raw samples and the other two opposite sections were submitted to cooking before analysis. It is also recommended that results be analyzed statistically so that the true meaning of the results can be appreciated.

References

Akhtar MH, Bryan M. 2008. Extraction and quantification of major carotenoids in processed foods and supplements by liquid chromatography. *Food Chem* 111:255–61.

Aman R, Biehl J, Carle R, Conrad J, Beifuss U, Schieber A. 2005. Application of HPLC coupled with DAD, APcI-MS and NMR to the analysis of lutein and zeaxanthin stereoisomers in thermally processed vegetables. *Food Chem* 92:753–63.

Amorim-Carrilho KT, Cepeda A, Fente C, Regal P. 2014. Review of methods for analysis of carotenoids. *Trends Anal Chem* 56:49–73.

Azevedo-Meleiro CH, Rodriguez-Amaya DB. 2004. Confirmation of the identity of the carotenoids of tropical fruits by HPLC-DAD and HPLC-MS. *J Food Compos Anal* 17:385–96.

Azevedo-Meleiro CH, Rodriguez-Amaya DB. 2007. Qualitative and quantitative differences in carotenoid composition among *Cucurbita moschata*, *Cucurbita maxima*, and *Cucurbita pepo*. *J Agric Food Chem* 55:4027–33.

Azevedo-Meleiro CH, Rodriguez-Amaya DB. 2009. Qualitative and quantitative differences in the carotenoid composition of yellow and red peppers determined by HPLC-DAD-MS. *J Sep Sci* 32:3652–8.

Baranska M, Baranski R, Schulz H, Nothnagel T. 2006a. Tissue-specific accumulation of carotenoids in carrot roots. *Planta* 224:1028–37.

Baranska M, Schütze W, Schulz H. 2006b. Determination of lycopene and β-carotene content in tomato fruits and related products: comparison of FT-Raman, ATR-IR, and NIR spectroscopy. *Anal Chem* 78:8456–61.

Barba AIO, Hurtado MC, Mata MCS, Ruiz VF, de Tejada MLS. 2006. Application of UV-vis detection-HPLC method for a rapid determination of lycopene and β-carotene in vegetables. *Food Chem* 95:328–36.

Barth MM, Zhou C, Kute KM, Rosenthal GA. 1995. Determination of optimum conditions for supercritical fluid extraction of carotenoids from carrot (*Daucus carota* L.) tissue. *J Agric Food Chem* 43:2876–8.

Berardo N, Brenna OV, Amato A, Valoti P, Pisacane V, Motto M. 2004. Carotenoids concentration among maize genotypes measured by near infrared reflectance spectroscopy (NIRS). *Innov Food Sci Emerg Technol* 5:393–8.

Berger TA, Berger BK. 2013. Separation of natural food pigments in saponified and unsaponified paprika oleoresin by ultra high performance supercritical fluid chromatography (UHPSFC). *Chromatographia* 76:591–601.

Bhosale P, Ermakov IV, Ermakova MR, Gellermann W, Bernstein PS. 2004. Resonance Raman quantification of nutritionally important carotenoids in fruits, vegetables, and their juices in comparison to high-pressure liquid chromatography analysis. *J Agric Food Chem* 52:3281–5.

Bicanic DD. 2011. On the photoacoustic, photothermal and colorimetric quantification of carotenoids and other phytonutrients in some foods: a review. *J Mol Struct* 993:9–14.

Bicanic D, Dimitrovski D, Luterotti S, Markovic K, van Twisk C, Buijnsters JG, Dóka O. 2010. Correlation of *trans*-lycopene measurements by the HPLC method with the optothermal and photoacoustic signals and the color readings of fresh tomato homogenates. *Food Biophys* 5:24–33.

Blake CJ. 2007. Status of methodology for the determination of fat-soluble vitamins in foods, dietary supplements, and vitamin premixes. *J AOAC Int* 90:897–910.

Bohoyo-Gil D, Dominguez-Valhondo D, García-Parra JJ, González-Gómez D. 2012. UHPLC as a suitable methodology for the analysis of carotenoids in food matrix. *Eur Food Res Technol* 235:1055–61.

Bonierbale M, Grüneberg W, Amoros W, Burgos G, Salas E, Porras E, Felde TZ. 2009. Total and individual carotenoid profiles in *Solanum phureja* cultivated potatoes: II. Development and application of near-infrared reflectance spectroscopy (NIRS) calibrations for germplasm characterization. *J Food Comp Anal* 22:509–16.

Breithaupt DE. 2004. Simultaneous HPLC determination of carotenoids used as food coloring additives: applicability of accelerated solvent extraction. *Food Chem* 86:449–56.

Breithaupt DE, Wirt U, Bamedi A. 2002. Differentiation between lutein monester regioisomers and detection of lutein diesters from marigold flowers (*Tagetes erecta* L.) and several fruits by liquid chromatography-mass spectrometry. *J Agric Food Chem* 50:66–70.

Brenna OV, Berardo N. 2004. Application of near-infrared reflectance spectroscopy (NIRS) to the evaluation of carotenoids content in maize. *J Agric Food Chem* 52:5577–82.

Britton G. 1991. Carotenoids. *Methods Plant Biochem* 7:473–518.

Britton G. 1995. UV/visible spectroscopy. In: Britton G, Liaaen-Jensen S, Pfander H. editors. *Carotenoids: spectroscopy*, vol 1B. Basel: Birkhäuser Verlag, p 13–63.

Chauveau Duriot B, Doreau M, Nozière P, Graulet B. 2010. Simultaneous quantification of carotenoids, retinol, and tocopherols in forages, bovine plasma, and milk: validation of a novel UPLC method. *Anal Bioanal Chem* 397:777–90.

Chávez AL, Ceballos H, Rodriguez-Amaya DB, Pérez JC, Sánchez T, Calle F, Morante, N. 2008. Sampling variation for carotenoids and dry matter contents in cassava roots. *J Root Crops* 34:43–9.

Chen JP, Tai C, Chen BH. 2004. Improved liquid chromatographic method for determination of carotenoids in Taiwanese mango (*Mangifera indica* L.). *J Chromatogr A* 1054:261–8.

Chen S, Kord A. 2009. Theoretical and experimental comparison of mobile phase consumption between ultra-high-performance liquid chromatography and high performance liquid chromatography. *J Chromatogr* A:6204–9.

Clément A, Dorais M, Vernon M. 2008. Nondestructive measurement of fresh tomato lycopene content and other physicochemical characteristics using visible-NIR spectroscopy. *J Agric Food Chem* 56: 9813–8.

Cortés C, Esteve MJ, Frígola A, Torregrosa F. 2004. Identification and quantification of carotenoids including geometrical isomers in fruit and vegetable juices by liquid chromatography and ultraviolet-diode array detection. *J Agric Food Chem* 52:2203–12.

Craft NE. 1992. Carotenoid reversed-phase high-performance liquid chromatography methods: reference compendium. *Methods Enzymol* 213:185–205.

Craft NE, Soares JH Jr. 1992. Relative solubility stability, and absorptivity of lutein and β-carotene in organic solvents. *J Agric Food Chem* 40:431–4.

Craft NE, Wise SA, Soares JH Jr. 1992. Optimization of an isocratic high-performance liquid chromatographic separation of carotenoids. *J Chromatogr* 589:171–6.

Craft NE, Wise SA, Soares JH Jr. 1993. Individual carotenoid content of SRM 1548 total diet and influence of storage temperature, lyophilization, and irradiation on dietary carotenoids. *J Agric Food Chem* 41:208–13.

Dachtler M, Glaser T, Kohler K, Albert K. 2001. Combined HPLC-MS and HPLC-NMR on-line coupling for the separation and determination of lutein and zeaxanthin stereoisomers in spinach and in the retina. *Anal Chem* 73:667–74.

Darrigues A, Schwartz SJ, Francis DM. 2008. Optimizing sampling of tomato fruit for carotenoid content with application to assessing the impact of ripening disorders. *J Agric Food Chem* 56:483–7.

Darwin ME, Gersonde I, Albrecht HA, Sterry W, Lademann J. 2007. Resonance Raman spectroscopy for the detection of carotenoids in foodstuffs. Influence of the nutrition on the antioxidative potential of the skin. *Laser Phys Lett* 4:452–6.

Davey MW, Keulemans J, Swennen R. 2006. Methods for the efficient quantification of fruit provitamin A contents. *J Chromatogr A* 1136:176–84.

Davey MW, Mellidou I, Keulemans W. 2009a. Considerations to prevent the breakdown and loss of fruit carotenoids during extraction and analysis in *Musa*. *J Chromatogr A* 1216:5759–62.

Davey MW, Saeys W, Hof E, Ramon H, Swennen RL, Keulemans J. 2009b. Application of visible and near-infrared reflectance spectroscopy (Vis/NIRS) to determine carotenoid contents in banana (*Musa* spp.) fruit pulp. *J Agric Food Chem* 57:1742–51.

Davey MW, Stals E, Ngoh-Newilah G, Tomekpe K, Lusty C, Markham R, Swennen R, Keulemans, J. 2007. Sampling strategies and variability in fruit pulp micronutrient contents of West and Central African bananas and plantains (*Musa* species). *J Agric Food Chem* 55:2633–44.

Dias MG, Camões MFGFC, Oliveira L. 2008. Uncertainty estimation and in house method validation of HPLC analysis of carotenoids for food composition data production. *Food Chem* 109:815–24.

Dugo P, Herrero M, Giuffrida D, Kumm T, Dugo G, Mondello L. 2008. Application of comprehensive two-dimensional liquid chromatography to elucidate the native carotenoid composition in red orange essential oil. *J Agric Food Chem* 56:3478–85.

Enzell CR, Back S. 1995. Mass spectrometry. In: Britton G, Liaaen-Jensen S, Pfander H. editors. *Carotenoids: spectroscopy*, vol 1B. Basel: Birkhäuser Verlag, p 261–320.

Epler KS, Sander LC, Ziegler RG, Wise SA, Craft NE. 1992. Evaluation of reversed-phase liquid chromatographic columns for recovery and selectivity of selected carotenoids. *J Chromatogr* 595:89–101.

Eugster CH. 1995. Chemical derivatization: Microscale tests for the presence of common functional groups in carotenoids. In: Britton G, Liaaen-Jensen S, Pfander H. editors. *Carotenoids: isolation and analysis*, vol 1A. Basel: Birkhäuser Verlag, p 71–80.

Felicissimo MP, Bittencourt C, Houssiau L, Pireaux J-J. 2004. Time-of-flight secondary ion mass spectrometry and x-ray photoelectron spectroscopy analyses of *Bixa orellana* seeds. *J Agric Food Chem* 52:1810–4.

Feltl L, Pacáková V, Stulik K, Volka K. 2005. Reliability of carotenoid analyses: a review. *Curr Anal Chem* 1:93–102.

Fraser PD, Enfissi EMA, Goodfellow M, Eguchi T, Bramley PM. 2007. Metabolite profiling of plant carotenoids using the matrix-assisted laser desorption ionization time-of-flight mass spectrometry. *Plant J* 49:552–64.

Frenich AG, Torres MEH, Vega AB, Vidal JLM, Bolaños PP. 2005. Determination of ascorbic acid and carotenoids in food commodities by liquid chromatography with mass spectrometry detection. *J Agric Food Chem* 53:7371–6.

Gama JJT, Sylos CM de. 2007. Effect of thermal pasteurization and concentration on carotenoid composition of Brazilian Valencia orange juice. *Food Chem* 100:1686–90.

Gentili A, Caretti F. 2011. Evaluation of a method based on liquid chromatography-diode array detector-tandem mass spectrometry for a rapid and comprehensive characterization of the fat-soluble vitamin and carotenoid profile of selected plant foods. *J Chromatogr A* 1218:684–97.

Giuffrida D, Salvo F, Salvo A, la Pera L, Dugo G. 2007. Pigments composition in monovarietal virgin olive oils from various Sicilian olive varieties. *Food Chem* 101:833–7.

Glaser T, Lienau A, Zeeb D, Krucker M, Dachtler M, Albert K. 2003. Qualitative and quantitative determination of carotenoid stereoisomers in a variety of spinach samples by use of MSPD before HPLC-UV, HPLC-APCI-MS, and HPLC-NMR on-line coupling. *Chromatographia* 57:S19–S25.

Godoy HT, Rodriguez-Amaya DB. 1994. Occurrence of cis isomers of provitamin A in Brazilian fruits. *J Agric Food Chem* 42:1306–13.

Godoy HT, Rodriguez-Amaya DB. 1998. Occurrence of cis isomers of provitamins A in Brazilian vegetables. *J Agric Food Chem* 46:3081–6.

Gómez-Prieto MS, Caja MM, Herraiz M, Santa-María G. 2003. Supercritical fluid extraction of all-trans-lycopene from tomato. *J Agric Food Chem* 51:3–7.

Griffiths DW, Dale MFB, Morris WL, Ramsay G. 2007. Effects of season and postharvest storage on the carotenoid content of *Solanum phureja* potato tubers. *J Agric Food Chem* 55:379–85.

Guzman I, Yousef GG, Brown AF. 2012. Simultaneous extraction and quantitation of carotenoids, chlorophylls, and tocopherols in *Brassica* vegetables. *J Agric Food Chem* 60:7238–44.

Hart DJ, Scott KJ. 1995. Development and evaluation of an HPLC method for the analysis of carotenoids in foods, and the measurement of the carotenoid content of vegetables and fruits commonly consumed in the UK. *Food Chem* 54:101–11.

Herrero-Martínez JM, Eeltink S, Schoenmakers PJ, Kok WT, Ramis-Ramos G. 2006. Determination of major carotenoids in vegetables by capillary electrochromatography. *J Sep Sci* 29:660–5.

Hiranvarachat B, Devahastin S, Chiewchan N, Vijaya Raghavan GS. 2013. Structural modification by different pretreatment methods to enhance microwave-assisted extraction of β-carotene from carrots. *J Food Eng* 115:190–7.

Hollywood K, Brison DR, Goodacre R. 2006. Metabolomics: current technologies and future trends. *Proteomics* 6:4716–23.

Hung PV, Hatcher DW. 2011. Ultra-performance liquid chromatography (UPLC) quantification of carotenoids in durum wheat: influence of genotype and environment in relation to the colour of yellow alkaline noodles (YAN). *Food Chem* 125:1510–6.

Kaulmann A, Jonville M-C, Schneider Y-J, Hoffman L, Bohn T. 2014. Carotenoids, polyphenols and micronutrient profiles of *Brassica oleraceae* and plum varieties and their contribution to measures of total antioxidant capacity. *Food Chem* 155:240–50.

Khachik F, Beecher GR, Whitaker NF. 1986. Separation, identification, and quantification of the major carotenoid and chlorophyll constituents in extracts of several green vegetables by liquid chromatography. *J Agric Food Chem* 34:603–16.

Kimura M, Kobori CN, Rodriguez-Amaya DB, Nestel P. 2007. Screening and HPLC methods for carotenoids in sweetpotato, cassava and maize for plant breeding trials. *Food Chem* 100:1734–46.

Kimura M, Rodriguez-Amaya DB. 1999. Sources of errors in the quantitative analysis of food carotenoids by HPLC. *Archiv Latinoam Nutr* 49:58S–66S.

Kimura M, Rodriguez-Amaya DB. 2002. A scheme for obtaining standards and HPLC quantification of leafy vegetable carotenoids. *Food Chem* 78:389–98.

Kimura M, Rodriguez-Amaya DB, Godoy HT. 1990. Assessment of the saponification step in the quantitative determination of carotenoids and provitamin A. *Food Chem* 35:187–95.

Kiss GAC, Forgács E, Cserháti T, Mota T, Morais H, Ramos A. 2000. Optimisation of the microwave-assisted extraction of pigments from paprika (*Capsicum annuum* L.) powders. *J Chromatogr A* 889:41–9.

Kobori CN, Rodriguez-Amaya DB. 2008. Uncultivated Brazilian green leaves are richer sources of carotenoids than are commercially produced leafy vegetables. *Food Nutr Bull* 29:333–41.

Kobori CN, Rodriguez-Amaya DB. 2013. Intralaboratory assessment of analyts' performance in carotenoid analysis using certified reference material. *Rev Inst Adolfo Lutz* 72(2):1–10.

Konings, EJM, Roomans, HHS. 1997. Evaluation and validation of an LC method for the analysis of carotenoids in vegetables and fruit. *Food Chem* 59:599–603.

Lessin WJ, Catigani GL, Schwartz SJ. 1997. Quantification of cis-trans isomers of provitamin A carotenoids in fresh and processed fruits and vegetables. *J Agric Food Chem* 45:3728–32.

Li H, Deng Z, Liu R, Loewen S, Tsao R. 2012. Ultra-performance liquid chromatographic separation of geometric isomers of carotenoids and antioxidant activities of 20 tomato cultivars and breeding lines. *Food Chem* 132:508–17.

Li H, Deng Z, Liu R, Loewen S, Tsao R. 2013. Carotenoid composition of coloured tomato cultivars and contribution to antioxidant activities and protection against H_2O_2-induced cell death in H9c2. *Food Chem* 136:878–88.

Liaan-Jensen S. 2004. Basic carotenoid chemistry. In: Krinsky NI, Mayne ST, Sies H. editors. *Carotenoids in health and disease*. New York: Marcel Dekker, p 1–30.

Lianfu Z, Zelong L. 2008. Optimization and comparison of ultrasound/microwave assisted extraction (UMAE) and ultrasonic assisted extraction (UAE) of lycopene from tomatoes. *Ultrason Sonochem* 15:731–7.

Lin CH, Chen BH. 2003. Determination of carotenoids in tomato juice by liquid chromatography. *J Chromatogr* A:103–9.

López M, Arce L, Garrido J, Ríos A, Valcárcel M. 2004. Selective extraction of astaxanthin from crustaceans by use of supercritical carbon dioxide. *Talanta* 64:726–31.

Luterotti S, Bicanic D, Kljak K, Grbesa D, Martinez ESM, Spruijt R. 2011. Assaying total carotenoids in flours of corn and sweetpotato by laser photoacoustic spectroscopy. *Food Biophys* 6:12–9.

Luterotti S, Markovic K, Franko M, Bicanic D, Madzgalj A, Kljak K. 2013. Comparison of spectrometric and HPLC methods for determination of carotenoids in foods. *Food Chem* 140:390–7.

Marsili R, Callahan D. 1993. Comparison of a liquid solvent extraction technique and supercritical fluid extraction for the determination of α- and β-carotene in vegetables. *J Chromatogr Sci* 31:422–8.

Marx M, Schieber A, Carle R. 2000. Quantitative determination of carotene stereoisomers in carrot juices and vitamin supplemented (ATBC) drinks. *Food Chem* 70:403–8.

Mathiasson L, Turner C, Berg H, Dahlberg L, Theobald A, Anklam E, Ginn R, Sharman M, Ulberth F, Gabernig R. 2002. Development of methods for the determination of vitamins A, E and β-carotene in processed food based on supercritical fluid extraction: a collaborative study. *Food Addit Contam* 19:632–46.

Matsumoto H, Ikoma Y, Kato M, Kuniga T, Nakajima N, Yoshida T. 2007. Quantification of carotenoids in citrus fruit by LC-MS and comparison of patterns of seasonal changes for carotenoids among citrus varieties. *J Agric Food Chem* 55:2356–68.

McEwen CN, McKay RG, Larsen BS. 2005. Analysis of solids, liquids, and biological tissues using solids probe introduction at atmospheric pressure on commercial LC/MS instruments. *Anal Chem* 77:7826–31.

Mellado-Ortega E, Hornero-Méndez D. 2012. Isolation and identification of lutein esters, including regioisomers, in tritordium (x *Tritordeum* Ascherson et Graebner) grains: evidence for a preferential acyltransferase activity. *Food Chem* 135:1344–52.

Morris WL, Ducreux L, Griffiths DW, Stewart D, Davies HV, Taylor MA. 2004. Carotenogenesis during tuber development and storage in potato. J. *Exp Bot* 55:975–82.

Murphy EW, Criner PE, Gray BC. 1975. Comparisons of methods for calculating retentions of nutrients in cooked foods. *J Agric Food Chem* 23:1153–7.

Nardo T de, Shiroma-Kian C, Halim Y, Francis D, Rodriguez-Saona LE. 2009. Rapid and simultaneous determination of lycopene and β-carotene contents in tomato juice by infrared spectroscopy. *J Agric Food Chem* 57:1105–12.

Niizu PY, Rodriguez-Amaya DB. 2005. The flowers and leaves of *Tropaeolum majus* as rich sources of lutein. *J Food Sci* 70:S605–9.

Oliveira GPR de, Rodriguez-Amaya DB. 2007. Processed and prepared corn as sources of lutein and zeaxanthin. *J Food Sci* 72:S79–S85.

Oliver J, Palou A. 2000. Chromatographic determination of carotenoids in foods. *J Chromatogr A* 881:543–55.

O'Neil CA, Schwartz SJ. 1995. Photoisomerization of β-carotene by photosensitization with chlorophyll derivatives as sensitizers. *J Agric Food Chem* 43:631–5.

Pedro AMK, Ferreira MMC. 2005. Nondestructive determination of solids and carotenoids in tomato products by near-infrared spectroscopy and multivariate calibration. *Anal Chem* 77:2505–11.

Periago MJ, Rincón F, Agüera MD, Ros G. 2004. Mixture approach for optimizing lycopene extraction from tomato and tomato products. *J Agric Food Chem* 52:5796–802.

Periago MJ, Rincón F, Jacob K, García-Alonso J, Ros G. 2007. Detection of key factors in the extraction and quantification of lycopene from tomato and tomato products. *J Agric Food Chem* 55:8825–9.

Phillips KM, Wolf WR, Patterson KY, Sharpless KE, Holden JM. 2007. Reference materials to evaluate measurement systems for the nutrient composition of foods: results from USDA's National Food and Nutrient Analysis Program (NFNAP). *Anal Bioanal Chem* 389:219–29.

Pinho FGR de, Lima Reis JM. 2012. Some developments regarding functional food products (functional foods). *Curr Nutr Food Sci* 8:102–11.

Pop RM, Weesepoel Y, Socaciu C, Pintea A, Vincken J-P, Gruppen H. 2014. Carotenoid composition of berries and leves from six Romanian sea buckthorn (*Hippophae rhamnoides* L.) varieties. *Food Chem* 147:1–9.

Pott I, Breithhaupt DE, Carle R. 2003. Detection of unusual carotenoid esters in fresh mango (*Mangifera indica* L. cv. 'Kent'). *Phytochem* 64:825–9.

Prasain JK, Moore R, Hurst JS, Barnes S, van Kuijk FJGM. 2005. Electrospray tandem mass spectrometric analysis of zeaxanthin and its oxidation products. *J Mass Spectrom* 40:916–23.

Quirós ARB de, Costa HS. 2006. Analysis of carotenoids in vegetable and plasma samples: a review. *J Food Comp Anal* 19:97–111.

Riso P, Porrini M. 1997. Determination of carotenoids in vegetable foods and plasma. *Int J Vitam Nutr Res* 67:47–54.

Rivera S, Canela R. 2012. Influence of sample processing on the analysis of carotenoids in maize. *Molecules* 17:11255–68.

Rivera, SM, Canela-Garayoa R. 2012. Analytical tools for the analysis of carotenoids in diverse materials. *J Chromatrogr A* 1224:1–10.

Rivera SM, Vilaró F, Zhu C, Bai C, Ferré G, Christou P, Canela-Garayoa, R. 2013. Fast quantitative method for the analysis of carotenoids in transgenic maize. J. *Agric Food Chem* 61:5279–85.

Rodriguez-Amaya DB. 1999. *A guide to carotenoid analysis in foods*. Washington DC: International Life Sciences Institute (ILSI) Press.

Rodriguez-Amaya DB. 2008. Reliability of carotenoid analysis. *Int Rev Food Sci Technol* 5:83–9.

Rodriguez-Amaya DB. 2010. Quantitative analysis, *in vitro* assessment of bioavailability and antioxidant activity of food carotenoids: A review. *J Food Compos Anal* 23:726–40.

Rodriguez-Amaya DB. 2015. Status of carotenoid analytical methods and *in vitro* assays for the assessment of food quality and health effects. *Curr Opin Food Sci* 1:56–63.

Rodriguez-Amaya DB, Kimura M. 2004. *HarvestPlus handbook for carotenoid analysis*. Washington DC: International Food Policy Research Institute.

Rodriguez-Amaya DB, Kimura M, Godoy HT, Amaya-Farfan J. 2008. Updated Brazilian database on food carotenoids: factors affecting carotenoid composition. *J Food Compos Anal* 21:445–63.

Rodriguez-Amaya DB, Kimura M, Godoy HT, Arima HK. 1988. Assessment of provitamin A determination by open column chromatography/visible absorption spectrophotometry. *J Chromatogr Sci* 26:624–9.

Rodriguez-Amaya DB, Kimura M, Kobori CN, Nestel P. 2012. International interlaboratory evaluation of laboratory's proficiency for carotenoid analysis in sweetpotato and cassava. Paper presented at the 16th World Congress of Food Science and Technology, Foz do Iguaçu, Brazil.

Rodriguez-Amaya DB, Rodriguez EB, Amaya-Farfan J. 2006. Advances in food carotenoid research: chemical and technological aspects, implications in human health. *Mal J Nutr* 12:101–21.

Rubio-Diaz DE, Francis DM, Rodriguez-Saona LE. 2011. External calibration models for the measurement of tomato carotenoids by infrared spectroscopy. *J Food Compos Anal* 24:121–6.

Sá MC de, Rodriguez-Amaya DB. 2004. Optimization of HPLC quantification of carotenoids in cooked green vegetables: Comparison of analytical and calculated data. *J Food Compos Anal* 17:37–51.

Sander LC, Sharpless KE, Craft NE, Wise SA. 1994. Development of engineered stationary phases for the separation of carotenoid isomers. *Anal Chem* 66:1667–74.

Sander LC, Sharpless KE, Pursch M. 2000. C_{30} stationary phases for the analysis of food by liquid chromatography. *J Chromatogr A* 880:189–202.

Schiedt K, Liaaen-Jensen S. 1995. Isolation and analysis. In: Britton G, Liaaen Jensen S, Pfander H. editors. *Carotenoids, vol. 1A: Isolation and analysis*. Basel: Birkhaüser Verlag, p 81–108.

Schoefs B. 2002. Chlorophyll and carotenoid analysis in food products. Properties of the pigments and methods of analysis. *Trends Food Sci Technol* 13:361–71.

Schüep W, Schierle J. 1997. Determination of β-carotene in commercial foods: interlaboratory study. *J AOAC Int* 80:1057–64.

Schulz H, Baranska M, Baranski R. 2005. Potential of NIR-FT-Raman spectroscopy in natural carotenoid analysis. *Biopolymers* 77:212–21.

Scott KJ. 1992. Observations on some problems associated with the analysis of carotenoids in foods by HPLC. *Food Chem* 45:357–64.

Scott KJ, Finglas PM, Seale R, Hart DJ, de Froidmont-Görtz I. 1996. Interlaboratory studies of HPLC procedures for the analysis of carotenoids in foods. *Food Chem* 57:85–90.

Sharpless KE, Arce-Osuna M, Thomas JB, Gill LM. 1999. Value assignment of retinol, retinyl palmitate, tocopherol, and carotenoid concentrations in standard reference material 2383 (baby food composite). *J AOAC Int* 82:288–96.

Sharpless KE, Margolis S, Thomas JB. 2000. Determination of vitamins in food matrix standard reference materials. *J Chromatogr A* 881:171–81.

Slavin M, Cheng Z, Luther M, Kenworthy W, Yu L. 2009. Antioxidant properties and phenolic, isoflavone, tocopherol and carotenoid composition of Maryland grown soybean lines with altered fatty acid profiles. *Food Chem* 114:20–7.

Su Q, Rowley KG, Balazs NDH. 2002. Carotenoids: separation methods applicable to biological samples. *J Chromatogr B* 781:393–418.

Sun H, Ge X, Lv Y, Wang A. 2012. Application of accelerated solvent extraction in the analysis of organic contaminants, bioactive and nutritional compounds in food and feed. *J Chromatogr A* 1237:1–23.

Sun T, Xu Z, Godber JS. 2006. Ultrasound assisted extraction in quantifying lutein from chicken liver using high-performance liquid chromatography. *J Chromatogr B* 830:158–60.

Taungbodhitham AK, Jones GP, Wahlqvist ML, Briggs DR. 1998. Evaluation of extraction method for the analysis of carotenoids in fruits and vegetables. *Food Chem* 63:577–84.

Tavares CA, Rodriguez-Amaya DB. 1994. Carotenoid composition of Brazilian tomatoes and tomato products. *Lebensm-Wissen Technol* 27:219–24.

Thompson M, Ellison SLR, Wood R. 2006. The International Harmonized Protocol for the Proficiency Testing of Analytical Chemistry Laboratories. *Pure Appl Chem* 78:145–96.

Tiziani S, Schwartz SJ, Vodovotz Y. 2006. Profiling of carotenoids in tomato juice by one- and two-dimensional NMR. *J Agric Food Chem* 54:6094–100.

Tonucci LH, Holden JM, Beecher GR, Khachik F, Davis CS, Mulokozi G.1995. Carotenoid content of thermally processed tomato-based food products. *J Agric Food Chem* 43:579–586.

van Breemen RB. 1995. Electrospray liquid chromatography-mass spectrometry of carotenoids. *Anal Chem* 67:2004–9.

van Breemen RB. 1997. Liquid chromatography/mass spectrometry of carotenoids. *Pure Appl Chem* 69:2061–6.

van Meulebroek L, Vanhaecke L, de Swaef T, Steppe K, de Brabander H. 2012. UHPLC-MS/MS to quantify liposoluble antioxidants in red-ripe tomatoes, grown under different salt stress levels. *J Agric Food Chem* 60:566–73.

Weller P, Breithaupt DE. 2003. Identification and quantification of zeaxanthin esters in plants using liquid chromatography-mass spectrometry. *J Agric Food Chem* 51:7044–9.

Xiao X, Song W, Wang J, Li G. 2012. Microwave-assisted extraction performed in low temperature and in vacuo for the extraction of labile compounds in food samples. *Anal Chim Acta* 712:85–93.

Yue X, Xu Z, Prinyawiwatkul W, King JM. 2006. Improving extraction of lutein from egg yolk using an ultrasound-assisted solvent method. *J Food Sci* 71:C239–41.

4 In vitro assays of bioaccessibility and antioxidant capacity

4.1 INTRODUCTION

Quantitative compositional analysis will continue to have a fundamental role in carotenoid research and applications, but biologically relevant in vitro assays are also needed to assess functional properties.

4.2 IN VITRO ASSESSMENT OF BIOACCESSIBILITY

With the great emphasis on the health effects of food components, it becomes evident that aside from the quantitative composition, information on bioavailability is needed. Bioavailability is defined as the fraction of an ingested nutrient or bioactive compound that becomes available to the body for utilization in physiological functions or for storage. It includes gastrointestinal digestion, absorption, metabolism, tissue distribution, and bioactivity. Bioaccessibility (i.e., matrix release and micellarization) refers to the amount of ingested compound that is released from the food matrix during the digestion process and becomes available for intestinal absorption.

It is widely recognized that carefully controlled studies with human subjects are ultimately required for accurate determination of the bioavailability and bioconversion of carotenoids. These studies are, however, laborious, expensive, time-consuming, and complex, limiting their use to a few food samples. Moreover, there are ethical issues (Biehler and Bohn, 2010) and it is well known that interindividual responses are highly variable. Some animal models are available, but no model appears ideal as their physiology differs considerably from humans (e.g., intestinal flora, conversion of provitamin A to retinol, distribution among lipoprotein fractions in blood plasma) and costs and ethical considerations also limit their use (Lee et al., 1999; Biehler and Bohn, 2010).

Evaluation of a large number of food samples is necessary in breeding experiments to select breeding lines for agricultural production; in research on the effects of the different home preparation and industrial processing technologies, including detailed

Food Carotenoids: Chemistry, Biology, and Technology, First Edition. Delia B. Rodriguez-Amaya.

appraisal of cooking/processing conditions; and in providing bioavailability information on carotenogenic foods that make up the existing or potential food supply.

4.2.1 Static gastrointestinal digestion assays

Simple, inexpensive, rapid, reproducible, and noninvasive in vitro methods have been developed and widely employed to evaluate bioaccessibility of carotenoids (Garrett et al., 1999a; Hedrén et al., 2002; C.-S. Liu et al., 2004; Granado-Lorencio et al., 2007; Colle et al., 2010; Cilla et al., 2012). These methods mimic the physiologic conditions and the sequence of events that occurs during gastrointestinal digestion in humans. The quantity of micellarized carotenoids is used as an estimate of carotenoid bioaccessibility, calculated as the amount of the compound in the final micellar fraction compared to its initial content in the food (expressed in percentage).

Although the method proponents have tried to simulate as much as possible the physiological conditions in the human gastrointestinal tract, the methods differ in several aspects, such as the preparation of the food samples, inclusion or not of an oral phase, choice and concentration of enzymes, pH, duration of the gastric and small intestine phases, and isolation of the micellar fraction (Rodriguez-Amaya, 2010; Carbonell-Capella et al., 2014). These differences can have significant variable influence on the results. Evaluating the impact of several digestion parameters on carotenoid bioaccessibility from pasta, for example, Werner and Böhm (2011) observed that the estimated bioaccessibility values were highly dependent on the amount of bile extract in the digestive medium and, to a lesser extent, on the simulated gastric pH and the incubation time with digestive enzymes. Method standardization and interlaboratory validation are therefore warranted and advocated. (Biehler and Bohn, 2010; Rodriguez-Amaya, 2010; van Buggenhout et al., 2010; Etcheverry et al., 2012).

Since in vitro assays often begin with a fine grinding of the food to be tested, Degrou et al. (2013) argued that the models used currently do not deal with the release of the carotenoids from the food matrix to the lipid phase, considering that plant foods are often ingested as large particles (Borel, 2003; Jalabert-Malbos et al., 2007).

Veda et al. (2006) examined the suitability of membrane filtration and dialysis to separate the micellar fraction. The values obtained for β-carotene bioaccessibility with membrane filtration were similar to those obtained by ultracentrifugation. Equilibrium dialysis was found unsuitable for this purpose.

The method of Garrett et al. (1999a) is the most widely used assay, with or without slight modifications. Aside from that of the starting material, the carotenoid concentrations of the digesta and the micelle fraction are determined by HPLC to appraise digestive stability and micellarization, respectively. The method has been used by Failla's group extensively to investigate the effects of chemical speciation, food matrix, food processing, and various other dietary factors. Modifications have been introduced to better reflect physiological conditions (Figure 4.1). Porcine pancreatic lipase was added in the small intestine phase for a test material containing corn oil to facilitate lipid digestion (Ferruzzi et al., 2006). For high starch cassava, an oral digestion phase with α-amylase was included (Thakkar et al., 2007). Moreover, the pH of gastric digestion was adjusted to 2.5 instead of 2.0 and that of small intestinal digestion was adjusted to 6.5 instead of 7.0. The micelle fraction was isolated from the digesta by centrifugation

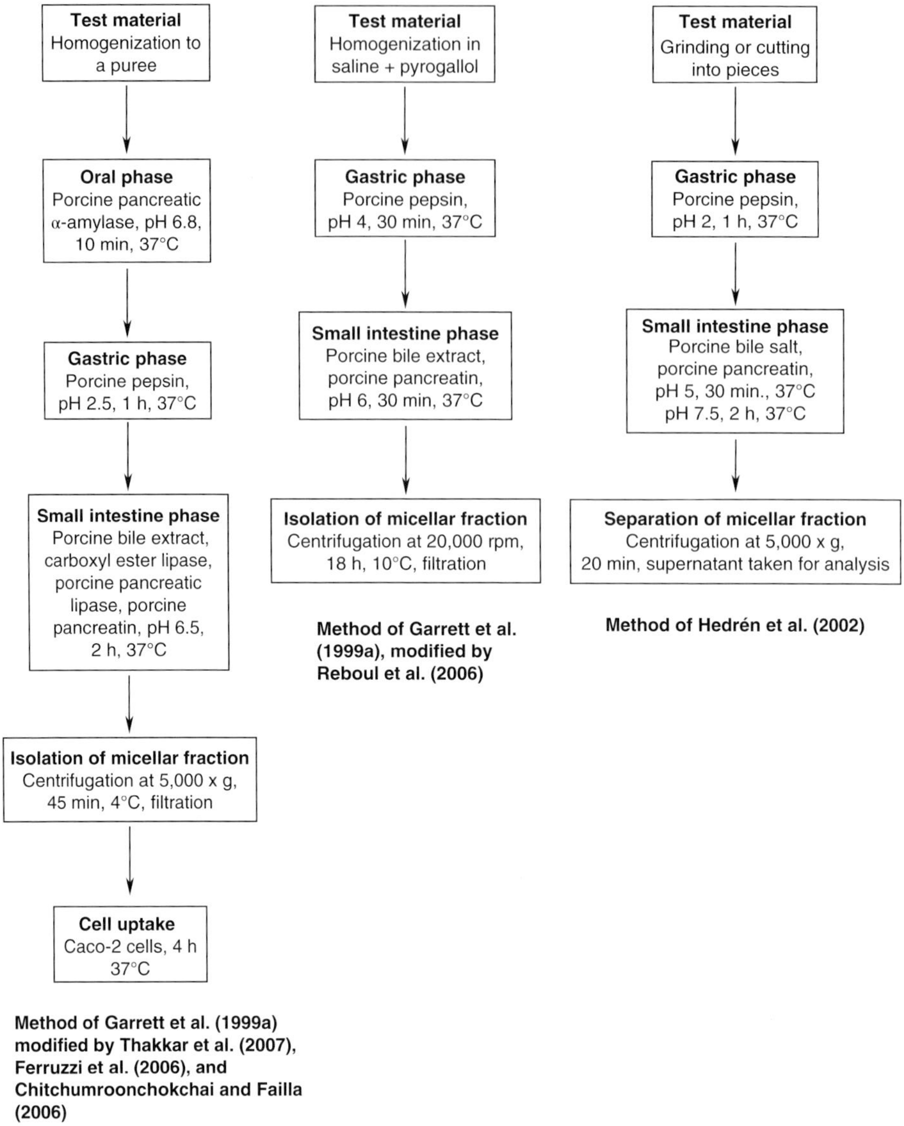

Figure 4.1 Widely used methods for the in vitro assessment of bioaccessibility.

at 5000 × g for 45 min instead of the previous high-speed centrifugation at 167,000 × g for 35 min. Carboxyl ester lipase was added in the intestinal phase (Chitchumroonchokchai and Failla, 2006), especially for fruits containing carotenol esters, because this enzyme was shown to catalyze the hydrolysis of diverse substrates, including the esters of the xanthophylls lutein, capsanthin, β-cryptoxanthin (Breithaupt et al., 2002), and zeaxanthin (Chitchumroonchokchai and Failla, 2006). Human pancreatic lipase accepted only retinyl palmitate as substrate; carotenoid mono- and diesters were not hydrolyzed (Breithaupt et al., 2002).

Taking into consideration data on lipid digestion and carotenoid processing in the human gastrointestinal tract obtained by Tyssandier et al. (2003), Reboul et al. (2006) made the following modifications of the method of Garrett et al. (1999a) (Figure 4.1): (a) BHT (butylated hydroxytoluene) was replaced by the water-soluble pyrogallol; (b) the pH of the gastric medium was adjusted to 4 instead of 2 because the mean pH measured in the human stomach after ingestion of vegetable-rich meals ranged between 5.8 just after meal intake to 3 at 3 h later; (c) the pH of the duodenal medium was set at 6 instead of 7.5 to match the pH measured in the human duodenum during digestion; (d) the duration of incubation in duodenal conditions was set at 30 min instead of 2 h to approximate the digestive transit time of a food particle in the human duodenum; and (e) bile salt concentrations in the duodenal conditions were increased because lycopene was barely soluble in the micellar phase at the original concentrations, and preliminary experiments showed that an increase in bile salt led to accurate detection of lycopene in the micellar fraction. The modified method was validated, determining α-carotene, β-carotene, lycopene, and lutein bioaccessibility from main dietary sources. The bioaccessibility as assessed with the in vitro method correlated well with human-derived bioaccessibility values ($r = 0.90$, $p < .05$), as well as with published relative mean bioavailability values in healthy human groups ($r = 0.98$, $p < .001$).

Another widely used assay for in vitro bioaccessibility (called in vitro accessibility) is that of Hedrén et al. (2002). This method employs a lower pH and longer incubation in the gastric phase compared to the other assays in Figure 4.1. The intestinal phase starts with a lower pH and ends with a higher pH than those of the other assays.

Recently, 29 researchers published an international consensus paper, proposing a general (not specific to carotenoids) standardized and practical static digestion method, based on physiologically relevant conditions that can be amended to accommodate further specific requirements (Minekus et al., 2014). They recommended pH 3 and 2 h incubation for the gastric phase, and pH 7 and 2 h incubation for the intestinal phase.

As discussed in detail in Chapter 9, findings of in vitro assessment of bioaccessibility are generally coherent with those of bioavailability studies in humans. For example, both in vitro assay (Schweiggert et al., 2012) and a randomized crossover study in humans (Schweiggert et al., 2014) showed β-carotene from papaya more bioaccessible/bioavailable than that of carrot and tomato. Moreover, the bioaccessibility/bioavailability of β-cryptoxanthin was superior to that of the carotenes. Xanthophylls have been shown to be more efficiently micellarized than carotenes in fruits and vegetables (Goñi et al., 2006), a blended fruit juice (Rodríguez-Roque et al., 2013), and dried chilli peppers (Pugliese et al., 2014), in agreement with results of human studies.

Also consistent with many human studies, bioaccessibility is enhanced by a small amount of oil, the increase varying with different types of oil (Colle et al., 2012; Moelants et al., 2012; Gleize et al., 2013).

Researchers in the area support the use of the bioaccessibility in vitro model to assess food-related factors affecting bioavailability of carotenoids from foods (Granado-Lorencio et al., 2009), particularly as a high throughput screening tool (Biehler and Bohn, 2010; van Buggenhout et al., 2010). Fernández-García et al. (2012) consider this assay an excellent analytical resource, allowing a detailed analysis of the influence of the food matrix composition on the digestive process.

In the method of Garrett et al. (1999a), digestion was coupled with uptake by Caco-2 cells to simulate absorption, confirming that the micellarized carotenoids were accessible for uptake by absorptive small intestine cells (Failla and Chitchumronchkchai, 2005). Although some characteristics of Caco-2 cells differ from those of epithelial cells lining the intestinal mucosa, they exhibit some similar morphological and functional characteristics (Sambruy et al., 2001). The Caco-2 cells were found to accumulate carotenoids from micelles generated during in vitro digestion (Garrett et al., 1999b). Under conditions mimicking the in vivo postprandial state, these cells took up carotenoids and secreted them incorporated into chylomicrons (During and Harrison, 2005). The Caco-2 cell uptake is therefore considered a relevant model to study the intestinal absorption of carotenoids (Liu et al., 2004; During and Harrison, 2005).

The in vitro bioaccessiblity assay coupled with Caco-2 cell uptake can be extended up to incorporation into chylomicrons and other lipoproteins, using the in vitro model of During and Harrison (2005), as suggested by During (2008).

4.2.2 Dynamic gastrointestinal models

Static models do not mimic the mechanical and physiological processes that occur in vivo, such as pH change and peristalsis. To provide a better simulation of the physical and chemical processes and closely mimic the transit time and the luminal environment within the human stomach, dynamic gastric models of digestion have been proposed (Blanquet-Diot et al., 2009; Déat et al., 2009; Kong and Singh, 2008, 2010). The dynamic, computer-controlled TNO gastrointestinal tract model (TIM), for example, closely simulates the in vitro dynamic physiological processes occurring within the lumen of the stomach and small intestine of humans (Blanquet-Diot et al., 2009). The main parameters of digestion (pH; body temperature; peristaltic mixing and transport; gastric, biliary, and pancreatic secretion; and passive absorption of small molecules and water) are reproduced. However, because of increased complexity (Biehler and Bohn, 2010) and requirement for equipment, they have had limited use.

4.3 IN VITRO ASSESSMENT OF ANTIOXIDANT ACTIVITY

The health effects of carotenoids and other bioactive compounds have been widely attributed to antioxidant activity; thus, numerous papers reporting the antioxidant activity/capacity of foods measured in vitro have been published. Many in vitro assays have been developed and applied to a diversity of foods. Review articles discuss these methods, including their shortcomings and advantages (Frankel and Meyer, 2000; Sínchez-Moreno, 2002; Arouma 2003; Becker et al., 2004; Huang et al., 2005; Prior et al., 2005; Roginsky and Lissi, 2005; MacDonald-Wicks et al., 2006; Singh and Singh, 2008; Moon and Shibamoto, 2009).

Based on the reactions involved, Huang et al. (2005) classified the antioxidant capacity assays into two types: those based on hydrogen atom transfer reactions and those based on electron transfer. Assays of the first group usually use a competitive reaction scheme, in which the antioxidant and substrate compete for peroxyl radicals that are generated through the decomposition of azo compounds. Examples are the oxygen radical absorbance capacity (ORAC) (Cao et al., 1993; Cao & Prior, 1999) and the total radical trapping antioxidant parameter (TRAP) (Wayner et al., 1985) methods. Assays of the second group measure the antioxidant's capacity in reducing an oxidant that changes color when reduced. The degree of color change is correlated with the sample's antioxidant concentrations. These assays include the total phenol by Folin-Ciocalteu reagent (Singleton et al., 1999), trolox equivalent antioxidant capacity (TEAC) (Miller et al., 1993; Re et al., 1999), ferric reducing antioxidant power (FRAP) (Benzie and Strain, 1996), and the 2,2-diphenyl-1-picrylhydrazyl (DPPH) (Brand-Williams et al., 1995) methods. The assays differ in substrate/probe, free radical source, underlying chemical reaction, and measurement technique. The results obtained are inconsistent, often conflicting, and difficult to compare. There have been increasing strong criticisms of these methods, especially of their lack of biological relevance.

The most widely employed in foods are the ORAC, FRAP, TEAC (or ABTS), and DPPH assays. The ORAC method is considered more physiologically relevant because it measures the peroxyl radical, which is the most abundant free radical in biological systems (Prior and Cao, 2000). It is based on the inhibition of the peroxyl radical-induced oxidation initiated by thermal decomposition of azo-compounds, such as 2,2′-azobis (2-amidino propane) dihydrochloride (AAPH). The antioxidant reacts with the peroxyl radicals and delays the degradation of fluorescin, a fluorescent probe. The FRAP assay measures the ability of antioxidants to reduce a ferric tripyridyltriazine complex. The main limitation of this method is that the measured reducing capacity does not necessarily reflect antioxidant activity (Frankel and Meyer, 2000). Operationally simple, the TEAC and DPPH assays are very popular. The TEAC method is based on the ability of antioxidants to scavenge the radical 2,2′-azonobis(3-ethylbenzothiazoline-6-sulphonate) ($ABTS^{\bullet+}$) while the DPPH assay is based on the scavenging of the chromogen radical $DPPH^{\bullet}$. The absorption spectra of the stable free radicals change when the molecule is reduced by an antioxidant. Both methods are criticized for using nonphysiological radicals, bearing no similarity to the highly reactive, transient radicals formed in lipid peroxidation.

Aside from the structural features of the carotenoid, the nature of the free radical and its environment affect the rate and mechanism of free radical scavenging (see Chapter 1). The nature of the radical species may have greater effect than the carotenoid structure (Mortensen et al., 1997; Martinez et al., 2009).

For a given assay, protocols are widely differing that discrepancies can be observed among the values obtained by different laboratories. For the simple and rapid DPPH method, for example, different DPPH concentrations, incubation time, reaction solvent, and pH of the reaction mixture are used (Sharma and Bhat, 2009).

Conflicting results can be observed in the literature even in the order or ranking of foods or phytochemicals according to their antioxidant activity obtained by different assays. For example, the antioxidant capacity of 18 Brazilian tropical fruits was determined by Rufino et al. (2010). Acerola ranked third with the ABTS and FRAP assays, but only 14th with DPPH. Cashew apple was second with the DPPH method but only 12th with the FRAP method and 13th with the ABTS assay. Analyzing a total of 927 freeze-dried vegetables, the ORAC and FRAP assays also gave different rankings in antioxidant activity (Ou et al., 2002).

Typically, a hydrophilic extract is obtained, the antioxidant activity is determined, and the result is correlated with the phenolic and vitamin C content. A lipophilic extract is also obtained, the antioxidant capacity determined, and result correlated with the carotenoid content. Since the assays are carried out with aqueous or organic solvent extracts of foods, aside from the use of nonphysiological substrate or radical/radical source, the chemical assays are criticized for not representing the physiological environment (Aruoma, 2003; Aliaga et al., 2009). They do not take into account bioavailability, uptake, and metabolism aspects, as well as location of the antioxidants within the cells (R.H. Liu and Finley, 2005).

As discussed in Chapter 1, the factors that may influence the antioxidant activity of carotenoids in biological systems are (a) the structure and physical form of the carotenoid molecule, (b) the location or site of action of the carotenoid molecule within the cell, (c) the potential for interaction with other carotenoids or antioxidants (especially vitamins C and E), (d) the concentration of the carotenoid, and (e) the partial pressure of oxygen (Britton, 1995; Young and Lowe, 2001).

An inherent limitation in these assays comes from the fact that antioxidants have different modes of action, including free radical and oxygen scavenging, singlet oxygen quenching, metal chelation, and inhibition of oxidative enzymes. Thus, Frankel and Meyer (2000) affirmed that the problem is using a rapid one-dimensional method to evaluate multifunctional food and biological antioxidants. They therefore suggested that several methods be used to include different mechanisms of inhibiting oxidation. Limiting the assay only to radical chain breaking might exclude important antioxidants in food and biology. The use of several methods has been supported by other authors (Arouma 2003; Singh and Singh 2008; Rodriguez-Amaya 2010; Carocho and Ferreira 2013).

Good to strong correlation between the total phenolic content and the antioxidant capacity has been consistently reported, and phenolic compounds are considered the major contributors to the antioxidant activity of foods. Since the assays measure the radical scavenging activity, the principal mode of action of these compounds, this finding is expected. In contrast, papers reporting the antioxidant activity of foods in relation to carotenoids are fewer and the results are inconsistent. Many papers did report that carotenoids contributed to or are correlated positively with the antioxidant capacity of foods (Arnao et al., 2001; Dewanto et al., 2002; Cano et al., 2003; Jaramillo-Flores et al., 2003; Sánchez-Moreno et al., 2003, 2004; George et al., 2004; Ishida and Chapman, 2004; Pinilla et al., 2005; Gliszczynska-Swiglo et al., 2006; Grassmann et al., 2007; Vaio et al., 2008; Díaz-Mula et al., 2009; Zanfini et al., 2010; Tlili et al., 2011; Divya et al., 2012; Singh et al., 2012; Legua et al., 2013; Li et al., 2012, 2013; Pereira et al., 2013; Korekar et al., 2014; Zlotek et al., 2014). However, others found no or poor correlation between the carotenoid content and the antioxidant capacity (Ancos et al., 2002; Choi et al., 2007; Teow et al., 2007; Lavelli et al., 2009; Hung and Hatcher, 2011) or the antioxidant contribution of carotenoids was negligible (Gardner et al., 2000) or lower than those of phenolic compounds (Gil et al., 2002) and/or vitamin C (Podsedek et al., 2003; Sánchez-Moreno et al., 2006; Valle et al., 2007). Thaipong et al. (2006) found negative correlation between antioxidant activity determined by the ABTS, DPPH, and FRAP of a methanol extract and total carotenoids extracted by ethanol-hexane in pink-fleshed guava.

Noting the discrepancy in the results of their own work, in which the carotenoid content correlated well with the antioxidant activity (measured in a chloroform extract prepared for HPLC analysis), and those of Gil et al. (2002), in which correlation was found with polyphenols but not with carotenoids, Vaio et al. (2008) raised the possibility that this discrepancy could be due to correlating the carotenoid levels with the hydrophilic antioxidant activity. Indeed, the low or lack of correlation between the antioxidant capacity values obtained and the carotenoid content of the food sample may be due at least in part to incomplete extraction of the carotenoids in the lipophilic extract submitted to the antioxidant assay. In some papers the extract submitted to the quantification of the carotenoids is different from that submitted to the antioxidant assay, using solvents that are known to be efficient for carotenoid extraction for the former analysis and solvents of doubtful efficiency to extract the carotenoids completely for the latter.

On the other hand, the assay assumes that the hydrophilic extract is composed only of vitamin C and phenolics and the lypophilic extract only of carotenoids. Moreover, it does not provide data for individual compounds when it is known that members of a class of bioactives differ in their antioxidant efficacy.

Corral-Aguayo et al. (2008) analyzed eight agricultural crops (guava, avocado, black sapote, mango, papaya, prickly pear fruit, cladodes, and strawberry) using six different assays: DPPH, N,N-dimethyl-*p*-phenylendiamine (DMPD), FRAP, ORAC, TEAC, and total oxidant scavenging capacity (TOSC). β-carotene content had high correlation with total antioxidant capacity only in the DMPD assay.

Considering the mode of action, it is evident that the antioxidant activity of carotenoids is grossly underestimated by current assays. Carotenoids are known to be excellent quenchers of singlet oxygen and can, in fact, prevent its formation by quenching excited sensitizers (Krinsky, 1989; Beutner et al., 2001). They are not so efficient as free radical scavengers, but they have the ability to interact with and quench various radical species that can be generated within the cells, aside from the peroxyl radical (Edge et al., 1997). In the Chinese herb *Lycium barbarum* L., for example, Wang et al. (2010) found that the flavonoid fraction was the most effective in scavenging the DPPH and ABTS free radicals, but the zeaxanthin fraction showed the most pronounced effect in scavenging hydroxyl radicals. Thus, to account for carotenoids' antioxidant activity, the development, validation, and standardization of a biologically relevant set of methods for the in vitro assessment of the antioxidant capacity of foods, supplements, and the carotenoids themselves have yet to be done. The assays should include quenching of singlet oxygen, aside from scavenging of peroxyl radicals and other biologically important radicals.

The antioxidant effect in the food itself can be more easily shown. The relevance of simple in vitro assays as indicator of in vitro antioxidant activity is much more difficult to demonstrate. Becker et al. (2004) concluded that the screening of antioxidant capacity using simple assays to predict positive health effects of foods was not scientifically justified. They suggested that different protocols be used for the evaluation of food quality and of health effects of antioxidants. Likewise, Huang et al. (2005) contended that the current assays are strictly based on chemical reactions in vitro and bear no similarity to biological systems. Since the human body is equipped with powerful antioxidant defense systems that are enzymatic and dietary phytochemicals undergo uptake and metabolism, Sies (2007) contends that extrapolation of what is called total antioxidant capacity to health effects is not appropriate and should be discouraged.

The USDA developed an extensive database for total antioxidant capacity in foods, using the ORAC method (Wu et al., 2004a, b). The hydrophilic extract was obtained with acetone:water:acetic acid, 70:29.5:0.5, and the lipophilic extract with hexane: dichloromethane, 1:1. Total antioxidant capacity was calculated as the sum of the hydrophilic and lipophilic ORAC values. This USDA ORAC database has now been removed from the USDA website "due to mounting evidence that the values indicating antioxidant capacity have no relevance to the effects of specific bioactive compounds, including polyphenols on human health." This is a serious move, considering that the ORAC method has been considered the most biologically relevant of the existing chemical assays.

In a recent comprehensive review, Prior (in press) justified the use of the ORAC method, especially in terms of polyphenols. An important development is what is termed oxygen radical absorbance capacity using multiple radicals ($ORAC_{MR}$), which is the sum of the antioxidant capacity against six of the most predominant reactive species found in the human body: peroxyl radical, hydroxyl radical, superoxide anion, singlet oxygen, peroxynitrite, and hypochlorite.

Standardization of existing assays, as advocated by many researchers (Frankel and Meyer 2000; Arouma 2003; Prior et al., 2005; Frankel and Finley, 2008) will resolve problems with method performance, especially measurement accuracy and comparability of analytical results. The development of assays relevant to human health is much more difficult and needs the concerted effort of researchers in the field.

References

Aliaga C, Rezende MC, Arenas A. 2009. How meaningful is the assessment of antioxidant activities in microheterogeneous media? *Food Chem* 113:1083–7.

Ancos B de, Sgroppo S, Plaza L, Cano MP. 2002. Possible nutritional and health-related value promotion in orange juice preserved by high-pressure treatment. *J Sci Food Agric* 82:790–6.

Arnao MB, Cano A, Acosta M. 2001. The hydrophilic and lipophilic contribution to total antioxidant activity. *Food Chem* 73:239–44.

Arouma OI. 2003. Methodological considerations for characterizing potential antioxidant actions of bioactive components in plant foods. *Mutation Res* 523/524:9–20.

Becker EM, Nissen LR, Skibsted LH. 2004. Antioxidant evaluation protocols: food quality or health effects. *Eur Food Res Technol* 219:561–71.

Benzie IFF, Strain JJ. 1996. The ferric reducing ability of plasma (FRAP) as a measure of "antioxidant power": the FRAP assay. *Anal Biochem* 239:70–6.

Beutner S, Bloedorn B, Frixel S, Blanco IH, Hoffmann T, Martin H-D, Mayer B, Noack P, Ruck C, Schmidt M, Schülke I, Sell S, Ernst H, Haremza S, Seybold G, Sies H, Stahl W, Walsh R. 2001. Quantitative assessment of antioxidant properties of natural colorants and phytochemicals: carotenoids, flavonoids, phenols and indigoids. The role of β-carotene in antioxidant functions. *J Sci Food Agric* 81:559–68.

Biehler E, Bohn T. 2010. Methods for assessing aspects of carotenoid bioavailability. *Curr Nutr Food Sci* 6:44–69.

Blanquet-Diot S, Soufi M, Rambeau M, Rock E, Alric M. 2009. Digestive stability of xanthophylls exceeds that of carotenes as studied in a dynamic gastrointestinal system. *J Nutr* 139:876–83.

Borel P. 2003. Factors affecting intestinal absorption of highly lipophilic food microconstituents (fat-soluble vitamins, carotenoids and phytosterols). *Clin Chem Lab Med* 41:979–94.

Brand-Williams W, Cuvelier ME, Berset C. 1995. Use of a free radical method to evaluate antioxidant activity. *Lebens Wissen Tecnol* 28:25–30.

Breithaupt DE, Bamedi A, Wirt U. 2002. Carotenol fatty acid esters: easy substrates for digestive enzymes? *Comp Biochem Physiol B* 132:721–8.

Britton G. 1995. Structure and properties of carotenoids in relation to functions. *FASEB J* 9:1551–8.

Cano A, Acosta M, Arnao MB. 2003. Hydrophilic and lipophilic antioxidant activity changes during on-vine ripening of tomatoes (*Lycopersicum esculentum* Mill.). *Postharvest Biol Technol* 28:59–65.

Cao G, Alessio HM, Cutler RG. 1993. Oxygen-radical absorbance capacity assay for antioxidant. *Free Radic Biol Med* 14:303–11.

Cao G, Prior RL. 1999. Measurement of oxygen radical absorbance capacity in biological samples. *Meth Enzymol* 299:50–62.

Carbonell-Capella JM, Buniowska M, Barba FJ, Esteve MJ, Frigola A. 2014. Analytical methods for determining bioavailability and bioaccessibility of bioactive compounds from fruits and vegetables: a review. *Comp Rev Food Sci Food Safety* 13:155–71.

Carocho M, Ferreira ICFR. 2013. A review on antioxidants, prooxidants and related controversy: Natural and synthetic compounds, screening and analysis methodologies and future perspectives. *Food Chem Toxicol* 51:15–25.

Chitchumroonchokchai C, Failla ML. 2006. Hydrolysis of zeaxanthin esters by carboxyl ester lipase during digestion facilitates micellarization and uptake of the xanthophyll by caco-2 human intestinal cells. *J Nutr* 136:588–94.

Choi Y, Jeong H-S, Lee J. 2007. Antioxidant activity of methanolic extracts from some grains consumed in Korea. *Food Chem* 103:130–8.

Cilla A, Alegría A, Ancos B de, Sanchez-Moreno C, Cano MP, Plaza L, Clemente G, Lagarda MJ, Barberá R. 2012. Bioaccessibility of tocopherols, carotenoids and ascorbic acid from milk- and soy-based fruit beverages: influence of food matrix and processing. *J Agric Food Chem* 60: 7282–90.

Colle IJP, van Buggenhout S, Lemmens L, van Loey AM, Hendrickx ME. 2012. The type and quantity of lipids present during digestion influence the in vitro bioaccessibility of lycopene from raw tomato pulp. *Food Res Int* 45:250–5.

Colle IJP, van Buggenhout S, van Loey AM, Hendrickx ME. 2010. High-pressure homogenization followed by thermal processing of tomato pulp: Influence on microstructure and lycopene in vitro bioaccessibility. *Food Res Int* 45:250–5.

Corral-Aguayo RD, Yahia EM, Carrillo-Lopez A, González-Aguilar G. 2008. Correlation between some nutritional components and total antioxidant capacity measured with six different assays in eight horticultural crops. *J Agric Food Chem* 56:10498–504.

Déat E, Blanquet-Diot S, Jarrige J-F, Denis S, Beyssac E, Alric M. 2009. Combining the dynamic TNO-gastrointestinal tract system with a Caco-2 cell culture model: application to the assessment of lycopene and α-tocopherol bioavailability from a whole food. *J Agric Food Chem* 57:11314–20.

Degrou A, Georgé S, Renard CMGC, Page D. 2013. Physicochemical parameters that influence carotenoids bioaccessibility from a tomato juice. *Food Chem* 136:435–41.

Dewanto V, Wu X, Adom KK, Liu RH. 2002. Thermal processing enhances the nutritional value of tomatoes by increasing total antioxidant activity. *J Agric Food Chem* 50:3010–4.

Díaz-Mula HM, Zapata PJ, Guillén F, Martínez-Romero D, Castillo S, Serrano M, Valero D. 2009. Changes in hydrophilic and lipophilic antioxidant activity and related bioactive compounds during postharvest storage of yellow and purple plum cultivars. *Postharvest Biol Technol* 51:354–63.

Divya P, Puthusseri B, Neelwarne B. 2012. Carotenoid content, its stability during drying and the antioxidant activity of commercial coriander (*Coriandrum sativum* L.) varieties. *Food Res Int*. 45:342–350.

During A. 2008. Bioavailability of natural pigments. In: Socaciu C. editor. *Food colorants: chemical and functional properties*. Boca Raton: Taylor and Francis Goup. p 147–175.

During A, Harrison EH. 2005. An in vitro model to study the intestinal absorption of carotenoids. *Food Res Int* 38:1001–8.

Edge R, McGarvey DJ, Truscott TG. 1997. The carotenoids as anti-oxidants: a review. *J Photochem Photobiol B: Biol* 41:189–200.

Etcheverry P, Gruzak MA, Fleiger LE. 2012. Application of in vitro bioaccessibility and bioavailability methods for calcium, carotenoids, folate, iron, magnesium, polyphenols, zinc, and vitamins B_6, B_{12}, D, and E. Front Physiol 06 August 2012 doi: 10.3389/fphys.2012.00317.

Failla ML, Chitchumronchokchai C. 2005. In vitro models as tools for screening the relative bioavailabilities of provitamin A carotenoids in foods. *HarvestPlus Technical Monograph Series 3*. Washington DC: International Food Policy Research Institute.

Fernández-García E, Carvajal-Lérida I, Jarén-Galán M, Garrido-Fernández J, Pérez-Gálvez A, Hornero-Méndez D. 2012. Carotenoid bioavailability from foods: from plant pigments to efficient biological activities. *Food Res Int* 46:438–50.

Ferruzzi MG, Lumpkin JL, Schwartz SJ, Failla M. 2006. Digestive stability, micellarization, and uptake of β-carotene isomers by Caco-2 human intestinal cells. *J Agric Food Chem* 54:2780–5.

Frankel EN, Finley JW. 2008. How to standardize the multiplicity of methods to evaluate natural antioxidants. *J Agric Food Chem* 56:4901–8.

Frankel EN, Meyer AS. 2000. The problems of using one-dimensional methods to evaluate multifunctional food and biological antioxidants. *J Sci Food Agric* 80:1925–41.

Gardner PT, White TAC, McPhail DB, Duthie GG. 2000. The relative contributions of vitamin C, carotenoids and phenolics to the antioxidant potential of fruit juices. *Food Chem* 68:471–4.

Garrett DA, Failla ML, Sarama RJ. 1999a. Development of an in vitro digestion method to assess carotenoid bioavailability from meals. *J Agric Food Chem* 47:4301–9.

Garrett DA, Failla ML, Sarama RJ, Craft N. 1999b. Accumulation and retention of micellar β-carotene and lutein by Caco-2 human intestinal cells. *J Nutr Biochem* 10:573–81.

George B, Kaur C, Khurdiya DS, Kapoor HC. 2004. Antioxidants in tomato (*Lycopersicum esculentum*) as a function of genotype. *Food Chem* 84:45–51.

Gil MI, Tomás-Barberán FA, Hess-Pierce B, Kader AA. 2002. Antioxidant capacities, phenolic compounds, carotenoids, and vitamin C contents of nectarine, peach, and plum cultivars from California. *J Agric Food Chem* 50:4976–82.

Gleize B, Tourniaire F, Depezay L, Bott R, Nowicki M, Albino L, Lairon D, Kesse-Guyot E, Galan P, Hercberg S, Borel P. 2013. Effect of type of TAG fatty acids on lutein and zeaxanthin bioavailability. *Brit J Nutr* 110:1–10.

Gliszczynska-Swiglo A, Ciska E, Pawlak-Lemanska K, Chmielewski J, Borkowski T, Tyrakowska B. 2006. Changes in the content of health-promoting compounds and antioxidant activity of broccoli after domestic processing. *Food Addit Contam* 23, 1088–98.

Goñi I, Serrano J, Saura-Calixto F. 2006. Bioaccessibility of β-carotene, lutein, and lycopene from fruits and vegetables. *J Agric Food Chem* 54:5382–7.

Granado-Lorencio F, Herrero-Barbudo C, Blanco-Navarro I, Pérez-Sacristán B, Olmedilla-Alonso B. 2009. Bioavailability of carotenoids and α-tocopherol from fruit juices in the presence of absorption modifiers: *in vitro* and *in vivo* assessment. *Brit J Nutr* 101:576–582.

Granado-Lorencio F, Olmedilla-Alonso B, Herrero-Barbudo C, Blanco-Navarro I, Pérez-Sacristán B, Blázquez-García S. 2007. In vitro bioaccessibility of carotenoids and tocopherols from fruits and vegetables. *Food Chem* 102:641–8.

Grassmann J, Schnitzler WH, Habegger R. 2007. Evaluation of different coloured carrot cultivars on antioxidative capacity based on their carotenoid and phenolic contents. *Int J Food Sci Nutr* 58:603–11.

Hedrén E, Diaz V, Svanberg U. 2002. Estimation of carotenoid accessibility from carrots determined by an in vitro digestion method. *Eur J Clin Nutr* 56:425–30.

Huang D, Ou B, Prior RL. 2005. The chemistry behind antioxidant capacity assays. *J Agric Food Chem* 53:1841–56.

Hung PV, Hatcher DW. 2011. Ultra-performance liquid chromatography (UPLC) quantification of carotenoids in durum wheat: influence of genotype and environment in relation to the colour of yellow alkaline noodles (YAN). *Food Chem* 125:1510–6.

Ishida BK, Chapman MH. 2004. A comparison of carotenoid content and total antioxidant activity in catsup from several commercial sources in the United States. *J Agric Food Chem* 52:8017–20.

Jalabert-Malbos M-L, Mishellany-Dutour A, Woda A, Peyron M-A. 2007. Particle size distribution in the food bolus after mastication of natural foods. *Food Qual Prefer* 18:803–12.

Jaramillo-Flores ME, González-Cruz L, Cornejo-Mazón M, Dorantes-Álvarez L, Gutiérrez-López GF, Hernández-Sánchez H. 2003. Effect of thermal treatment on the antioxidant activity and content of carotenoids and phenolic compounds of cactus pear cladodes (*Opuntia ficus-indica*). *Food Sci Tech Int* 9:271–8.

Kong F, Singh RP. 2008. A model stomach system to investigate disintegration kinetics of solid foods during gastric digestion. *J Food Sci* 73:E202–10.

Kong FB, Singh RP. 2010. A human gastric simulator (HGS) to study food digestion in human stomach. *J Food Sci* 75:E627–35.

Korekar G, Dolkar P, Singh H, Srivasta RB, Stobdan T. 2014. Variability and the genetic effect on antioxidant activity, total phenolics, carotenoids and ascorbic acid content in seventeen natural populations of Seabuckthorn (*Hippophae rhamnosides* L.) from trans-Himalaya. *LWT: Food Sci Technol* 55.157–162.

Krinsky NI. 1989. Antioxidant functions of carotenoids. *Free Radic Biol Med* 7:617–35.

Lavelli V, Hidalgo A, Pompei C, Brandolini A. 2009. Radical scavenging activity of einkorn (*Triticum monococcum* L. subsp. monococcum) whole meal flour and its relationship to soluble phenolic and lipophilic antioxidant content. *J Cereal Sci* 49:319–21.

Lee CM, Boileau AC, Boileau TWM, Williams AW, Swanson KS, Heintz KA, Erdman JW Jr. 1999. Review of animal models in carotenoid research. *J Nutr* 129:2271–7.

Legua P, Serrano M, Melgarejo P, Valero D, Martínez JJ, Martínez R, Hernández F. 2013. Quality parameters, biocompounds and antioxidant activity in fruits of nine quince (*Cydonia oblonga* Miller) accessions. *Sci Hort* 154:61–5.

Li H, Deng Z, Liu R, Loewen S, Tsao R. 2012. Ultra-performance liquid chromatographic separation of geometric isomers of carotenoids and antioxidant activities of 20 tomato cultivars and breeding lines. *Food Chem* 132:508–17.

Li H, Deng Z, Liu R, Loewen S, Tsao R. 2013. Carotenoid compositions of coloured tomato cultivars and contribution to antioxidant activities and protection against H_2O_2-induced cell death in H9c2. *Food Chem* 136:878–88.

Liu C-S, Glahn RP, Liu RH. 2004. Assessment of carotenoid bioavailability of whole foods using a Caco-2 cell culture model coupled with an in vitro digestion. *J Agric Food Chem* 52:4330–7.

Liu RH, Finley J. 2005. Potential cell culture models for antioxidant research. *J Agric Food Chem* 53:4311–4.

MacDonald-Wicks LK, Wood LG, Garg ML. 2006. Methodology for the determination of biological antioxidant capacity in vitro: a review. *J Sci Food Agric* 86:2046–56.

Martinez A, Vergas R, Galano A. 2009. What is important to prevent oxidative stress? A theoretical study on electron-transfer reactions between carotenoids and free radicals. *J Phys Chem B* 113:12113–20.

Miller NJ, Rice-Evans CA, Davies MJ, Gopinathan V, Milner A. 1993. A novel method for measuring antioxidant capacity and its application to monitoring the antioxidant status in premature neonates. *Clin Sci* 84:407–12.

Minekus M, Alminger M, Alvito P, Ballance S, Bohn T, Bourlieu C, Carrière F, Boutrou R, Corredig M, Dupont D, Dufour C, Egger L, Golding M, Karakaya S, Kirkhus B, Le Feunteun S, Lesmes U, Macierzanka A, Mackie A, Marze S, McClements DJ, Ménard O, Recio I, Santos CN, Singh RP, Vegarud GE, Wickham MSJ, Weitschies W, Brodkorb A. 2014. A standardized static in vitro digestion method suitable for food: an international consensus. *Food Funct* 5:1113–24.

Moelants KRN, Lemmens L, Vandebroeck M, van Buggenhout S, van Loey AM, Hendrickx ME. 2012. Relation between particle size and carotenoid bioaccessibility in carrot- and tomato-derived suspensions. *J Agric Food Chem* 60:11995–2003.

Moon J-K, Shibamoto T. 2009. Antioxidant assays for plant and food components. *J Agric Food Chem* 57:1655–66.

Mortensen A, Skibsted LH, Sampson J, Rice-Evans C, Everett SA. 1997. Comparative mechanisms and rates of free radical scavenging by carotenoid antioxidants. *FEBS Lett* 418:91–7.

Ou B, Huang D, Hampsch-Woodill M, Flanagan JA, Deemer EK. 2002. Analysis of antioxidant activities of common vegetables employing oxygen radical absorbance capacity (ORAC) and ferric reducing antioxidant power (FRAP) assays: a comparative study. *J Agric Food Chem* 50:3122–8.

Pereira MC, Steffens RS, Jablonski A, Hertz PF, Rios AO, Vizzoto M, Flôres SH. 2013. Characterization, bioactive compounds and antioxidant potential of three Brazilian fruits. *J Food Compos Anal* 29:19–24.

Pinilla MJ, Plaza L, Sánchez-Moreno C, de Ancos B, Cano MP. 2005. Hydrophilic and lipophilic antioxidant capacities of commercial Mediterranean vegetable soups (gazpachos). *J Food Sci* 70:S60–5.

Prior RL. in press. Oxygen radical absorbance capacity (ORAC): new horizons in relating dietary antioxidants/bioactives and health benefits. J Funct Foods.

Prior RL, Cao G. 2000. Analysis of botanicals and dietary supplements for antioxidant capacity: a review. *J AOAC Int* 83:950–6.

Prior RL, Wu X, Schaich K. 2005. Standardized methods for the determination of antioxidant capacity and phenolics in foods and dietary supplements. *J Agric Food Chem* 53:4290–302.

Podsedek A, Sosnowska D, Anders B. 2003. Antioxidative capacity of tomato products. *Eur Food Res Technol* 217:296–300.

Pugliese A, O'Callaghan Y, Tundis R, Galvin K, Menichini F, O'Brien N, Loizzo MR. 2014. In vitro assessment of the bioaccessibility of carotenoids from sun-dried chilli peppers. *Plant Food Hum Nutr* 69:8–17.

Re R, Pellegrini N, Proteggente A, Pannala A, Yang M, Rice-Evans C. 1999. Antioxidant activity applying an improved ABTS radical cation decolorization assay. *Free Radic Biol Med* 26:1231–7.

Reboul E, Richelle M, Perrot E, Desmoulins-Malezet C, Pirisi V, Borel P. 2006. Bioaccessibility of carotenoids and vitamin E from their main dietary sources. *J Agric Food Chem* 54:8749–55.

Rodriguez-Amaya DB. 2010. Quantitative analysis, in vitro assessment of bioavailability and antioxidant activity of food carotenoids: a review. *J Food Compos Anal* 23:726–40.

Rodríguez-Roque MJ, Rojas-Graü MA, Elez-Martínez P, Martín-Belloso O. 2013. Changes in vitamin C, phenolic, and carotenoid profiles throughout in vitro gastrointestinal digestion of blended fruit juice. *J Agric Food Chem* 61:1859–67.

Roginsky V, Lissi EA. 2005. Review of methods to determine chain-breaking antioxidant activity in food. *Food Chem* 92:235–54.

Rufino MSM, Alves RE, Brito ES de, Pérez-Jiménez J, Saura-Calixto F, Mancini-Filho J. 2010. Bioactive compounds and antioxidant capacities of 18 non-traditional tropical fruits from Brazil. *Food Chem* 121:996–1002.

Sambruy Y, Ferruzza S, Ranaldi G, De Angelis I. 2001. Intestinal cell culture models. *Cell Biol Toxicol* 17:301–17.

Sánchez-Moreno C. 2002. Review: methods used to evaluate the free radical scavenging activity in foods and biological systems. *Food Sci Technol Int* 8:121–37.

Sánchez-Moreno C, Plaza L, Ancos B de, Cano MP. 2003. Quantitative bioactive compounds assessment and their relative contribution to the antioxidant capacity of commercial orange juices. *J Sci Food Agric* 83:430–9.

Sánchez-Moreno C, Plaza L, Ancos B de, Cano MP. 2004. Effect of combined treatments of high-pressure and natural additives on carotenoid extractability and antioxidant activity of tomato puree (*Lycopersicum esculentum* Mill.) *Eur Food Res Technol* 219:151–60.

Sánchez-Moreno C, Plaza L, Ancos B de, Cano MP. 2006. Nutritional characterization of commercial traditional pasteurized tomato juices: carotenoids, vitamin A and radical-scavenging capacity. *Food Chem* 98:749–56.

Schweiggert RM, Kopec RE, Villalobos-Gutierrez MG, Högel J, Quesada S, Esquivel P, Schwartz SJ, Carle R. 2014. Carotenoids are more bioavailable from papaya than from tomato and carrot in humans: a randomised cross-over study. *Brit J Nutr* 111:490–8.

Schweiggert RM, Mezger D, Schimpf F, Steingass CB, Carle R. 2012. Influence of chromoplast morphology on carotenoid bioaccessibility of carrot, mango, papaya, and tomato. *Food Chem* 135:2736–42.

Sharma OP, Bhat TK. 2009. DPPH antioxidant assay revisited. *Food Chem* 113:1202–5.

Sies H. 2007. Total antioxidant capacity: appraisal of a concept. *J Nutr* 137:1493–5.

Singh S, Singh RP. 2008. In vitro methods of assay of antioxidants: an overview. *Food Rev Int.* 24:392–415.

Singh DR, Singh S, Salim KM, Srivastava RC. 2012. Estimation of phytochemicals and antioxidant activity of underutilized fruits of Andaman Islands (India). *Int J Food Sci Nutr* 63:446–52.

Singleton VL, Orthofer R, Lamuela-Raventos RM. 1999. Analysis of total phenols and other oxidation substrates and antioxidants by means of the Folin-Ciocalteu reagent. *Meth Enzymol* 299:152–78.

Teow CC, Truong V-D, McFeeters RF, Thompson RL, Pecota KV, Yencho GC. 2007. Antioxidant activities, phenolic and β-carotene contents of sweet potato genotypes and varying flesh colours. *Food Chem* 103:829–38.

Thaipong K, Boonprakob U, Crosby K. 2006. Comparison of ABTS, DPPH, FRAP, and ORAC assay for estimating antioxidant activity from guava fruit extracts. *J Food Compos Anal* 19:669–75.

Thakkar SK, Maziya-Dixon B, Dixon AGO, Failla ML. 2007. β-carotene micellarization during in vitro digestion and uptake by Caco-2 cells is directly proportional to β-carotene content in different genotypes of cassava. *J Nutr* 137:2229–33.

Tlili I, Hdider C, Lenucci MS, Ilahy R, Jebari H, Dalessando G. 2011. Bioactive compounds and antioxidant activities during fruit ripening of watermelon cultivars. *J Food Comp Anal* 24:923–8.

Tyssandier V, Reboul E, Dumas J-F, Bouteloup-Demange C, Armand M, Marcand J, Sallas M, Borel P. 2003. Processing of vegetable-borne carotenoids in the human stomach and duodenum. *Am J Physiol: Gastrointest Liver Physiol* 284:G913–23.

Vaio C, Graziani G, Marra L, Cascone A, Ritieni A. 2008. Antioxidant capacities, carotenoids and polyphenols evaluation of fresh and refrigerated peach and nectarine cultivars from Italy. *Eur Food Res Technol* 227:1225–31.

Valle AZD, Mignani I, Spinardi A, Galvano F, Ciappellano S. 2007. The antioxidant profile of three different peach cultivars (*Prunus persica*) and their short-term effect on antioxidant status in human. *Eur Food Res Technol* 225:167–72.

van Buggenhout S, Alminger M, Lemmens L, Colle I, Knockaert G, Moelants K, van Loey A, Hendrickx M. 2010. In vitro approaches to estimate the effect of food processing on carotenoid bioavailability need thorough understanding of process induced microstructural changes. *Trends Food Sci Technol* 21:607–18.

Veda S, Kamath A, Platel K, Begum K, Srinivasan K. 2006. Determination of bioaccessibility of β-carotene in vegetables by in vitro methods. *Mol Nutr Food Res* 50:1047–52.

Wang CC, Chang SC, Inbaraj BS, Chen BH. 2010. Isolation of carotenoids, flavonoids and polysaccharides from *Lycium barbarum* L. and evaluation of antioxidant activity. *Food Chem* 120:184–92.

Wayner DDM, Burton GW, Ingold KU, Locke S. 1985. Quantitative measurement of the total, peroxyl radical-trapping antioxidant capability of human blood plasma by controlled peroxidation. *FEBS Lett* 187:33–7.

Werner S, Böhm V. 2011. Bioaccessibility of carotenoids and vitamin E from pasta: evaluation of an in vitro digestion model. *J Agric Food Chem* 59:1163–70.

Wu X, Beecher GR, Holden JM, Haytowitz DB, Gebhardt SE, Prior RL. 2004a. Lipophilic and hydrophilic antioxidant capacities of common foods in the United States. *J Agric Food Chem* 52:4026–37.

Wu X, Gu L, Holden J, Haytowitz DB, Gebhardt SE, Beecher G, Prior RL. 2004b. Development of a database for total antioxidant capacity in foods: a preliminary study. *J Food Compos Anal* 17:407–22.

Young AJ, Lowe GM. 2001. Antioxidant and prooxidant properties of carotenoids. *Arch Biochem Biophys* 385:20–7.

Zanfini A, Corbini G, La Rosa C, Dreassi E. 2010. Antioxidant activity of tomato lipophilic extracts and interactions between carotenoids and α-tocopherol in synthetic mixtures. *LWT-Food Sci Technol* 43:67–72.

Zlotek U, Swieca M, Jabubczyk A. 2014. Effect of abiotic elicitation on main health-promoting compounds, antioxidant activity and commercial quality of butter lettuce (*Lactuca sativa* L.). *Food Chem* 148:253–60.

5 Composition and influencing factors

5.1 INTRODUCTION

In the preface of the 1981 book edited by Bauernfeind on carotenoids as colorants and vitamin A precursors, Chichester wrote, "The volume illustrates the imperfect state of knowledge on the qualitative and quantitative distribution of carotenoids in natural foods, and calls for a renewed effort in applying modern analytical methodology to carotenoid determination in currently used cultivars of fruits, vegetables, and cereal grains, and in dairy, egg, fish, and poultry products so that in the future date one may have more reliable tables of individual carotenoids in the many food products around the world." Today, after a little over 30 years, his wish has been amply fulfilled. Progress in quantitative analysis of carotenoids has given the expertise and incentive that made the determination of the carotenoid composition the most active endeavor in the carotenoid field worldwide. The United States and Brazil have comprehensive databases on food carotenoids (Holden et al., 1999; Rodriguez-Amaya et al., 2008b), but there are also smaller databases (Muller, 1997; Murkovic et al., 2000; O'Neil et al., 2001; Furtado et al., 2004; Reif et al., 2013b). Moreover, the different factors affecting carotenoid composition have been extensively investigated.

Plants are able to synthesize carotenoids de novo; thus, their carotenoid composition is enriched by small or trace amounts of biosynthetic precursors, along with derivatives of the main components (Rodriguez-Amaya, 1999). Often thought of as plant pigments, carotenoids are also encountered in animal foods, albeit with a more limited occurrence and at lower levels. Animals are incapable of carotenoid biosynthesis; thus, their carotenoids are diet derived, selectively or unselectively absorbed, and accumulated (unchanged or modified slightly) to become typical animal carotenoids.

Food Carotenoids: Chemistry, Biology, and Technology, First Edition. Delia B. Rodriguez-Amaya.

5.2 COMPOSITION OF LEAFY AND NONLEAFY GREEN VEGETABLES

Carotenoids are universally encountered in photosynthetic tissues. Located in chloroplasts, with the xanthophylls unesterified and their color masked by chlorophyll, carotenoids of green vegetables have a defined qualitative pattern, with lutein, β-carotene, violaxanthin, and neoxanthin as the main carotenoids (Kimura and Rodriguez-Amaya, 2002; Kobori and Rodriguez-Amaya, 2008). The absolute concentrations differ considerably. The major carotenoids of a leafy vegetable are indicated in Figure 5.1 and the carotenoid levels of some leafy vegetables are presented in Table 5.1. Lettuce (*Lactuca sativa*), exceptionally, also has lactucaxanthin as a major carotenoid. α-Carotene, α- or β-cryptoxanthin, zeaxanthin, antheraxanthin, and lutein-5,6-epoxide may also be found as minor pigments (Figure 5.2).

5.3 COMPOSITION OF FRUITS AND FRUIT VEGETABLES

In contrast to green vegetables, fruits, including those used as vegetables, are known for their variable and often complex carotenoid composition. The compositions of some fruits and fruit vegetables are shown in Table 5.2, demonstrating pronounced qualitative

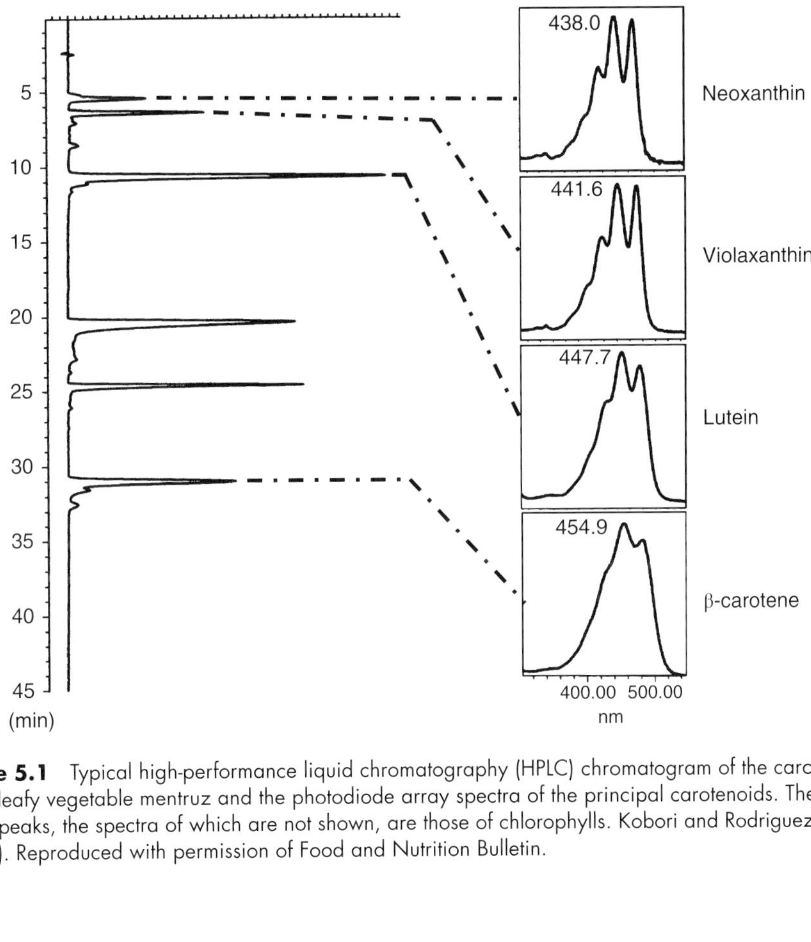

Figure 5.1 Typical high-performance liquid chromatography (HPLC) chromatogram of the carotenoids of the leafy vegetable mentruz and the photodiode array spectra of the principal carotenoids. The other major peaks, the spectra of which are not shown, are those of chlorophylls. Kobori and Rodriguez-Amaya (2008). Reproduced with permission of Food and Nutrition Bulletin.

Table 5.1 Concentrations (μg/g) of major carotenoids in some leafy vegetables.

Vegetable	n	α-Carotene	β-Carotene	Lactucaxanthin	Lutein	Violaxanthin	Neoxanthin
Beldroega (*Portulaca oleracea*)	5	nd	32	nd	34	22	9
Caruru (*Amaranthus viridis*)	5	5	114	nd	119	62	26
Chicory (*Cichorium intybus* L.)							
Conventional	6	nd	35	nd	54	32	20
Hydroponic, winter	5	nd	36	nd	57	21	15
Coriander (*Coriandrum sativum*)	5	nd	55	nd	74	37	18
Endive (*Cichorium endivia* L.)							
Minimally processed							
Summer	5	nd	31	nd	43	23	16
Winter	5	nd	25	nd	35	18	12
Stir-fried	5	nd	12	nd	23	7	7
Kale (*Brassica oleracea* var. *acephala*)							
Young leaves	3	nd	35	nd	46	40	13
Mature leaves	5	nd	41	nd	50	30	15
Minimally processed							
Summer	5	nd	34	nd	52	27	20
Winter	5	nd	33	nd	44	17	9
Stir-fried	15	nd	23	nd	31	6	6
Lettuce (*Lactuca sativa*)							
Curly, conventional	6	nd	16	7	14	19	8
Curly, hydroponic, winter	5	nd	17	8	15	14	6
French, hydroponic, winter	5	nd	25	12	23	20	11
Boston, conventional	6	nd	15	8	14	18	8
Boston, hydroponic, winter	5	nd	23	12	21	19	10
Freelice, hydroponic, winter	5	nd	10	7	10	8	5

Mentruz (*Lepidium pseudodidymun*)	5	nd	97	nd	111	58	31
New Zealand spinach (*Tetragonia expansa*)							
Minimally processed							
Summer	5	nd	55	nd	68	31	22
Winter	5	nd	40	nd	52	24	20
Parsley (*Petroselium crispum*)	5	nd	65	nd	88	36	22
Rucula (*Eruca sativa*)							
Conventional	6	nd	28	nd	50	30	18
Hydroponic, winter	5	nd	33	nd	52	21	12
Serralha (*Sonchus oleraceus*	5	nd	72	nd	87	53	25
Taioba (*Xanthosoma sp*)	5	7	66	nd	104	38	28
Watercress (*Nasturtium officinale*)							
Conventional	6	nd	27	nd	56	26	18
Hydroponic, winter	5	nd	37	nd	75	26	17

n = number of different sample lots analyzed individually; nd = not detected.
Compiled from Sá and Rodriguez-Amaya (2003), Kimura and Rodriguez-Amaya (2003), Azevedo and Rodriguez-Amaya (2005). Azevedo-Meleiro and Rodriguez-Amaya (2005), Niizu and Rodriguez-Amaya (2005a), Kobori and Rodriguez-Amaya (2008). Only papers with the individual major carotenoids quantified by high-performance liquid chromatography (HPLC) and in which three or more different sample lots were analyzed individually are included in the table.

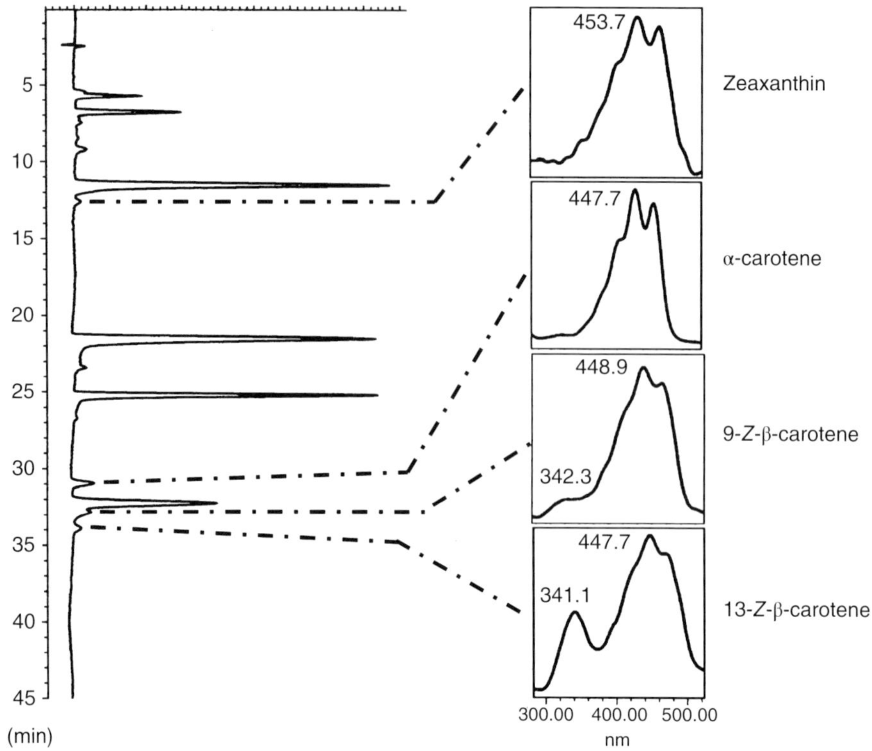

Figure 5.2 Typical HPLC chromatogram of the carotenoids of the leafy vegetable taioba and photodiode array spectra of the minor carotenoids. Kobori and Rodriguez-Amaya (2008). Reproduced with permission of Food and Nutrition Bulletin.

and quantitative variations. The chromatograms in Figure 5.3 also illustrate the variability of fruit carotenoids, the chromatogram of the carotenoids of tomato (*Lycopersicon esculentum*) being much simpler than that of pitanga (*Eugenia uniflora*), although both have lycopene as the main carotenoid.

Notwithstanding the variation in carotenoid composition of fruits, seven major patterns can be discerned (Gross, 1987; Rodriguez-Amaya et al., 2008a): (a) insignificant levels of carotenoids, e.g., apple (*Malus domestica*), cashew-apple (*Anacardium occidentale*), plum (*Prunus domestica*), and Bulgarian berries (Assunção and Mercadante, 2003; Kim et al., 2007; Marinova and Ribarova, 2007); (b) small amounts generally of chloroplast carotenoids, e.g., date (*Phoenix dactylifera*), grape (*Vitis vinifera*), and camu-camu (*Myrciaria dubia*) (C. Oliveira et al., 2003; Boudries et al., 2007; Zanatta and Mercadante, 2007); (c) predominance of lycopene, e.g., pink-fleshed guava (*Psidium guajava*), pitanga, red-fleshed papaya (*Carica papaya*), sarsaparilla (*Smilax aspera*), and watermelon (*Citrullus lanatus*) (Perkins-Veazie et al., 2001; Chandrika et al., 2003; Niizu and Rodriguez-Amaya, 2003; Azevedo-Meleiro and Rodriguez-Amaya, 2004; Tadmor et al., 2005; Yano et al., 2005; Wall, 2006; Rodriguez-Amaya et al., 2007; Sentanin and Rodriguez-Amaya, 2007; Porcu and Rodriguez-Amaya, 2008); (d) predominance of β-carotene, e.g., acerola (*Malpighia emarginata*), marolo (*Annona coriaceae*), apricot (*Prunus armeniaca*), tucumã (*Astrocaryum vulgare*), cantaloupe (*Cucumis melo*), jackfruit (*Artocarpus heterophyllus*), loquat (*Eriobotrya japonica*), and buriti (*Mauritia*

Table 5.2 Concentrations (μg/g) of major carotenoids in some fruits and nonleafy vegetables.

Fruit/vegetable	Origin	n	Principal Carotenoid	Other Major Carotenoids	Reference
Acerola (*Malpighia emarginata*) 'Olivier'	Brazil	3	β-carotene (38)	α-carotene (0.7), β-cryptoxanthin (1.2), lutein (1.1), violaxanthin (3.1), neoxanthin (0.2)	Porcu and Rodriguez-Amaya, 2006
Apricot (*Prunus armeniaca*), 'Harlayne'	U.S.	3	β-carotene (17)	β-cryptoxanthin (0.1), lutein (0.1)	Campbell et al., 2013
Carrot (*Daucus carota*), 'Nantes'	Brazil	6	β-carotene (62)	α-carotene (35), lutein (5.1)	Niizu and Rodriguez-Amaya, 2005a
Papaya (*Carica papaya*)	Brazil				
'Formosa'		5	total lycopene (23), all-*E*-lycopene (20)	all-*E*-β-carotene (1.2), total β-cryptoxanthin (7.0) all-*E*-β-cryptoxanthin (6.7)	Sentanin and Rodriguez-Amaya, 2007
'Sunrise'		5	total lycopene (24), all-*E*-lycopene (21)	all-*E*-β-carotene (0.5), total β-cryptoxanthin (8.2) all-*E*-β-cryptoxanthin (7.6)	
'Golden'		5	total lycopene (18), all-*E*-lycopene (16)	all-*E*-β-carotene (1.2), total β-cryptoxanthin (8.7) all-*E*-β-cryptoxanthin (8.1)	
Papaya (*Carica papaya*)	U.S.				
'Sunrise'		6	lycopene (37)	β-carotene (4.1), β-cryptoxanthin (9.2), lutein (1.3)	Wall, 2006
'SunUp'		6	lycopene (17)	β-carotene (1.0), β-cryptoxanthin (2.9), lutein (0.9)	
Pepper (*Capsicum annuum*)	Brazil				
Yellow hybrid F1 Amanda		5	all-*E*-violaxanthin (31)	all-*E*-β-carotene (2.3), all-*E*-lutein (7.8)	Azevedo-Meleiro and Rodriguez-Amaya, 2009
Red hybrid F1 Magali		5	all-*E*-capsanthin (33)	all-*E*-β-carotene (5.8), all-*E*-lutein (7.5), all-E-violaxanthin (2.7)	
Pepper (*Capsicum annuum* var *annuum*)	US				
'Bell Captain'		3	capsanthin (41)	β-carotene (1.4), β-cryptoxanthin (1.5), zeaxanthin (5.9)	Russo and Howard, 2002
'Ranger'		3	capsanthin (26)	β-carotene (6.8), β-cryptoxanthin (4.3), zeaxanthin (4.0)	
'Red Beauty'		3	capsanthin (9.3)	β-carotene (1.4), β-cryptoxanthin (1.8), zeaxanthin (4.3)	

(*Continued*)

Table 5.2 (*Continued*)

Fruit/vegetable	Origin	n	Principal Carotenoid	Other Major Carotenoids	Reference
Pitanga (*Eugenia uniflora*)	Brazil	5	all-*E*-lycopene (71)	all-*E*-β-carotene (3.2), all-*E*-β-cryptoxanthin (12), all-*E*-γ-carotene (3.8), 13-*Z*-lycopene (5.0), all-*E*-lutein (1.2), all-*E*-rubixanthin (9.4), *Z*-rubixanthin (5.3), all-*E*-violaxanthin (2.3)	Porcu and Rodriguez-Amaya, 2008
Sarsaparilla (*Smilax aspera*)	Spain	4	all-*E*-lycopene (242)	all-*E*-β-carotene (66), all-*E*-β-cryptoxanthin (7.4), all-*E*-β-cryptoxanthin caprate (7.3), all-*E*-β-cryptoxanthin laurate (8.9), all-*E*-β-cryptoxanthin myristate (8.9), all-*E*-β-cryptoxanthin oleate (1.0), all-*E*-β-cryptoxanthin palmitate (5.3), all-*E*-β-cryptoxanthin stearate (3.4), all-*E*-lutein (0.7), *Z*-lutein (0.3), all-*E*-zeaxanthin (4.4), *Z*-zeaxanthin (0.2), all-*E*-zeaxanthin monomyristate (4.0), lycophyll (14), all-*E*-antheraxanthin (0.6)	Delgado-Pelayo and Hornero-Méndez, 2012
Squashes and pumpkins	Brazil				
Cucurbita moschata					
'Menina verde'		5	β-carotene (67)	α-carotene (27), lutein (17), neoxanthin (7.8)	Azevedo-Meleiro and Rodriguez-Amaya, 2007
'Goianinha'		5	β-carotene (57)	α-carotene (24), lutein (18), neoxanthin (6.3)	
Cucurbita maxima					
'Exposição'		5	violaxanthin (21)	β-carotene (15), lutein (11), neoxanthin (9.8)	
Hybrid 'Tetsukabuto'		5	lutein (57)	β-carotene (30), violaxanthin (22), neoxanthin (14)	
Cucurbita pepo					
'Mogango'		5	lutein (9.8)	β-carotene(5.4), violaxanthin (6.9), neoxanthin (3.6)	
Tomato (*Lycopersicon esculentum*)	Brazil	6	lycopene (35)	β-carotene (3.2), lutein (1.0)	Niizu and Rodriguez-Amaya, 2005a

n = number of different sample lots analyzed individually.
Only foods for which the major carotenoids were quantified by HPLC, three or more different sample lots were analyzed individually, and the total carotenoid content is 15 μg/g or more are included in the table.

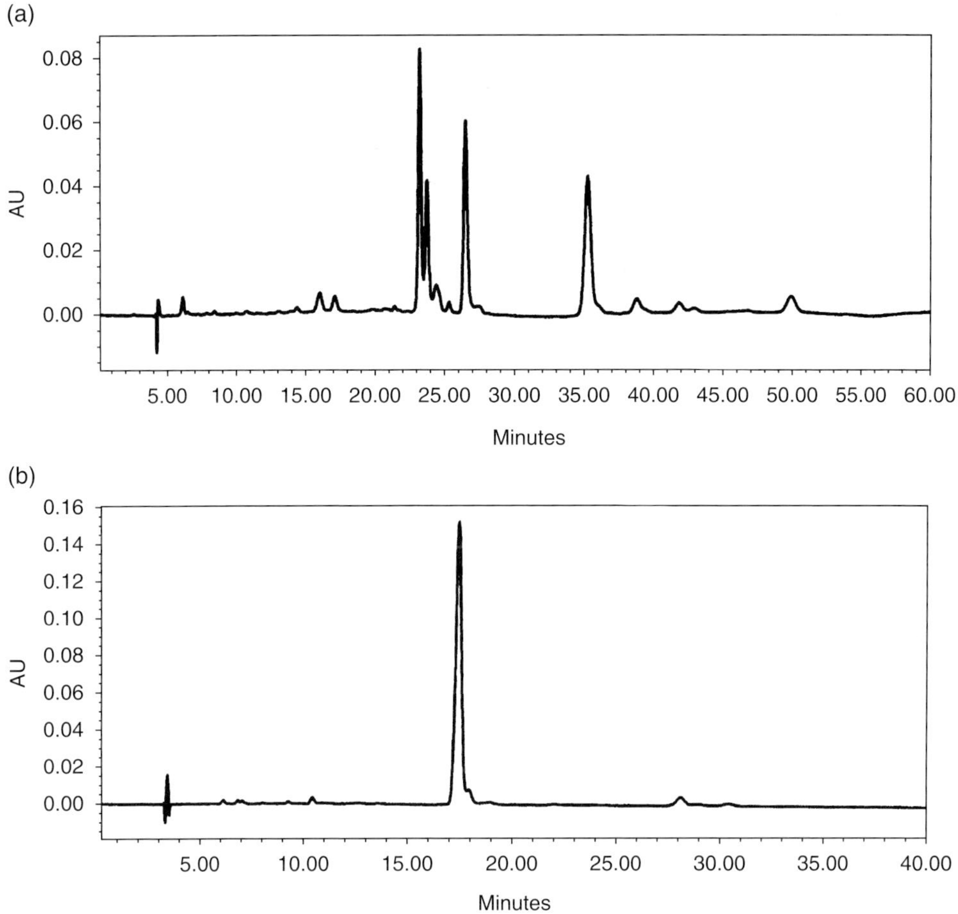

Figure 5.3 HPLC chromatograms of the carotenoids of (a) pitanga and (b) tomato.

vinifera) (Godoy and Rodriguez-Amaya, 1995a,b; Azevedo-Meleiro and Rodriguez-Amaya, 2004; Furtado et al., 2004; Mezadri et al., 2005; Rosso and Mercadante, 2005; Sass-Kiss et al., 2005; Yano et al., 2005; Porcu and Rodriguez-Amaya, 2006; Dragovic-Uzelac et al., 2007; Mercadante and Rosso, 2007; Faria et al., 2009; Campbell et al., 2013); (e) β-cryptoxanthin as the principal carotenoid, e.g., nectarine (*Prunus persica nectarina*), yellow- or orange-fleshed papaya, mandarin (*Citrus reticulata*), peach (*Prunus persica*), and tree tomato (*Solanum betaceum*) (Lin and Chen 1995; Ben-Amotz and Fishler 1998; Godoy and Rodriguez-Amaya, 1998; Chandrika et al., 2003;Yano et al., 2005; Sentanin and Rodriguez-Amaya, 2007; Mertz et al., 2009, 2010); (f) violaxanthin as the main carotenoid, e.g., piquí (*Caryocar brasiliense*), mango (*Mangifera indica*), and orange (*Citrus sinensis*) (Mercadante and Rodriguez-Amaya 1998; Lee and Castle, 2001; Azevedo-Meleiro and Rodriguez-Amaya, 2004; Dhuique-Mayer et al., 2005); and finally, (g) other carotenoids predominating, e.g., yellow passion fruit (*Passiflora edulis* flavicarpa), rose hips (*Rosa mosqueta*), and seabuckthorn berries (*Hippophae rhamnoides*) with ζ-carotene, rubixanthin, and zeaxanthin, respectively, as principal carotenoids (Mercadante et al., 1998; Homero-Méndez and Minguéz-Mosquera, 2000; Silva and

Mercadante, 2002; Raffo et al., 2004; Pop et al., 2014). Some merging of these patterns is seen in some fruits, and cultivars of the same fruit may have different patterns.

In ripe fruits, the hydroxycarotenoids are mostly esterified with fatty acids. In jalapeño peppers (*Capsicum annuum*), for example, the content of esterified carotenoids represented 26%, 40%, and 44%, respectively, of the total carotenoid content at three intermediate ripening stages: brown, 50% red, and 75% red fruits (Cervantes-Paz et al., 2014). In ripe sarsaparilla berries, of a total of 42 μg/g of β-cryptoxanthin, only 7.4 μg/g refer to free β-cryptoxanthin (Delgado-Pelayo and Hornero-Méndez, 2012).

5.4 COMPOSITION OF ROOTS, SEEDS, AND FLOWERS

Carotenoids are not widely distributed in root crops. Carrot (*Daucus carota*), in which β-carotene and α-carotene predominate, and yellow to orange sweet potatoes (*Ipomoea batatas*), with β-carotene as the main carotenoid, are well-known carotenoid-rich roots.

Corn (*Zea mays*) is an example of a carotenogenic seed, with lutein and zeaxanthin as the major carotenoids. In commercial samples of pistachio (*Pistacia vera*) nuts from Greece, Iran, Italy, and Turkey, lutein was also the main carotenoid, ranging from 18 to 52 μg/g (Bellomo and Fallico, 2007). The Italian samples had the highest concentration. Canaryseed (*Phalaris canariensis*), a specialty crop grown in Western Canada, has β-carotene, lutein, and zeaxanthin as the major carotenoids (Li and Beta, 2012). In 19 glabrous brown and yellow varieties, the carotenoid content ranged from 7.6 to 12 μg/g.

Although the carotenoid concentration of wheat (*Triticum aestivum*) is low, there is high daily consumption of wheat-based products in some populations, making it an important dietary source (Lachman et al., 2013). Wheat germ contains about 5.5 μg/g dry weight of total carotenoid (Panfili et al., 2004), comprising mainly hydroxylated xanthophylls, especially lutein.

The edible yellow and brownish nasturtium (*Tropaeolum majus*) flowers have very high contents of lutein (450 and 350 μg/g, respectively) (Niizu and Rodriguez-Amaya, 2005b). In flowers of daylily (*Hemerocallis distichia*), which is commonly used in Chinese cuisine, zeaxanthin predominates (Tai and Chen, 2000).

5.5 COMPOSITION OF PROCESSED FOODS

Some homogenization is done during processing; thus, within-sample variation is usually low. However, between-sample variation can be substantial. The composition of processed foods depends not only on the amount of the carotenoid-containing ingredients and their carotenoid contents but also on the effects of processing. Alterations during processing are discussed in detail in Chapter 6.

For comparison, the carotenoid compositions of commercial common corn and tomato products, manufactured in Brazil and the United States, are presented in Table 5.3. The corn products from Brazil tended to have higher carotenoid contents, especially of the principal carotenoid zeaxanthin. On the other hand, while the lycopene content of ketchup produced in the United States is within the range found in Brazilian ketchup, those of the tomato puree and especially of the tomato paste are markedly higher in the U.S. products. However, even U.S. products can differ substantially.

Table 5.3 Concentrations (μg/g) of major carotenoids in processed corn and tomato.

Product	Origin	n	Mean Carotenoid Concentration	Reference
Canned corn (4 brands)	Brazil	20	All-*E*-β-carotene (1.1 to 1.6), all-E-β-cryptoxanthin (1.9 to 3.1), all-*E*-lutein (0.6 to 2.3), all-*E*-zeaxanthin (10 to 15)	G.P.R. Oliveira and Rodriguez-Amaya, 2007
Corn meal (3 brands)		15	All-*E*-β-carotene (0.8 to 1.0), all-*E*-β-cryptoxanthin (1.0 to 1.8), all-*E*-lutein (3.1 to 6.8), all-*E*-zeaxanthin (5.4 to 9.5)	
Corn flour, coarse (2 brands)		10	All-*E*-β-carotene (0.4, 0.7), all-*E*-β-cryptoxanthin (0.6, 1.2), all-*E*-lutein (1.7, 4.6), all-*E*-zeaxanthin (3.4, 8.4)	
Corn flour, precooked, fine (2 brands)		10	All-*E*-β-carotene (0.6, 0.7), all-*E*-β-cryptoxanthin (1.0, 1.2), all-*E*-lutein (4.2, 4.7), all-*E*-zeaxanthin (7.2, 7.3)	
Corn flakes, cereal (3 brands)		15	All-*E*-β-carotene (0.7 to 0.9), all-*E*-β-cryptoxanthin (1.2 to 1.9), all-*E*-lutein (1.3 to 3.2), all-*E*-zeaxanthin (7.4 to 9.5)	
Canned corn	U.S.	5	β-carotene (0.1), β-cryptoxanthin (0.4), α-cryptoxanthin (1.0), lutein (3.4), zeaxanthin (2.2)	Scott and Eldridge, 2005
Frozen corn		5	β-carotene (0.2), β-cryptoxanthin (0.3), α-cryptoxanthin (1.1), lutein (3.6), zeaxanthin (2.1)	
Corn flakes, cereal	U.S.	2	β-cryptoxanthin (0.1), all-*E*-lutein (0.4), *Z*-lutein (0.2), all-*E*-zeaxanthin (0.5), *Z*-zeaxanthin (0.1)	Perry et al., 2009
Corn meal, yellow		2	All-*E*-β-carotene (0.3), β-cryptoxanthin (0.5), all-*E*-lutein (trace), *Z*-lutein (0.6), all-*E*-zeaxanthin (5.3), *Z*-zeaxanthin (0.2)	
Catsup (3 brands	Brazil	15	All-*E*-β-carotene (3.5 to 5.2), *Z*-β-carotene (1.5 to 1.8), all-*E*-lycopene (104-192), *Z*-lycopene (6.6 to11)	Kobori and Rodriguez-Amaya, 2008
Tomato paste (3 brands)		15	All-*E*-β-carotene (6.5 to 9.2), *Z*-β-carotene (2.8 to 3.6), all-*E*-lycopene (179-248), *Z*-lycopene (9.6 to14)	
Tomato puree (3 brands)		15	All-*E*-β-carotene (3.0 to 5.1), *Z*-β-carotene (1.4 to 2.1), all-*E*-lycopene (72-110), *Z*-lycopene (5.0 to 6.7)	
Catsup	U.S.	9	β-carotene (5.9), γ-carotene (30), ζ-carotene (3.3), lycopene (172), neurosporene (26), phytoene (34), phytofluene (15), lycopene-5,6-diol (1.8)	Tonucci et al., 1995
Tomato paste		9	β-carotene (13), γ-carotene (100), ζ-carotene (8.4), lutein (3.4), lycopene (554), neurosporene (70), phytoene (84), phytofluene (36), lycopene-5,6-diol (4.4)	
Tomato puree		9	β-carotene (4.1), γ-carotene (29), ζ-carotene (2.5), lutein (0.9), lycopene (167), neurosporene (21), phytoene (24), phytofluene (11), lycopene-5,6-diol (1.7)	

n = number of different sample lots analyzed individually.

In samples of ketchup from 13 commercial sources, representing at least 10 U.S. manufacturers, the lycopene content ranged from 59 to 183 μg/g (Ishida and Chapman, 2004). In Hungarian ketchup, lycopene ranged from 64 to 234 μg/g, with an average of 153 μg/g (Lugasi et al., 2003).

5.6 RICH SOURCES OF THE MAJOR FOOD CAROTENOIDS

It is now widely known that the carotenoids most commonly encountered in foods and in human serum are β-carotene, α-carotene, β-cryptoxanthin, lycopene, lutein, and zeaxanthin. Understandably, these are also the most investigated carotenoids in terms of human health. In Brazil, violaxanthin is also found as a major food carotenoid (Rodriguez-Amaya et al., 2008b). This carotenoid may have a wider occurrence, but it is often underestimated because it can degrade easily during analysis. Rich sources of the major food carotenoids around the world are discussed below. Although there are some exceptions, there is remarkable coincidence regarding the richest sources identified in different countries.

Carrot is recognized worldwide as the rich dietary source of β-carotene. It is also widely consumed in Brazil, but it is surpassed by the palm fruits buriti (*Mauritia vinifera*), umari (*Poraqueiba sericea*), tucumã, and bocaiúva (*Acrocomia aculeata*), with average β-carotene concentrations of 360, 99, 99, and 59 μg/g, respectively (Rodriguez-Amaya et al., 2008b). Squashes (*Cucurbita moschata*), such as the cultivars 'Baianinha','Menina Brasileira', and 'Goianinha', are also rich sources, with mean β-carotene concentrations of 235, 67, and 57 μg/g, respectively (Table 5.2).

Among 40 common fruits and vegetables in the Costa Rican diet, cooked celery leaves and stalk (*Apium graveolens*), carrot, cantaloupe, cooked cilantro (coriander, *Coriandrum sativum*), and cooked broccoli (*Brassica oleracea italica*) have the highest all-*E*-β-carotene contents (138, 69, 34, 28, and 25 μg/g, respectively) (Furtado et al., 2004).

Out of 38 U.S. fruits and vegetables, β-carotene is highest in cooked spinach (*Spinacia oleracea*) (88 μg/g), cilantro (55 μg/g), romaine lettuce (27 μg/g), parsley (*Petroselinum crispum*) (23 μg/g), and dried apricot (22 μg/g) (Perry et al., 2009). From the extensive USDA database, carrot A-plus cultivar, grape leaves, canned and drained mango, kale (*Brassica oleracea acephala*), and sweet potato have the highest β-carotene contents (182, 162, 131, 92, and 92 μg/g, respectively) (Holden et al., 1999).

Among Fijian fruits and vegetables, the richest sources of β-carotene in descending order are the leaves of *Moringa oleifera* (drumstick), *Amaranthus viridis* (amaranth), *Ipomoea aquatica* (kangkong), sweet potato, and *Colocasia esculenta* (taro) (Lako et al., 2007).

β-carotene is sometimes accompanied by α-carotene, as in carrot and *C. moschata* (Table 5.2). In the USDA database, cooked carrot A-plus cultivar, cooked carrot, canned pumpkin, and cooked/baked butternut winter squash have the highest α-carotene concentrations (150, 55, 48, and 11 μg/g, respectively) (Holden et al., 1999). The Brazilian database has buriti, *C. moschata* 'Baianinha', carrot 'Nantes', *C. moschata* 'Menina', *C. moschata* 'Goianinha', and carrot (80, 47, 35, 25, and 24 μg/g, respectively) as the richest sources of this carotenoid (Rodriguez-Amaya et al., 2008b).

β-cryptoxanthin is the main carotenoid of many orange-fleshed fruits, but at concentrations comparatively lower than those of β-carotene, lycopene, and lutein as principal carotenoids. Breithaupt and Bamedi (2001) analyzed 20 samples of selected fruits and vegetables for free and esterified β-cryptoxanthin and found 0.1 to 8.9 μg/g free β-cryptoxanthin, 0.1 to 8.9 μg/g β-cryptoxanthin laurate, 0.2 to 4.2 μg/g β-cryptoxanthin myristate and 0.2 to 2.9 μg/g β-cryptoxanthin palmitate, the highest values being obtained from red (sharp) pepper, papaya, and loquat from Spain. Yellow and red tree tomato have 14 and 16 μg/g β-cryptoxanthin, respectively (Mertz et al., 2009). In the USDA database, the highest β-cryptoxanthin levels were obtained from frozen tangerine juice (*Citrus reticulata*), sweet red pepper, canned and drained mango, and Japanese persimmon (*Diospyros kaki*) (28, 22, 16, and 14 μg/g, respectively) (Holden et al., 1999).

Among 75 fruits produced in Japan, the highest concentrations of β-cryptoxanthin were obtained from papaya 'Sunrise' (32 μg/g), satsuma mandarin (29 μg/g), mandarin 'Saga' (14 μg/g), and loquat (11 μg/g) (Yano et al., 2005).

Tomato and tomato products are the main dietary sources of lycopene in many countries. In Brazil, there is high intake of tomatoes and tomato products, but the fruit sources with the highest concentrations of lycopene are pitanga (71 μg/g) and guava 'Paluma' (66 μg/g) and 'Ogawa' (57 μg/g) (Table 5.2). In the United States, 'Crimson Trio' watermelon also presented 71 μg/g of lycopene (Perkins-Veazie et al., 2001). In the USDA database, the highest lycopene contents were obtained from tomato products: canned tomato paste, 293 μg/g; ketchup, 170 μg/g; canned tomato puree, 167 μg/g; pasta/spaghetti sauce, 160 μg/g; and canned tomato sauce, 159 μg/g (Holden et al., 1999). Of 75 fruits from Japan, the highest levels of lycopene were found in watermelon (62 μg/g), guava (44 μg/g), and papaya 'Fruit tower' (25 μg/g) (Yano et al., 2005).

The richest sources of lycopene, however, are the Asian gac (*Momordica cochinchinensis*) fruit and the Spanish sarsaparilla. Lycopene is concentrated in the bright red seed membrane (aril) of the ripe gac fruit, which is used primarily in the preparation of *xoi gac* (red rice) in Vietnam (Vuong et al., 2006). The lycopene concentration exceeds that of β-carotene by a factor of about five (408 vs. 83 μg/g). An earlier paper presented the following composition for the gac aril in μg/g: 1342 all-*E*-lycopene, 204 *Z*-lycopene, 597 all-*E*-β-carotene, 39 *Z*-β-carotene, and 107 α-carotene (Ishida et al., 2004). Sarsaparilla was found to have 242 μg/g all-*E*-lycopene, along with 66 μg/g all-*E*-β-carotene and 42 μg/g total β-cryptoxanthin (free + esters) (Delgado-Pelayo and Hornero-Méndez, 2012).

Corn and corn products are the major dietary sources of zeaxanthin/lutein and leafy green vegetables the major sources of lutein in the United States. Of 38 U.S. fruits and vegetables, cooked spinach, cooked kale, cilantro, parsley, and romaine lettuce have the highest all-*E*-lutein content (126, 89, 77, 43, and 38 μg/g, respectively) (Perry et al., 2009). In another study on commonly consumed fruits, vegetables, and pasta products in the United States, 9 green vegetables have the highest concentrations of lutein, especially kale (130 μg/g), parsley (99 μg/g), spinach (84 μg/g), and collard (*Brassica oleracea*) (49 μg/g) (Humphries and Khachik, 2003). Ten commonly consumed yellow-orange fruits and vegetables, with the exception of squash (butternut variety), presented much lower levels of lutein but contained higher concentrations of zeaxanthin.

Among 21 selected Indian vegetables, the highest lutein levels were obtained from pumpkin (*Cucurbita maxima*) (106 μg/g), chili (19 μg/g), and brinjal (*Solanum melongena*) (18 μg/g) (Aruna et al., 2009). Of seven leafy vegetables commonly consumed by the rural population, *Peucedanum sowa*, spinach, and *Basella rubra* presented the highest lutein concentrations (93,78, and 68 μg/g dry weight, respectively) (Lakshminarayana et al., 2005). Of 26 Indian spices, curry leaves (*Murraya koenigii*), spearmint (*Mentha spicata*), green chili, and coriander leaves have the highest lutein levels (272, 177, 133, and 99 μg/g dry weight, respectively) (Aruna and Baskaran, 2010). *Chenopodium album*, *Commelina benghalensis*, and *Solanum nigrum* were found to contain higher levels of both lutein (840–1870 μg/g dry weight) and β-carotene (500–1150 μg/g dry weight) among 30 medicinally important Indian green leafy vegetables (Raju et al., 2007).

Of 13 Sri Lankan green leafy vegetables, wel kohila (*Syngonium angustatum*), sweet potato, cassava (*Manihot esculenta*), pumpkin (*Cucurbita maxima*), and pitasudu sarana (*Boerhavia diffusa*) have the highest lutein concentrations (Chandrika et al., 2010).

Characterizing the carotenoid contents of selected components of the Mediterranean diet commonly eaten by Greek migrants in Melbourne, Su et al. (2002) found that the wild green vegetables sow thistle (*Sonchus oleraceus*) and amaranth contained lutein (150 and 130 μg/g, respectively) and β-carotene (33 and 40 μg/g, respectively) at concentrations greater than those of commercially available species of chicory (*Chicorium intybus*) and endive (*Chicorium endivia*). Similarly, in Brazil, the uncultivated native green leaves caruru (*Amaranthus viridis*), mentruz (*Lepidium pseudodidymus*), taioba (*Xanthosoma* sp.), and serralha (*Sonchus oleraceus*) have higher contents of lutein and β-carotene than commercially produced leafy vegetables (Table 5.1) (Kobori and Rodriguez-Amaya, 2008). Of the commercial leaves, the richest sources of these carotenoids in decreasing order are parsley, New Zealand spinach (*Tetragonia expansa*), coriander leaves, kale, rucula (*Eruca sativa*), and chicory.

Among 29 Austrian vegetables, dill (*Anethum graveolens*) (138 μg/g), basil (*Ocimum basilicum*) (70 μg/g), parsley (64 μg/g), sage (64 μg/g), and spinach (59 μg/g) have the highest lutein/zeaxanthin contents (Murkovic et al., 2000). Carrot (88 μg/g), dill (54 μg/g), basil (48 μg/g), spinach (48 μg/g), and parsley (46 μg/g) have the highest β-carotene concentrations.

Of 107 different vegetable cultivars (mostly leafy vegetables) commonly produced and eaten in Switzerland, *Brassica rapa* 'pak choi Amur' and 'pak choi Tatsoi Red', *Chicorium intybus* 'catalogna Selvatica da Campo', and summer spinach have the highest lutein contents (105, 86, 84, and 83 μg/g, respectively) (Reif et al., 2013b). Garlic chives (*Chicorium intybus*) 'Kobold', summer spinach, *Brassica rapa* L. 'pak choi Amur', and 'pak choi Tatsoi Red' presented the highest β-carotene levels (81, 73, 66, and 58 μg/g, respectively).

In Germany, of a total of 22 species of vegetables and 28 species of fruits, carrot, kale, parsley, red paprika, and spinach have the highest β-carotene levels (90, 73, 55, 32, and 32 μg/g, respectively) (Muller, 1997). Kale, parsley, Lamb's lettuce, spinach (186, 138, 96 and 95, respectively) have the highest lutein contents.

In traditional Portuguese fruits and vegetables (10 varieties of five fruit species and five varieties of four species of vegetables), the analyzed leafy vegetables were found to be good sources of lutein (5.2–72 μg/g) and β-carotene (4.6–64 μg/g)

(Dias et al., 2009). The fruits have considerably lower carotenoid content (0.03–1.6 μg/g lutein, 0.1–1.7 μg/g β-carotene) and a complex and variable qualitative and quantitative carotenoid composition.

Zeaxanthin is not as widely distributed in foods. In the Brazilian database (Rodriguez-Amaya et al., 2008b), only buriti and canned corn have appreciable amounts of this carotenoid (20 and 13 μg/g, respectively). The East Asian fruit goji (*Lycium barbarium*) and seabuckthorn appear to be the best sources. The goji cultivars Inner Mogolia and Ning Xia had 43 and 36 μg/g, respectively, of zeaxanthin (Lam and But, 1999). Nine *Lycium* species have zeaxanthin palmitate as the main carotenoid, comprising 31%–56% of the total carotenoid content (Peng et al., 2005). *Lycium* fruits are used as health food and herbal medicine in China. Three German cultivars of seabuckthorn have 30–150 μg/g of zeaxanthin, the principal carotenoid (Raffo et al., 2004). Six Romanian seabuckthorn varieties have zeaxanthin dipalmitate as their principal carotenoid component, varying from 64 to 183 μg/g dry weight (Pop et al., 2014).

5.7 GENETIC AND ENVIRONMENTAL FACTORS AFFECTING CAROTENOID COMPOSITION

The carotenoid composition is highly influenced by genetic and environmental factors and postharvest handling. In a given food, qualitative and quantitative variations in the carotenoid composition exist because of factors such as cultivar/variety, stage of maturity, climate/geographic site of production, season, part of the plant used, agronomic conditions and agricultural practices, postharvest handling, processing, and storage conditions.

5.7.1 Cultivar/variety

Differences among cultivars of the same food can be both qualitative and quantitative or only quantitative, with essentially the same carotenoids being found in the different varieties.

Varietal differences have been demonstrated in numerous fruits. In the Brazilian acerola 'Waldy Cati 30' and 'Olivier', β-carotene (2.7–17 μg/g), lutein (0.4–1.0 μg/g), β-cryptoxanthin (0.2–0.6 μg/g), and α-carotene (0.1–0.6 μg/g) were found to be the major carotenoids (Rosso and Mercadante, 2005). In fruits of two harvests, β-carotene, β-cryptoxanthin, and α-carotene were higher in 'Olivier', whereas the lutein content was higher in the 'Waldy Cati 30.'

Eleven apricot varieties produced in Hungary had 15 to 38 μg/g of β-carotene (Sass-Kiss et al., 2005). Four cultivars of commercial ripe U.S. apricot had 6.9 to 17 μg/g β-carotene (Campbell et al., 2013).

In 16 cultivars of Micronesian bananas (*Musa* spp.), β-carotene ranged from 0.6 to 28 μg/g and α-carotene from 0.1 to 8.3 μg/g (Englberger et al., 2003a,b). Lutein was also quantified in seven cultivars and it varied from <0.1 to 2.3 μg/g. Twelve banana cultivars produced in Australia had concentrations of all-*E*-β-carotene, α-carotene, and lutein ranging from 0.5 to 14, 0.6 to 11, and 0.1 to 1.5 μg/g, respectively (Englberger et al., 2006c).

In 14 Marshallese pandanus (*Pandanus tectorius*), β-carotene, zeaxanthin, and lutein varied from 0.3 to 6.7, 0.3 to 3.4, and 0.1 to 2.1 μg/g, respectively (Englberger et al., 2006b). Four of these cultivars had β-carotene as the major carotenoid, whereas zeaxanthin predominated in three cultivars and lutein in two. Ten cultivars of the pandanus from Kiribati had 0.6 to 9.0 μg/g β-carotene and 0.1 to 0.9 μg/g α-carotene (Englberger et al., 2006a). Four cultivars were also analyzed for β-cryptoxanthin and a range of 0.4 to 2.4 μg/g was obtained.

The carotenoid composition of citrus fruits is known to be very complex and diverse, consisting of a large number of carotenoids (Lee, 2001; Cortés et al., 2004; Xu et al., 2006; Dugo et al., 2008; Meléndez-Martínez et al., 2007, 2008). Citrus genotypes belonging to eight cultivated citrus species presented different carotenoid profiles with 25 distinct compounds isolated (Fanciullino et al., 2006). As would be expected, interspecific variability was greater than intraspecific variation. Two carotenoids, *Z*- violaxanthin and β-cryptoxanthin, strongly determined the classification based on the qualitative data. The general evolution of cultivated citrus was found to be the main factor of the organization of carotenoid diversity among citrus varieties. In another study (Matsumoto et al., 2007), 39 citrus species were classified into five clusters in terms of the flavedo carotenoids: carotenoid-poor, phytoene-abundant, violaxanthin-abundant, β,β-xanthophylls violaxanthin– and β-cryptoxanthin-abundant, and phytoene-, violaxanthin-, and β-cryptoxanthin-abundant. In terms of the carotenoids of the juice sac (pulp), they were classified into four clusters: carotenoid-poor, violaxanthin-abundant, violaxanthin- and phytoene-abundant, and violaxanthin-, phytoene-, and β-cryptoxanthin-abundant. Among eight varieties of Mediterranean oranges, three cultivars (Pera, Sanguinelli, and Shamouti) and two Mandarin species had high retinol equivalents due to high content of β-cryptoxanthin (Dhuique-Mayer et al., 2005).

In the four principal mango cultivars produced in southern China, the β-carotene content varied from 26 to 61 μg/g (Liu et al., 2013). Keitt mangoes had significantly higher β-carotene concentrations, whereas JinHwang mangoes had lower β-carotene content and antioxidant activity.

Three red-fleshed papaya cultivars produced in São Paulo, Brazil, had all-*E*-lycopene content varying from 16 to 21 μg/g (Table 5.2) (Sentanin and Rodriguez-Amaya, 2007). In three Brazilian peach cultivars, the main carotenoid all-*E*-β-cryptoxanthin varied from 0.1 to 5.9 μg/g.

The lycopene content of 11 red-fleshed watermelon cultivars grown at one location, representing seedless, open-pollinated, and hybrid types, and in commercially shipped hybrid and seedless melons, representing seasonal production periods, ranged from 36 to 71 μg/g (Perkins-Veazie et al., 2001). In three red watermelon mutants, lycopene varied from 39 to 49 μg/g, while prolycopene (8.2 μg/g) was the major carotenoid of an orange mutant (Tadmor et al., 2005). A later study determined the lycopene content of 50 commercial U.S. cultivars of seeded and seedless red-fleshed watermelons (Perkins-Veazie et al., 2006). Based on the total lycopene, the watermelon cultivars were separated into low (<50 μg/g), average (50–70 μg/g), high (70–90 μg/g), and very high (>90 μg/g). The lycopene content ranged from 33 to 100 μg/g. Most of the seeded hybrid cultivars had average lycopene contents. Sixteen of the 33 seedless types had lycopene contents in the high and very high ranges. All-*trans*-lycopene was the predominant carotenoid (84%–97%). In Brazil, the cv. Crimson Sweet had almost exclusively all-*E*-lycopene (36 μg/g), with a very small amount of *Z*-lycopene and 4.7 μg/g β-carotene (Niizu and Rodriguez-Amaya, 2003).

Eleven cultivars of red tomatoes purchased from retail outlets in the United Kingdom had 0.5 to 1.9 μg/g of lutein, 12 to 50 μg/g of all-*E*-lycopene and 3.5 to 17 μg/g of all-*E*-β-carotene (Hart and Scott, 1995). Three of nine commercial tomato varieties produced in Spain had >50 μg/g lycopene, while the concentration in the other varieties was between 30 and 50 μg/g, with the exception of one variety that had less than 20 μg/g (Martínez-Valverde et al., 2002. In 12 tomato genotypes from India, lycopene varied from 20 to 69 μg/g in the pulp and from 48 to 141 μg/g in the peel (George et al., 2004). Cherry tomatoes had the highest lycopene contents. In Hungary, six processing varieties of tomato grown in open fields and seven table varieties from greenhouses had lycopene ranges of 93–111 μg/g and 49–80 μg/g, respectively (Sass-Kiss et al., 2005). In an earlier study, Abushita et al. (2000) did not find great differences between cultivars for fresh consumption (salad tomatoes), but processing cultivars had significant differences not only in the total carotenoid content but also in the qualitative distribution of some pigments such as lycopene, β-carotene, and lutein. The lycopene content of 14 cultivars of cherry tomatoes produced in southern Italy ranged from 43 to 120 μg/g (Lenucci et al., 2006). Tomato cultivars containing the Crimson gene (og) were usually found to have higher lycopene content (51 to 58 μg/g) than those lacking the gene (26 to 43 μg/g) (Thompson et al., 2000).

In 57 cultivars of six *Capsicum* species in 1996, β-carotene in the ripe fruit varied from not detected to 166 μg/g and the total carotenoid content from 1 to 896 μg/g (Wall et al., 2001). The range for β-carotene was similar in 1997, but that of the total carotenoid was wider (4–1173 μg/g). The other carotenoids were not quantified. Another study on 12 varieties of *Capsicum* cultivars belonging to three species (*C. chinense, C. annuum, C. frutescens*) demonstrated considerable qualitative and quantitative variation in the carotenoid composition (Giuffrida et al., 2013). Among the red cultivars, some had high contents of capsanthin and β-carotene, whereas others showed high capsanthin levels but no detectable β-carotene. A golden-yellow and a yellow cultivar had high lutein, α-carotene, and β-carotene concentrations; an orange cultivar was rich in antheraxanthin, capsanthin, and zeaxanthin. Among 10 pungent and nonpungent peppers, the Ancho type had the most β-cryptoxanthin, α-carotene, β-carotene, and total carotenoid (Russo and Howard, 2002). Red cherry had the most capsanthin and zeaxanthin while Bell Captain had the most lutein. Notably, differences in the capsanthin (769–1270), capsolutein (171–278), capsorubin (40–67), violaxanthin (50–101), zeaxanthin (213–462), and β-cryptoxanthin (113–166) concentrations (in μg/g dry matter) of the ripe fruits of five *C. annuum* cultivars cultivated in Turkey were not found to be statistically significant (Topuz and Ozdemir, 2007). Only the β-carotene level (70–124 μg/g) was statistically different among the cultivars.

The all-*E*-lutein concentration (μg/g dry weight) in 10 green, yellow, orange, and red varieties of pepper varied from 5.1 in Green Italian to 802 in Red Italian; zeaxanthin ranged from not detected in four varieties to 97 μg/g dry weight in Red Italian (Guil-Guerrero et al., 2006). In seven landraces of Italian hot pepper, the capsanthin content varied from 7.9 to 18.8 μg/g (Masi et al., 2007). In Brazil, a yellow hybrid had violaxanthin (31 μg/g) as the main carotenoid, whereas capsanthin (33 μg/g) predominated in the red hybrid (Table 5.2) (Azevedo-Meleiro and Rodriguez-Amaya, 2009).

Twelve selected pepper cultivars, bred for mechanical harvesting and adaptation to different cultivation cycles (short or long) were characterized by their carotenoid composition with the aim of producing high-quality paprika (Hornero-Méndez et al., 2002). The MA1 cultivar showed the highest carotenoid content (12,698 μg/g dry weight), followed by DN5 and RN2 cultivars with 11,087 and 10,393 μg/g dry weight, respectively. Most of the cultivars had a total carotenoid content of 7000–9700 μg/g dry weight.

β-carotene varied from 0.6 to 72 μg/g, α-carotene from not detected to 75 μg/g, and lutein + zeaxanthin from 0.8 to 75 μg/g in 21 Austrian varieties of three species of squashes and pumpkins (*C. pepo*, *C. maxima*, *C. moschata*) (Murkovic et al., 2002).

The Brazilian *C. moschata* 'Menina Brasileira' and 'Goianinha' have similar profiles, with β-carotene, α-carotene, and lutein as the major carotenoids (Table 5.2). (Azevedo-Meleiro and Rodriguez-Amaya, 2007). *C. maxima* 'Exposição' exhibits the predominance of violaxanthin, followed by β-carotene and lutein. The hybrid 'Tetsukabuto' has lutein, β-carotene, and violaxanthin as the principal carotenoids.

The carotenoid content in 20 varieties of carrot, produced in one location in France, varied from 30 to 170 μg/g (Nicolle et al., 2004). In yellow and purple carrots, lutein represented nearly half of the total carotenoids. In orange carrots, β-carotene was the major carotenoid (65%). In six genotypes of the Nantes type carrots organically grown in two locations, the concentrations differed among genotypes and between the sites of production, both in terms of α-carotene (20–42 μg/g for location 1, 9–26 for location 2) and β-carotene (47–88 μg/g for location 1, 29–78 for location 2) (Kidmose et al., 2004). In carrots sown in the same location in the United Kingdom, the purple carrots contained 2.2 and 2.3 times more α- and β-carotenes, respectively, than orange carrots (Alasalvar et al., 2001). These carotenoids were in trace amounts in yellow carrot and not detected in white carrot. In contrast, in carrots field-grown in Germany, the purple cultivar, along with the white and yellow carrots, had low carotenoid contents, although it had the most phenolic compounds (Grassman et al., 2007).

Profiling the carotenoids in 60 potato cultivars, Fernandez-Orozco et al. (2013) segregated them into three groups according to the main pigments: violaxanthin (37 cultivars, especially those with higher carotenoid content), lutein (16 cultivars), and neoxanthin (16 cultivars). The total carotenoid content ranged from 5.0 to 15 μg/g dry weight. Xanthophyll esters were present in most cultivars, mainly as diesters. A direct correlation was observed between carotenoid content and the esterified fraction, suggesting that esterification facilitates the accumulation of these lipophilic compounds within the plastids.

The mean all-*E*-β-carotene content, which varied over the geographical sites, ranged from 51 to 165 μg/g in orange-fleshed sweet potato produced in South Africa (Laurie et al., 2012). In Hawaiian sweet potatoes, β-carotene ranged from 67 to 128 μg/g in seven orange-fleshed varieties, from 1 to 6 μg/g in seven yellow/white varieties, and from 1 to 5 μg/g in purple-fleshed varieties (Huang et al., 1999).

In nine Micronesian giant swamp taro (corms) (*Cyrtosperma chamissonis*) cultivars, the concentration ranges for β-carotene, α-carotene, and lutein were 3.3–20, 2.0–8.3, and 0.1–1.5 μg/g, respectively (Englberger et al., 2003b). Of 34 cultivars of giant swamp taro from the Federated States of Micronesia and the Republic of Palau, β-carotene concentration varied from 0.5 to 45 μg/g (Englberger et al., 2008). The yellow-fleshed cultivars generally had higher carotenoid levels.

In 44 sweet and dent corn lines, the concentration ranges in μg/g dry weight were as follows: α-carotene, not detected–0.7; β-carotene, 0.1–7.6; β-cryptoxanthin, 0.1–2.4, lutein, not detected–28; zeaxanthin, trace–7.7 (Kurilich and Juvik, 1999). In 64 corn genotypes, the prevalent carotenoids lutein and zeaxanthin ranged, respectively, from not detectable to 30 μg/g and from 0.5 to 38 μg/g (Berardo et al., 2004).

Twenty-three kale cultigens were field-grown under similar fertility over two years (Kopsell et al., 2004). Lutein ranged from 48 to 134 μg/g and β-carotene from 38 to 100 μg/g. Carotenoid concentrations differed significantly, but the rank order among the cultigens for both lutein and β-carotene did not change between years. The lutein concentration ranged from 38 to 105 μg/g and the β-carotene content from 21 to 68 μg/g in 12 Japanese *Brassica* greens grown under different conditions (Reif et al., 2013a). The *Brassica rapa* subsp. *chinensis* had significantly more carotenoids than the other green leafy vegetables. The effect of growing conditions was less pronounced, with slightly higher β-carotene contents observed in the summer. In 12 collard, 2 mustard (*Brassica juncea*), and 2 turnip green (*Brassica rapa*) genotypes, the lutein concentration varied from 51 to 154 μg/g (Farnham et al., 2012).

In six organically grown spinach genotypes after frozen storage (−24°C for 6 months), the β-carotene concentration did not vary significantly, but the lutein and neoxanthin contents differed significantly between genotypes (Kidmose et al., 2001). The highest values were found in the dark green genotype. In a total of 16 cultivars of lettuce, the β-carotene content varied from 19 to 42 μg/g (López et al., 2014). Lactucaxanthin ranged from 4.0 to 9.3 μg/g. Caldwell and Britz (2006) noted a 10-fold cultivar-specific difference in the carotenoid levels of eight green leaf and eight red leaf lettuce cultivars grown under identical conditions.

Fifty accessions of broccoli presented ranges of not detected–0.7 μg/g for α-carotene and 3.7–24 μg/g for β-carotene (Kurilich et al., 1999). Fernández-León et al. (2012) obtained 8.0 μg/g β-carotene and 6.0 μg/g lutein in the 'Pathenon' cultivar and 7.1 μg/g β-carotene and 5.4 μg/g lutein in the 'Monaco' cultivar of this vegetable.

Significant genotype effects on the carotenoid contents were found in wheat, with einkorn differing from emmer and spring wheats (Lackman et al., 2013). The year of cultivation had less effect. The β-carotene and lutein contents ranged from not detected to 2.4 and from not detected to 14 μg/g dry weight, respectively. Earlier studies showed the lutein content varying from 1.2 to 5.8 μg/g dry weight in 3 varieties (Leenhardt et al., 2006), from 0.3 to 1.4 μg/g in 11 soft and hard wheat varieties (Adom et al., 2003), and from 0.8 to 1.1 μg/g in 8 soft wheat varieties (Moore et al., 2005).

5.7.2 Stage of maturity

In fruits in which the color at the ripe stage is due to anthocyanins and in fruits that retain their green color when ripe, such as kiwi (*Actinidia chinensis*) and avocado (*Persea americana*) (Gross 1987; Ashton et al., 2006), the carotenoid concentrations decrease with ripening. The same trend is seen with some fruits that undergo yellowing simply by unmasking the carotenoids through chlorophyll degradation (Gross 1987). In general, however, maturation of a vegetable or ripening of a fruit is usually accompanied by enhanced carotenoid biosynthesis, the number of carotenoids and their concentrations increasing markedly (Gross, 1987, 1991).

In the Brazilian acerola 'Olivier', β-carotene increased from 12 to 38 μg/g, violaxanthin from 0.7 to 3.1 μg/g, lutein from 0.7 to 1.1 μg/g, β-cryptoxanthin from 0.3 to 1.2 μg/g, and α-carotene 0.3 to 0.7 μg/g from the partially ripe to the ripe fruits (Porcu and Rodriguez-Amaya, 2006).

In Croatian apricot, the β-carotene content increased from 0.5 to 5.8 μg/g in 'Keckemetska Ruza', 1.8 to 11 μg/g in 'Madjarska Najbolja', and 1.1 to 8.3 μg/g in 'Velika Rana', from the immature to the commercial mature stage in one location (Dragovic-Uzelac et al., 2007). The corresponding increases were 0.7 to 8.0, 2.0 to 14 and 1.5 to 9.5 in another location. In 25 citrus genotypes, variability in carotenoid composition was found to be more interspecific than intraspecific (Fanciullino et al., 2006). *Z*-violaxanthin and β-cryptoxanthin strongly determined the classification based on qualitative data.

In three Algerian palm date varieties at three ripening stages (stage 1—khallal, stage 2—rutab, stage 3—tamr), the carotenoid trend during ripening was somewhat different (Boudries et al., 2007). In one variety, lutein and β-carotene had the highest level at the rutab stage, whereas in the other two varieties, these two carotenoids had the highest concentrations at the khallal stage, declining thereafter.

In mangos produced in Japan, β-carotene rose from 2.9 to 9.7 μg/g and violaxanthin from 2.6 to 11.3 μg/g during the 2 weeks before harvest (Ogawa et al., 2005). In Brazilian-produced 'Keitt' mangos, all-*E*-β-carotene, all-*E*-violaxanthin, and 9-*Z*-violaxanthin increased from 1.7, 5.4, and 1.7 μg/g in the mature-green fruits to 6.7, 18 and 7.2 μg/g, respectively, in the ripe fruits (Mercadante and Rodriguez-Amaya, 1998). In the 'Tommy Atkins' cultivar, these carotenoids went from 2.0, 6.9, and 3.3 μg/g to 5.8, 22, and 14 μg/g, respectively. Rubixanthin, β-cryptoxanthin, and lycopene increased from 4.7, 7.6, and 34 μg/g to 9.4, 12, and 71 μg/g, respectively, from the partially ripe to ripe Brazilian pitanga (Porcu and Rodriguez-Amaya, 2008).

In *Fructus lycii* fruits analyzed at seven different ripening stages, as the fruits matured, the total amount of carotenoids increased while the amount of chlorophyll decreased (Piao et al., 2005). In the fully matured fruit, 65% of total carotenoids was zeaxanthin and 13% was lutein.

Ripening of five red pepper cultivars showed the typical carotenoid biosynthesis pattern for the *Capsicum* genus (Hornero-Méndez et al., 2000). Lutein and neoxanthin, both characteristic of chloroplast pigments, decreased with ripening and eventually disappeared. β-carotene, antheraxanthin, and violaxanthin increased, whereas zeaxanthin, β-cryptoxanthin, capsanthin, capsorubin, capsanthin-5,6-epoxide, and cucurbitaxanthin A were biosynthesized de novo. In six commercial pepper cultivars, β-cryptoxanthin, α-carotene, β-carotene, capsanthin, and zeaxanthin increased considerably, whereas lutein declined to not detectable levels, from the immature to the mature stage (Howard et al., 2000). On the other hand, in a yellow bell cultivar, lutein increased as the color changed from green to yellow. In jalapeño peppers harvested at the intermediate ripening stage, the concentrations of free, mono-, and diesterified carotenoids increased continuously during ripening, from 250 to 584, 29 to 219, and 66 to 306 μg/g dry weight, respectively (Cervantes-Paz et al., 2014). In red pepper (paprika) (*Capsicum annuum*

L. var. Km-622), harvest at unripe stages (color break or faint red) resulted in a high accumulation of dehydroascorbic acid in the overripe fruits, whereas de novo biosynthesis of carotenoids was partially retarded (Márkus et al., 1999).

Although not as pronounced as in fruits, carotenoids in leaves are also affected by maturity. In five different lots of kale, β-carotene and lutein tended to be significantly higher in the mature leaves, whereas violaxanthin tended to be significantly higher in the young leaves (Table 5.1) (Azevedo and Rodriguez-Amaya, 2005). Generally, no significant difference in neoxanthin was observed between young and mature leaves. In endive and lettuce, β-carotene, lutein, violaxanthin, and neoxanthin were all significantly higher in the mature leaves (Azevedo-Meleiro and Rodriguez-Amaya, 2005). Exceptionally, these four major carotenoids were significantly higher in the young leaves than in the mature leaves in New Zealand spinach.

In all three cultivars of lettuce, the β-carotene, neoxanthin, lutein, and violaxanthin contents were significantly lower in the inner leaves than in the outer leaves (Baslam et al., 2013). In another study, however, lutein concentrations were in general significantly higher in younger (lower) leaves of collard, turnip green, and mustard green (Farnham et al., 2012). In 10 commercial varieties of coriander leaves, β-carotene was consistently higher in the mature leaves (507–823 μg/g dry weight) than in the young leaves (323–586 μg/g dry weight) (Divya et al., 2012). The outer leaves of savoy cabbage were found to contain 150 times more lutein and up to 200 times more β-carotene than the average for the inner leaves (Hart and Scott, 1995).

In three types of waxy corn (white, yellow, and black) and normal corn (yellow) grains, lutein generally increased from maturation stage M1 to M2 then declined at complete maturity (Hu and Xu, 2011). Zeaxanthin had the same pattern for white waxy corn but progressively decreased in the other three types as the seed went to full maturity. In four cultivars of yellow-endosperm sorghum (Kean et al., 2007), large increases in total carotenoid occurred between 10 and 30 days after half bloom, resulting in peak accumulation between 6.0 and 28 μg per thousand kernels. Significant decreases were then noted from 30 to 50 days after full bloom, resulting in a final total carotenoid content of 2.6 to 15 μg per thousand kernels. Zeaxanthin, lutein, and β-carotene followed the same trend.

On a dry weight basis, total carotenoid levels were at a maximum early in potato tuber development (Morris et al., 2004). In *S. phureja* total carotenoid remained at a high level throughout tuber development, whereas in *S. tuberosum*, the carotenoid content decreased as the dry weight increased. The major carotenoids in the former were zeaxanthin, antheraxanthin, and violaxanthin, whereas violaxanthin, lutein, and neoxanthin predominated in the latter.

Using nondestructive reflectance spectroscopy, Solovchenko et al. (2005) found that apple fruit detachment triggered, after a lag period of a few days, a sharp increase in the carotenoid content. This increase as a result of 3–4 weeks of off-tree ripening composed 40% of the on-tree level.

In two tomato genotypes, considerable carotenoid accumulation occurred both in vine and postharvest ripening, but at the end of the experiment (after 16 days), the lycopene and β-carotene concentrations in postharvest-ripened tomatoes were almost twice those reached in vine-ripened tomatoes (Giovanelli et al., 1999).

5.7.3 Climate, season, geographic site, and year of production

Geographic and climatic effects can be pronounced. Higher temperature and greater exposure to sunlight increase carotenogenesis in fruits, but excessive sunlight may cause photodegradation. As discussed below, in general, fruits produced in warmer locations have distinctly higher carotenoid contents than those of the same fruits of the same cultivars produced in temperate or colder places. In leafy vegetables produced in open fields, photodegradation appears to prevail, the carotenoid levels being lower in the summer than in the winter. In leaves produced in greenhouses or protected by plastic roofings, however, the carotenoid concentrations tend to be higher in the summer than in the winter.

A dwarf Brazilian banana cultivar produced at seven different locations in Hawaii (on four different islands) had 0.6 to 1.3 μg/g of β-carotene and 1.1 to 1.9 μg/g of lutein (Wall, 2006). Rainbow papaya from four locations varied from 4.2 to 10 μg/g in β-cryptoxanthin, the major carotenoid. In Hamlin, Earlygold, and Budd Blood orange juices, analyzed in the United States from mid-September to mid-January of two consecutive years, lutein and violaxanthin were the predominant carotenoids throughout the season (Lee and Castle, 2001). However, lutein tended to decrease while β-cryptoxanthin and, to a lesser extent, zeaxanthin increased during the season.

Geographic effects were shown by fruits produced in Brazilian states with different climates. Formosa papaya from the temperate São Paulo state had lower β-carotene (1.4 vs. 6.1 μg/g), β-cryptoxanthin (5.3 vs. 8.6 μg/g), and lycopene (19 vs. 26 μg/g) concentrations than those produced in the hot state of Bahia (Kimura et al., 1991). All-*E*-β-carotene was twice as high in Keitt mango from Bahia compared to Keitt mango from São Paulo, and all-*E*-violaxanthin and 9-*Z*-violaxanthin were also higher in the Bahian mangos (Mercadante and Rodriguez-Amaya, 1998). These differences were greater than those observed between cultivars Keitt and Tommy Atkins mangos both produced in São Paulo, indicating that for carotenoids, climatic effects could surpass cultivar differences. Pitanga produced in Campinas had higher all-*E*-lycopene (71 vs. 14 μg/g), 13-*Z*-lycopene (5.0 vs. 1.1 μg/g), and all-*E*-γ-carotene (3.8 vs. 1.6 μg/g) contents than those produced in the colder Medianeira (Porcu and Rodriguez-Amaya, 2008).

With the vitamin C–rich Brazilian fruit camu-camu (*Myrciaria dubia*), fruits from Mirandópolis had higher violaxanthin (1.2 vs. 0.1 μg/g), luteoxanthin (0.6 vs. 0.2 μg/g), lutein (6.0 vs. 1.6 μg/g), zeaxanthin (0.4 vs. 0.2 μg/g), β-carotene (1.4 vs. 0.7 μg/g), and total carotenoid (11 vs. 3.5 μg/g) contents than those of camu-camu from Iguape (Zanatta and Mercadante, 2007). Both municipalities are from the state of São Paulo, but to explain higher carotenoid levels of the former place, higher temperature and light exposure were raised as possible explanation for the higher carotenoid levels of camu-camu from Mirandópolis. With greater sunlight exposure, acerola fruits harvested in 2004 had higher total carotenoid content than those of the 2003 harvest (Rosso and Mercadante, 2005).

In general, the carotenoid levels were higher in the red than in the yellow cashew apples (*Anacardium occidentale* L.) from both northeastern and southeastern regions of Brazil (Assunção and Mercadante, 2003). α-carotene and β-carotene, for example, were about 1.8 and 1.3 times higher in red than in yellow fruits. Yellow fruits from the northeast presented 1.7 times higher provitamin A levels than those from the southeast, but the values were similar for the red fruits.

Total carotenoid was higher in Valencia orange juice from Spain (17 mg/L) than Valencia juice from Belize (4.8 mg/L) (Mouly et al., 1999a). Phytoene was lower and ζ-carotene higher in the Spanish Valencia orange juice. In another study, juices from oranges grown in Mediterranean regions (Israel and Spain) had higher carotenoid content, compared with those of tropical and subtropical regions (Cuba, Belize, and Florida) (Mouly et al., 1999b). The quantitative data allowed differentiation of Valencia oranges according to geographical origins.

Five cultivars of Thai mangoes differed substantially in their β-carotene content between two years of production (Vásquez-Caicedo, 2005); even the ranking was changed. The all-*E*-β-carotene concentrations varied from 14 to 79 μg/g dry weight in 2001 and from 21 to 107 μg/g dry weight in 2002.

Spanish tomatoes were found to be generally superior in carotenoid content and bioaccessibility in comparison with Irish tomatoes, suggesting that geographical location has greater influence than variety (Aherne et al., 2009). A comparison of three processing tomato cultivars grown in four Californian counties during three seasons showed that the mean lycopene concentration was significantly greater in 2000 (106 μg/g) and 1999 (101 μg/g) than in 2001 (88 μg/g) (Garcia and Barrett, 2006).

Notably, the lycopene content of tomato decreased significantly when the temperature of the fruit exceeded 30°C (Brandt et al., 2006). The average lycopene content was the lowest (36 μg/g) when the average temperature of the greenhouse preceding the harvest ranged from 28°C to 32°C. Fruits gathered at two other periods when the temperature was lower had approximately the same higher lycopene level, 65 and 69 μg/g.

In greenhouse cherry tomatoes ('Pomodoro di Pachino', cv. Naomi F1) harvested at six different times of the year, carotenoids (83–151 μg/g) did not show definite seasonal trends or correlation with solar radiation or average temperature (Raffo et al., 2006). Nevertheless, tomatoes harvested in mid-summer were characterized by lowered lycopene levels.

Another study indicated that the antioxidant components of tomatoes could vary considerably with changes in environmental conditions within the greenhouse (Toor et al., 2006). The lycopene content of three commercial New Zealand tomato cultivars studied over a period of 8 months varied from 190 to 730 μg/g dry matter. The mean lycopene content of the three cultivars was 31% lower in the summer months than at other times of the study.

In red pepper (paprika), a rainy and cool season yielded fruits with more β-carotene but less diesters of red xanthophylls as compared with those produced in a relatively dry and warm season (Márkus et al., 1999).

Wu et al. (2008) found a large effect of growing site on the content of β-carotene of the same variety of sweet potato (as much as double), ascribed possibly to sunlight, soil type, and other environmental factors. With the variety Yanshu No. 5, the β-carotene contents in sweet potato grown in different farming sites in the same area ranged from 53 to 84 μg/g.

In potato tubers from 38 lines grown in field plots over three years, a significant difference in total carotenoid content was noted, but the ranking was similar from year to year, and the interaction season and variety was small (Griffiths et al., 2007).

5.7.4 Farming practice and conditions

Studies on the effects of agronomic practices and conditions are still limited, and the results (e.g., open-field vs. greenhouse, conventional vs. organic farming) are somewhat inconsistent.

A two-year study in greenhouse tomato showed that β-carotene, lycopene, and lutein responded negatively to light and positively to temperature (Ehret et al., 2013). None of 10 genes involved with antioxidant biosynthesis/metabolism were affected by salinity in ripe fruit, but the expression of three of them (ζ-carotene desaturase, carotene β-hydroxylase 1, and 9-*Z*-epoxycarotenoid dioxygenase) varied with the stage of fruit development. The carotenoid content was previously shown to increase in cherry tomato produced under the influence of moderate salt stress (Leonardi et al., 2000).

In 13 varieties of *C. annuum* and *C. chinense*, greenhouse-grown peppers contained more carotenoids (particularly lutein) than field-grown peppers (Lee et al., 2005). In another study, levels of most carotenoids in 10 pungent and nonpungent pepper cultivars were significantly higher in glasshouse-grown plants than in plants grown in the field (Russo and Howard 2002). Significantly higher lycopene content was also observed in tomato harvested in greenhouse (83 μg/g) than in the field (59 μg/g) (Brandt et al., 2003). The lycopene content was also shown to be higher in fruits supplied with 50% optimal water intake (86 μg/g) than those supplied with 100% of optimal water intake (62 μg/g).

Conventional Rio Red grapefruit was better colored and higher in lycopene, and the juice was less tart, lower in the bitter principle naringin, and better accepted by the consumer panel than the organic fruit (Lester et al., 2007). On the other hand, in three tomato varieties, when the results were expressed on a fresh weight basis, organic tomatoes had significantly higher lycopene and β-carotene contents than conventional tomatoes (Caris-Veyrat et al., 2004). When expressed on a dry matter basis and in purees made from these tomatoes, no significant difference in carotenoid content was found between the two modes of culture. In mandarin oranges, organic farming resulted in juices with higher contents of carotenoids, containing a total concentration of 14 mg/L compared to 10 mg/L in conventional juice (Beltrán-González et al., 2008). The lycopene content was not statistically different between organic and conventional samples, whereas the level of all-*E*-β-carotene was higher in the conventional marinara pasta sauces (Koh et al., 2008). To the authors, the results suggested that any beneficial differences in levels of carotenoids gained through cultivation practices was not measurable at the consumer level in processed tomato products.

Organic bell pepper contained significantly more dry matter, vitamin C, total carotenoid, β-carotene, α-carotene, *Z*-β-carotene, total phenolic acids, and flavonoids than the conventional fruits (Hallman and Rembialkowska 2012). On the other hand, organic acerola fruit had significantly lower β-carotene content (25 vs. 63 μg/g) than conventionally produced fruits (Cardoso et al., 2011), although carotenoids of persimmon (lycopene and β-carotene) and strawberry (β-carotene) had no significant differences between organic and conventional farming. In general, the nonorganic berry-based desserts (baby foods) contained more carotenoids than the organic type (Jiwan et al., 2010).

In a black grapevine variety, the total carotenoid content of the grapes was similar, with or without irrigation, with higher water retention capacity (C. Oliveira et al., 2003).

With lower retention capacity soil, the levels of carotenoids were approximately 60% lower with irrigation than without irrigation. Soil characteristics had larger influence than irrigation on the concentration of carotenoids in grapes.

Application of Se and Zn (90 to 810 kg/ha) to the soil stimulated an increase of α-carotene and lutein synthesis and a decrease of β-carotene with slight increase in the total carotenoid content of carrots (Biacs et al., 1995). With Mo, the highest dose resulted in a significant decrease in the carotenoid content of the roots. In tomatoes, the type of soil (sand, brown earth) and K treatment did not show a significant effect on lycopene content (Sass-Kiss et al., 2005).

Comparing curly lettuce taken from neighboring farms, the hydroponic lettuce had significantly lower lutein, β-carotene, violaxanthin, and neoxanthin contents than the conventionally produced lettuce (Kimura and Rodriguez-Amaya, 2003). Because the hydroponic farm had a polyethylene covering, less exposure to sunlight and lower temperatures might have decreased carotenoid biosynthesis.

Eight green leaf lettuce and eight red leaf lettuce cultivars grown in a greenhouse (under identical conditions) received supplemental UV-A (320–400 nm) and supplemental UV-A plus UV-B (290–320 nm) radiation (Caldwell and Britz, 2006). Aside from up to 10-fold cultivar-specific differences, supplemental UV-B radiation increased the lutein, β-carotene, and neoxanthin concentrations in green lettuce but reduced the levels of these carotenoids in red lettuce. Field-grown spinach had significantly higher levels of 9-Z-β-carotene and significantly lower 9,13-di-Z-β-carotene compared to greenhouse-grown spinach (Heymann et al., 2014).

The effects of N rate and form on the accumulation of lutein, β-carotene, and chlorophyll pigments were investigated in the leaf tissues of greenhouse grown Winterbor, Toscano, and Redbor kale cultivars (Kopsell et al., 2007). On a fresh weight basis, plant pigment concentrations were not affected by N rate. When calculated on a dry weight basis, however, carotenoid pigments increased linearly in response to increasing N rate. Increasing NO_3-N resulted in increases in both lutein and β-carotene concentrations.

Differences among durum wheat cultivars were observed in their response to water deficit and sulfur fertilization (Fratianni et al., 2013). Simeto cultivar showed a significant effect of water deficit (occurring under a Mediterranean environment) on whole meal and semolina carotenoids, with 20% and 15% increases, respectively. Sulfur fertilization positively impacted mainly Ofanto whole-grain and semolina carotenoids.

Split foliar fertilization and the fertilizer type significantly increased saffron yield, number of flowers, and crocin of the saffron stigma (Rabani-Foroutagheh et al., 2013). The fertilizer Agrimel had the greatest effect, compared to Prolex and Multipurplex.

5.8 CAROTENOID DISTRIBUTION IN A FRUIT OR VEGETABLE

Carotenoids are not uniformly distributed in a fruit, root, or bunch of leafy vegetable. Most fruits have higher carotenoid levels in the peel than in the pulp. Peeled ripe acerola 'Olivier', for example, had 30 μg/g of β-carotene, compared to 38 μg/g in the whole ripe fruits (Porcu and Rodriguez-Amaya, 2006). The total carotenoid content was significantly higher in the peel (25 vs. 8.1 μg/g) than in the pulp of the Amazonian fruit arazá (*Eugenia stipitata* McVaugh) (Garzón et al., 2012), with lutein, β-cryptoxanthin, and zeinoxanthin as the major carotenoids. An exception is pink-fleshed guava, in which lycopene is concentrated in the pulp, compensating the greater amounts of other carotenoids in the peel.

In the Asian fruit gac (*Momordica cochinchinensis*), while the seed membrane contained 101 μg/g β-carotene and 380 μg/g lycopene, the fruit flesh had only 22 and 0.9 μg/g, respectively, of these carotenoids (Aoki et al., 2002). In three species of citrus fruits, *Citrus unshiu*, *C. reticulata*, and *C. sinensis*, the total carotenoid content was significantly higher in the juice sac than in the segment and segment membrane (Abeysinghe et al., 2007). In Yuhuan pummelo, the total carotenoid content of the peel was reported to be 250 times higher than that of juice vesicle (Xu et al., 2006).

Noncorn and corn cereals were hand dissected into endosperm, germ, and aleurone fractions to compare the distribution of carotenoids across the grain (Ndolo and Beta, 2013). Endosperm fractions had total carotenoid ranging from 0.9 to 2.3 μg/g in non-corn cereals (barley, oat, and wheat) and 14 to 31 μg/g in corn cereals. Lutein and zeaxanthin contents were higher in the germs of noncorn cereals but lower in noncorn cereal endosperm. The aleurone layer had zeaxanthin levels 2- to 5-fold higher than lutein among the cereals.

The pale green kohlrabi (turnip cabbage) had 9.5 μg/g β-carotene and 6.7 μg/g lutein in the skin but only 1.3 μg/g β-carotene and 0.8 μg/g lutein in the flesh (Park et al., 2012). The corresponding values for the purple kohlrabi were 6.2 μg/g β-carotene and 5.5 μg/g lutein in the skin and only 0.5 μg/g β-carotene and 0.3 μg/g lutein in the flesh. All values are expressed on a dry weight basis.

In cassava, the carotenoid content was higher in the part of the root closest to its attachment to the stem (proximal section), gradually decreasing toward the opposite end (distal section) (Chávez et al., 2008). Across the root, carotenoid content was higher in the core, lower toward the periphery.

5.9 METABOLIC ENGINEERING OF CAROTENOID BIOSYNTHESIS

Advances in knowledge of plant biochemical pathways, cloning of the genes that code the enzymes responsible for carotenoid biosynthesis, and availability of gene transfer techniques have paved the way for genetic engineering of the biosynthetic pathway in crop plants and in microorganisms to achieve higher content or better composition of carotenoids. Numerous reviews have been published on the underlying principles and potential applications of this modern technique for this purpose (Hirschberg, 1999; van den Berg et al., 2000; Guiliano et al., 2000, 2008; Sandmann, 2001a,b; Matthews et al., 2003; Fraser and Bramley, 2004; Botella-Pavía and Rodríguez-Concepción, 2006; Zhu et al., 2009; Farré et al., 2011; V.M. Ye and Bhatia 2012; Shumskaya and Wurtzel, 2013).

As shown with sweet corn and broccoli, improving carotenoid content in vegetable crops by conventional breeding is feasible (Ibrahim and Juvik, 2009). However, advantages of genetic engineering over conventional breeding include the ability to transfer genes in a faster and targeted manner. In addition to the transfer of genes and cDNAs from the same species, modern recombinant technology permits the introduction of genetic material from diverse plants and unrelated species such as microorganisms.

To increase the carotenoid contents of foods, two strategies can be followed: (a) fermentative production in a microorganism, followed by isolation and addition to processed food, (b) the desired carotenoid can be biosynthesized in food plants and consumed directly (Sandmann, 2001b). The first approach is employed in preparing carotenoid food and feed additives, discussed in Chapter 8.

Different approaches have been followed to modify the carotenoid content in plants to enhance the nutritional value (Sandmann, 2001a):

- Modification of the carotenoid pathway to enhance formation of a specific carotenoid (e.g., β-carotene, as in maize).
- Increasing the amounts of preexisting carotenoids, as in rapeseed (Shewmaker et al., 1999).
- Engineering a carotenoid pathway in tissue that is completely devoid of carotenoids, such as rice endosperm (X. Ye et al., 2000).

In engineering corn plants to accumulate higher levels of β-carotene, an initial concern was that such a strategy could reduce lutein and zeaxanthin, which are also important for human health. Available evidence suggests that diverting flux specifically toward β-carotene by conventional and/or biotechnological means can result in enhanced production of lutein and zeaxanthin as well as other carotenoids (Farré et al., 2011).

Overexpression of a bacterial phytoene synthase gene increased the carotenoid content of mature rapeseed by up to 50-fold (Shewmaker et al., 1999). Considered a great achievement, this tremendous increase in β-carotene concentration in modified rapeseeds yields β-carotene-enriched oils.

The rice grain is devoid of carotenoids but is able to synthesize geranylgeranyl diphosphate. Genetic modification to establish a β-carotene biosynthestic pathway in rice endosperm was achieved by introducing the genes that code for phytoene synthase and lycopene β-cyclase, both from daffodil (*Narcissus pseudonarcissus*), together with a gene from the bacteria *Erwinia uredovora*, which codes for a desaturase that catalyzes desaturation from phytoene to lycopene (X. Ye et al., 2000; Beyer et al., 2002). Further studies revealed that the presence of the cyclase was not necessary as phytoene synthase and desaturase alone were able to drive β-carotene synthesis. The genetically modified rice, which became known as Golden Rice, had a maximum level of 1.6 μg/g total carotenoids. Subsequent studies had shown that the source of the PSY gene had a significant impact on the level of carotenoid accumulation. Substitution of the daffodil gene with that of corn resulted in Golden Rice 2, which accumulated 23-fold more carotenoids (maximum of 37 μg/g) than the original Golden Rice (Paine et al., 2005).

Sandmann (2001b) pointed out three basic problems for the successful manipulation of a pathway for higher metabolite levels or novel compounds:

- Precursors are consumed at the expense of existing pathways.
- Interference with a well-balanced regulation pathway might occur.

- Product storage, especially when highly lipophilic compounds such as carotenoids are generated, must be ensured. A major problem for reaching high yields is the storage capacity of the hosts.

The final barrier of all these efforts in genetic engineering of the carotenoid pathway to achieve higher content or a better composition of carotenoids is approval of the resulting genetically modified (GM) foods for commercialization and consumer acceptance. The safety of GM foods is still a hotly debated issue. Food components are significantly affected by various genetic and environmental factors, such that it can be very difficult to detect potential adverse effects caused by the introduction of a transgene (Kitta, 2013). The very nature of foods as complex, multicomponent systems makes the application of traditional toxicological testing not necessarily appropriate for GM foods. A comparative approach focusing on the identification of differences between GM foods and their conventional counterparts is considered the most appropriate strategy for the safety assessment of GM foods (OECD, 1993; WHO, 1995). This concept of substantial equivalence for evaluation of food safety and nutritional quality in GM foods is widely shared by authorities in many countries. Botella-Pavía and Rodríguez-Concepción (2006) suggested the development of genomic and metabolomic approaches to carefully analyze the molecular and biochemical consequences of metabolic engineering of carotenoid biosynthesis in plants and ascertain that the expected nutritional improvement of the derived foods is achieved without affecting the metabolic pathways negatively.

5.10 CAROTENOIDS OF ANIMAL-DERIVED FOODS

Raw milk (4.4% fat) from the Netherlands contains an average of 40 μg retinol and 20 μg carotenoids per 100 g, 90% of which is β-carotene (Hulshof et al., 2006). Compared to summer milk, winter milk contains 20% less retinol and β-carotene. Retention of retinol and β-carotene per gram fat in hard cheese is one-third to one-half in relation to the corresponding raw milk. In liquid and semiliquid dairy products (pasteurized milk, buttermilk, vanilla custard, and yogurt), retention of both compounds is above 80%.

Among ruminants, only bovines accumulate high concentrations of carotenoids, mainly β-carotene and, to a lesser extent, lutein (Nozière et al., 2006). β-carotene concentration in milk depends on its dietary supply, and that of cheese is highly linked to milk concentration. Gentili et al. (2013) found 243 μg/L of β-carotene and 7.0 μg/L of β-cryptoxanthin in cow's milk but did not detect these carotenoids in the milk samples of buffalo, sheep, goat, and donkey. Lutein was encountered at 10 μg/L in cow's milk, 9.9 μg/L in sheep's milk, and trace level in goat's milk but was not detected in buffalo's or donkey's milk.

Human milk samples from Northern Ireland mothers had lutein and zeaxanthin concentrations of 0.42 to 9.98 nmol/g fat and undetected to 1.70 nmol/g fat, respectively (Jewell et al., 2004). Five of six formula milks also contained lutein and zeaxanthin with concentrations of 0.7–9.7 and 0.1–1.2 nmol/g fat, respectively, the probable source being egg yolk.

Egg yolk from California, Illinois, Massachusetts, and Mexico had average lutein concentrations of 9.8, 8.8, 6.4, and 15 μg/g, respectively (Rasmussen et al., 2012). The corresponding values for zeaxanthin were 6.7, 6.8, 8.5, and 9.6 μg/g.

Astaxanthin is the red pigment of salmon, trout, and Arctic char, as well as of cooked shrimp, lobster, and crab. It may be found free, esterified in one or both hydroxyl groups with different fatty acids, or as a complex with proteins (carotenoproteins) or lipoproteins (carotenolipoproteins) (Shahidi and Brown, 1998). The total carotenoid content of the major marine crab (*Charybdis cuciata*) (3.4 μg/g in the meat and 11 μg/g in the shell) and freshwater crab (*Potamon potamon*) (4.1 μg/g in the meat and 6.9 in the shell) from Indian waters was low (Sachindra et al., 2005). Astaxanthin and its esters were the major carotenoids in the marine crab; zeaxanthin was the main carotenoid of the freshwater crab.

References

Abeysinghe DC, Li X, Sun CD, Zhang WS, Zhou CH, Chen KS. 2007. Bioactive compounds and antioxidant capacities in different edible tissues of citrus fruit of four species. *Food Chem* 104:1338–44.

Abushita AA, Daood HG, Biacs PA. 2000. Change in carotenoids and antioxidant vitamins in tomato as a function of varietal and technological factors. *J Agric Food Chem* 48:2075–81.

Adom KK, Sorrells ME, Liu RH. 2003. Phytochemical profiles and antioxidant activity of wheat varieties. *J Agric Food Chem* 51:7825–34.

Aherne SA, Jiwan MA, Daly T, O'Brien NM. 2009. Geographical location has greater impact on carotenoid content and bioaccessibility from tomatoes than variety. *Plant Food Hum Nutr* 64:250–6.

Alasalvar C, Grigor JM, Zhang D, Quantick PC, Shahidi F. 2001. Comparison of volatiles, phenolics, sugars, antioxidant vitamins, and sensory quality of different colored carrot varieties. *J Agric Food Chem* 49:1410–6.

Aoki H, Kieu NTM, Kuze N, Tomisaka K, Chuyen NV. 2002. Carotenoid pigments in GAC fruit (*Momordica cochinchinensis* Spreng). *Biosci Biotechnol Biochem* 66:2479–82.

Aruna G, Baskaran V. 2010. Comparative study on the levels of carotenoids lutein, zeaxanthin and β-carotene in Indian spices of nutritional and medicinal importance. *Food Chem* 123:404–9.

Aruna G, Mamatha BS, Baskaran V. 2009. Lutein content of selected Indian vegetables and vegetable oils determined by HPLC. *J Food Compos Anal* 22:632–6.

Ashton OBO, Wong M, McGhie TK, Vather R, Wang Y, Requejo-Jackman C, Ramankutty P, Woolf AB. 2006. Pigments in avocado tissue and oil. *J Agric Food Chem* 54:10151–8.

Assunção RB, Mercadante AZ. 2003. Carotenoids and ascorbic acid from cashew apple (*Anacardium occidentale* L.): variety and geographic effects. *Food Chem* 81:495–502.

Azevedo CH, Rodriguez-Amaya DB. 2005. Carotenoid composition of kale as influenced by maturity, season and minimal processing. *J Sci Food Agric* 85:591–7.

Azevedo-Meleiro CH, Rodriguez-Amaya DB. 2004. Confirmation of the identity of the carotenoids of tropical fruits by HPLC-DAD and HPLC-MS. *J Food Compos Anal* 17:385–96.

Azevedo-Meleiro CH, Rodriguez-Amaya DB. 2005. Carotenoids of endive and New Zealand spinach as affected by maturity, season and minimal processing. *J Food Compos Anal* 18:845–55.

Azevedo-Meleiro CH, Rodriguez-Amaya DB. 2007. Qualitative and quantitative differences in carotenoid composition among *Cucurbita moschata, Cucurbita maxima* and *Cucurbita pepo*. *J Agric Food Chem* 55:4027–33.

Azevedo-Meleiro CH, Rodriguez-Amaya DB. 2009. Qualitative and quantitative differences in the carotenoid composition of yellow and red peppers determined by HPLC-DAD-MS. *J Sep Sci* 32:3652–8.

Baslam M, Morales F, Garmendia I, Goicoechea N. 2013. Nutritional quality of outer and inner leaves of green and red pigmented lettuces (*Lactuca sativa* L.) consumed as salads. *Sci Hort* 151:103–11.

Bauernfeind JC (ed). 1981. *Carotenoids as colorants and vitamin A precursors*. New York: Academic Press.

Bellomo MG, Fallico B. 2007. Anthocyanins, chlorophylls and xanthophylls in pistachio nuts (*Pistacia vera*) of different geographic origin. *J Food Compos Anal* 20:352–9.

Beltrán-González F, Pérez-López AJ, López-Nicolás JM, Carbonell-Barrachina AA. 2008. Effects of agricultural practices on instrumental color, mineral content, carotenoid composition, and sensory quality of mandarin orange juice, cv. Hernandina. *J Sci Food Agric* 88:1731–8.

Ben-Amotz A, Fishler R. 1998. Analysis of carotenoids with emphasis on 9-*cis*-β-carotene in vegetables and fruits commonly consumed in Israel. *Food Chem* 62:515–20.

Berardo N, Brenna OV, Amato A, Valoti P, Pisacane V, Motto M. 2004. Carotenoids concentration among maize genotypes measured by near infrared reflectance spectroscopy (NIRS). *Innov Food Sci Emerg Technol* 5:393–8.

Beyer P, Al-Babili S, Ye X, Lucca P, Schaub P, Welsch R, Potrykus I. 2002. Golden rice: introducing the β-carotene biosynthesis pathway into rice endosperm by genetic engineering to defeat vitamin A deficiency. *J Nutr* 132:506S–10S.

Biacs PA, Daood HG, Kádár I. 1995. Effect of Mo, Se, Zn, and Cr treatments on the yield, element concentration and carotenoid content of carrot. *J Agric Food Chem* 43:589–91.

Botella-Pavía P, Rodríguez-Concepción M. 2006. Carotenoid biotechnology in plants for nutritionally improved foods. *Physiol Plant* 126:369–81.

Boudries H, Kefalas P, Hornero-Méndez D. 2007. Carotenoid composition of Algerian date varieties (*Phoenix dactylifera*) at different edible maturation stages. *Food Chem* 101:1372–7.

Brandt S, Lugasi A, Barna E, Hóvári J, Pék Z, Helyes L. 2003. Effects of the growing methods and conditions on the lycopene content of tomato fruits. *Acta Aliment* 32:269–78.

Brandt S, Pék Z, Barna E, Lugasi A, Helyes L. 2006. Lycopene content and colour of ripening tomatoes as affected by environmental conditions. *J Sci Food Agric* 86:568–72.

Breithaupt DE, Bamedi A. 2001. Carotenoid esters in vegetables and fruits: A screening with emphasis on β-cryptoxanthin esters. *J Agric Food Chem* 49:2064–70.

Caldwell CR, Britz SJ. 2006. Effect of supplemental ultraviolet radiation on the carotenoid and chlorophyll composition of green house-grown leaf lettuce (*Lactuca sativa* L.) cultivars. *J Food Compos Anal* 19:637–44.

Campbell OE, Merwin IA, Padilla-Zakour OI. 2013. Characterization and the effect of maturity at harvest on the phenolic and carotenoid content of Northeast USA apricot (*Prunus armenica*) varieties. *J Agric Food Chem* 61:12700–10.

Cardoso PC, Tomazini APB, Stringheta PC, Ribeiro SMR, Pinheiro-Sant'Ana HM. 2011. Vitamin C and carotenoids in organic and conventional fruits grown in Brazil. *Food Chem* 126:411–6.

Caris-Veyrat C, Amiot M-J, Tyssandier V, Grasselly D, Buret M, Mikolajczak M, Guilland J-C, Bouteloup-Demange C, Borel P. 2004. Influence of organic versus conventional agriculture practice on the antioxidant microconstituent content of tomatoes and derived purees: consequences on antioxidant plasma status in humans. *J Agric Food Chem* 52:6503–9.

Cervantes-Paz B, Yahia EM, Ornelas-Paz JJ, Victoria-Campos CI, Ibarra-Junguera V, Pérez-Martínez JD, Escalante-Minakata P. 2014. Antioxidant activity and content of chlorophylls and carotenoids in raw and heat-processed jalapeño peppers at intermediate stages of ripening. *Food Chem* 146:188–96.

Chandrika UG, Basnayake BMLB, Athukorala I, Colombagama PWNM, Goonetilleke A. 2010. Carotenoid content and *in vitro* bioaccessibility of lutein in some leafy vegetables popular in Sri Lanka. *J Nutr Sci Vitaminol* 56:203–7.

Chandrika UG, Jansz ER, Wickramasinghe SMDN, Warnasuriya N. 2003. Carotenoids in yellow- and red-fleshed papaya (*Carica papaya* L). *J Sci Food Agric* 83:1279–82.

Chávez AL, Ceballos H, Rodriguez-Amaya DB, Pérez JC, Sánchez T, Calle F, Morante, N. 2008. Sampling variation for carotenoids and dry matter contents in cassava roots. *J Root Crops* 34:43–9.

Cortés C, Esteve MJ, Frígola A, Torregosa F. 2004. Identification and quantification of carotenoids including geometrical isomers in fruit and vegetable juices by liquid chromatography with ultraviolet-diode array detection. *J Agric Food Chem* 52: 2203–12.

Delgado-Pelayo R, Hornero-Méndez D. 2012. Identification and quantitative analysis of carotenoids and their esters from sarsaparilla (*Smilax aspera* L.) berries. *J Agric Food Chem* 60:8225–32.

Dhuique-Mayer C, Caris-Veyrat C, Ollitrault P, Curk F, Amiot MJ. 2005. Varietal and interspecific influence on micronutrient contents in citrus from the Mediterranean area. *J Agric Food Chem* 53:2140–5.

Dias MG, Camões MFGFC, Oliveira L. 2009. Carotenoids in traditional Portuguese fruits and vegetables. *Food Chem* 113:808–15.

Divya P, Puthusseri B, Neelwarne B. 2012. Carotenoid content, its stability during drying and the antioxidant activity of commercial coriander (*Coriandrum sativum* L.) varieties. *Food Res Int* 45:342–350.

Dragovic-Uzelac V, Levaj B, Mrkic V, Bursac D, Boras M. 2007. The content of polyphenols and carotenoids in three apricot cultivars depending on stage of maturity and geographical region. *Food Chem* 102:966–75.

Dugo P, Herrero M, Giuffrida D, Ragonese C, Dugo, G, Mondello L. 2008. Analysis of native carotenoid composition in orange juice using C30 columns in tandem. *J Sep Sci* 31:2151–60.

Ehret DL, Usher K, Helmer T, Block G, Steinke D, Frey B, Kuang T, Diarra M. 2013. Tomato fruit antioxidants in relation to salinity and greenhouse climate. *J Agric Food Chem* 61:1138–45.

Englberger L, Aalbersberg W, Dolodolotawake U, Schierle J, Humphries J, Luta T, Marks GC, Fitzgerald MH, Rimon B, Kaiririete M. 2006a. Carotenoid content of pandanus fruit cultivars and other foods of the Republic of Kiribati. *Public Health Nutr* 9:633–43.

Englberger L, Aalbersberg W, Ravi P, Bonnin E, Marks GC, Fitzgerald MH, Elymore J. 2003a. Further analyses on Micronesian banana, taro, breadfruit and other food for provitamin A carotenoids and minerals. *J Food Compos Anal* 16:219–36.

Englberger L, Aalbersberg W, Schierle J, Marks GC, Fitzgerald MH, Muller F, Jekkein A, Alfred J, Velde NV. 2006b. Carotenoid content of different edible pandanus cultivars of the republic of the Marshall Islands. *J Food Compos Anal* 19:484–94.

Englberger L, Schierle J, Kraemer K, Aalbersberg W, Dolodolotawake U, Humpries J, Graham R, Reid AP, Lorens A, Albert K, Levendusky A, Johnson E, Paul Y, Sengebau F. 2008. Carotenoid and mineral content of Micronesian giant swamp taro (*Cyrtosperma*) cultivars. *J Food Compos Anal* 21:93–106.

Englberger L, Schierle J, Marks GC, Fitgerald MH. 2003b. Micronesian banana, taro and other foods: newly recognized sources of provitamin A and other carotenoids. *J Food Compos Anal* 16:3–19.

Englberger L, Wills RBH, Blades B, Dufficy L, Daniells JW, Coyne T. 2006c. Carotenoid content and flesh color of selected banana cultivars growing in Australia. *Food Nutr Bull* 27:281–91.

Fanciullino A-L, Dhuique-Mayer C, Luro F, Casanova J, Morillon R, Ollitrault P. 2006. Carotenoid diversity in cultivated citrus is highly influenced by genetic factors. *J Agric Food Chem* 54:4397–406.

Faria AF de, Rosso VV de, Mercadante AZ. 2009. Carotenoid composition of jackfruit (*Artocarpus heterophyllus*), determined by HPLC-PDA-MS/MS. *Plant Foods Hum Nutr* 64:108–15.

Farnham MW, Lester GE, Hassel R. 2012. Collard, mustard and turnip greens: effects of genotypes and leaf position on concentrations of ascorbic acid, folate, β-carotene, lutein and phylloquinone. *J Food Compos Anal* 27:1–7.

Farré G, Bai C, Twyman RM, Capell T, Christou P, Zhu C. 2011. Nutritious crops producing multiple carotenoids: a metabolic balancing act. *Trends Plant Sci* 16:532–40.

Fernández-León MF, Fernández-León AM, Lozano M, Ayuso MC, González-Gómez D. 2012. Identification, quantification and comparison of the principal bioactive compounds and external quality parameters of two broccoli cultivars. *J Funct Foods* 4:465–73.

Fernandez-Orozco R, Gallardo-Guerrero L, Hornero-Méndez D. 2013. Carotenoid profiling in tubers of different potato (*Solanum* sp.) cultivars: accumulation of carotenoids mediated by xanthophyll esterification. *Food Chem* 141:2864–72.

Fraser PD, Bramley PM. 2004. The biosynthesis and nutritional uses of carotenoids. *Prog Lipid Res* 43:228–65.

Fratianni A, Giuzio L, Di Criscio T, Zina F, Panfili G. 2013. Response of carotenoids and tocols of durum wheat in relation to water stress and sulfur fertilization. *J Agric Food Chem* 61:2583–90.

Furtado JD, Siles X, Campos H. 2004. Carotenoid concentrations in vegetables and fruits common to the Costa Rican diet. *Int J Food Sci Nutr* 55:101–13.

Garcia E, Barrett DM. 2006. Assessing lycopene content in California processing tomatoes. *J Food Process Preserv* 30:56–70.

Garzón GA, Narváez-Cuenca C-E, Kopec RE, Barry AM, Riedl KM, Schwartz SJ. 2012. Determination of carotenoids, total phenolic content, and antioxidant activity of arazá (*Eugenia stipitata* McVaugh), an Amazonian fruit. *J Agric Food Chem* 60:4709–17.

Gentili A, Caretti F, Bellante S, Ventura S, Canepari S, Curini R. 2013. Comprehensive profiling of carotenoids and fat-soluble vitamins in milk from different animal species by LC-DAD-MS/MS hyphenation. *J Agric Food Chem* 61:1628–39.

George B, Kaur C, Khurdiya DS, Kapoor HC. 2004. Antioxidants in tomato (*Lycopersicum esculentum*) as a function of genotype. *Food Chem* 84:45–51.

Giovanelli G, Lavelli V, Peri C, Nobili S. 1999. Variation in antioxidant components of tomato during vine and post-harvest ripening. *J Sci Food Agric* 79:1583–1588.

Giuffrida D, Dugo P, Torre G, Bignardi C, Cavazza A, Corradini C, Dugo G. 2013. Characterization of 12 *Capsicum* varieties by evaluation of their carotenoid profile and pungency determination. *Food Chem* 140:794–802.

Giuliano G, Aquilani R, Dharmapuri S. 2000. Metabolic engineering of plant carotenoids. *Trends Plant Sci* 5:406–9.

Giuliano G, Tavazza R, Diretto G, Beyer P, Taylor MA. 2008. Metabolic engineering of carotenoid biosynthesis in plants. *Trends Biotechnol* 26:139–145.

Godoy HT, Rodriguez-Amaya DB. 1995a. Buriti (*Mauritia vinifera* Mart), uma fonte riquíssima de pró-vitamina A. *Arquiv Biol Tecnol* 38:109–120.

Godoy HT, Rodriguez-Amaya DB. 1995b. Carotenoid composition and vitamin A value of Brazilian loquat (*Eriobotrya japonica* Lindl.). *Archiv Latinoamer Nutr* 45:336–9.

Godoy HT, Rodriguez-Amaya DB. 1998. Composição de carotenóides em nectarina (*Prunus persica*) brasileira. *Rev Inst Adolfo Lutz* 57:73–9.

Grassmann J, Schnitzler WH, Habegger R. 2007. Evaluation of different coloured carrot cultivars on antioxidative capacity based on their carotenoid and phenolic contents. *Int J Food Sci Nutr* 58:603–11.

Griffiths DW, Dale MFB, Morris WL, Ramsay G. 2007. Effects of season and postharvest storage on the carotenoid content of *Solanum phureja* potato tubers. *J Agric Food Chem* 55:379–85.

Gross J. 1987. *Pigments in fruits*. London: Academic Press.

Gross J. 1991. *Pigments in vegetables: chlorophylls and carotenoids*. New York: Van Nostrand Reinhold.

Guil-Guerrero JL, Martínez-Guirado C, Rebolloso-Fuentes MM, Carrique-Pérez A. 2006. Nutrient composition and antioxidant activity of 10 pepper (*Capsicum annuum*) varieties. *Eur Food Res Technol* 224:1–9.

Hallmann E, Rembialkowska E. 2012. Characterization of antioxidant compounds in sweet bell pepper (*Capsicum annuum* L.) under organic and conventional growing systems. *J Sci Food Agric* 92: 2409–2415.

Hart DJ, Scott KJ. 1995. Development and evaluation of an HPLC method for the analysis of carotenoids in foods, and the measurement of the carotenoid content of vegetables and fruits commonly consumed in the UK. *Food Chem* 54:101–11.

Heyman T, Westphal L, Weesjohann L, Glomb MA. 2014. Growing and processing conditions lead to changes in the carotenoid profile of spinach. *J Agric Food Chem* 62:4960–7.

Hirschberg J. 1999. Production of high-value compounds: carotenoids and vitamin E. *Curr Opin Biotechnol* 10:186–91.

Holden JM, Eldridge AL, Beecher GR, Buzzard IM, Bhagwat S, Davis CS, Douglass LW, Gebhardt S, Haytowitz D, Schakel S. 1999. Carotenoid content of US foods: an update of the database. *J Food Compos Anal* 12:169–96.

Hornero-Méndez D, Costa-García J, Mínguez-Mosquera MI. 2002. Characterization of carotenoid high-producing *Capsicum annuum* cultivars selected for paprika production. *J Agric Food Chem* 50:5711–6.

Hornero-Méndez D, de Guevara RGL, Mínguez-Mosquera MI. 2000. Carotenoid biosynthesis changes in five red pepper (*Capsicum annuum* L.) cultivars during ripening. Cultivar selection for breeding. *J Agric Food Chem* 48:3857–64.

Hornero-Méndez A, Mínguez-Mosquera MI. 2000. Carotenoid pigments in *Rosa mosqueta* hips, an alternative source for foods. *J Agric Food Chem* 48:825–8.

Howard LR, Talcott ST, Brenes CH, Villalon B. 2000. Changes in phytochemical and antioxidant activity of selected pepper cultivars (*Capsicum* species) as influenced by maturity. *J Agric Food Chem* 48:1713–20.

Hu Q-P, Xu J-G. 2011. Profiles of carotenoids, anthocyanins, phenolics, and antioxidant activity of selected color waxy corn grains during maturation. *J Agric Food Chem* 59:2026–33.

Huang AS, Tanudjaja L, Lum D. 1999. Content of alpha-, beta-carotene, and dietary fiber in 18 sweetpotato varieties grown in Hawaii. *J Food Compos Anal* 12:147–151.

Hulshof PJM, van Roekel-Jansen T, van de Bovenkamp P, West CE. 2006. Variation in retinol and carotenoid content of milk and milk products in The Netherlands. *J Food Compos Anal* 19:67–75.

Humphries JM, Khachik F. 2003. Distribution of lutein, zeaxanthin, and related geometrical isomers in fruit, vegetables, wheat, and pasta products. *J Agric Food Chem* 51:1322–7.

Ibrahim KE, Juvik JA. 2009. Feasibility for improving phytonutrient content in vegetable crops using conventional breeding strategies: case study with carotenoids and tocopherols in sweet corn and broccoli. *J Agric Food Chem* 57:4636–44.

Ishida BK, Chapman MH. 2004. A comparison of carotenoid content and total antioxidant activity in catsup from several commercial sources in the United States. *J Agric Food Chem* 52:8017–20.

Ishida BK, Turner C, Chapman MH, McKeon TA. 2004. Fatty acid and carotenoid composition of gac (*Momordica cochinchinensis* Spreng) fruit. *J Agric Food Chem* 52:274–9.

Jewell VC, Mayes CBD, Tubman TRJ, Northrop-Clewes CA, Thurnham DI. 2004. A comparison of lutein and zeaxanthin concentrations in formula and human milk samples from Northern Ireland mothers. *Eur J Clin Nutr* 58:90–7.

Jiwan MA, Duane P, O'Sullivan L, O'Brien NM, Aherne SA. 2010. Content and bioaccessibility of carotenoids from organic and non-organic baby foods. *J Food Compos Anal* 23:346–52.

Kean EG, Ejeta G, Hamaker BR, Ferruzzi MG. 2007. Characterization of carotenoid pigments in mature and developing kernels of selected yellow-endosperm sorghum varieties. *J Agric Food Chem* 55:2619–26.

Kidmose U, Hansen SL, Christensen LP, Edelenbos M, Larsen E, Norbaek R. 2004. Effects of genotype, root size, storage, and processing on bioactive compounds in organically grown carrots (*Daucus carota* L.). *J Food Sci* 69:S388–94.

Kidmose U, Knuthsen P, Edelenbos M, Justesen U, Hegelund E. 2001. Carotenoids and flavonoids in organically grown spinach (*Spinacia oleracea* L.) genotypes after deep frozen storage. *J Sci Food Agric* 81:918–23.

Kim Y-N, Giraud DW, Driskell JA. 2007. Tocopherol and carotenoid contents of selected Korean fruits and vegetables. *J Food Compos Anal* 20:458–65.

Kimura M, Rodriguez-Amaya DB. 2002. A scheme for obtaining standards and HPLC quantification of leafy vegetable carotenoids. *Food Chem* 78:389–98.

Kimura M, Rodriguez-Amaya DB. 2003. Carotenoid composition of hydroponic leafy vegetables. *J Agric Food Chem* 51:2603–7.

Kimura M, Rodriguez-Amaya DB, Yokoyama SM. 1991. Cultivar differences and geographic effects on the carotenoid composition and vitamin A value of papaya. *Lebensm Wissen Technol* 24:415–8.

Kitta K. 2013. Availability and utility of crop composition data. *J Agric Food Chem* 61:8304–11.

Kobori CN, Rodriguez-Amaya DB. 2008. Uncultivated green leaves are richer sources of carotenoids than are commercially produced leafy vegetables. *Food Nutr Bull* 29:333–41.

Koh E, Wimalasiri K, Renaud E, Mitchell AE. 2008. A comparison of flavonoids, carotenoids and vitamin C in commercial organic and conventional marinara paste sauce. *J Sci Food Agric* 88:344–54.

Kopsell DA, Kopsell DE, Curran-Celentano J. 2007. Carotenoid pigments in kale are influenced by nitrogen concentration and form. *J Sci Food Agric* 87:900–7.

Kopsell DA, Kopsell DE, Lefsrud MG, Curran-Celentano J, Dukach LE. 2004. Variation in lutein, β-carotene, and chlorophyll concentrations among *Brassica oleracea* cultigens and seasons. *HortSci* 39:361–4.

Kurilich AC, Juvik JA. 1999. Quantification of carotenoid and tocopherol antioxidants in *Zea mays*. *J Agric Food Chem* 47:1948–55.

Kurilich AC, Tsau GJ, Brown A, Howard L, Klein BP, Jeffery EH, Kushad M, Wallig MA, Juvik JA. 1999. Carotene, tocopherol, and ascorbate contents in subspecies of *Brassica oleracea*. *J Agric Food Chem* 47:1576–81.

Lachman J, Hejtmánková K, Kotíková Z. 2013. Tocols and carotenoids of einkorn, emmer and spring wheat varieties: selection for breeding and production. *J Cereal Sci* 57:207–14.

Lako J, Trenerry VC, Wahlqvist M, Wattanapenpaiboon N, Sotheeswaran S, Premier R. 2007. Phytochemical flavonols, carotenoids and the antioxidant properties of a wide selection of Fijian fruit, vegetables and other readily available foods. *Food Chem* 101:1727–1741.

Lakshminarayana R, Raju M, Krishnakantha TP, Baskaran V. 2005. Determination of major carotenoids in a few Indian leafy vegetables by high-performance liquid chromatography. *J Agric Food Chem* 53:2838–42.

Lam K-W, But P. 1999. The content of zeaxanthin in Gou Qi Zi, a potential health benefit to improve visual acuity. *Food Chem* 67:173–6.

Laurie SM, van Jaarsveld PJ, Faber M, Philpott MF, Labuschagne MT. 2012. *Trans*-β-carotene, selected mineral content and potential nutritional contribution of 12 sweetpotato varieties. *J Food Compos Anal* 27:151–9.

Lee HS. 2001. Characterization of carotenoids in juice of red navel orange (Cara Cara). *J Agric Food Chem* 49:2563–8.

Lee HS, Castle WS. 2001. Seasonal changes of carotenoid pigments and color in Hamlin, Earlygold, and Budd Blood orange juices. *J Agric Food Chem* 49:877–82.

Lee JJ, Crosby KM, Pike LM, Yoo KS, Leskovar DI. 2005. Impact of genetic and environmental variation on development of flavonoids and carotenoids in pepper (*Capsicum* spp.). *Sci Hort* 106:341–52.

Leenhardt F, Lyan B, Rock E, Boussard A, Potus J, Chanliaud E, Remesy C. 2006. Genetic variability of carotenoid concentration, and lipoxygenase and peroxidase activities among cultivated wheat species and bread wheat varieties. *Eur J Agron* 25:170–6.

Lenucci MS, Cadinu D, Taurino M, Piro G, Dalessandro G. 2006. Antioxidant composition in cherry and high-pigment tomato cultivars. *J Agric Food Chem* 54:2606–13.

Leonardi C, Ambrosino P, Esposito F, Fogliano V. 2000. Antioxidative activity and carotenoid and tomatine contents in different typologies of French consumption tomatoes. *J Agric Food Chem* 48:4723–7.

Lester GE, Manthey JA, Buslig BS. 2007. Organic vs conventionally grown Rio Red whole grapefruit and juice: comparison of production inputs, market quality, consumer acceptance, and human health-bioactive compounds. *J Agric Food Chem* 55:4474–80.

Li W, Beta T. 2012. An evaluation of carotenoid levels and composition of glabrous canaryseed. *Food Chem* 133:782–6.

Lin SD, Chen AO. 1995. Major carotenoids in juices of ponkan mandarin and liucheng orange. *J Food Biochem* 18:273–83.

Liu F-X, Fu S-F, Bi X-F, Chen F, Liao X-J, Hu X-S, Wu J-H. 2013. Physico-chemical and antioxidant properties of four mango (*Mangifera indica* L.) cultivars in China. *Food Chem* 138:396–405.

López A, Javier G-A, Fenoll J, Hellín P, Flores P. 2014. Chemical composition and antioxidant capacity of lettuce: comparative study of regular-sized (Romaine) and baby-sized (Little Gem and Mini Romaine) types. *J Food Compos Anal* 33:39–48.

Lugasi A, Bíró L, Hóváre J, Sági KV, Brandt S, Barna E. 2003. Lycopene content of foods and lycopene intake in two groups of the Hungarian population. *Nutr Res* 23:1035–44.

Marinova D, Ribarova F. 2007. HPLC determination of carotenoids in Bulgarian berries. *J Food Compos Anal* 20:370–4.

Márkus F, Daood HG, Kapitány J, Biacs PA. 1999. Change in the carotenoid and antioxidant content of spice red pepper (paprika) as a function of ripening and some technological factors. *J Agric Food Chem* 47:100–7.

Martínez-Valverde I, Periago MJ, Provan G, Chesson A. 2002. Phenolic compounds, lycopene and antioxidant activity in commercial varieties of tomato (*Lycopersicum esculentum*). *J Sci Food Agric* 82:323–30.

Masi L de, Siviero P, Castaldo D, Cautela D, Esposito C, Laratta B. 2007. Agronomic, chemical and genetic profiles of hot peppers (*Capsicum annuum* ssp.). *Mol Nutr Food Res* 51:1053–62.

Matsumoto H, Ikoma Y, Kato M, Kuniga T, Nakajima N, Yoshida T. 2007. Quantification of carotenoids in citrus fruit by LC-MS and comparison of patterns of seasonal changes for carotenoids among citrus varieties. *J Agric Food Chem* 55:2356–68.

Matthews PD, Luo RB, Wurtzel ET. 2003. Maize phytoene desaaturase and ζ-carotene desaturase catalyse a poly-*Z* desaturase pathway: implications for genetic engineering of carotenoid content among cereal crops. *J Exp Bot* 54:2215–30.

Meléndez-Martínez AJ, Britton G, Vicario IM, Heredia FJ. 2008. The complex carotenoid pattern of orange juices from concentrate. *Food Chem* 109:546–53.

Meléndez-Martínez AJ, Vicario IM, Heredia FJ. 2007. Review: analysis of carotenoids in orange juice. *J Food Compos Anal* 20:638–49.

Mercadante AZ, Britton G, Rodriguez-Amaya DB. 1998. Carotenoids from yellow passion fruit (*Passiflora edulis*). *J Agric Food Chem* 46:4102–6.

Mercadante AZ, Rodriguez-Amaya DB. 1998. Effects of ripening, cultivar differences, and processing on the carotenoid composition of mango. *J Agric Food Chem* 46:128–30.

Mercadante AZ, Rosso VV de. 2007. Identification and quantification of carotenoids, by HPLC-PDA-MS/MS, from Amazonian fruits. *J Agric Food Chem* 55:5062–72.

Mertz C, Brat P, Caris-Veyrat C, Z. Gunata Z. 2010. Characterization and thermal lability of carotenoids and vitamin C of tamarillo fruit (*Solanum betaceum* Cav.). *Food Chem* 119:653–9.

Mertz C, Gancel A-L, Gunata Z, Alter P, Dhuique-Mayer C, Vaillant F, Perez AM, Ruales, J., Brat, P. 2009. Phenolic compounds, carotenoids and antioxidant capacity of three tropical fruits. *J Food Compos Anal* 22:381–7.

Mezadri T, Perez-Galvez A, Hornero-Mendez D. 2005. Carotenoid pigments in acerola fruits (*Malpighia emarginata* DC.) and derived products. *Eur Food Res Technol* 220:63–9.

Moore J, Hao Z, Zhou K, Luther M, Costa J, Yu LL. 2005. Carotenoid, tocopherol, phenolic acid, and antioxidant properties of Maryland-grown soft wheat. *J Agric Food Chem* 53:6649–57.

Morris WL, Ducreux L, Griffiths DW, Stewart D, Davies HV, Taylor MA. 2004. Carotenogenesis during tuber development and storage in potato. *J. Exp Bot* 55:975–82.

Mouly PP, Gaydou EM, Corsetti J. 1999a. Determination of the geographical origin of valencia orange juice using carotenoid liquid chromatographic profiles. *J Chromatogr A* 844:149–59.

Mouly PP, Gaydou EM, Lapierre L, Corsetti J. 1999b. Differentiation of several geographical origins in single-strength Valencia orange juices using quantitative comparison of carotenoid profiles. *J Agric Food Chem* 47:4038–45.

Muller H. 1997. Determination of the carotenoid content in selected vegetables and fruit by HPLC and photodiode array detection. *Z Lebensm Unters Forsch A* 204:88–94.

Murkovic M, Gams K, Draxl S, Pfannhauser W. 2000. Development of an Austrian carotenoid database. *J Food Compos Anal* 13:435–40.

Murkovic M, Mülleder U, Neunteufl H. 2002. Carotenoid content in different varieties of pumpkins *J Food Compos Anal* 15:633–8.

Ndolo VU, Beta T. 2013. Distribution of carotenoids in endosperm, germ, and aleurone fractions of cereal grain kernels. *Food Chem* 139:663–71.

Nicolle C, Simon G, Rock E, Amouroux P, Rémésey C. 2004. Genetic variability influences carotenoid, vitamin, phenolic, and mineral content in white, yellow, purple, orange, and dark-orange carrot cultivars. *J Am Soc Hort Sci* 129:523–9.

Niizu PY, Rodriguez-Amaya DB. 2003. Watermelon as source of lycopene. *Rev Inst Adolfo Lutz* 62:195–9.

Niizu PY, Rodriguez-Amaya DB. 2005a. New data on the carotenoid composition of raw salad vegetables. *J Food Compos Anal* 18:739–49.

Niizu PY, Rodriguez-Amaya DB. 2005b. Flowers and leaves of *Tropaeolum majus* L. as rich sources of lutein. *J Food Sci* 70:S605–9.

Noziére P, Graulet B, Lucas A, Martin B, Grolier P, Doreau M. 2006. Carotenoids for ruminants: from forages to dairy products. *Anim Feed Sci Technol* 131:418–50.

Ogawa K, Fukamachi H, Kato H. 2005. Evaluation of predominant carotenoid contents in domestic 'Irwin' mango cultivated in plastic greenhouses at different sites in Japan. *J Jpn Soc Hort Sci* 74:414–6.

Oliveira GPR de, Rodriguez-Amaya DB. 2007. Processed and prepared products of corn as sources of lutein and zeaxanthin. Compositional variation in the food chain. *J Food Sci* 72:S79–85.

Oliveira C, Silva Ferreira AC, Mendes Pinto M, Hogg T, Alves F, Guedes de Pinho P. 2003. Carotenoid compounds in grapes and their relationship to plant water status. *J Agric Food Chem* 51:5967–71.

O'Neill ME, Carroll Y, Corridan B, Olmedilla B, Granado F, Blanco I, van den Berg H, Hininger I, Rousell A-M, Chopra M, Southon S, Thurnham DI. 2001. A European carotenoid database to assess carotenoid intakes and its use in a five-country comparative study. *Brit J Nutr* 85:499–507.

Organization of Economic Cooperation and Development (OECD). 1993. *Safety evaluation of foods derived by modern biotechnology: concepts and principles*. Paris: OECD.

Paine JA, Shipton CA, Chaggar S, Howells RM, Kennedy MJ, Vernon G, Wright SY, Hinchliffe E, Adams JL, Silverstone AL, Drake R. 2005. Improving the nutritional value of Golden Rice through increased pro-vitamin A content. *Nat Biotech* 23:482–7.

Panfili G, Fratianni A, Irano M. 2004. Improved normal-phase high-performance liquid chromatography procedure for the determination of carotenoids in cereals. *J Agric Food Chem* 52:6373–7.

Park WT, Kim JK, Park S, Lee S-W, Li X, Kim YB, Uddin MR, Park NI, Kim S-J, Park SU. 2012. Metabolic profiling of glucosinolates, anthocyanins, carotenoids, and other secondary metabolites in kohlrabi (*Brassica oleracea* var. *gongylodes*). *J Agric Food Chem* 60:8111–6.

Peng Y, Ma C, Li Y, Leung KS-Y, Jiang Z-H, Zhao Z. 2005. Quantification of zeaxanthin dipalmitate and total carotenoids in *Lycium* fruits (*Fructus lycii*). *Plant Foods Hum Nutr* 60:161–4.

Perkins-Veazie P, Collins JK, Davis AR, Warren Roberts W. 2006. Carotenoid content of 50 watermelon cultivars. *J Agric Food Chem* 54:2593–7.

Perkins-Veazie P, Collins JK, Pair SD, Roberts W. 2001. Lycopene content differs among red-fleshed watermelon cultivars. *J Sci Food Agric* 81:983–7.

Perry A, Rasmussen H, Johnson EJ. 2009. Xanthophyll (lutein, zeaxanthin) content in fruits, vegetables and corn and egg products. *J Food Compos Anal* 22:9–15.

Piao M, Murata Y, Zhu B, Shimoishi Y, Tada M. 2005. Changes in the carotenoid content and its composition during maturation of *Fructus lycii* fruits. *Jpn J Food Chem* 12:35–39.

Pop RM, Weesepoel Y, Socaciu C, Pintea A, Vincken J-P. 2014. Carotenoid composition of berries and leaves from six Romanian sea buckthorn (*Hippophae rhamnoides* L.) varieties. *Food Chem* 147:1–9.

Porcu OM, Rodriguez-Amaya DB. 2006. Variation in the carotenoid composition of acerola and its processed products. *J Sci Food Agric* 86:1916–20.

Porcu OM, Rodriguez-Amaya DB. 2008. Variation in the carotenoid composition of the lycopene-rich Brazilian fruit *Eugenia uniflora* L. *Plant Food Hum Nutr* 63:195–9.

Rabani-Foroutagheh M, Hamidoghli Y, Mohajeri SA. 2013. Effect of split foliar fertilisation on the quality and quantity of active constituents in saffron (*Crocus sativus* L.). *J Sci Food Agric* 94:1872–8.

Raffo A , la Malfa G, Fogliano V, Maiani G, Quaglia G. 2006. Seasonal variations in antioxidant components of cherry tomatoes (*Lycopersicon esculentum* cv. Naomi F1). *J Food Compos Anal* 19:11–9.

Raffo A, Paoletti F, Antonelli M. 2004. Changes in sugar, organic acid, flavonol and carotenoid composition during ripening of berries of three seabuckthorn (*Hippophae rhamnoides* L.) cultivars. *Eur Food Res Technol* 219:360–8.

Raju M, Varakumar S, Lakshminaravana R, Krishnakantha TP, Baskaran V. 2007. Carotenoid composition and vitamin A activity of medicinally important green leafy vegetables. *Food Chem* 101:1598–605.

Rasmussen HM, Muzhingi T, Eggert EMR, Johnson EJ. 2012. Lutein, zeaxanthin, *meso*-zeaxanthin content in egg yolk and their absence in fish and seafood. *J Food Compos Anal* 27:139–44.

Reif C, Arrigoni E, Berger F, Baumgartner D, Nyström L. 2013a. Lutein and β-carotene content of green leafy *Brassica* species grown under different conditions. *LWT Food Sci Technol* 53:378–81.

Reif C, Arrigoni E, Schärer H, Nyström L, Hurrell RF. 2013b. Carotenoid databse of commonly eaten Swiss vegetables and their estimated contribution to carotenoid intake. *J Food Compos Anal* 29:64–72.

Rodriguez-Amaya DB. 1999. *A guide to carotenoid analysis in foods*. Washington DC: International Life Sciences Institute Press.

Rodriguez-Amaya DB, Amaya-Farfan J, Rodriguez EB. 2008a. Carotenoids in fruits: biology, chemistry, technology and health benefits. In: Francesco E. editor. *Trends in phytochemistry*. Kerala: Research Signpost, p 167–88.

Rodriguez-Amaya DB, Kimura M, Godoy HT, Amaya-Farfan J. 2008b. Updated Brazilian database on food carotenoids: factors affecting carotenoid composition. *J Food Compos Anal* 21:445–63.

Rodriguez-Amaya DB, Porcu OM, Azevedo-Meleiro CH. 2007. Variation in the carotenoid composition of fruits and vegetables along the food chain. *Acta Hort* 744:387–94.

Rosso VV de, Mercadante AZ. 2005. Carotenoid composition of two Brazilian genotypes of acerola (*Malpighia punicifolia* L.) from two harvests. *Food Res Int* 38:1073–7.

Russo VM, Howard LR. 2002. Carotenoids in pungent and non-pungent peppers at various developmental stages grown in the field and glasshouse. *J Sci Food Agric* 82:615–24.

Sá MC de, Rodriguez-Amaya DB. 2003. Carotenoid composition of cooked green vegetables from restaurants. *Food Chem* 83:595–600.

Sachindra NM, Bhaskar N, Mahendrakar NS. 2005. Carotenoids in crabs from marine and fresh waters of India. *LWT* 38:221–5.

Sandmann G. 2001a. Carotenoid biosynthesis and biotechnological application. *Arch Biochem Biophys* 385:4–12.

Sandmann, G. 2001b. Genetic manipulation of carotenoid biosynthesis: strategies, problems and achievements. *Trends Plant Sci* 6:14–17.

Sass-Kiss A, Kiss J, Milotay P, Kerek MM, Toth-Markus M. 2005. Differences in anthocyanin and carotenoid content of fruits and vegetables. *Food Res Int* 38:1023–29.

Scott CE, Eldridge AL. 2005. Comparison of carotenoid content in fresh, frozen and canned corn. *J Food Comp Anal* 18:551–9.

Sentanin MA, Rodriguez-Amaya DB. 2007. Teores de carotenóides em mamão e pêssego determinados por cromatografia líquida de alta eficiência. *Ciênc Tecnol Aliment* 27:13–9.

Shahidi F, Metusalach, Brown JA. 1998. Carotenoid pigments in seafoods and aquaculture. *Crit Rev Food Sci Nutr* 38:1–67.

Shewmaker CK, Sheehy JA, Daley M, Colburn S, Ke DY. 1999. Seed-specific overexpression of phytoene synthase: increase in carotenoids and other metabolic effects. *Plant J* 20:401–12.

Shumskaya M, Wurtzel ET. 2013. The carotenoid biosynthetic pathway: thinking in all dimentions. *Plant Sci* 208:58–63.

Silva SR da, Mercadante AZ. 2002. Composição de carotenoides de maracujá-amarelo (*Passiflora edulis* flavicarpa) in natura. *Cienc Tecnol Aliment* 22:254–8.

Solovchenko AE, Chivkunova OB, Merzlyak MN, Gudkovsky VA. 2005. Relationship between chlorophyll and carotenoid pigments during on- and off-tree ripening of apple fruit as revealed non-destructively with reflectance spectroscopy. *Postharvest Biol Technol* 38:9–17.

Su Q, Rowley KG, Itsiopoulos C, O'Dea K. 2002. Identification and quantitation of major carotenoids in selected components of the Mediterranean diet: green leafy vegetables, figs and olive oil. *Eur J Clin Nutr* 56:1149–54.

Tadmor Y, King S, Levi A, Davis A, Meir A, Wasserman B, Hirschberg J, Lewinsohn, E. 2005. Comparative fruit colouration in watermelon and tomato. *Food Res Int* 38:837–41.

Tai CY, Chen BH. 2000. Analysis and stability of carotenoids in the flowers of daylily (*Hemerocallis distichia*) as affected by various treatments. *J Agric Food Chem* 48:5962–8.

Thompson KA, Marshall MR, Sims CA, Wei CI, Sargent SA, Scott, JW. 2000. Cultivar, maturity, and heat treatment on lycopene content in tomatoes. *J Food Sci* 65:791–795.

Tonucci LH, Holden JM, Beecher GR, Khachik F, Davis CS, Mulokozi G. 1995. Carotenoid content of thermally processed tomato-based food products. *J Agric Food Chem* 43:579–86.

Toor RK, Savage GP, Lister CE. 2006. Seasonal variations in the antioxidant composition of greenhouse grown tomatoes. *J Food Compos Anal* 19:1–10.

Topuz A, Ozdemir F. 2007. Assessment of carotenoids, capsaicinoids and ascorbic acid composition of some selected pepper cultivars (*Capsicum annuum* L.) grown in Turkey. *J Food Compos Anal* 20:596–602.

van den Berg H, Faulks R, Granado HF, Hirschberg J, Olmedilla B, Sandmann G, Southon S, Stahl W. 2000. The potential for the improvement of carotenoid levels in foods and the likely systemic effects. *J Sci Food Agric* 80:880–912.

Vásquez-Caicedo AL, Sruamsiri P, Carle R, Neidhart S. 2005. Accumulation of all-*trans*-β-carotene and its 9-*cis* and 13-*cis* stereoisomers during postharvest ripening of nine Thai mango cultivars. *J Agric Food Chem* 53:4827–35.

Vuong LT, Franke AA, Custer LJ, Murphy SP. 2006. *Momordica cochinchinensis* Spreng. (gac) fruit carotenoids reevaluated. *J Food Compos Anal* 19:664–668.

Wall MM. 2006. Ascorbic acid, vitamin A, and mineral composition of banana (*Musa* sp.) and papaya (*Carica papaya*) cultivars grown in Hawaii. *J Food Comp Anal* 19:434–45.

Wall MM, Waddell CA, Bosland PW. 2001. Variation in β-carotene and total carotenoid content in fruits of *Capsicum. HorstSci* 36:746–9.

World Health Organization (WHO). 1995. Application of the principles of substantial equivalence to the safety evaluation of foods or food components from plants derived by modern biotechnology. Report of a WHO workshop. Geneva: WHO.

Wu X, Sun C, Yang L, Zeng G, Liu Z, Li Y. 2008. β-carotene content in sweet potato varieties from China and the effect of preparation on β-carotene retention in the Yanshu No. 5. *Innov Food Sci Emerg Technol* 9:581–6.

Xu C-J, Fraser PD, Wang W-J, Bramley PM. 2006. Differences in the carotenoid content of ordinary citrus and lycopene-accumulating mutants. *J Agric Food Chem* 54:5474–81.

Yano M, Kato M, Ikoma Y, Kawasaki A, Fukawaza Y, Sugiura M, Matsumoto Y, Oohara Y, Nagao A, Ogawa K. 2005. Quantitation of carotenoids in raw and processed fruits in Japan. *Food Sci Technol Res* 11:13–18.

Ye VM, Bhatia SK. 2012. Metabolic engineering strategies for the production of beneficial carotenoids in plants. *Food Sci Biotechnol* 21:1511–7.

Ye X, Al-Babili S, Klöti A, Zhang J, Lucca P, Beyer P, Potrykus I. 2000. Engineering the provitamin A (β-carotene) biosynthetic pathway into (carotenoid-free) rice endosperm. *Science* 287:303–5.

Zanatta CF, Mercadante AZ. 2007. Carotenoid composition from the Brazilian tropical fruit camu-camu (*Myrciaria dubia*). *Food Chem* 101:1526–32.

Zhu C, Naqvi S, Capell T, Christou P. 2009. Metabolic engineering of ketocarotenoid biosynthesis in higher plants. *Arch Biochem Biophys* 483:182–90.

6 Effects of processing and storage

6.1 INTRODUCTION

Fruits and vegetables are the main dietary sources of carotenoids. These foods are, however, highly perishable, and many are seasonal. Processing at peak harvest is necessary to reduce postharvest losses, provide a year-round supply of a variety of plant foods, and permit distribution to places far removed from agricultural production. Processing can have both positive and negative effects on carotenoids. A good understanding of processing effects could lead to measures that would accentuate desirable effects while minimizing those that are undesirable. Processing and storage conditions should be optimized to guarantee maximum retention of health-promoting compounds.

Earlier papers on the effects of processing and storage on food carotenoids were reviewed by Rodriguez-Amaya (1997). Ruiz-Rodriguez et al. (2008) and Palermo et al. (2014) focused on the influence of domestic processing on bioactive compounds, including carotenoids, while Calvo (2005) discussed lutein specifically. Processing and storage effects on food carotenoids per se were reviewed by Rodriguez-Amaya (1999, 2002) and were included in the comprehensive reviews of Maiani et al. (2009) and Namitha and Negi (2010). Undoubtedly, tomato (I. Shi and Le Maguer, 2000), carrot (Hager and Howard, 2006), and pepper have been the most investigated foods on this topic.

Because of the individual influence and interplay of many factors, such as the carotenoid concerned (carotene or xanthophyll, *E*- or *Z*-isomer, esterified or unesterified), the nature of the food (fruit, root, leaf, juice, puree) and disruption (peeled, sliced, shredded) of the food matrix, presence of oxygen, exposure to light, processing method and condition (especially temperature and duration), and storage condition and duration, appraisal of the results of the numerous studies on the effects of home and industrial processing is not straightforward. Variations in the raw material and of the processing and storage conditions make comparisons difficult. Moreover, in spite of the great progress in carotenoid analytical capability, existence of some errors in the analysis and in the calculation of retention or loss, as discussed in Chapter 3, cannot be ruled out.

Food Carotenoids: Chemistry, Biology, and Technology, First Edition. Delia B. Rodriguez-Amaya.

Isomerization and oxidation of carotenoids during analysis and/or during storage of samples may also be attributed erroneously to the processing and storage of foods.

6.2 POSTHARVEST STORAGE

Carotenoid biosynthesis continues after harvest in fruits and fruit vegetables, provided that they are kept intact and the enzymes responsible for carotenogenesis are not inactivated (Rodriguez-Amaya, 1997). This is well illustrated in 'Navalina' oranges harvested at two maturation stages, before color break (breaker stage) and with a light orange coloration, and stored at 2°C and 12°C and 90%–95% relative humidity for up to 7 weeks (Carmona et al., 2012). At 12°C, the total carotenoid content increased considerably and coloration was enhanced in both flavedo and pulp. β-cryptoxanthin increased two and three times in the pulp of the breaker and colored fruit, respectively, after 7 weeks of storage. At 2°C, coloration and carotenoid content remained almost unchanged. The expression of the genes for phytoene synthase, phytoene desaturase, ζ-carotene desaturase, β-lycopene cyclase, and β-carotene hydroxylase increased during storage at 12°C. In contrast, at 2°C, expression of these genes was maintained or slightly declined, a clear demonstration that ripening and carotenogeneses are retarded by low temperature.

Under an ethylene-free atmosphere, storage at 20°C rapidly increased the carotenoid content in the flavedo while maintaining the carotenoid level in the juice sacs of Satsuma mandarin (Matsumoto et al., 2009). Storage at 5°C and 30°C slowly increased the carotenoid content of the flavedo but gradually decreased that of the juice sacs. Under an ethylene atmosphere, storage at 20°C enhanced the carotenoid accumulation in the flavedo more dramatically, with distinct changes in the carotenoid composition, but did not noticeably change the content and composition in juice sacs. Storage at 5°C under an ethylene atmosphere repressed carotenoid accumulation of the flavedo. Degreening with ethylene did not have a significant effect on β-carotene and lycopene levels in 'Star Ruby' grapefruit (Chaudhary et al., 2012).

In nine Thai mango cultivars, β-carotene accumulated during postharvest ripening (Vásquez-Caicedo et al., 2005). Four cultivars developed a bright yellow-orange mesocarp at the fully ripe stage, acquiring total β-carotene contents of 65–112 μg/g dry weight. Five poorly colored cultivars reached total β-carotene contents of 10–22 μg/g dry weight. In 'Ataulfo' and 'Manila' mangos obtained from a Mexican market, the main carotenoids were all-*E*-β-carotene and the dibutyrates of all-*E*-violaxanthin and 9-*Z*-violaxanthin (Ornelas-Paz et al., 2008). The concentrations of these carotenoids increased in an exponential manner during ripening in 'Ataulfo' and in an exponential or second-order polynomial manner in 'Manila'.

Carotenoids of 'Maradol' papayas stored at 25°C had more carotenoids than those stored at 1°C. The low temperature negatively affected the content of major carotenoids, except β-carotene (Rivera-Pastrana et al., 2010). Storage of eight plum cultivars (four yellow and four dark purple) at 2°C for 35 days followed by 4 days at 20°C resulted in no significant loss of carotenoids and antioxidant activity (Díaz-Mula et al., 2009).

The carotenoids behaved differently in two banana cultivars stored at 13°C for 15 days, then increased to 19°C to complete the ripening process (Facundo et al., 2015).

In 'Prata', all-*E*-α-carotene and all-*E*-β-carotene were significantly affected by the low temperature, the concentrations tending to decrease. In 'Nanicão', no carotenoid was significantly affected by cold storage.

Room temperature–stored tomatoes showed significant increase in lycopene, whereas storage at 5°C inhibited lycopene formation (Javanmardi and Kubota, 2006). Similarly, Toor and Savage (2006) reported that storage at 7°C inhibited the accumulation of lycopene, but the lycopene level of light-red tomatoes can be increased up to three-fold by storing at 15°C–25°C.

Mature green tomatoes (breaker stage) were exposed to different levels of UV-C radiation (1.0, 3.0, and 12.2 kj/m^2) and stored at room temperature for 8 days (Bravo et al., 2012). The lycopene content increased almost twofold while the β-carotene level decreased in the breaker tomatoes following UV light treatments. *Z*-lycopene also increased when the tomatoes were treated with UV light for more than 3 h.

Studies on carotenoid behavior during postharvest storage of carrots gave mixed results. Storing carrots at either 4°C to simulate long-term storage or 20°C to simulate marketing practices resulted in increases of 20% in all-*E*-β-carotene after 3 days at 4°C and 34% after 14 days at 20°C, respectively (Imsic et al., 2010). The levels of *Z*-isomers were low with 13-*Z*-β-carotene and 9-*Z*-β-carotene accounting for less than 2% of the total β-carotene present. 9-*Z*-β-Carotene decreased during storage at either temperature, whereas storage at 4°C resulted in a 109% increase in 13-*Z*-β-carotene after 56 days.

On the other hand, the total carotenoid content of lycopene-containing Kintoki carrots was reduced by about 30% during 8 weeks of storage at 1°C with 97% relative humidity (Mayer-Miebach and Spieβ, 2003). Lycopene decreased about 60% while 20% of β-carotene was lost. In another study, cold storage of carrots (0°C, 85%–90% relative humidity) did not affect the β-carotene, α-carotene, and total carotenoid levels; lutein, however, showed a 38% loss (Koca and Karadeniz, 2008). According to Kopas-Lane and Warthesen (1995), neither lighted nor dark cold storage affected major carotenoids of carrots. However, light promoted degradative losses in the carotenoids of spinach, ranging from 22% for lutein to 60% for violaxanthin at 8 days. Dark, cold storage did not affect carotenoid levels except for all-*E*-β-carotene, which showed an 18% loss at 8 days.

Postharvest degradation prevails in broccoli and leafy vegetables. The lutein concentration of broccoli heads tended to decrease during storage for 21 days, this decrease being greater under standard atmospheric conditions (1°C–2°C, 85%–90% RH) than under controlled atmosphere condition (1°C–2°C, 85%–90% RH, 10% O_2 and 5% CO_2) (Fernández-León et al., 2013b). The β-carotene concentration was maintained during storage at controlled atmosphere conditions. Under standard atmospheric conditions, β-carotene declined towards the end of storage. Broccoli florets packed in polypropylene micro-perforated film bags showed significantly lower losses (4%) under refrigerated conditions (Nath et al., 2011).

Carotenoid losses were promoted by light in raw spinach; degradative losses at 8 days (4°C) ranged from 22% for lutein to 60% for violaxanthin (Kopas-Lane and Warthesen, 1995). Dark, cold storage did not affect carotenoid levels except for all-*E*-β-carotene, which showed an 18% loss at 8 days.

Controlled atmosphere (CA) and modified atmosphere packaging (MAP) have been found effective in maintaining the quality and extending the marketability of fresh produce. CA or MAP technologies offer the possibility to retard respiration, maintain bioactive compounds, and extend the shelf life of fruits and vegetables as compared with conventionally stored or packaged samples. While air-stored baby carrots showed a reduction of about 45% of the initial β-carotene content after 12 days, only a 15% loss was observed in baby carrots stored under CA containing low (2 kPa O_2 + 15 kPa CO_2) and moderate (5 kPa O_2 + 5 kPa CO_2) levels of O_2 (Simões et al., 2011).

6.3 EFFECTS OF HOME PREPARATION

Attention is often focused on industrial processing, but home preparation can also cause carotenoid losses, sometimes to a greater extent. Because the effects of home preparation or processing on a food are dependent on so many factors, sometimes with opposing consequences as well as their interactions, the findings of the various studies may appear at times inconsistent. The net effect will be due primarily to the prevailing factors.

Toor and Savage (2005) calculated that the skin and seeds of three cultivars of tomato had on average 48% of the total lycopene. Thus, removal of skin and seeds of tomato during home cooking and processing would result in significant losses of lycopene.

Food preparation operations such as boiling, addition of vegetable oil, chopping, and agitation were assessed in tomatoes (Nguyen et al., 2001). Significant amounts of all-*E*-β-carotene and all-*E*-lutein were converted to the *Z*-configurations. Electron microscopy indicated that heat treatment provoked changes in the physical ultrastructure, such as cell wall and organelle deformation, and differences in relative susceptibility to thermally induced isomerization might be due to differences in physical state and cellular localization.

Boiling and baking had a relatively small effect on lycopene of two New Zealand commercial cultivars of tomato (Sahlin et al., 2004). Frying significantly reduced the lycopene contents of both cultivars. Losses of all-*E*-β-carotene varied from 2% to 27% in sweet bell pepper, sweet potato, and tomato that were stir-fried for 0.5 to 3 min (Kidmose et al., 2006). Extraction of β-carotene into the frying oil was observed in low amounts only after 3 min frying of sweet potato shreds.

Free all-*E*-capsanthin, the most abundant pigment of the red jalapeño pepper, increased slightly while lutein, the major pigment of the green jalapeño pepper, decreased slightly as a consequence of boiling and grilling (Cervantes-Paz et al., 2012). Total carotenoid losses due to boiling were significantly higher in nonpungent (31%–53%) than in pungent peppers (3%–24%) (Ornelas-Paz et al., 2013). This difference was attributed to the antioxidant activity of capsaicinoids. For grilling, 2%–46% reduction of total carotenoid content occurred in most peppers, except for three varieties in which increases of 14%–52% were found. These increases were attributed to loss of water during the heat treatment. In terms of β-carotene, reduction was 16%–45%, except in green pungent peppers in which variable increases occurred. Grilling reduced the β-carotene content by 1%–40% in some pepper types but increased it in other peppers.

In jalapeño peppers at intermediate ripening stage, boiling and grilling consistently decreased the concentrations of most carotenoids, including violaxanthin, capsanthin-5,6-epoxide, antheraxanthin, capsanthin, zeaxanthin, α-cryptoxanthin, β-cryptoxanthin, and three unidentified carotenoids (Cervantes-Paz et al., 2014). Losses of monoesters

(1%–8%) tended to be lower than those of free (6%–17%) and diesterified carotenoids (2%–13%). In contrast, Márkuz et al. (1999) found lower thermolability in diesters than the free and monoesterified carotenoids in caramelized ground paprika.

On a fresh weight basis, the concentrations of β-carotene in boiled, stewed, steamed, and pressure steamed fresh red pepper, frozen broccoli, and frozen red pepper were lower than those obtained before cooking (Bernhardt and Schlich, 2006). The β-carotene level of cooked fresh broccoli, however, was higher than that obtained before cooking. β-carotene was reduced in Italian peppers 16%–60% by different styles of thermal processing but was unaffected or even increased by heat treatment in other pepper types (Greco et al., 2007).

Considerable loss of β-carotene occurred during two commonly used domestic cooking techniques in carrot, pumpkin, amaranth leaves, and drumstick leaves, the loss ranging from 27% to 71% during pressure cooking and 16% to 67% during open pan boiling (Gayathri et al., 2004). The spice turmeric and onion generally improved β-carotene retention in the four vegetables. Combinations of acidulants and antioxidant spices also improved retention. In another study, boiling frozen carrot maintained α-carotene but reduced β-carotene; steaming had the opposite effect (Mazzeo et al., 2011).

Lutein was slightly increased by boiling (+11%) but was significantly reduced (34% and 43%, respectively) during steaming and frying of carrots (Miglio et al., 2008). α-carotene decreased significantly after all cooking methods, especially after steaming and frying. β-carotene was not significantly affected by boiling but was reduced 10% by steaming and 24% by frying.

Simulated cooking (steaming in an autoclave at 100°C for 20 min) of pumpkin slices caused higher losses of carotenoids than simulated commercial sterilization (heat treatment in an autoclave at 121°C for 20 min) of pumpkin puree (Provesi et al., 2011). The major provitamin A carotenes (α- and β-carotene) of *C. moschata* 'Menina Brasileira' and β-carotene of *C. maxima* 'Exposição' had high retentions (>75%), while the xanthophylls (such as lutein and violaxanthin) had high losses.

Changes in carotenoid concentrations due to boiling varied significantly among native Andean potato accessions (Burgos et al., 2012). Violaxanthin and antheraxanthin were significantly reduced in all accessions, but the lutein and zeaxanthin concentrations were not affected or were higher than those of the raw tubers.

True retention of β-carotene, calculated as explained in Chapter 3, was 92% when medium-sized orange-fleshed sweet potatoes were boiled for 20 min covered with water in a pot with the lid on; without the lid, boiling took 30 min and true retention was 88% (van Jaarsveld et al., 2006). In another study (Bengtsson et al., 2008), retentions calculated on a dry weight basis were 78% for boiling for 20 min, 77% for steaming for 30 min, and 78% for deep-frying for 10 min. Also, determining true retention and appraising the effects of boiling, steaming, microwave cooking, and frying, Wu et al. (2008) found that steaming resulted in much more loss of β-carotene than boiling. Microwave cooking resulted in the biggest loss of β-carotene.

Boiling sweet potatoes of selected varieties (six orange- and yellow-fleshed varieties) appeared to result in a higher true retention of all-*E*-β-carotene than roasting, the retention seemingly dependent on the variety (42%–128%) (Kidmose et al., 2007). Preparation of chips by drying caused significant reduction (approximately 21%) of all-*E*-β-carotene, which was further reduced when flour was produced from chips.

Four cultivars of biofortified orange-fleshed sweet potatoes were subjected to four heat treatments (boiled, roasted, steamed, and flour) (Donado-Pestana et al., 2012). The flour presented the greatest losses of the major carotenoids, likely due to longer exposure to heat and air circulation. Boiling and steaming of the roots appeared to result in better retention of all-*E*-β-carotene.

Boiling yellow maize at 100°C for 30 min increased the carotenoid concentration, while baking at 450°F for 25 min resulted in almost 70% loss compared to the uncooked yellow maize flour (Muzhingi et al., 2008).

Leaves of savoy beet, amaranth, and fenugreek were blanched at 95°C in (a) water, (b) water followed by potassium metabisulphite dip, (c) salt solution, (d) salt solution followed by potassium metabisulphite dip, and (e) mixture of sodium bicarbonate, magnesium oxide, and potassium metabisulphite dip (Negi and Roy, 2000). Method "b" was found most suitable for blanching, resulting in better retention of β-carotene.

Boiling frozen spinach resulted in significant loss of total carotenoid content, mainly due to a substantial decrease of lutein; β-carotene was more stable (Mazzeo et al., 2011). Steaming caused a more limited reduction of lutein and an increase in β-carotene. In another study, neither boiling nor steaming reduced the lutein concentration of fresh, frozen, and canned green beans and spinach (Delchier et al., 2012).

The antioxidant components in broccoli were lost heavily during cooking, but total carotenoids were retained better compared to total phenolics and ascorbic acid (D. Zhang and Hamauzu, 2004). The florets cooked in microwave for 120 and 300 sec lost 17% and 22% of total carotenoids, respectively, while the microwaved stems lost 20%. Losses during conventional boiling for 30, 60, 90, 120, and 300 sec amounted to 3%, 12%, 14%, 17%, and 23% for the florets, while those of stems boiled for 60, 120, and 300 sec were 10%, 20%, and 20%. Miglio et al. (2008) reported that the carotenoids of broccoli increased on boiling and steaming, while drastic losses occurred during frying.

For fresh broccoli, steaming did not affect the carotenoid content, whereas microwaving resulted in a significant decrease of both lutein and β-carotene and boiling a significant decrease of lutein (Pellegrini et al., 2010). In the case of frozen broccoli, both carotenoids were negatively affected by the cooking methods applied, the least decrease occurring with boiling. Boiling resulted in a significant increase of lutein in fresh Brussels sprouts, while microwaving and steaming caused significant losses of β-carotene. Except for a significant decrease of β-carotene by steaming, the carotenoids were maintained during cooking of frozen Brussels sprouts.

Comparing the four major carotenoids of broccoli, boiling (5 min) resulted in higher true retention for lutein (96%–99%), and stir-frying provided higher retention for β-carotene (90%–94%) (Sá and Rodriguez-Amaya, 2004). The notoriously unstable violaxanthin had the lowest retentions (53%–56% for boiling and 52%–64% for stir-frying). Lutein was also the most stable in stir-fried kale (97%–98%); violaxanthin only had 33%–49% retention. Lutein can be erroneously considered unstable because it is often underestimated in carotenoid analysis by degradation or physical loss through adherence to walls of containers or removal with the washing water, as explained in Chapter 3.

Unlike the hydrophilic nutrients and bioactive compounds, the lipid-soluble carotenoids do not leach to the water medium; thus, boiling is not as detrimental. The conditions during frying might be more drastic than those of boiling and there could be some leaching of carotenoids to the oil, although, on the other hand, there is also some evaporation of water, concentrating the carotenoids (Sá and Rodriguez-Amaya, 2004). Miglio et al. (2008) also attributed the substantial loss of carotenoids during frying of broccoli to leaching into oil and to a higher temperature.

Retention of α-carotene, β-carotene, and lutein/zeaxanthin did not differ among vegetables (broccoli, carrots, green beans, and sweet potato) subjected to induction boiling, conventional boiling, and microwave steaming, with the exception of β-carotene, which had higher retention in broccoli and sweet potato that were induction boiled (90% and 86%, respectively) than those that were microwave steamed (62% and 66%, respectively) (Nunn et al., 2006).

For vegetables from northeastern Thailand (ivy gourd, amaranth, swamp cabbage, Chinese cabbage, pumpkin), blanching resulted in 7%–11% loss of β-carotene, while steaming, frying, and boiling showed losses of 15%, 18%, and 43%, respectively (Sungpuag et al., 1999). Traditional foods, such as bamboo shoot soup (Kang-nho-mai) and chicken organ soup (Om-kruang-nai-kai), exhibited β-carotene losses ranging from 6% to 21%. In contrast, boiling preserved the majority of carotenoids, whereas stir-frying and deep-frying significantly decreased the total carotenoid content and all-*E* forms of carotenoids (β-carotene, lutein, and zeaxanthin) of cilantro, sweet potato leaf, Thai basil leaf, and choy sum (Kao et al., 2012). These 4 vegetables had the highest total carotenoid contents among 25 fresh vegetables commonly consumed in Taiwan.

A meta-analysis of studies that evaluated the effects of cooking methods on carotenoids was conducted by Murador et al. (2014). The data search found 404 articles from 1992 to 2013, of which 18 articles that followed the inclusion criteria were selected. Significant reductions of carotenoid levels were observed after microwaving and frying but an increase after stewing. Carotenoids were degraded most in frying.

Using high β-carotene corn, the cumulative losses of β-carotene in the final cooked products were 24% and 25% for the fermented and unfermented porridges (Li et al., 2007). Thus, fermentation, a traditional African household processing, does not adversely affect the retention of β-carotene in porridges prepared with high β-carotene corn.

6.4 EFFECTS OF THERMAL PROCESSING

Thermal processing remains the most widely adopted food preservation technique. Carotenoid losses during this processing have been widely monitored for a long time. In reviewing earlier studies, Rodriguez-Amaya (1997) concluded:

- The stability of carotenoids differs in different foods (different matrices), even when the same processing and storage conditions are used. Optimum conditions for carotenoid retention during processing differ from one food to another. Carotenoids per se have different susceptibilities to degradation.
- The main cause of carotenoid degradation during processing and storage of foods is enzymatic or nonenzymatic oxidation. Isomerization of all-*E*-carotenoids to the *Z*-isomers, particularly during heat treatment, also lowers the vitamin A value of foods, but not to the same extent as oxidation. Enzymatic degradation of carotenoids may be a more serious problem than thermal decomposition in many foods.

- Whatever the processing method chosen, retention of carotenoids decreases with longer processing time, higher processing temperatures, and cutting or maceration of the food.
- The heat treatment in blanching may provoke some losses of carotenoids, but the inactivation of oxidative enzymes will prevent further and greater losses during processing and storage.
- Freezing (especially quick freezing) and frozen storage generally preserve carotenoids, but long-time thawing may be detrimental.
- Peeling and juicing result in substantial losses of carotenoids, often surpassing those of heat treatment.
- Exclusion of oxygen (through vacuum or hot filling, oxygen-impermeable packaging, or inert atmosphere), protection from light, and storage at low temperatures all protect carotenoids from decomposition.
- Reported increases in carotenoid concentrations during domestic or industrial thermal processing are not likely to be true increases but are consequences of the analytical procedure, such as loss of carotenoid in fresh samples due to enzymatic activity, greater extractability of carotenoids from processed samples, and unaccounted loss of water and leaching of soluble solids.

Recent studies continue to lend support to these conclusions. Greater emphasis is being given to the formation of *Z*-isomers.

6.4.1 Preliminary operations

Carotenoids are naturally protected in plant tissues. Peeling, cutting, or pulping of fruits and vegetables increases exposure to oxygen and releases enzymes that catalyze carotenoid oxidation. Thus, thermal treatment should be carried out immediately after these operations.

As mentioned above, peeling and juicing physically remove considerable amounts of carotenoids. In nectars produced from three peach varieties, within the same variety, carotenoid content was lower in nectars obtained from lye-peeled fruits than those from unpeeled fruits (Lavelli et al., 2009).

6.4.2 Thermal treatment

Thermal degradation of carotenoids in citrus juice revealed differences among the major provitamin A carotenoids and between these and other carotenoids of the xanthophyll family (Dhuique-Mayer et al., 2007). The main provitamin A carotenoids (β-carotene and β-cryptoxanthin) in citrus juice displayed a relative heat stability. Isomerization of the epoxide function at the 5,6 position into the 5,8 furanoxide function was a common reaction of several xanthophylls.

Several studies on the effect of pasteurization on the carotenoids of orange juice demonstrate the variable susceptibility of the constituent carotenoid to degradation, with violaxanthin showing the greatest instability. Pasteurization (95°C–105°C for 10 sec) of Valencia orange juice resulted in loss of violaxanthin (38%), lutein (20%), ζ-carotene (14%), α-carotene (13%), β-carotene (11%), and zeaxanthin (9%) (Gama and Sylos, 2007). Losses caused by the concentration process were 31% for violaxanthin, 29% for ζ-carotene, 24% for zeaxanthin, 17% for lutein, 12% for α-carotene, 5% for β-carotene, and 3% for β-carotene. This is in agreement with an earlier study on Valencia orange juice that reported losses of 46% for violaxanthin and 25% for antheraxanthin (Lee and Coates, 2003). With the decrease of violaxanthin and antheraxanthin, lutein became the major carotenoid, followed by zeaxanthin, in the pasteurized juice.

Pasteurization (90°C for 30 sec) of an orange juice–milk beverage resulted in significant reductions of 23% and 22%, respectively, of lutein and zeaxanthin, but no significant changes in α-carotene, β-carotene, and β-cryptoxanthin (Zulueta et al., 2010). Pasteurization (90°C for 30 sec) of Valencia orange juice, followed by rapid chilling in an ice water bath, had no significant effect on provitamin A carotenoids but provoked a 46% reduction in violaxanthin and 25% in antheraxanthin (Lee and Coates, 2003). In another study, pasteurization (90°C for 1 min) decreased the total carotenoid content by about 35% (Velázquez-Estrada et al., 2013). The reduction of individual carotenoids differed: α-carotene, 44%; β-carotene, 38%; β-cryptoxanthin, 32%; zeaxanthin, 23%; lutein, 21%. Lessin et al. (1997) observed losses of about 36% in the concentrations of provitamin A carotenoids of orange juice pasteurized at 80°C for 2 min.

In microwave heating of orange juice at 60°C and 70°C for 10 min, violaxanthin and antheraxanthin were the most unstable; lutein and provitamin A carotenoids were more stable (Fratianni et al., 2010). At 85°C a decrease of about 50% occurred for almost all carotenoids after 1 min of microwave heating.

In mango puree, although significant *E-Z* isomerization of β-carotene occurred, as shown by the formation of 13-*Z*-β-carotene, maximum vitamin A value reduction during pasteurization did not exceed 15% due to a total β-carotene retention of 93% (Vásquez-Caicedo et al., 2007). A protective effect of the matrix was thought to be responsible for the relatively high stability of β-carotene, which might be partly associated with the high pectin and fiber contents of mango fruits.

Microwave heating at 285, 570, and 850 W for 30 sec did not have a significant effect on the total xanthophyll and β-carotene contents of papaya puree (Ancos et al., 1999). At 475 W for 45 and 60 sec, a small but significant reduction of the xanthophyll level occurred.

In nectars produced from three peach varieties, carotenoids and phenolic contents were lower in nectars obtained from peeled fruits than those obtained from unpeeled fruits (Lavelli et al., 2009). Pasteurization (90°C, 5 min) of peach induced significant reduction of zeaxanthin and completely eliminated β-cryptoxanthin but maintained lutein and β-carotene (Oliveira et al., 2012).

In an extensive study of more than 20 commonly consumed vegetables in Finland, industrial blanching (95°C–99°C for 2–4 min) or freezer storage did not affect carotenoids and sterols (Puupponen-Pomiä et al., 2003). Vitamin C, folic acid, and phenolics turned out to be much more sensitive, substantial losses occurring during blanching. Mayer-Miebach and Spieβ (2003) confirmed high stability of lycopene in Kintoki carrot during blanching at high temperature (90°C) for 15 min.

Lycopene content of tomatoes remained unchanged during the multistep processing operations for the production of juice or paste and remained stable for up to 12 months of storage at ambient temperature (Agarwal et al., 2001). In tomato juice, hot-broken at 82°C, screened, and subjected to three processing treatments, the high-temperature, short-time treatment (121°C for 40 sec before canning) provided the highest yield of all-*E*- plus *Z*-forms of lutein and lycopene, followed by heating at 90°C for 5 min prior to canning, and heating in water at 100°C for 30 min after canning (Lin and Chen, 2005a). These treatments caused only a minor change in β-carotene.

Individual carotenoids and their isomeric forms behaved differently during production and storage of canned tomato juice (Rubio-Diaz et al., 2010). An apparent increase of carotenoids was noted after hot-break, due to improved extraction efficiency, accompanied by isomerization. Canning reduced all-*E*-lycopene, all-*E*-δ-carotene, all-*E*-β-carotene, and all-*E*-lutein by 30%, 34%, 43%, and 67%, respectively. Canning also caused a drastic reduction of tetra-*Z*-lycopene and promoted its isomerization to other geometric forms, including all-*E*-lycopene.

Homogenization and pasteurization at 98°C for 40 sec maintained the carotenoid content of tomato puree (Pérez-Conesa et al., 2009). Knockaert et al. (2012) also found no significant effect of mild (60°C, 1 min) and intense (90°C, 10 min) pasteurization, but the lycopene concentration decreased significantly during thermal (117°C, 1.5 or 3 min) and high-pressure sterilization (450 MPa, 15 min, 20°C; or 600 MPa, 20 min, 45°C), no significant difference being observed between the two sterilization processes.

The major effect of thermal processing of tomato puree was a significant decrease in the total lycopene content, which increased as the temperature was raised from 90°C to 150°C and the treatment time was prolonged (J. Shi et al., 2003). The level of Z-isomers increased as treatment time increased, but only for a short time at the beginning of the treatment. Lycopene was relatively stable when heated at temperatures below 100°C, but the duration of heating had serious effects.

In laboratory-formulated bush tomato sauce, lycopene and β-carotene increased by 48% and 14%, respectively (Sommano et al., 2013). Investigating samples of tomato sauce, tomato soup, baked tomato slices, and tomato juice taken at different times of heating, loss of water increased the lycopene and β-carotene contents on a wet weight basis (Seybold et al., 2004). On a dry weight basis, lycopene content increased or decreased depending on the origin of the tomatoes used. β-carotene decreased or was stable, and it isomerized due to thermal processing.

Comparison of carotenoid levels of samples of raw tomatoes, tomato juice after hot-break scalder, and final paste obtained from two different plants over 2 years indicated that lycopene losses during processing of tomatoes into final paste (25°Bx–30°Bx) ranged from 9% to 28% (Takeoka et al., 2001). The initial Brix level of raw tomatoes seemed to affect the amount of lycopene loss, possibly because of the processing time required to achieve the final desired degrees Brix of the paste. In general, no consistent changes were observed in the other carotenoids as a function of processing.

Industrial processing of fresh tomato into paste had no significant effect on lycopene and a slight significant effect on β-carotene (Chanforan et al., 2012). Transformation of the paste to sauce appeared to have a slight significant lowering of both carotenoids. Also working with industrial samples, Capanoglu et al. (2008) observed a gradual and significant decrease in carotenoids (final losses of 32%–75%) on processing from fruit to tomato paste.

During the first steps of processing into sauce, which included heating and juicing operations, a large decrease in tetra-*Z*-lycopene of tangerine tomatoes occurred, accompanied by increases in all-*E*- and other *Z*-lycopene isomers (Ishida et al., 2007).

In subsequent steps, consisting mostly of heating to concentrate the juice, degradation was much less, but isomerization increased.

Colle et al. (2010) found that 74% to 75% of lycopene was preserved after 30 min treatment of tomato pulp at 130°C and 140°C. Lycopene isomerization was limited, even at high temperature (140°C). Investigating the impact of pilot-scale aseptic processing on a model tomato soup, Colle et al. (2011) observed limited lycopene degradation with thermal processing. High-pressure homogenization caused additional losses and resulted in higher viscosity that was accompanied by a decrease in lycopene bioaccessibility. Lipids clearly enhanced lycopene isomerization and improved bioaccessibility.

For carrot juice, canning (121°C, 30 min) resulted in the highest destruction of carotenoids, followed by high-temperature short-time processing (120°C, 30 sec or 110°C, 30 sec), acidification plus heating at 105°C for 25 sec, and acidification (B.H. Chen et al., 1995). The effect of thermal processing on *E-Z* isomerization of β-carotene in carrot juice produced in pilot plant scale was studied by Marx et al. (2003). Pasteurization and sterilization at 121°C caused only minor isomerization, whereas sterilization at 130°C and blanching increased the levels of Z-isomers. Dissolution of crystalline carotenes by cellular lipids during blanching was identified as the prerequisite for isomerization. Addition of grape seed oil to the coarse mash enhanced isomerization in both unheated and heated-preserved juices.

Thermal processing of carrot puree over a broad temperature range (80°C–150°C) induced conversion of β-carotene into its *Z*-isomers until an equilibrium state was reached after prolonged heating (Lemmens et al., 2010). It could be concluded, however, that the retention of all-*E*-β-carotene in plain carrot puree was relatively high, which was most likely due to the presence of the protecting food matrix.

Three industrial varieties of carrot were submitted to heat treatment by boiling in water with or without citric acid or in a convection-type steam furnace (Borowska et al., 2003). The all-*E*-α-carotene and all-*E*-β-carotene contents decreased significantly, the loss during heat treatment in water being higher (up to 50%) than with the convection-type steam furnace.

NaCl and acetic acid concentrations and pasteurization conditions affected carotenoid retention in canned pickled carrots and jalapeño peppers (Guerra-Vargas et al., 2001). The optimal pasteurization conditions were 70°C for 12.45 min for carrot and 83°C for 5.2 min for pepper, 2% NaCl, and 2% acetic acid.

In several fruits and vegetables, processing (principally canning) produced an increase of 16%–50% of total provitamin A carotenoids relative to the fresh samples (Lessin et al., 1997). Possible explanations given for these increases were increased extraction efficiency, inactivation of enzymes capable of degrading carotenoids, and/or loss of soluble solids into the liquid canning medium. The percentage *Z*-isomers increased 10%–39% with canning.

Seven fruits and vegetables (apricot, cherry, nectarine, peach, plum, carrot, and pepper) purchased from local growers in New Zealand were subjected to heating (98°C, 10 min), freezing (–20°C), and freeze-drying (Leong and Oey, 2012). From the values presented on dry weight basis for the processed foods in comparison with the fresh produce, apricot appeared to be more prone to losing β-carotene and β-cryptoxanthin on heating and, to a lesser extent, on freeze-drying. Carrot and nectarine also tended to decrease in these carotenoids on heating. Carotenoids appeared to be stable during processing of the other foods. Notably, β-carotene, β-cryptoxanthin, α-carotene, and lutein increased in pepper during heating and freezing.

Thermal processing of broccoli (microwaved), corn (canned), kale (canned), green pea (canned), and spinach (canned) increased the *Z*-isomers of lutein and zeaxanthin up to 22% and 17%, respectively (Updike and Schwartz, 2003). Minimal preparation techniques, like blanching and boiling, and storage can significantly affect the level and stability of carotenoids in spinach, affecting all its major carotenoids, lutein, β-carotene, violaxanthin, and neoxanthin (Bunea et al., 2008).

Sterilization (T_{max} = 121°C, F = 5) of sweet corn and blanching (2 min, steam) of spinach resulted in decreases in total lutein content by 26% and 17%, respectively (Aman et al., 2005). In sweet corn, total zeaxanthin decreased by 29%, and the amount of *Z*-isomers of lutein and zeaxanthin increased from 12% to 30% and 7% to 25%, respectively. In spinach, lutein *Z*-isomers decreased from 21% to 14%.

Lime-cooking significantly decreased the lutein content in yellow, red, and high-carotenoid corns (La Parra et al., 2007). Further processing into tortilla and tortilla chips did not affect the lutein concentration significantly, except for yellow corn. The zeaxanthin level of yellow corn declined after lime-cooking and baking, and was further reduced by frying.

6.4.3 Drying

Drying slices of mango 'Kent' and 'Tommy Atkins' in an overflow tray dryer for 3.5 h (the fruit temperature rose within 2 h from ambient to more than 50°C), in the dark, resulted in losses of 7% and 31%, respectively, of all-*E*-β-carotene (Pott et al., 2003).

Freeze-drying significantly decreased the lycopene content of 'Rio Red' grapefruit pulp, the loss being greater in the freeze-dried pulp from the control fruit compared to that made from an irradiated sample (300 Gy) (Vanamala et al., 2005). Reduction of β-carotene was significant only in the control sample.

A combination of different techniques (osmotic dehydration, convection drying, and microwave-assisted air-drying) was used to dehydrate cherry tomatoes (Heredia et al., 2010). Osmotic pretreatment limited isomerization during the later stages of drying, whereas both the loss of total lycopene and the *E-Z* isomerization were favored by an increase in temperature and the microwave power. In a previous study, an increase in lycopene and β-carotene was observed in cherry tomato osmotically dehydrated at moderate temperatures (30°C and 40°C) with solutions that include sucrose in its composition (Heredia et al., 2009). In studying the effects of osmotic treatment, vacuum drying, air-drying, and their combination on tomato lycopene, J. Shi et al. (1999) suggested that osmotic solution (sugar) remaining on the surface layer of the tomato might have prevented oxygen from penetrating and oxidizing lycopene, reducing lycopene losses in comparison with the other dehydration methods. In the osmotic treatment, isomerization was found to be the predominating reaction. In the air-drying processing, both isomerization and oxidation were major reactions.

Lycopene decreased 8% to 21% during spray-drying of tomato pulp under various operating conditions (Goula and Adamopoulos, 2005). This loss increased with increasing air inlet temperature and both drying and compressed air flow rate. It was attributed to actual degradation of lycopene into colorless form, rather than to a progressive conversion of all-*E*-lycopene to less-colored *Z*-forms.

Simulating the traditional slow drying process of red pepper fruits for paprika production, the evolution of carotenoid concentration was monitored and found to directly depend on the existing physical conditions (Pérez-Gálvez et al., 2004). Three different stages could be observed during the process. In the first stage, corresponding to a physiological adaptation to the newly imposed conditions, a decrease (~20%) in the carotenoid content was indicated during the first 24 h. After that short period and during 5 days, a second stage recovering the biosynthetic (carotenogenic) capability of the fruits denoted an accommodation of the fruits to the new environmental conditions. During the following 48 h (third stage) a sharp increase in the carotenoid content was observed. The results demonstrated that a fine control of the temperature and moisture content would help to positively modulate carotenogenesis and minimize catabolism.

Korean red pepper was dried by two methods: (a) cut pods, 70°C, 6 h; and (b) whole pods, 80°C, 5 h, then 60°C, 18 h (S. Kim et al., 2004). Capsanthin stability was influenced by the drying method until 2 months of storage. Thereafter the temperature became the major factor.

Capsanthin, zeaxanthin, capsorubin, and β-cryptoxanthin esters showed comparable processing stability, higher than those of the unesterified counterparts, in chili powder and paprika (Schweiggert et al., 2007). This behavior might be related to the more lipophilic nature and hence the better integration of esterified carotenoids into membrane structures, thereby protecting them from thermal degradation. Susceptibility of the unesterified carotenoids differed, with capsanthin and β-cryptoxanthin retaining 69% and 78%, respectively, of the initial content in chili and 68% and 74%, respectively, in paprika. Only 48% and 58% of the initial zeaxanthin, and 20% and 21% of the initial β-carotene contents in chili and paprika, respectively, were retained.

The presence of capsaicinoids in pungent pepper had a favourable effect on the stability of carotenoids during thermal drying (Daood et al., 2006). The diesters of lutein and zeaxanthin and the monoester of β-cryptoxanthin were more stable than those of capsorubin and capsanthin. During storage in a refrigerator for 3 months, paprika showed high degradation of all the examined carotenoids, particularly in samples prepared from pods dried at high temperatures (90°C and 100°C), with the exception of β-cryptoxanthin monoester and violaxanthin diesters in a nonpungent variety.

Significant losses (12%–15%) of all-*E*-α-carotene and all-*E*-β-carotene occurred when pumpkin slices were dried without coating (Lago-Vanzela et al., 2013). Significant improvement in carotenoid retention was observed in dehydrated slices previously coated with a native maize starch solution at 90°C, with a modified maize starch solution at 30°C, or a modified cassava starch solution at 90°C.

Heating carrot homogenates at temperatures above 100°C under nonoxidizing conditions initiated isomerization of all-*E*-lycopene, manifested by a significant increase in 9-*Z*-lycopene (Mayer-Miebach et al., 2005). Isomerization at short treatment times was enhanced when sunflower oil was added prior to thermal treatment. Lycopene remained stable during convection drying in the range of 50°C–90°C and during microwave vacuum drying of blanched carrot slices. No isomerization took place during either drying process. About 20% of β-carotene was degraded, however, during convection drying at 90°C. In another study (Frias et al., 2010), loss of β-carotene in carrot occurred during blanching (92% retention), and convective air-drying resulted in further losses (73%–90% retentions). Ultrasound drying provided higher β-carotene retention (96%–98%), but retention was lower when carrot was blanched prior to dehydration by ultrasound (88%).

Vacuum drying and low-pressure superheated steam drying of diced carrot at the temperature range of 60°C–80°C and at a pressure of 7 kPa led to more conversion of all-*E*-β-carotene to 13-*Z*-β-carotene but less total β-carotene degradation than hot-air drying at the same temperatures (Hiranvarachat et al., 2008).

Carrot slices were dried by microwave vacuum until the moisture content reached about 20% (wet basis), and then by conventional air-drying (45°C–50°C) or conventional vacuum drying (55°C–60°C) or by continued microwave vacuum drying at a lower power level to a final moisture content of about 6% (Cui et al., 2004). The carotenoid retention of the carrot slices dried by these methods was very close to or even as much as those dried by freeze-drying and much better than those dried by conventional hot air.

In lycopene-containing carrots (*Daucus carota* L. 'Nutri Red'), β-carotene and lycopene remained unchanged on convection drying at temperatures below 70°C, independent of the drying medium (Regier et al., 2005). Freeze-drying did not show any advantage to convection-drying in terms of carotenoid retention. Microwave vacuum drying resulted in dry products with high carotenoid retention within very short drying times of about 2 h.

Microwaving for short time at high power was found effective in drying coriander leaves, without affecting *E-Z* isomerization of β-carotene and with negligible loss of pigments, providing all-*E*-β-carotene-rich dried foliage for direct use in processed foods and in culinary preparations (Divya et al., 2012).

With freeze-drying, only a minor change of each carotenoid was observed in the Chinese flower daylily; hot-air drying resulted in greater losses (Tai and Chen, 2000). Under both processing treatments, the amounts of most carotenoids were higher in samples previously soaked in a 1% sodium sulfite solution for 4 h.

An average of about 50% loss was observed for carotenoids at the end of the egg pasta–making process. The 13-*Z/E* ratio changed from about 12% in the mix to 32% in the final pastas (Fratianni et al., 2012). The degradation of carotenoids was mostly limited to the kneading step, where several physicochemical and enzymatic factors seemed to lead to degradation. The drying step did not induce significant changes.

Cold-smoking Atlantic salmon includes salting and drying. Extraction of protein-carotenoid complexes during processing might cause surface discoloration and lead to a smoked product of low quality. The use of excess water during dry salting may dilute salt at the surface and contribute in part to discoloration of salmon products (Birkeland and Bjerkeng, 2004). On the other hand, the high salt concentrations used during injection and brine salting may prevent protein-astaxanthin extraction.

6.5 EFFECTS OF SUN AND SOLAR DRYING

Traditional sun drying, although the cheapest and most accessible means of food preservation in developing regions, causes considerable carotenoid destruction (Rodriguez-Amaya, 1997). Drying in a solar dryer, even of simple and inexpensive design, can appreciably reduce carotenoid losses. Protecting the food from direct sunlight (e.g., drying in the shade) also has a positive effect.

Drying mango slices in a laboratory overflow dryer (drying air temperature of 75°C and maximum drying time of 3.5 h) resulted in complete degradation of xanthopylls and partial degradation of all-*E*-β-carotene (losses of 7% in Kent mango and 31% in Tommy Atkins mango) (Pott et al., 2003). Solar drying (average drying temperature between 60°C and 65°C) of Thai mangos 'Nam Dokmai' and 'Kaew' in a sunlit tunnel dryer (mango slices exposed to sunlight for about 7.5 h) led to greater losses, 34% and 42%, respectively.

Solar drying and open-air sun drying of orange-fleshed sweet potato slices to a moisture content of ≤10% resulted in all-*E*-β-carotene losses of 9% and 16%, respectively (Bengtsson et al., 2008). Drying orange-fleshed slices at 57°C in a forced-air oven for 10 hours reduced all-*E*-β-carotene by 12%. In another study (Bechoff et al., 2009), all-*E*-β-carotene losses in flour made from dried chips varied from 16% to 34% in different drying treatments. Hot air cross-flow drying retained significantly more provitamin A than sun drying. Solar and sun drying did not differ significantly in terms of provitamin A retention. The shape of the sweet potato pieces influenced provitamin A retention, the crimped slices retaining more provitamin A than chips. No significant increase in *Z*-isomers was observed after drying.

Oven drying, shadow drying, and boiling retained 72%, 59%, and 56% of cassava β-carotene (Chávez et al., 2007). Lower retention (34%) was obtained with gari, which is a popular method of cassava processing in West Africa, involving peeling, grating, packing in a perforated sack, pressing, and toasting. Higher retention was observed when the dried cassava was stored as chips rather than flour.

The amounts of all-*E*-β-carotene in eight Tanzanian green leafy vegetables (amaranth, cowpea, sweet potato, pumpkin, maimbe, mgagani, nsonga, and ngwiba) were substantially reduced by open sun drying while solar drying resulted in significantly more retention (Mulokozi and Svanberg, 2003). A previous study had already shown that sun drying resulted in significant reductions of total carotenoids, β-carotene, and α-carotene in all Tanzanian vegetables studied (amaranth, cowpea, peanut, pumpkin, and sweet potato leaves). All-*E*-α-carotene and 9-*Z*-β-carotene were similarly affected by the two drying methods. Mdziniso et al. (2006) found that vegetable type accounted for significant differences in dehydration rate and β-carotene content. β-carotene losses due to solar drying were 49%–67%, 4%–6%, and 2%–20% (dry basis) in carrot, sweet potato, and collard green, respectively.

Savoy beet, amaranth, and fenugreek leaves were dried in (a) sun, (b) shade, (c) solar drier, (d) cabinet drier, and (e) low-temperature drier (Negi and Roy, 2000). Method "e" had the least drastic effect on the β-carotene content of the processed product. In another study by the same authors (Negi and Roy, 2001a), greater loss of β-carotene was observed in solar drying as compared to cabinet drying of savoy beet and amaranth leaves.

Dried salted shrimp is made from raw shrimp that is cooked and dried under direct sunlight. During sun drying, most of the astaxanthin of the cooked shrimp was degraded (75%) (Hernández Becerra et al., 2014). Further degradation of astaxanthin occurred during storage (83%).

6.6 EFFECTS OF NONTHERMAL PROCESSING

Food technology has relied heavily on heat as the standard processing tool to ensure the safety and quality of food. While there is a high degree of confidence in using heat to kill pathogens and spoilage microflora, heat treatment inevitably causes some changes in the texture, aroma, flavour, or appearance of food. There are also concerns about the energy cost of heat processes and the possibility of damaging some of the nutrients in food.

In recent years, nonthermal processing technologies have been developed to avoid the adverse thermal effects on texture, aroma, and flavor, as well as losses of nutrients and bioactives. Some of these technologies have not reached commercial application, but others, such as minimal processing and high-pressure processing, have been accepted in the food industry.

6.6.1 Minimal processing

The market sales of ready-to-use fresh vegetables have grown rapidly in recent decades, especially of fresh-cut lettuce and carrot used in prepared salads. Ready-to-eat fresh-cut fruits and vegetables are defined as those that have been lightly or minimally processed, undergoing such operations as sorting, trimming, washing, peeling, coring, slicing or chopping, hygienization, dipping in stabilizer solution, or packaging under appropriate atmospheres.

Since drastic processing conditions, such as heating, are not employed, minimally processed products are expected to retain fresh or freshlike properties and retain good nutritive quality. However, as a result of peeling, cutting, and shredding, a large number of physiological phenomena, such as biochemical changes and microbiological spoilage, takes place and may result in degradation of color, texture, and flavor. The natural protection of the epidermis and compartmentation that separates enzymes from substrates is destroyed. Also, respiratory activity and ethylene emission are generally higher, especially during the first hours after the cutting operations. With such alterations, fresh-cut products are rendered more perishable than the intact original produce.

Loss of cellular integrity and of cell compartmentalization in fresh-cut products destroys the natural protection of carotenoids and exposes them to oxidative enzymes and oxygen. Carotenoid losses occur as enzymatic oxidation prevails over continued biosynthesis.

The total carotenoid content increased significantly for the whole orange fruits, but no significant change was observed in segments or peeled fruits during storage at 4°C for 12 days (Plaza et al., 2011a), indicating inactivation of carotenogenic enzymes in the latter samples. In general, the same pattern was observed with individual carotenoids (lutein, zeaxanthin, α-cryptoxanthin, β-cryptoxanthin, α-carotene and β-carotene); β-carotene presented a significant increase for all samples, the whole fruit showing the highest value.

In fresh-cut fruits kept at 5°C for 6 days, no losses in total carotenoids occurred in kiwi slices and watermelon cubes. On the other hand, a 25% loss in pineapple pieces and 10%–15% losses in cantaloupe cubes, mango cubes, and strawberry slices were observed (Gil et al., 2006). Except for watermelon, in which the lycopene content was similar for the whole and the fresh-cut fruits, and kiwi, in which the total, lutein, and β-carotene contents in the fresh-cut fruits were slightly higher after 9 days, the carotenoid levels of whole fruits were generally higher than those of fresh-cut fruits. The carotenoid contents of the whole fruits increased in strawberry throughout 9 days of storage and initially (up to 3 days) in pineapple and kiwi whole fruits; in mango the total carotenoid content decreased in 3 days but increased thereafter.

The effect of controlled atmospheres of 2% O_2, 12% CO_2 in air, and 2% O_2 + 12% CO_2 on the quality and carotenoid content was assessed in sliced persimmon held for 8 days and peach held for 7 days at 5°C (Wright and Kader, 1997). Peach slices stored in air + 12% CO_2 had lower β-carotene and β-cryptoxanthin contents. The different carotenoids in persimmon did not show a definite trend. In fresh-cut papaya 'Maradol' stored at 5°C, 10°C, or 20°C, loss of β-carotene was greater at higher temperature in both cubes and slices (Rivera-López et al., 2005). In both studies, the shelf life based on the visual quality ended before significant loss of carotenoids occurred.

Passive or active modified atmosphere packaging (MAP) with different concentrations of CO_2 and O_2 have been used to maintain the quality of fresh-cut tomato. Low levels of O_2 and high levels of CO_2 reduce respiration rate and ethylene production, resulting in delayed ripening and senescence, thus extending the storage life of the products. The modified atmosphere can be achieved passively (the package is sealed under normal air conditions) or actively (the package is flushed with a gas mixture before being closed). Once the package is closed, no further control of the gas composition is exercised. Because minimally processed fruits and vegetables are not heated, regardless of the use of additive or packaging, they must be stored at refrigeration temperatures to achieve sufficient shelf life and ensure microbiological safety.

Lycopene did not differ significantly between whole and just-processed fresh-cut tomatoes (six different cultivars) (Odriozola-Serrano et al., 2008a). The fresh-cut tomatoes in MAP (5% O_2 + 5% CO_2) retained their initial lycopene content for a period of 21 days at 4°C, except for cultivars 'Rambo' and 'Bodar'. For the first cultivar, the lycopene content was maintained for 14 days but decreased after 21 days. Lycopene of the second cultivar decreased slightly but continuously throughout storage.

In fresh-cut red sweet pepper (slices wrapped with polyvinyl chloride film), all the main carotenoids (capsanthin, cucurbitaxanthin A, zeaxanthin, β-carotene and β-cryptoxanthin) accumulated in samples stored at 8°C but decreased at 4°C (Raffo et al., 2008). Hot water treatment inhibited carotenoid accumulation. In minimally processed jalapeño pepper rings packed in perforated (air atmosphere) polyethylene bags and stored at 4.4°C for 12 days and an additional 3 days at 13°C, α-carotene and β-carotene decreased 48% and 32%, respectively, after 3 days (Howard and Hernandez-Brenes, 1998). With modified atmosphere (5% O_2, 4% CO_2), losses of these carotenoids amounted to only 8% and 13%, respectively.

The total carotenoid content was determined in ready-to-eat shredded carrot, packed in air (control) or in MAP (90% N_2 + 5% O_2 + 5% CO_2 and 95% O_2 + 5% CO_2) and stored chilled for up to 13 days (Alasalvar et al., 2005). In both orange and purple carrots, the main loss of total carotenoids occurred in the 95% O_2 + 5% CO_2 treatment.

Lutein and β-carotene decreased during storage of fresh-cut broccoli florets at 5°C for 12 days, but the decrease was lower in samples stored in modified atmosphere than in samples stored in air (Fernández-León et al., 2013a).

In minimally processed shredded kale packed in polyethylene bags and stored at 7°C–9°C for 5 days, β-carotene, lutein, violaxanthin, and neoxanthin were reduced by 14%, 27%, 20%, and 31%, respectively (Azevedo and Rodriguez-Amaya, 2005a). The corresponding losses were 42%, 32%, 20%, and 20% in whole New Zealand leaves and 18%, 19%, 12%, and 8% in endive strips, minimally processed and stored under the same conditions as kale (Azevedo-Meleiro and Rodriguez-Amaya, 2005b).

Carotenoid losses were lower in minimally processed kale strips packed in passive modified atmosphere (Kobori et al., 2011). Neoxanthin and violaxanthin did not change significantly after 15 days at 1°C in the dark; β-carotene and lutein decreased 11% and 7%, respectively. At 11°C in the dark, β-carotene, lutein, violaxanthin, and neoxanthin decreased 24%, 24%, 13%, and 16%, respectively, after 10 days. At 11°C under light, lutein and neoxanthin had a slight increase and β-carotene and violaxanthin were reduced 16% and 23% after 5 days. Fluctuations in carotenoid levels during storage might indicate that both biosynthesis and degradative oxidation might be occurring simultaneously, the concentration of the carotenoid at any one time reflecting which of these two opposing processes was predominating. More interestingly, zeaxanthin, which was not found in the leaves before minimal processing and in leaves stored in the dark, appeared under lighted storage, indicating that the xanthophyll cycle was functioning.

The total carotenoid content of minimally processed kale in packaging of different permeability to O_2 and CO_2 remained stable during storage at 1°C, 5°C, and 10°C for 15 days (Carnelossi et al., 2002). There was a slight increase when high permeability packaging was used at 1°C storage. Carotenoid stability was lower when the vegetable was packed in PET trays. Total carotenoid did not decline significantly in fresh-cut Swiss chard under dark or lighted storage for 12 days at 5°C (Ferrante et al., 2008), but it decreased in cut lamb's lettuce after 8 days of storage at 4°C in the dark (Ferrante et al., 2009).

6.6.2 High-pressure processing

High pressure processing (HPP) employs 400–1200 MPa to kill microorganisms and inactivate enzymes that cause undesirable changes in fruits and vegetables, reducing their shelf life. HPP is gaining popularity because of its potential to achieve desirable effects with minimum changes in sensory and nutritional attributes. The combination of high pressure and elevated temperature does considerably less damage to the product than conventional heat sterilization.

High-temperature short-time processing (HTST) at 110°C for 8.6 sec had no effect on total and individual carotenes of apricot nectars except for a significant decrease in α-carotene (Huang et al., 2013). HP treatments (300–500 MPa for 5–20 min) also showed no effect on total carotenoid and individual carotenoids, except that the treatment at 500 MPa, 20 min, significantly increased total carotenoid and β-carotene. HTST treatment gave a better impact on the quality of apricot nectar.

Reported higher concentrations of carotenoids in HP-processed fruit products are not due to increased formation of carotenoids but to greater extractability, brought about by

HPP's effect on macromolecular structures, such as proteins and polymer carbohydrates, facilitating the release of carotenoids from the food matrix.

The effects of HP treatments (50–350 MPa) at different temperatures (30°C and 60°C) and times (2.5, 5, and 15 min) on the carotenoids (β-carotene, α-carotene, zeaxanthin, lutein, and β-cryptoxanthin) of orange juice were investigated by Ancos et al. (2002). Some of the pressure/temperature/time combinations resulted in significant increase of extractable carotenoids. HP treatments of orange juice at 100 MPa/5 min/60°C, 350 MPa/2.5 min/30°C, 400 MPa/1 min/40°C led to equal or higher concentrations of individual carotenoids compared to the untreated juice. This effect increased with the pressure applied. Velázquez-Estrada et al. (2013) found no significant effect of HPP of orange juice at 100, 200, and 300 MPa on the lutein, zeaxanthin, β-cryptoxanthin, α-carotene, and β-carotene contents of orange juice. On the other hand, pasteurization (90C, 1 min) caused significant reductions: 44% for α-carotene, 38% for β-carotene, 32% for β-cryptoxanthin, 23% for zeaxanthin, and 21% for lutein.

HP-treated (400 MPa/40°C/1 min) orange juice had higher concentrations of all the carotenoids quantified (β-cryptoxanthin, α-cryptoxanthin, zeaxanthin, lutein, β-carotene, α-carotene) than did untreated orange juice and those subjected to traditional thermal processing (low pasteurization, 70°C/30 sec; high pasteurization, 90°C/1 min; freezing at −38°C/15 min) and pulsed electric field processing (35 $kVcm^{-1}$/750 μs) (Sánchez-Moreno et al., 2005). HP treatment at 400 MPa, 40°C, 1 min, produced significant increases in the carotenoid content of orange juice (varying from 30% in β-carotene to 75% in lutein). HP treatment at 350 MPa also produced significant increases (20%–43%) (Ancos et al., 2002). An increase in time (beyond 5 min) or temperature (above 30°C) did not improve the amount of carotenoids extracted.

HP treatments of orange juice at 100 MPa/5 min/60°C, 350 MPa/2.5 min/30°C, 400 MPa/1 min/40°C led to increased extraction of carotenoids. After 10 days of refrigerated storage (4°C), no significant change in total carotenoid content was observed with the first treatment, while small losses were observed with the other two treatments (Sánchez-Moreno et al., 2003). Moderate decrease (less than 11%) of the individual carotenoids occurred in orange juice subjected to 400 MPa/1 min/40°C toward the end of 20 days of storage at 4°C (Plaza et al., 2011b). In general, the carotenoids remained higher in HP juice than in low pasteurization (70°C, 30 sec) and pulsed electric field (35 kV cm^{-1}/730 μs) juices during refrigerated storage.

HPP of persimmons 'Rojo Brilhante' and 'Sharon' purees at 50, 150, 300, and 400 MPa/15 min/25°C generally caused no significant modifications of the individual carotenoids (Ancos et al., 2000). Isomerization and degradation of carotenoids as a consequence of the HP treatments were not detected. Instead, extractability of the carotenoids increased 9%–27%. The same group (Plaza et al., 2012) studied the effect of HPP on the carotenoid content of astringent and nonastringent persimmons at two maturity stages (III and V). In general, HPP at 200 MPa produced a statistically significant increase in extracted carotenoids for the astringent samples (up to 86% and 45% at maturity stages III and V, respectively). No significant difference or no decrease was observed with nonastringent samples or those treated at 400 MPa. The best result in terms of carotenoid extractability was obtained with astringent persimmon at 200 MPa, 25°C, 6 min.

In watermelon juice, HP treatments at 300–900 MPa, 5–60 min, 60°C, had small impact on the all-*E*-lycopene, total *Z*-lycopene, and total lycopene concentrations (C. Zhang et al., 2011). It had the least effect on the carotenoid levels, compared with thermal and ultraviolet-C treatments. In the latter treatments, the carotenoid concentrations were significantly lower with higher temperature and higher UV-C dose.

Even after 60 min of high pressure treatment (600 MPa), no change was observed in the total concentration of lycopene or β-carotene of tomato pulp (Butz et al., 2002). No isomers were detected. Even extreme temperature processing (95°C for 60 min) did not cause any loss. However, high pressure did induce structural changes that reduced carotene extractability and accessibility in carrots, as shown by simulated gastric digestion.

Thermal (60°C, 90°C) and high-pressure pasteurization (mild—15 min at 450 MPa, 20°C; intense—20 min at 600 MPa and 45°C) did not affect the total lycopene concentration of tomato puree (Knockaert et al., 2012). Only the formation of *Z*-lycopene during intense thermal pasteurization was observed. On the other hand, a significant decrease in total lycopene concentration was found after sterilization (thermal—117°C; high pressure—117°C, 600 MPa), no significant difference being observed between the two sterilization processes. Aside from degradation, significant isomerization was observed: all-*E*-lycopene was converted mainly to 9-*Z*- and 13-*Z*-lycopene. Significantly fewer *Z*-isomers were formed during HP sterilization compared to thermal sterilization. The formation of 5-*Z*-lycopene seemed to be favored by HP. The in vitro lycopene bioaccessibility of a HP homogenized tomato puree containing oil was decreased during subsequent thermal or HPP.

HPP (700 MPa) at ambient temperature and high-pressure sterilization (HPS) (one pulse, 700 MPa, 30 s, 90°C) did not affect the lycopene content of tomato puree, compared to a 40% loss after conventional sterilization (20 min at 118°C, after 15 min preheating) (Krebbers et al., 2003). Individual, total, and provitamin A carotenoids were significantly higher in tomato puree subjected to high pressure (400 MPa, 25°C, 15 min) than in untreated samples or those processed by low pasteurization (70°C, 30 sec), high pasteurization (90°C, 1 min), freezing (-38°C, 15 min), or high pasteurization plus freezing (Sánchez-Moreno et al., 2006).

Using pilot- and industrial-scale equipment and processing conditions that result in equivalent microbial safety, different HP and thermal treatments of carrots were evaluated (Vervoort et al., 2012). The total carotenoid content remained constant after mild and severe pasteurization, both for thermal and HP processing. No significant changes occurred in the individual α- and β-carotene concentrations. Substantial changes were observed only at the level of sterilization. At this intensity, thermal processing caused a decrease of 28% in α-carotene and 31% in β-carotene.

HP treatment at two pressure levels (400 MPa, 600 MPa) did not affect the total carotenoid content of three commonly consumed vegetables (carrot, green bean, and broccoli), although it differed between vegetables (McInerney et al., 2007).

The combined treatment of high pressure and mild heat could be used as an effective process for production of high-quality carrot juice (Y.S. Kim et al., 2001). The optimum process condition was estimated at 395 to 445 MPa, 70°C, for 8 to 11 min. α-Carotene and β-carotene were relatively stable during this combined process.

The carotenoid levels of commonly consumed vegetables (carrot, tomato, green and red pepper, broccoli, spinach) were not significantly influenced by HP (625 MPa, 5 min, 20°C) or high-pressure high-temperature (HPHT) treatments at 70°C and 117°C (625 MPa, 5 min) (Sánchez et al., 2014). An increase of lutein or β-carotene was observed in some cases (broccoli and spinach) after HP and HPHT at 70°C treatments, which was probably due to increased extractability of these carotenoids. Only minor carotenoid loss was noted in red and green pepper, respectively, after HPHT at 117°C. Isomerization (to 13-Z-β-carotene) was only found significant in red pepper after the more intense treatment.

6.6.3 High-intensity pulsed electric field processing

High-intensity pulsed electric field (HIPEF) (30kV/cm, 100 μs) processing did not provoke a significant decrease in the concentration of any of the carotenoids in comparison with the untreated orange juice (Cortés et al., 2006b). During refrigerated storage at 2°C and 10°C for 7 and 6 weeks, respectively, reduction in the total carotenoid content was greater in the untreated and pasteurized (90°C, 20 sec) orange juice than in the juice subjected to HIPEF. In another study, pasteurization (90°C, 20 sec) caused greater decrease in most of the carotenoids identified in orange juice than did HIPEF processing (Cortés et al., 2006a). The total carotenoid decreased 13% in pasteurized orange juice, as opposed to decreases of 10%, 6%, and 8% when fields of 15, 30, and 40 kV/cm were applied.

HIPEF processing (at 25, 30, 35 and 40 kV/cm, 30 to 340 μs) of an orange–carrot juice mixture was investigated by Torregrosa et al. (2005). HIPEF treatment at 25 and 30 kV/cm caused a significant increase in the concentrations of most of the 16 carotenoids quantified and provided higher RAE values than those of pasteurized juice (98°C, 21 sec).

There was high retention of lycopene in watermelon juice subjected to HIPEF at electric field strengths of 30–35 kV/cm, frequencies of 50–250 Hz, pulse widths of 1–7 μs, and treatment time of 50–2050 μs (Oms-Oliu 2009). Maximum relative lycopene content was obtained when HIPEF treatments were set at 35 kV/cm for 50 μs using 7 μs bipolar pulses at 200 Hz.

Optimization of the HIPEF treatment conditions was carried out with tomato juice, evaluating the effects of the variables: frequency, pulse width, and pulse polarity (Odriozola-Serrano et al., 2007). Maximal lycopene content was obtained with HIPEF treatment of 1 μs pulse duration applied at 250 Hz in bipolar mode.

HIPEF (35 kV/cm for 1500 μs with 4 μs bipolar pulse at 100 Hz) and thermal pasteurization (90°C, 30 sec and 90°C, 60 sec) resulted in tomato juice with higher total and individual carotenoids (lycopene, β-carotene, and phytofluene) and redder color than fresh juice, this effect being greater in the HIPEF-processed juice (Odriozola-Serrano et al., 2009). The carotenoids were also better maintained in the HIPEF-processed juice during storage than in thermally treated and untreated juices.

Pulsed electric fields (15, 25, 35, 40 kV/cm, from 40 to 700 μs) influenced the concentration of extracted carotenoids in an orange juice–milk beverage, resulting in a slight increase at 15 kV/cm and a slight decrease at 40 kV/cm (Zulueta et al., 2010). Pasterurization (90°C, 20 sec) caused a reduction of the total carotenoid content.

The effects of HIPEF (35 kV/cm, 4 μs bipolar pulses at 200 Hz for 800 or 1400 μs) and thermal (90°C, 60 sec) treatments on the carotenoids of a fruit juice (orange, kiwi, and pineapple)–soymilk beverage stored at 4°C for 56 days were evaluated and compared (Morales-de la Peña et al., 2011). Both treatments led to significant decreases, lutein, zeaxanthin, and β-cryptoxanthin being the most affected. However, the HIPEF-treated beverages had higher concentrations than the heat-processed beverages. The total carotenoid content decreased in all evaluated samples as storage time increased. Individual carotenoids suffered losses, remained without change, or even increased over time.

Tomato juice made of moderate-intensity pulsed electric field (MIPEF) (1 kV/cm, 16 monopolar pulses of 4 μs) processed tomatoes presented high concentrations of lutein, α-carotene, β-carotene, all-*E*-lycopene, 9-*Z*-lycopene, and 13-*Z*-lycopene (Vallverdú-Queralt et al., 2013). This was attributed by the authors to a MIPEF-induced stress response that could enhance metabolic activity and accumulation of secondary metabolites. The MIPEF-treated juices were then subjected to thermal (90°C, 60 sec) and HIPEF (35 kV/cm, 1500 μs) processing. HIPEF-treated tomato juice maintained higher carotenoid levels (10%–20%) through the storage time (under refrigeration for 56 days) than heat-treated and untreated juices. Thus, the combination of MIPEF and HIPEF treatments could be proposed as strategy for producing and preserving tomato juice with high carotenoid content.

6.6.4 Irradiation

Carotenoids tend to be stable to radiation. The total carotenoid level of coriander leaves was unaffected by exposure to 1 kGy dose; a dose-dependent enhancement in their extractability was observed in irradiated leaves (Kamat et al., 2003). Radiation of 1 and 2 kGy had no significant effects on the carotenoid contents of dew gram, chickpea (Nagar et al., 2012), green gram, and garden pea sprouts (Hajare et al., 2007). Moreover, storage did not alter the total carotenoid contents in irradiated samples.

All-*E*-β-carotene decreased during storage (5°C for 13 days) in arugula treated with 1 or 2 kGY, but the decrease was statistically significant only with the samples treated with 2 kGY (Nunes et al., 2013). In general, the minor provitamin A carotenoids were not significantly affected by exposure to both irradiation doses.

Sun-dried and dehydrated paprika samples were irradiated in a ^{60}Co γ-irradiator at five doses (0, 2.5, 5.0, 7.5, and 10 kGy) in polyethylene bags and stored for 10 months at ambient temperature (Topuz and Ozdemir, 2003). Higher irradiation doses and a longer storage period resulted in a significant ($p < .01$) reduction of all the carotenoids, except capsorubin, for which there was no significant ($p < .05$) effect of irradiation dose. The decrease of red carotenoids, for all irradiation treatments, was less than that of the storage period. The highest irradiation dose, 10 kGy, caused 11% capsanthin reduction; 10 months of storage at ambient temperature caused 42% reduction of capsanthin. Yellow pigments of paprika (zeaxanthin, capsolutein, violaxanthin, β-carotene, and β-cryptoxanthin) were significantly decreased by all treatments.

6.7 STORAGE OF PROCESSED FOODS

Of 14 identified carotenoids, only antheraxanthin and the mixture of violaxanthin and neoxanthin decreased in mixed orange and carrot juice, packaged in lightweight paperboard cartons, and stored at −40°C for 132 days (Cortés et al., 2005).

Freshly squeezed orange juice was treated by HP (400 MPa, 40°C, 1 min), pulsed electric field (PEF) (35 kV/cm, 750 μs), and low pasteurization (LP) (70°C, 30 sec) and stored at 4°C for 40 days (Plaza et al., 2011b). The concentrations of the major carotenoids were maintained during the refrigerated storage, except for a slight decrease during the last 20 days in lutein in LP- and PEF-treated juices, in zeaxanthin in PEF-treated juice, and in α-cryptoxanthin in all three treated juices, the reduction being statistically significant only with α-cryptoxanthin. In general, the carotenoids remained higher in HP juice than in LP and PEF juices during refrigerated storage. Moderate decrease (less than 11%) of the carotenoids occurred in orange juice subjected to 400 MPa/1 min/40°C during the last 20 days of storage at 4°C. In orange-carrot juice stored at −40°C for 132 days, of the 14 carotenoids identified, only antheraxanthin, 9-Z-violaxanthin, and neoxanthin decreased during the storage period (Cortés et al., 2005).

Lee and Coates (2002) observed more than 20% loss of lycopene and about 7% loss of β-carotene in red grapefruit juice concentrate stored in plastic container at −23°C for 12 months. In metal can, the same trends were observed, but pigment losses were slightly smaller.

During 1 year of frozen storage of watermelon chunks stored in zip-closure plastic bags or puree stored in centrifuge tubes, lycopene suffered losses of ~30%–40% at −20°C and ~5%–10% at -80°C over a year's storage (Fish and Davis 2003). Lycopene was slightly more stable in the puree than in diced watermelon at −20°C but not at −80°C. β-carotene appeared to be more stable than lycopene during storage at −20°C. In fresh-cut watermelon held for 7 or more days at 2°C, a slight loss of lycopene was observed, probably due to senescence (Perkins-Veazie and Collins, 2004).

Fresh-cut papaya cubes and slices stored at 5°C did not have any change in the β-carotene content during 10 days of storage (Rivera-López et al., 2005). At 14 and 18 days of storage, this carotenoid decreased by an average of 18% and 22%, respectively, for both the cubes and slices. At 10°C, there was no change up to 6 days, but after 14 days of storage, there was reduction of 62% for cubes and 63% for slices. At 20°C, losses of 57% for the cubes and 61% for the slices were observed.

In tomato products (pulp, puree, and paste) subjected to accelerated aging (30, 40, and 50°C for 3 months), β-carotene decreased even at 30°C (Lavelli and Giovanelli, 2003). Lycopene was stable in all samples.

In tomato puree pressurized at 100 to 600 MPa at 20°C for 12 min and stored at refrigerator temperature (4°C) and ambient temperature (24°C), the higher the storage temperature, the greater the loss of total lycopene and the higher the percentage of 13-Z-lycopene (Qiu et al., 2006). The highest stability of lycopene was found when the puree was pressurized at 500 MPa and stored at 4°C.

Just after processing, HIPEF (35 kV/cm, 1500 μs in bipolar 4 μs pulses at 100 Hz) and heat-treated (90°C, 1 min or 30 sec) tomato juices showed higher lycopene levels than the untreated juice (Odriozola-Serrano et al., 2008b). During storage at 4°C, lycopene of both treated and untreated samples decreased exponentially following first-order kinetics.

The lycopene and β-carotene levels were significantly lower in the HPP and thermally processed grapefruit juices compared to the control after 7 days of storage at 4°C (Uckoo et al., 2013). However, after 21 days, the treated and the control grapefruit juices had significantly lower contents of these carotenoids than those found initially, no significant difference being observed in the carotenoid concentrations of the three types of samples.

In juice processed by hot-breaking of tomatoes at 82°C, screening, heating at 121°C for 40 sec, and storing for 12 weeks, 15-*Z*-lycopene was the major isomer formed during dark storage at 4°C, while 9-*Z*- and 13-*Z*-lycopene were favored at 25°C (Lin and Chen, 2005b). 5-*Z*- and 13-*Z*-lycopene dominated at 35°C. Under lighted storage, 9-*Z*- and di-*Z*-lycopene were the main isomers at 35°C, whereas 13-*Z*- and 15-*Z*-lycopene prevailed at 4°C and 25°C.

Thermal stability and isomerization of lycopene in oleoresins prepared from three tomato varieties were studied at 4 temperatures in the dark (Hackett et al., 2004). As the storage temperature increased from 25°C to 100°C, the degradation of total lycopene in all samples increased significantly. At 25°C and 50°C, lycopene might degrade mainly through oxidation without isomerization. Isomerization of lycopene increased at 75°C and 100°C. The red color of tomato oleoresin began to lighten into orange-yellow as the all-*E*-lycopene was converted into *Z*-forms. On the other hand, the orange-colored tangerine tomato turned into more intense red due to the transformation of the tetra-*Z*-lycopene, typical of this tomato variety, into the all-*E*- and other *Z*-isomers.

Lycopene degradation during storage of two types of spray-dried tomato powders (hot break and cold break) proceeded to the same extent, 60% of lycopene being degraded at 45°C after 6 weeks (Anguelova and Warthesen, 2000). At lower temperature, losses were about 30% after the same period. Mechanisms of loss appeared to be both isomerization and oxidation. In both blanched and unblanched batches of freeze-dried carrots, the rate of carotenoid degradation was at a minimum over the water activity range 0.31–0.54 (Lavelli et al., 2007).

During storage for 4 months at ambient temperature, carotenoid contents dropped by 17% and 10% in chili and by 40% and 39% in paprika powders, with and without illumination, respectively (Schweiggert et al., 2007).

There was an overall loss of pigmentation in paprika oleoresins during storage, which was more marked with increasing temperature (Jarén-Galán and Mínguez-Mosquera, 1999). At temperatures below 60°C, the rate of destruction of the yellow pigment fraction was higher than that of the red pigments. Above 60°C, the red pigment fraction became more unstable.

During ambient storage, β-carotene decreased in both unblanched and blanched dehydrated carrot, but loss was greater in the unblanched product (Negi and Roy, 2001b). Reduction of β-carotene was gradual during the first 6 months of storage, but a sharp decline was noted after 9 months. Higher retention was observed under cold storage (7.5°C–8.5°C).

The efficacy of double packed and cold stored samples over other combinations was shown in two green leafy vegetables, savoy beets, and fenugreek, dehydrated in a low-temperature drier and stored for 9 months packed in high-density polyethylene in single or double layers (Negi and Roy, 2001c). Nevertheless, double packed and cold stored samples of fenugreek retained only 67% β-carotene, whereas savoy beet leaves retained only 57%.

Lycopene underwent significant losses in commercial gazpachos throughout storage (3 months at 4°C) (Vallverdú-Queralt et al., 2012). *Z*-lycopene isomers decreased slightly, except 5-*Z*-lycopene, which increased slightly.

After 6 months of storage, the contents of all main carotenoids (all-*E*-canthaxanthin, all-*E*-lutein, all-*E*-zeaxanthin, 9-*Z*-canthaxanthin, and β-apo-8′-carotenoic acid ethyl ester) in egg yolk powder were significantly lower (Wenzel et al., 2010). The synthetic carotenoids canthaxanthin and β-apo-8′-carotenoic acid ethyl ester showed higher retention, and the greatest losses occurred within the first 8 weeks. After 26 weeks, the egg yolk powders stored at −18°C showed only a slightly higher retention of carotenoids when compared to the powders stored at 20°C.

6.8 MICROENCAPSULATION AND NANOENCAPSULATION

The utilization of carotenoids as colorant additives and functional ingredients in food and beverage can be problematic because of their insolubility in water, instability, and low bioavailability. The first two problems have been addressed by the formulation of water-dispersable market products, as colloidal suspensions, emulsions, or dispersions in suitable colloids. In recent years, attention has centered on microencapsulation and nanoencapsulation.

6.8.1 Microcapsules

Microencapsulation is defined as a process in which tiny particles or droplets are surrounded by a coating, or embedded in a homogenous or heterogenous matrix, to give small capsules with many useful properties (Gharsallaoui et al., 2007).

Shahidi and Han (1993) cited the following reasons for the application of microencapsulation in the food industry: to reduce the reactivity of the core in relation to the outside environment (e.g., light, oxygen, and water), to decrease the evaporation or transfer rate of the core material to the outside environment, to promote easier handling of the core material, to control the release of the core material in order to achieve the proper delay until the right stimulus, to mask the core taste, and to dilute the core material when it is used in only very small amounts but achieve uniform dispersion in the host material.

Microencapsulation provides a means of protecting sensitive food components, such as carotenoids, during processing and storage. It has been applied to synthetic or extracted/isolated natural carotenoids or to oleoresins and juices, using different coating materials. Spray-drying has been the most commonly used microencapsulation method.

Lycopene was microencapsulated by spray-drying, using a modified starch as encapsulating agent. Encapsulation efficiency varied from 21% to 29% (Rocha et al., 2011). Lycopene microcapsules were also prepared by spray-drying with gelatin and sucrose as coating material (Shu et al., 2006). Encapsulation yield and efficiency were significantly affected by ratio of core and wall materials, ratio of gelatin and sucrose, homogenization pressure, inlet temperature, feed temperature, and lycopene purity. The microcapsules had regular spherical shape, were varied in size, and had a rounded outer surface with the formation of concavities. The stability test revealed that microencapsulation offered greater protection to lycopene compared to its free form.

β-carotene was microencapsulated by spray-drying with acid-modified tapioca starch, native tapioca starch, and maltodextrin (Loksuwan, 2007). The total β-carotene content was highest for modified tapioca starch and lowest for maltodextrin. The surface β-carotene was lowest for modified tapioca starch and highest for native tapioca starch. The modified tapioca starch was more effective than its native starch in β-carotene retention and was therefore considered as potential wall material for the encapsulation of this carotenoid.

Bixin was encapsulated with gum arabic or maltodextrin by spray-drying, and the stability was evaluated in aqueous solution under illumination or in the dark at 21°C (Barbosa et al., 2005). Bixin encapsulated with gum arabic was 3 to 4 times more stable than that encapsulated with maltodextrin. Greater bixin stability was noted in the microcapsules stored in the dark than those stored under illumination. Moreover, 10 times greater stability was observed for encapsulated bixin compared to unencapsulated bixin in the dark. Encapsulation by spray-drying warm aqueous ethanol solution with dissociated sodium caseinate and dissolved bixin resulted in transparent dispersions upon hydration of the spray-dried powder (Y. Zhang and Zhong, 2013). The stability of bixin was much improved and a consistent yellow color was obtained.

Water-in-oil-in-water multiple emulsions with 25% and 35% solid contents were spray-dried, producing microcapsules with 3.9:1, 2.6:1, and 1.4:1 biopolymers blend to primary emulsion ratios and 0.25% theoretical carotenoid concentration (Rodriguez-Huezo et al., 2004). Microcapsules obtained from higher biopolymers blend to primary emulsion ratios and solid content had better morphology, encapsulation efficiency, and larger particle size but showed relatively higher carotenoids degradation kinetics than microcapsules made with lower biopolymers blend to primary emulsion ratios and solid content, which exhibited poorer morphology, encapsulation efficiency, and smaller particle size. Microcapsules stored at different water activities showed maximum carotenoid degradation at a water activity (a_w) of 0.628, with lower degradation occurring at lower or higher a_w.

The spray-drying conditions for the encapsulation of gac oil with whey protein concentrate and gum arabic were optimized using the response surface methodology (Kha et al., 2014). The optimally encapsulated oil powder was found to have high quality and could be used as a nutrient supplement and natural food colorant due to its contents of unsaturated fatty acids, β-carotene, and lycopene, and its attractive red-yellow color. It was expected that the powder could be stored for a long time because of its low a_w and good protective structure of particles against light, oxidation, and unwanted release of the oil droplets and carotenoids.

Microcapsules of paprika oleoresin with gum arabic and soy protein isolate were prepared by high-pressure homogenization and spray-drying (Rascón et al., 2011). Maximal carotenoid stability was achieved at a_w of 0.274 and 0.710 for microcapsules prepared with gum arabic and soy protein isolate, respectively. In contrast to the soy protein microcapsules, those of gum arabic were unable to retain their structural integrity at a_ws above 0.743.

Oleoresin of rosa mosqueta (*Rosa rubiginosa*) was encapsulated with starch or gelatin by spray-drying (Robert et al., 2003). Gelatin provided greater protection of the main pigments, as shown by the lower degradation rate constants and longer half-lives. Degradation of all-*E*-rubixanthin, all-*E*-lycopene, and all-*E*-β-carotene occurred at the same rate in the starch microcapsules. In the gelatin microcapsules, all-*E*-β-carotene had a lower degradation rate.

The influence of process conditions on microcapsules of extract of pequi (Brazilian fruit) pulp produced by spray-drying using gum arabic as microencapsulating agent was studied by Santana et al. (2013). Tween 80 was used as a secondary emulsifier. Only powder moisture content, hygroscopicity, water activity, and vitamin C content were statistically influenced by independent variables. Spray-drying was optimized for maximum vitamin C and carotenoids content and minimal water content and hygroscopicity. The powder was characterized as to particle morphology, bulk, absolute density, and particle size distribution.

Astaxanthin oleoresin from *Haematococcus pluvialis* was dispersed in aqueous solutions with soy lecithin as dispersant agent and encapsulated by spray-drying using gum arabic and whey protein, alone or combined with maltodextrin or inulin (Bustos-Garza et al., 2013). Whey protein alone or combined with gum arabic presented the best encapsulation yield (61%–70%). The microcapsules with 100% whey protein also exhibited the highest temperature stability.

The effects of storage temperature and water activity on degradation of carotenoids contained in spray-dried microcapsules of nonaqueous chili extracts with gum arabic–maltodextrin DE (dextrose equivalent) 20 was investigated (Guadarrama-Lezama et al., 2014). Total carotenoid content decreased over time, but degradation was lower in microcapsules stored at 25°C than those stored at 35°C or 40°C. The morphology of microcapsules was altered at $a_w > 0.6$, including swelling of the polysaccharide matrix and possible subsequent dissolution of the wall material, which indicated a high rate of carotenoid degradation. When the microcapsules were stored with 0.2–0.6 of a_w, the highest glass transition temperatures were achieved. In this range, the wall materials of the microcapsules suffered less microstructural modifications, associated with the minimum level of carotenoid degradation.

Lyophilization appears to be the second-most used mode of microencapsulation for carotenoids. Lycopene extracted from red-fleshed guava was encapsulated with gum arabic or gum arabic + maltodextrin by spray-drying or lyophilization (Matioli and Rodriguez-Amaya, 2002). The powders were packed in polyethylene bags and stored at room temperature for 40 days in the presence or absence of light. The encapsulated lycopene had two periods of degradation, more rapid in the beginning and slower after 15 days. Greater lycopene stability was observed with lycopene encapsulated by lyophilization with gum arabic, together with maltodextrin.

Stored at different conditions (under light, in the dark, at different temperatures), β-carotene microencapsulated with native pinhão (*Araucaria angustifolia* seeds) starch by freeze-drying exhibited lower stability than those microencapsulated with 12 DE hydrolyzed starch (Spada et al., 2012).

Gelatin and poly(γ-glutamic acid) (γ-PGA) were used as coating materials for the encapsulation of lycopene extract from tomato pulp waste (Chiu et al., 2007). Lycopene was extracted with supercritical CO_2. A 24% loss occurred during freeze-drying. During storage of the microencapsulated powder, the concentrations of *Z*-, all-*E*-, and total lycopene decreased with increasing time and temperature.

Sousdaleff et al. (2013) evaluated the stability of potassium norbixinate microencapsulated with maltodextrin DE 20 by freeze-drying, as a function of light, air, and different pH. The best results were obtained with microencapsulated potassium norbixinate 1:20, which, when vacuum-packed and in the presence of natural light, showed color retention of 78%. The microencapsulated colorant could be used in a wide range of pH and food applications.

Lycopene was microencapsulated by complex coacervation using gelatin and gum arabic as the encapsulating agents (Rocha-Selmi 2013). Most of the systems studied presented spherical microcapsules with defined walls. The encapsulation efficiency was above 90% and the microencapsulated lycopene was more stable than the free form.

To enhance stability and bioavailability of lycopene, ultrasonic emulsification was used to prepare lycopene microcapsules (Guo et al., 2014). Technological parameters were optimized by the response surface methodology. Encapsulation efficiency of the lycopene microcapsules under the optimized conditions approached 64%.

Solid lipid microparticles were produced by adding β-carotene to melted lipid (30% sunflower oil + 70% stearic acid), followed by mixing with polysorbate 80 (employed to stabilize the stearic acid microparticles) and ultra-agitation (Gomes et al., 2013). For stearic acid microparticles with α-tocopherol, more than 90% of the initial amount of β-carotene was maintained after 7 months under refrigerated storage in the dark. Significant microstructural alterations were detected in the microparticles without α-tocopherol.

For bixin, Marcolino et al. (2011) considered coprecipitation as the best method of complexation with β-cyclodextrin. Complexation with β-cyclodextrin promoted an intensification of color, increased water solubility, and stabilization in the presence of light. Application of bixin-β-cyclodextrin in curd did not alter the initial characteristics of the product, which were sensorially well accepted.

The purple Brazilian cherry juice was encapsulated by lyophilization in xanthan, tara, and xanthan-tara hydrogel matrices (Rutz et al., 2013). The highest encapsulation efficiency was obtained with xanthan gum. Stored microparticles showed carotenoid degradation at 4°C and 25°C; xanthan and hydrogel provided greater stability.

Encapsulation of saffron water-soluble carotenoids (mainly crocin) in three amorphous matrices (pullulan and two polyvinylpyrrolidone, PVP, differing in molecular weight) improved their stability to oxidation (Selim et al., 2000). PVP 40 was the most effective wall material under the storage conditions studied. Estimation of T_g of the polymer used as wall material was not a useful predictor of colorant stability, indicating that molecular mobility might not be rate limiting even when the polymer existed in the glassy state. Other factors such as microstructure and porosity of the polymer might be more important modifiers of reaction kinetics. Porosity also had a major effect on the stability of β-carotene encapsulated in freeze-dried maltodextrin-emulsion systems (Harnkarnsujarit et al., 2012). As with the encapsulated saffron carotenoid described above, the highest stability was found in fully plasticized and collapsed solids. The latter system was prepared from emulsions of β-carotene in sunflower oil dispersed in maltodextrin systems, prefrozen at various freezing conditions prior to freeze-drying to control nucleation and subsequent pore size and structural collapse of freeze-dried solids.

Lycopene formed complexes with β- and γ-cyclodextrins, but not with α-cyclodextrin (Matioli and Rodriguez-Amaya, 2003). After 180 days of storage at refrigeration temperature, lycopene level remained constant in the lycopene-γ-cyclodextrin complex but was reduced 80% in the lycopene-β-cyclodextrin complex. The complex was dispersible in water, maintaining the red color of lycopene. Stability under light exposure was excellent, retention being 100% during 40 days at ambient temperature.

Microencapsulation by molecular inclusion was applied, using β-cyclodextrin, to reduce the degradation of carotenoids in the habanera chili oleoresin (Domínguez-Cañedo, 2015). The complex in the ratio 30:70 oleoresin:β-cyclodextrin stored at 25°C had greater retention of total carotenoid, showed greater shelf life, and had a lower degradation constant, compared to the 20:80 ratio.

Direct evidence was provided for the formation of 1:1 inclusion complex between β-caroten-8′-oic acid and β-cyclodextrin (Polyakov et al., 2004). Cyclodextrin protected the carotenoid from reactive oxygen species. However, complexation with cyclodextrin resulted in considerable decrease in the antioxidant ability of the carotenoid. This result differs with that of another study with antioxidants, including β-carotene, apo-8′-carotenal, and apo-12′-carotenal, in gum arabic and maltodextrin microcapsules. Enhancement of the antioxidant activity due to the incorporation of antioxidant molecules was observed, more pronounced in gum arabic microcapsules (Rodrigues et al., 2012). The empty microcapsules could scavenge all the studied reactive oxygen and nitrogen species, gum arabic being a more potent antioxidant than maltodextrin. Apo-8′-carotenal incorporation promoted the highest increase in scavenging capacities, varying from 50% to 132% and from 39% to 85% for gum arabic and maltodextrin microcapsules, respectively.

Synthetic astaxanthin was microencapsulated in a chitosan matrix cross-linked with glutaraldehyde using the multiple emulsion/solvent evaporation method (Higuera-Ciapara et al., 2004). The microencapsulated pigment did not suffer isomerization nor degradation during storage at 25°C, 35°C, and 45°C for 8 weeks.

6.8.2 Nanocapsules and nanodispersions

Different nano-delivery systems have been developed during the last years to protect carotenoids from degradation and to enhance their bioavailability. Gutiérrez et al. (2013) reviewed nanoencapsulation techniques compatible with labile compounds, such as β-carotene, including nanoencapsulation using lipid nanoparticles, supercritical fluids, casein micelles by self-assembling, and β-lactoglobulin complexes. The need for a careful toxicological safety evaluation was also addressed.

Oxidation of β-carotene of synthetic and natural origins was investigated after dispersion in Tween micelles or polylactic acid particles, using auto-oxidation and oxidation by xanthine oxidase-generated-reactive oxygen species (Cao-Hoang et al., 2011). Encapsulation of β-carotene in polylactic acid particles gave rise to a more stable supramolecular organization which offered better protection against oxidation.

To provide information for designing effective nanoemulsion-based delivery systems that retard the degradation of encapsulated carotenoids during long-term storage, Qian et al. (2012a) examined the impact of antioxidants on β-carotene incorporated into oil-in-water nanoemulsions stabilized by either a globular protein (β-lactoglobulin) or a nonionic surfactant (Tween 20). The rate of β-carotene degradation decreased with the addition of water-soluble or oil-soluble antioxidants. EDTA was more effective than ascorbic acid, and Coenzyme Q10 was more effective than vitamin E acetate. A combination of water-soluble EDTA and oil-soluble vitamin E acetate was less effective than using them individually. β-carotene degraded considerably slower in β-lactoglobulin-stabilized nanoemulsions than in those stabilized by Tween 20 (Qian et al., 2012b). Degradation increased with increasing storage temperature and was faster at pH 3 than pH 4–8 and largely independent of ionic strength.

Casein micelles can be used as nanostructures to encapsulate, stabilize, and protect β-carotene from degradation during food processing. Self-assembly method is applied to reassemble nanomicelles containing β-carotene. Casein micelles protected β-carotene during sterilization, pasteurization, high hydrostatic pressure processing, and baking (Sáiz-Abajo et al., 2013).

β-carotene molecules were successfully encapsulated within protein (ferritin) cages with a β-carotene:protein molar ratio of 12.4:1 (L. Chen et al., 2014). These nanocomposites were water soluble and had markedly improved thermal stability.

The retention of β-carotene in oil-in-water nanoemulsions stabilized by food-grade biopolymer emulsifiers (modified starches) was significantly higher compared to that of β-carotene dispersed in bulk oil (Liang et al., 2013). Nanoencapsulation also increased the in vitro bioaccessibility from 3.1% to 36%.

Lipid nanoparticles were prepared by homogenizing lipid (cocoa butter and/or hydrogenated palm oil), surfactant (Tween 80), and water together at a temperature exceeding the melting point of the lipid phase (~60°C), then cooling the oil-in-water nanoemulsions formed (Qian et al., 2013). Liquid lipid nanoparticles had better stability to droplet aggregation and β-carotene degradation than solid lipid nanoparticles after storage for 8 days. These effects were attributed to the ability of the fat crystals within the lipid nanoparticles to promote partial coalescence and expulsion of the carotenoids to the particle exterior.

Bixin nanocapsules were produced by the interfacial deposition of preformed poly-ε-caprolactone (Lobato et al., 2013). Poly-ε-caprolactone, capric/caprylic triacylglycerol, sorbitan monostearate, and bixin were dissolved in a mixture of acetone and ethanol under stirring. This organic solution was added to an aqueous solution containing Tween 80. Encapsulation efficiency was around 100% and the nanocapsules were considered physically stable during 119 days of storage at ambient temperature.

β-carotene in canola stearin solid lipid nanoparticle dispersions and canola oil-in-water emulsions with Poloxamer 188 and Tween 20 was investigated (Nik et al., 2012). Less β-carotene degradation was observed for the solid lipid nanodispersions versus canola oil–in-water emulsions and during storage at 4°C versus 20°C.

Nanodispersion is a promising approach to overcome bioavailability problems. The increase in bioavailability is attributed to special characteristics of nanodispersions, such as increasing the surface areas and dissolution velocities of poorly soluble compounds (Cheong et al., 2014). A top-down approach based on an emulsification-evaporation technique was used to prepare nanodispersions of astaxanthin (Anarjan et al., 2010). Response surface methodology was employed to study the effect of the main processing conditions. Astaxanthin nanodispersions displayed significantly better stability in food systems (orange juice and skimmed milk) compared to the control (deionized water) (Anarjan and Tan, 2013). The cellular (human colon carcinoma HT-29 cell line) uptake of astaxanthin nanodispersions in skimmed milk was significantly higher than that of these nanodispersions in orange juice and deionized water.

Encapsulation of fucoxanthin in chitosan-sodium tripolyphosphate-glycolipid prepared by ionic gelation method produced smooth and spherical nanogels with extensive hydrogen bonding between fucoxanthin and chitosan (Ravi and Baskaran, 2015). Encapsulation efficiency was 90% with glycolipids, significantly higher than that of nanogels without glycolipids. Glycolipid offered enhanced fucoxanthin stability. The bioavailability of fucoxanthin in vitro from the chitosan nanogels with glycolipid was higher (68%) compared with that from the chitosan nanogels without glycolipid (51%), fucoxanthin with glycolipid (36%), and control (22%).

6.9 UTILIZATION OF INDUSTRIAL BY-PRODUCTS

It has been increasingly shown that the processing wastes (e.g., peel) of the fruit and vegetable industry are richer in carotenoids and other bioactives than the processed products themselves, demonstrating the need for better utilization of by-products for food and feed. This is best exemplified by the tomato processing industry, which generates a considerable amount of waste (called pomace) consisting of peel, seeds, and a part of the pulp. The tomato peel by-product was found to contain 734 μg/g lycopene on a dry weight basis (Knoblich et al., 2005). Significant amounts of lutein, β-carotene, and *Z*-β-carotene were also present. The seed by-product contained 130 μg lycopene per kg of dry matter.

Two products have been proposed to utilize the tomato industry by-products: lycopene extract and tomato skin powder. Extraction of lycopene from tomato waste has been carried out, employing enzymes (Choudhari and Ananthanarayan, 2007; Cuccolini et al., 2013), solvents (Kaur et al., 2008), and especially supercritical CO_2 (Baysal et al., 2000; Rozzi et al., 2002; Sabio et al., 2003; Topal et al., 2006; Vági et al., 2007; Kassama et al., 2008; Nobre et al., 2009; J. Shi et al., 2009). Ground tomato peel was used to enrich tomato paste, increasing lycopene and β-carotene bioavailability in men (Reboul et al., 2005). Tomato skin powder was included in the formulation of ketchup, improving its textural properties (Farahnaky et al., 2008), and tomato peel was added directly to dry fermented sausages to obtain a product enriched with lycopene with good textural properties (Calvo et al., 2008). Lavelli and Torresani (2011) demonstrated that, aside from well-known factors affecting oxidation rate of lycopene-rich products, such as light and oxygen exposure, control of water activity also has a remarkable effect on high-lycopene powders.

In Malaysia, nearly 25% of pink guava fruits is discarded as by-product of the puree processing industry. Utilization of this lycopene-rich waste as functional ingredient is suggested (Amin and Mukhrizah, 2006; Kong et al., 2010). Other materials are being targeted for the recovery of β-carotene, such as apricot pomace (Sanal et al., 2004, 2005) and carrot pulp residue (Vega et al., 1996; B.H. Chen and Tang, 1998). Mango peel, a major by-product of mango processing, can be used for the production of extract (Ajila et al., 2007) or powder for macaroni preparations (Ajila et al., 2010).

In Brazil, wide-scale production of cashew is done for the nuts, which represent only 10% of the total fruit weight. Large quantities of the nutritious juicy pseudofruit (called cashew apple) are discarded as waste, although cashew apple juice is a popular drink. The Brazilian Northeast has an annual production of about two million tons of cashew apple, 90% of which is lost or underutilized. Moreover, about 20% to 25% of the pseudofruit used in the cashew juice processing industry is almost entirely discarded or used as animal feed. Greater utilization of the pseudofruit and the by-product of juice processing is warranted. Abreu et al. (2013) obtained an aqueous extract by pressing followed by concentration through microfiltration, resulting in a final extract reaching 54 µg/g total carotenoids.

Shrimp waste (head and body carapace) compose 45%–60% of the whole shrimp. Sachindra and Mahendrakar (2005) determined extraction yield of shrimp waste in different vegetable oils. The highest yield was obtained by extraction using refined sunflower oil compared to groundnut, gingelly, mustard, soy, coconut, and rice oils. Supercritical extraction of the carotenoid fraction of pink shrimp residue was also investigated, the highest astaxanthin yield being obtained with CO_2 at 300 bar/333.15K (Mezzomo et al., 2013). Mechanical cell disruption of shrimp shell wastes pretreated by optimized microbial fermentation gave 66% more astaxanthin compared to the control (Cheong et al., 2014).

References

Abreu FP de, Dornier M, Dionisio AP, Carail M, Caris-Veyrat C, Dhuique-Mayer C. 2013. Cashew apple (*Anacardium occidentale* L.) extract from by-product of juice processing: a focus on carotenoids. *Food Chem* 138:25–31.

Agarwal A, Shen H, Agarwal S, Rao AV. 2001. Lycopene content of tomato products: its stability, bioavailability and in vivo antioxidant properties. *J Med Food* 4:9–15.

Ajila CM, Aalami M, Leelavathi K, Presada Rao UJS. 2010. Mango peel powder: a potential source of antioxidant and dietary fiber in macaroni preparations. *Innov Food Sci Emerg Technol* 11:219–24.

Ajila CM, Naidu KA, Bhat SG, Prasada Rao UJS. 2007. Bioactive compounds and antioxidant potential of mango peel extract. *Food Chem* 105:982–8.

Alasalvar C, Al-Farsi M, Quantick PC, Shahidi F, Wiktorowicz R. 2005. Effect of chill storage and modified atmosphere packaging (MAP) on antioxidant activity, anthocyanins, carotenoids, phenolics and sensory quality of ready-to-eat shredded orange and purple carrots. *Food Chem* 89:69–76.

Aman R, Biehl J, Carle R, Conrad J, Beifuss U, Schieber A. 2005. Application of HPLC coupled with DAD, APcI-MS and NMR to the analysis of lutein and zeaxanthin stereoisomers in thermally processed vegetables. *Food Chem* 92:753–63.

Amin I, Mukhrizah O. 2006. Antioxidant capacity of methanolic and water extracts prepared from food-processing by-products. *J Sci Food Agric* 86:778–84.

Anarjan N, Mirhosseini H, Baharin BS, Tan CP. 2010. Effect of processing conditions on physicochemical properties of astaxanthin nanodispersions. *Food Chem* 123:477–83.

Anarjan N, Tan CP. 2013. Chemical stability of astaxanthin nanodispersions in orange juice and skimmed milk as model food systems. *Food Chem* 139:527–31.

Ancos B de, Cano MP, Hernandez A, Monreal M. 1999. Effects of microwave heating on pigment composition and colour of fruit purees. *J Sci Food Agric* 79:663–70.

Ancos B de, Gonzalez E, Cano MP. 2000. Effect of high-pressure treatment on the carotenoid composition and the radical scavenging activity of persimmon fruit purees. *J Agric Food Chem* 48:3542–8.

Ancos B de, Sgroppo S, Plaza L, Cano MP. 2002. Possible nutritional and health-related value promotion in orange juice preserved by high-pressure treatment. *J Sci Food Agric* 82:790–6.

Anguelova T, Warthesen J. 2000. Lycopene stability in tomato powders. *J Food Sci* 65:67–70.

Azevedo CH, Rodriguez-Amaya DB. 2005. Carotenoid composition of kale as influenced by maturity, season and minimal processing. *J Sci Food Agric* 85:591–7.

Azevedo-Meleiro CH, Rodriguez-Amaya DB. 2005. Carotenoids of endive and New Zealand spinach as affected by maturity, season and minimal processing. *J Food Compos Anal* 18:845–55.

Barbosa MIMJ, Borsarelli CD, Mercadante AZ. 2005. Light stability of spray-dried bixin encapsulated with different edible polysaccharide preparations. *Food Res Int* 38:989–94.

Baysal T, Ersus S, Starmans DAJ. 2000. Supercritical CO_2 extraction of β-carotene and lycopene from tomato paste waste. *J Agric Food Chem* 48:5507–11.

Bechoff A, Dufour D, Dhuique-Mayer C, Marouzé C, Reynes M, Westby A. 2009. Effect of hot air, solar and sun drying treatments on provitamin A retention in orange-fleshed sweetpotato. *J Food Eng* 92:164–71.

Bengtsson A, Namutebi A, Alminger ML, Svanberg U. 2008. Effects of various traditional processing methods on the all-*trans*-β-carotene content of orange-fleshed sweet potato. *J Food Compos Anal* 21:134–43.

Bernhardt S, Schlich E. 2006. Impact of different cooking methods on food quality: retention of lipophilic vitamins in fresh and frozen vegetables. *J Food Eng* 77:327–33.

Birkeland S, Bjerkeng B. 2004. Extractabilities of astaxanthin and protein from muscle tissue of Atlantic salmon (*Salmo salar*) as affected by brine concentration and pH. *Food Chem* 85:559–68.

Borowska J, Kowalska M, Czaplicki S, Zadernowski R. 2003. Effect of hydrothermal processing on carrot carotenoids changes and interactions with dietary fiber. *Nahrung/Food* 47:46–8.

Bravo S, García-Alonso J, Martín-Pozuelo G, Gómez V, Santaella M, Navarro-González I, Periago MJ. 2012. The influence of postharvest UV-C hormesis on lycopene, β-carotene, and phenolic content and antioxidant activity of breaker tomatoes. *Food Res Int* 49:296–302.

Bunea A, Andjelkovic M, Socaciu C, Bobis O, Neacsu M, Verhe R, van Camp J. 2008. Total and individual carotenoids and phenolic acids content in fresh, refrigerated and processed spinach (*Spinacia oleracea* L.). *Food Chem* 108:649–56.

Burgos G, Amoros W, Salas E, Muñoa L, Sosa P, Díaz C, Bonierbale M. 2012. Carotenoid concentrations of native Andean potatoes as affected by cooking. *Food Chem* 133:1131–7.

Bustos-Garza C, Yáñez-Fernández J, Barragán-Huerta BE. 2013. Thermal and pH stability of spray-dried encapsulated astaxanthin oleoresin from *Haematococcus pluvialis* using several encapsulation wall materials. *Food Res Int* 54:641–9.

Butz P, Edenharder R, Fernández Garcia A, Fister H, Merkel C, Taucher B. 2002. Changes in the functional properties of vegetables induced by high pressure treatment. *Food Res Int* 35:295–300.

Calvo MM. 2005. Lutein: a valuable ingredient of fruit and vegetables. *Crit Rev Food Sci Nutr* 45:671–96.

Calvo MM, Garcia ML, Selgas MD. 2008. Dry fermented sausages enriched with lycopene from tomato peel. *Meat Sci* 80:167–72.

Cao-Hoang L, Fougère R, Waché Y. 2011. Increase in stability and change in supramolecular structure of β-carotene through encapsulation into polylactic acid nanoparticles. *Food Chem* 124:42–9.

Capanoglu E, Beekwilder J, Boyacioglu D, Hall R, de Vos R. 2008. Changes in antioxidant and metabolite profiles during production of tomato paste. *J Agric Food Chem* 56:964–73.

Carmona L, Zacarías L, Rodrigo MJ. 2012. Simulation of coloration and carotenoid biosynthesis during postharvest storage of 'Navelina' orange fruit at 12°C. *Postharvest Biol Technol* 74:108–17.

Carnelossi MAG, Silva EO, Campos RS, Soares NFF, Minim VPR, Puschmann R. 2002. Conservação de folhas de couve minimamente processadas. *Rev Bras Prod Agroind* 4:149–55.

Cervantes-Paz B, Yahia EM, Ornelas-Paz JJ, Gardea-Béjar AA, Ibarra-Junquera V, Pérez-Martínez JD. 2012. Effect of heat processing on the profile of pigments and antioxidant capacity of green and red jalapeño peppers. *J Agric Food Chem* 60:10822–33.

Cervantes-Paz B, Yahia EM, Ornelas-Paz JJ, Victoria-Campos CI, Ibarra-Junquera V, Pérez-Martínez JD, Escalante-Minakata P. 2014. Antioxidant activity and content of chlorophylls and carotenoids in raw and heat-processed jalapeño peppers at intermediate stages of ripening. *Food Chem* 146:188–96.

Chanforan C, Loonis M, Mora N, Caris-Veyrat C, Dufour C. 2012. The impact of industrial processing on health-beneficial tomato micronutrients. *Food Chem* 134:1786–95.

Chaudhary P, Jayaprakasha GK, Porat R, Patil BS. 2012. Degreening and postharvest storage influences 'Star Ruby' grapefruit (*Citrus paradisi* Macf.) bioactive compounds. *Food Chem* 135:1667–75.

Chávez AL, Sánchez T, Ceballos H, Rodriguez-Amaya DB, Nestel P, Tohme J, Ishitani M. 2007. Retention of carotenoids in cassava roots submitted to different processing methods. *J Sci Food Agric* 87:388–93.

Chen BH, Peng HY, Chen HE. 1995. Changes of carotenoids, color, and vitamin A contents during processing of carrot juice. *J Agric Food Chem* 43:1912–8.

Chen BH, Tang YC. 1998. Processing and stability of carotenoid powder from carrot pulp waste. *J Agric Food Chem* 46:2312–8.

Chen L, Bai G, Yang R, Zang J, Zhou T, Zhao G. 2014. Encapsulation of β-carotene within ferritin nanocages greatly increases its water solubility and thermal stability. *Food Chem* 149:307–12.

Cheong JY, Azwady AAN, Rusea G, Noormasshela UA, Shaziera AGN, Azleen AA, Muskhazli M. 2014. The availability of astaxanthin from shrimp shell wastes through microbial fermentations, *Aeromonas hydrophila* and cell disruptions. *Int J Agric Biol* 16:277–84.

Chiu YT, Chiu CP, Chien JT, Ho GH, Yang J, Chen BH. 2007. Encapsulation of lycopene extract from tomato pulp waste with gelatin and poly(γ-glutamic acid) as carrier. *J Agric Food Chem* 55:5123–30.

Choudhari SM, Ananthanarayan L. 2007. Enzyme aided extraction of lycopene from tomato tissues. *Food Chem* 102:77–81.

Colle IJP, Andrys A, Grundelius A, Lemmens L, Löfgren A, van Buggenhout S, van Loey A, Hendrickx M. 2011. Effect of pilot-scale aseptic processing on tomato soup quality parameters. *J Food Sci* 76:C714–23.

Colle I, Lemmens L, van Buggenhout S, van Loey A, Hendrickx M. 2010. Effect of thermal processing on the degradation, isomerization, and bioaccessibility of lycopene in tomato pulp. *J Food Sci* 75:C753–9.

Cortés C, Esteve MJ, Frígola A, Torregrosa F. 2005. Changes in carotenoids including geometrical isomers and ascorbic acid content in orange-carrot juice during frozen storage. *Eur Food Res Technol* 221:125–31.

Cortés C, Esteve MJ, Rodrigo D, Torregrosa F, Frígola A. 2006a. Changes of colour and carotenoids contents during high intensity pulsed electric field treatment in orange juices. *Food Chem Toxicol* 44:1932–9.

Cortés C, Torregrosa F, Esteve MJ, Frígola A. 2006b. Carotenoid profile modification during refrigerated storage in untreated and pasteurized orange juice and orange juice treated with high-intensity pulsed electric fields. *J Agric Food Chem* 54:6247–54.

Cuccolini S, Aldini A, Visai L, Daglia M, Ferrari D. 2013. Environmentally friendly lycopene purification from tomato peel waste: enzymatic assisted aqueous extraction. *J Agric Food Chem* 61:1646–51.

Cui Z-W, Xu S-Y, Sun D-W. 2004. Effect of microwave-vacuum drying on the carotenoids retention of carrot slices and chlorophyll retention of Chinese chive leaves. *Dry Technol* 22:563–75.

Daood HG, Kapitány J, Biacs P, Albrecht K. 2006. Drying temperature, endogenous antioxidants and capsaicinoids affect carotenoid stability in paprika (red pepper spice). *J Sci Food Agric* 86:2450–7.

Delchier N, Reich M, Renard CMGC. 2012. Impact of cooking methods on folates, ascorbic acid and lutein in green beans (*Phaseolus vulgaris*) and spinach (*Spinacea oleracea*). LWT—Food *Sci Technol* 49:197–201.

Dhuique-Mayer C, Tbatou M, Carail M, Caris-Veyrat C, Dornier M, Amiot MJ. 2007. Thermal degradation of antioxidant micronutrients in citrus juice: Kinetics and newly formed components. *J Agric Food Chem* 55:4209–16.

Díaz-Mula HM, Zapata PJ, Guillén F, Martínez-Romero D, Castillo S, Serrano M, Valero D. 2009. Changes in hydrophilic and lipophilic antioxidant activity and related bioactive compounds during postharvest storage of yellow and purple plum cultivars. *Postharvest Biol Technol* 51:354–63.

Divya P, Puthusseri B, Neelwarne B. 2012. Carotenoid content, its stability during drying and the antioxidant activity of commercial coriander (*Coriandrum sativum* L.) varieties. *Food Res Int* 45:342–50.

Domínguez-Cañedo IL, Beristain-Guevara CI, Díaz-Sobac R, Vásquez-Luna A. 2015. Degradation of carotenoids and capsaicin in the molecular inclusion complex of habanero chili oleoresin (*Capsicum chinense*) in β-cyclodextrin. *CYTA—J Food* 13:151–8.

Donado-Pestana CM, Salgado JM, Rios AO, dos Santos PR, Jablonski A. 2012. Stability of carotenoids, total phenolics and in vitro antioxidant capacity in the thermal processing of orange-fleshed sweet potato (*Ipomoea batatas* Lam.) cultivars grown in Brazil. *Plant Foods Hum Nutr* 67:262–70.

Facundo HVV, Gurak PD, Mercadante AZ, Lajolo FM, Cordenunsi BR. 2015. Storage at low temperature differentially affects the colour and carotenoid composition of two cultivars of banana. *Food Chem* 170:102–9.

Farahnaky A, Abbasi J, Jamalian J, Mesbahi G. 2008. The use of tomato pulp powder as a thickening agent in the formulation of tomato ketchup. *J Texture Stud* 39:169–82.

Fernández-León MF, Fernández-León AM, Lozano M, Ayuso MC, Amodio ML, Colelli G, González-Gómez D. 2013a. Retention of quality and functional values of broccoli ‘Parthenon’ stored in modified atmosphere packaging. *Food Cont* 31:302–13.

Fernández-León MF, Fernández-León AM, Lozano M, Ayuso MC, González-Gómez D. 2013b. Altered commercial controlled atmosphere storage conditions for ‘Parthenon’ broccoli plants (*Brassica oleracea* L. var. *italica*). Influence on the outer quality parameters and on the health-promoting compounds. LWT—Food *Sci Technol* 50:665–72.

Ferrante A, Incrocci L, Serra G. 2008. Quality changes during storage of fresh-cut or intact Swiss chard leafy vegetables. *Food Agr Environ* 6:60–2.

Ferrante A, Martinetti L, Maggiore T. 2009. Biochemical changes in cut vs. intact lamb's lettuce (*Valerianella olitoria*) leaves during storage. *Int J Food Sci Technol* 44:1050–6.
Fish WW, Davis AR. 2003. The effects of frozen storage conditions on lycopene stability in watermelon tissue. *J Agric Food Chem* 51:3582–5.
Fratianni A, Cinquanta L, Panfili G. 2010. Degradation of carotenoids in orange juice during microwave heating. LWT—Food *Sci Technol* 43:867–71.
Fratianni A, Di Criscio T, Mignogna R, Panfili G. 2012. Carotenoids, tocols and retinols evolution during egg pasta–making processes. *Food Chem* 131:590–5.
Frias J, Peñas E, Ullate M, Vidal-Valverde C. 2010. Influence of drying by convective air dryer or power ultrasound on the vitamin C and β-carotene content of carrots. *J Agric Food Chem* 58:10539–44.
Gama JJT, de Sylos CM. 2007. Effect of thermal pasteurization and concentration on carotenoid composition of Brazilian Valencia orange juice. *Food Chem* 100:1686–90.
Gayathri GN, Platel K, Prakash J, Srinivasan K. 2004. Influence of antioxidant spices on the retention of β-carotene in vegetables during domestic cooking processes. *Food Chem.* 84:35–43.
Gharsallaoui A, Roudaut G, Chambin O, Voilley A, Saurel R. 2007. Applications of spray-drying in microencapsulation of food ingredients: an overview. *Food Res Int* 40:1107–21.
Gil MI, Aguayo E, Kader AA. 2006. Quality changes and nutrient retention in fresh-cut versus whole fruits during storage. *J Agric Food Chem* 54:4284–96.
Gomes GVL, Borrin TR, Cardoso LP, Souto E, de Pinho SC. 2013. Characterization and shelf-life of β-carotene loaded solid lipid microparticles produced with stearic acid and sunflower oil. *Braz Arch Biol Technol* 56:663–71.
Goula AM, Adamopoulos KG. 2005. Stability of lycopene during spray drying of tomato pulp. LWT—Food *Sci Technol* 38:479–87.
Greco L, Riccio R, Bergero S, del Re AAM, Trevisan M. 2007. Total reducing capacity of fresh sweet peppers and five different Italian pepper recipes. *Food Chem* 103:1127–33.
Guadarrama-Lezama AY, Jaramillo-Flores E, Gutiérrez-López GF, Pérez-Alonso C, Dorantes-Álvarez L, Liliana Alamilla-Beltrán L. 2014. Effects of storage temperature and water activity on the degradation of carotenoids contained in microencapsulated chili extract. *Dry Technol* 32:1435–1447.
Guerra-Vargas M, Jaramillo-Flores ME, Dorantes-Alvarez L, Hernández-Sánchez H. 2001. Carotenoid retention in canned pickled jalapeño peppers and carrots as affected by sodium chloride, acetic acid, and pasteurization. *J Food Sci* 66:620–6.
Guo H, Huang Y, Qian J-Q, Gong Q-Y, Tang, Y. 2014. Optimization of technological parameters for preparation of lycopene microcapsules. *J Food Sci Technol* 51:1318–25.
Gutiérrez FJ, Albillos SM, Casas-Sanz E, Cruz Z, García-Estrada C, García-Guerra A, García-Reverter J, García-Suárez M, Gatón P, González-Ferrero C, Olabarrieta I, Olasagati M, Rainieri S, Rivera-Patiño D, Rojo R, Romo-Hualde A, Sáiz-Abajo M-J, Mussons M-L. 2013. Methods for nanoencapsulation of β-carotene in the food sector. *Trends Food Sci Technol* 32:73–83.
Hackett MM, Lee JH, Francis D, Schwartz SJ. 2004. Thermal stability and isomerization of lycopene in tomato oleoresins from different varieties. *J Food Sci* 69:C536–41.
Hager TJ, Howard LR. 2006. Processing effects on carrot phytonutrients. *HortSci* 41:74–9.
Hajare SN, Saroj SD, Dhokane VS, Shashidhar R, Bandekar JR. 2007. Effect of radiation processing on nutritional and sensory quality of minimally processed green gram and garden pea sprouts. *Radiat Phys Chem* 76:1642–9.
Harnkarnsujarit N, Charoenrein S, Roos YH. 2012. Reversed phase HPLC analysis of stability and microstructural effects on degradation kinetics of β-carotene encapsulated in freeze-dried maltodextrin-emulsion systems. *J Agric Food Chem* 60:9711–8.
Heredia A, Peinado I, Barrera A, Grau A. 2009. Influence of process variables on colour changes, carotenoids retention and cellular tissue alteration of cherry tomato during osmotic dehydration. *J Food Compos Anal* 22:285–94.
Heredia A, Peinado I, Rosa E, Andrés A. 2010. Effect of osmotic pre-treatment and microwave heating on lycopene degradation and isomerization in cherry tomato. *Food Chem* 123:92–8.
Hernández Becerra JA, Ochoa Flores AA, Valerio-Alfaro G, Soto-Rodriguez I, Rodríguez-Estrada MT, García HS. 2014. Cholesterol oxidation and astaxanthin degradation in shrimp during sun drying and storage. *Food Chem* 145:832–9.
Higuera-Ciapara I, Felix-Valenzuela L, Goycoolea FM, Argüelles-Monal W. 2004. Microencapsulation of astaxanthin in chitosan matrix. *Carbohyd Polym* 56:41–5.
Hiranvarachat B, Suvarnakuta P, Devahastin S. 2008. Isomerization kinetics and antioxidant activities of β-carotene in carrots undergoing different drying techniques and conditions. *Food Chem* 107:1538–46.

Howard LR, Hernandez-Brenes C. 1998. Antioxidant content and market quality of jalapeño rings as affected by minimal processing and modified atmosphere packaging. *J Food Qual* 21:317–27.

Huang W, Bi X, Zhang X, Liao X, Hu X, Wu J. 2013. Comparative study of enzymes, phenolics, carotenoids and color of apricot nectars treated by high hydrostatic pressure and high temperature short time. *Innov Food Sci Emerg Technol* 18:74–82.

Imsic M, Winkler S, Tomkins B, Jones R. 2010. Effect of storage and cooking on β-carotene isomers in carrots (*Daucus carota* L. cv. 'Stefano'). *J Agric Food Chem* 58:5109–13.

Ishida BK, Roberts JS, Chapman MH, Burri BJ. 2007. Processing tangerine tomatoes: Effects on lycopene-isomer concentrations and profile. *J Food Sci* 72:C307–12.

Jarén-Galán M, Mínguez-Mosquera MI. 1999. Quantitative and qualitative changes associated with heat treatments in the carotenoid content of paprika oleoresins. *J Agric Food Chem* 47:4379–83.

Javanmardi J, Kubota C. 2006. Variation of lycopene, antioxidant activity, total soluble solids and weight loss of tomato during postharvest storage. *Postharvest Biol Technol* 41:151–5.

Kamat A, Pingulkar K, Bhushan B, Gholap A, Thomas P. 2003. Potential application of low dose gamma irradiation to improve the microbiological safety of fresh coriander leaves. *Food Cont* 14:529–37.

Kao FJ, Chiu YS, Tsou MJ, Chiang WD. 2012. Effects of Chinese domestic cooking methods on the carotenoid composition of vegetables in Taiwan. LWT—Food *Sci Technol* 46:485–92.

Kassama LS, Shi J, Mittal GS. 2008. Optimization of supercritical fluid extraction of lycopene from tomato skin with central composite rotatable design model. *Sep Purif Technol* 60:278–84.

Kaur D, Wani AA, Oberoi DPS, Sogi DS. 2008. Effect of extraction conditions on lycopene extractions from tomato processing waste skin using response surface methodology. *Food Chem* 108:711–8.

Kha TC, Nguyen MH, Roach PD, Stathopoulos CE. 2014. Microencapsulation of Gac oil: optimization of spray drying conditions using response surface methodology. *Powder Technol* 264:298–309.

Kidmose U, Christensen LP, Agili SM, Thilsted SH. 2007. Effect of home preparation practices on the content of provitamin A carotenoids in coloured sweet potato varieties (*Ipomoea batatas* Lam.) from Kenya. *Innov Food Sci Emerg Technol* 8:399–406.

Kidmose U, Yang R-Y, Thilsted SH, Christensen LP, Brandt K. 2006. Contents of carotenoids in commonly consumed Asian vegetables and stability and extractability during frying. *J Food Compos Anal* 19:562–71.

Kim YS, Park SJ, Cho YH, Park J. 2001. Effects of combined treatment of high hydrostatic pressure and mild heat on the quality of carrot juice. *J Food Sci* 66:1355–60.

Kim S, Park J, Hwang IK. 2004. Composition of main carotenoids in Korean red pepper (*Capsicum annuum*, L.) and changes of pigment stability during drying and storage process. *J Food Sci* 69:FCT39–44.

Knoblich M, Anderson B, Latshaw D. 2005. Analyses of tomato peel and seed byproducts and their use as a source of carotenoids *J Sci Food Agric* 85:1166–70.

Knockaert G, Pulissery SK, Colle I, van Buggenhout S, Hendrickx M, van Loey A. 2012. Lycopene degradation, isomerization and in vitro bioaccessibility in high pressure homogenized tomato puree containing oil: effect of additional thermal and high pressure processing. *Food Chem* 135:1290–7.

Kobori CN, Huber LS, Sarantópoulos CIGL, Rodriguez-Amaya DB. 2011. Behavior of flavonols and carotenoids of minimally processed kale leaves during storage in passive modified atmosphere packaging. *J Food Sci* 76:H31–7.

Koca N, Karadeniz F. 2008. Changes of bioactive compounds and anti-oxidant activity during cold storage of carrots. *Int J Food Sci Technol* 43:2019–25.

Kong K-W, Rajab NF, Prasad KN, Ismail A, Markom M, Tan C-P. 2010. Lycopene-rich fractions derived from pink guava by-product and their potential activity towards hydrogen peroxide-induced cellular and DNA damage. *Food Chem* 123:1142–8.

Kopas-Lane LM, Warthesen JJ. 1995. Carotenoid photostability in raw spinach and carrots during cold storage. *J Food Sci* 60:773–6.

Krebbers B, Matser AM, Hoogerwerf SW, Moezelaar R, Tomassen MMM, van den Berg RW. 2003. Combined high-pressure and thermal treatments for processing of tomato puree: evaluation of microbial inactivation and quality parameters. *Innov Food Sci Emerg Technol* 4:377–85.

Lago-Vanzela ES, do Nascimento P, Fontes EAF, Mauro MA, Kimura M. 2013. Edible coating from native and modified starches retain carotenoids in pumpkin during drying. LWT—Food *Sci Technol* 50:420–5.

La Parra C de, Saldivar SOS, Liu RH. 2007. Effect of processing on the phytochemical profiles and antioxidant activity of corn for the production of masa, tortillas and tortilla chips. *J Agric Food Chem* 55:4177–83.

Lavelli V, Giovanelli G. 2003. Evaluation of heat and oxidative damage during storage of processed tomato products: II. Study of oxidative damage indices. *J Sci Food Agric* 83:966–71.

Lavelli V, Pompei C, Casadei MA. 2009. Quality of nectarine and peach nectars as affected by lye-peeling and storage. *Food Chem* 115:1291–8.

Lavelli V, Torresani MC. 2011. Modelling the stability of lycopene-rich by-products of tomato processing. *Food Chem* 125:529–35.

Lavelli V, Zanoni B, Zaniboni A. 2007. Effect of water activity on carotenoid degradation in dehydrated carrots. *Food Chem* 104:1705–11.

Lee HS, Coates GA. 2002. Characterization of color fade during frozen storage of red grapefruit juice concentrates. *J Agric Food Chem* 50:3988–91.

Lee HS, Coates GA. 2003. Effect of thermal pasteurization on Valencia orange juice color and pigments. *Lebens-Wiss Technol* 36:153–6.

Lemmens L, de Vleeschouwer K, Moelants KRN, Colle IJP, van Loey AM, Hendrickx ME. 2010. β-Carotene isomerization kinetics during thermal treatments of carrot puree. *J Agric Food Chem* 58:6816–24.

Leong SY, Oey I. 2012. Effects of processing on anthocyanins, carotenoids and vitamin C in summer fruits and vegetables. *Food Chem* 133:1577–87.

Lessin WJ, Catigani GL, Schwartz SJ. 1997. Quantification of *cis-trans* isomers of provitamin A carotenoids in fresh and processed fruits and vegetables. *J Agric Food Chem* 45:3728–32.

Li S, Tayie FAK, Young MF, Rocheford T, White WS. 2007. Retention of provitamin A carotenoids in high β-carotene maize (*Zea mays*) during traditional African household processing. *J Agric Food Chem* 55:10744–50.

Liang R, Shoemaker CF, Yang X, Zhong F, Huang Q. 2013. Stability and bioaccessibility of β-carotene in nanoemulsions stabilized by modified starches. *J Agric Food Chem* 61:1249–57.

Lin CH, Chen BH. 2005a. Stability of carotenoids in tomato juice during processing. *Eur Food Res Technol* 221:274–80.

Lin CH, Chen BH. 2005b. Stability of carotenoids in tomato juice during storage. *Food Chem* 90:837–46.

Lobato KBS, Paese K, Forgearini JC, Guterres SS, Jablonski A, Rios AO. 2013. Characterization and stability evaluation of bixin nanocapsules. *Food Chem* 141:3906–12.

Loksuwan J. 2007. Characteristics of microencapsulated β-carotene formed by spray drying with modified tapioca starch, native tapioca starch and maltodextrin. *Food Hydrocoll* 21:928–35.

Maiani G, Castón MJP, Catasta G, Toti E, Cambrodón IG, Bysted A, Granado-Lorencio F, Olmedilla-Alonso B, Knuthsen P, Valoti M, Böhm V, Mayer-Miebach E, Behsnilian D, Schlemmer U. 2009. Carotenoids: actual knowledge on food sources, intakes, stability and bioavailability and their protective role in humans. *Mol Nutr Food Res* 53:S194–218.

Marcolino VA, Zanin GM, Durrant LR, Benassi MT, Matioli G. 2011. Interaction of curcumin and bixin with β-cyclodextrin: complexation methods, stability, and applications in food. *J Agric Food Chem* 59:3348–57.

Márkuz F, Daood HG, Kapitány J, Biacs PA. 1999. Change in the carotenoid and antioxidant content of spice red pepper (paprika) as a function of ripening and some technological factors *J Agric Food Chem* 47:100–7.

Marx M, Stuparic M, Schieber A, Carle R. 2003. Effects of thermal processing on *trans-cis*-isomerization of β-carotene in carrot juice and carotene-containing preparations. *Food Chem* 83:609–17.

Matioli G, Rodriguez-Amaya DB. 2002. Lycopene encapsulated with gum arabic and maltodextrin: stability study. *Braz J Food Technol* 5:197–203.

Matioli G, Rodriguez-Amaya DB. 2003. Microencapsulation of lycopene with cyclodextrins. *Cienc Tecnol Aliment* 23(Suppl):102–5.

Matsumoto H, Ikoma Y, Kato M, Nakajima N, Hasegawa Y. 2009. Effect of postharvest temperature and ethylene on carotenoid accumulation in the flavedo and juice sacs of satsuma mandarin (*Citrus unshiu* Marc.) fruit. *J Agric Food Chem* 57:4724–32.

Mayer-Miebach E, Behsnilian D, Regier M, Schuchmann HP. 2005. Thermal processing of carrots: lycopene stability and isomerization with regard to antioxidant potential. *Food Res Int* 38:1103–8.

Mayer-Miebach E, Spieβ WEL. 2003. Influence of cold storage and blanching on the carotenoid content of *Kintoki* carrots. *J Food Eng* 56:211–3.

Mazzeo T, N'Dri D, Chiavaro E, Visconti A, Fogliano V, Pellegrini N. 2011. Effect of two cooking procedures on phytochemical compounds, total antioxidant capacity and colour of selected frozen vegetables. *Food Chem* 128:627–33.

McInerney JK, Seccafien CA, Stewart CM, Bird AR. 2007. Effects of high pressure processing on antioxidant activity, and total carotenoid content and availability, in vegetables. *Innov Food Sci Emerg Technol* 8:543–8.

Mdziniso P, Hinds MJ, Bellmer DD, Brown B, Payton ME. 2006. Physical quality and carotene content of solar-dried green leafy and yellow succulent vegetables. *Plant Food Hum Nutr* 61:13–21.
Mezzomo N, Martínez J, Maraschin M, Ferreira SRS. 2013. Pink shrimp (*P. brasiliensis* and *P. paulensis*) residue: supercritical extraction of carotenoid fraction. *J Supercrit Fluid* 74:22–33.
Miglio C, Chiavaro E, Visconti A, Fogliano V, Pellegrini N. 2008. Effects of different cooking methods on nutritional and physicochemical characteristics of selected vegetables. *J Agric Food Chem* 56:139–47.
Morales-de la Peña M, Salvia-Trujillo L, Rojas-Graü M A, Martín-Belloso O. 2011. Changes on phenolic and carotenoid composition of high intensity pulsed electric field and thermally treated fruit juice-soymilk beverages during refrigerated storage. *Food Chem.* 129:982–90.
Mulokozi G, Svanberg U. 2003. Effect of traditional open sun-drying and solar cabinet drying on carotene content and vitamin A activity of green leafy vegetables. *Plant Food Hum Nutr* 58:1–15.
Murador DC, da Cunha DT, de Rosso VV. 2014. Effects of cooking techniques on vegetable pigments: a meta-analytic approach to carotenoid and anthocyanin levels. *Food Res Int* 65:177–83.
Muzhingi T, Yeum K-J, Russell RM, Johnson EJ, Qin J, Tang G. 2008. Determination of carotenoids in yellow maize, the effects of saponification and food preparations. *Int J Vitam Nutr Res* 78:112–120.
Nagar V, Hajare SN, Saroj SD, Bandekar JR. 2012. Radiation processing of minimally processed sprouts (dew gram and chick pea): effect on sensory, nutritional and microbiological quality. *Int J Food Sci Technol* 47:620–6.
Namitha KK, Negi PS. 2010. Chemistry and biotechnology of carotenoids. *Crit Rev Food Sci Nutr* 50:728–60.
Nath A, Bagchi B, Misra LK, Deka BC. 2011. Changes in the post-harvest phytochemical qualities of broccoli florets during ambient and refrigerated storage. *Food Chem* 127:1510–4.
Negi PS, Roy SK. 2000. Effect of blanching and drying methods on β-carotene, ascorbic acid and chlorophyll retention of leafy vegetables. *Lebens Wissen Technol* 33:295–8.
Negi PS, Roy SK. 2001a. Effect of drying conditions on quality of green leaves during long term storage. *Food Res Int* 34:283–7.
Negi PS, Roy SK. 2001b. The effects of blanching on quality attributes of dehydrated carrots during long term storage. *Eur Food Res Technol* 212:445–8.
Negi PS, Roy SK. 2001c. Retention of quality characteristics of dehydrated green leaves during storage. *Plant Food Hum Nutr* 56:285–95.
Nguyen M, Francis D, Schwartz S. 2001. Thermal isomerization susceptibility of carotenoids in different tomato varieties. *J Sci Food Agric* 81:910–7.
Nik AM, Langmaid S, Wright AJ. 2012. Nonionic surfactant and interfacial structure impact crystallinity and stability of β-carotene loaded lipid nanodispersions. *J Agric Food Chem* 60:4126–35.
Nobre BP, Palavra AF, Pessoa FLP, Mendes RL. 2009. Supercritical CO_2 extraction of *trans*-lycopene from Portuguese tomato industrial waste. *Food Chem* 116:680–5.
Nunes TP, Martins CG, Faria AF, Biscola V, Souza KLO, Mercadante AZ, Cordenunsi BR, Landgraf M. 2013. Changes in total ascorbic acid and carotenoids in minimally processed irradiated arugula (*Eruca sativa* Mill) stored under refrigeration. *Radiat Phys Chem* 90:125–30.
Nunn MD, Giraud DW, Parkhurst AM, Hamouz FL, Driskell JA. 2006. Effects of cooking methods on sensory qualities and carotenoid retention in selected vegetables. *J Food Qual* 29:445–57.
Odriozola-Serrano I, Aguiló-Aguayo I, Soliva-Fortuny R, Gimeno-Añó V, Martín-Belloso O. 2007. Lycopene, vitamin C, and antioxidant capacity of tomato juice as affected by high-intensity pulsed electric fields critical parameters. *J Agric Food Chem* 55:9036–42.
Odriozola-Serrano I, Soliva-Fortuny, R, Hernández-Jover T, Martín-Belloso O. 2009. Carotenoid and phenolic profile of tomato juices processed by high intensity pulsed electric fields compared with conventional thermal treatments. *Food Chem* 112:258–66.
Odriozola-Serrano I, Soliva-Fortuny R, Martín-Belloso O. 2008a. Effect of minimal processing on bioactive compounds and color attributes of fresh-cut tomatoes. LWT—Food *Sci Technol* 41:217–26.
Odriozola-Serrano I, Soliva-Fortuny R, Martín-Belloso O. 2008b. Changes of health-related compounds throughout cold storage of tomato juice stabilized by thermal or high intensity pulsed electric field treatments. *Innov Food Sci Emerg Technol* 9:272–9.
Oliveira A, Pintado M, Almeida DPF. 2012. Phytochemical composition and antioxidant activity of peach as affected by pasteurization and storage duration. LWT—Food *Sci Technol* 49:202–7.
Oms-Oliu G, Odriozola-Serrano I, Soliva-Fortuny R, Martín-Belloso O. 2009. Effects of high-intensity pulsed electric field processing conditions on lycopene, vitamin C and antioxidant capacity of watermelon juice. *Food Chem* 115:1312–9.

Ornelas-Paz JJ, Cira-Chávez LA, Gardea-Béjar AA, Guevara-Arauza JC, Sepúlveda DR, Reyes-Hernández J, Ruiz-Cruz S. 2013. Effect of heat treatment on the content of some bioactive compounds and free radical-scavenging activity in pungent and non-pungent peppers. *Food Res Int* 50:519–25.

Ornelas-Paz JJ, Yahia EM, Gardea AA. 2008. Changes in external and internal color during postharvest ripening of 'Manila' and 'Ataulfo' mango fruit and relationship with carotenoid content determined by liquid chromatopgraphy-APcI$^+$-time-of-flight mass spectrometry. *Postharvest Biol Technol* 50:145–52.

Palermo M, Pellegrini N, Fogliano V. 2014. The effect of cooking on the phytochemical content of vegetables. *J Sci Food Agric* 94:1057–70.

Pellegrini N, Chiavaro E, Gardana C, Mazzeo T, Contino D, Gallo M, Riso P, Fogliano V, Porrini M. 2010. Effect of different cooking methods on color, phytochemical concentration, and antioxidant capacity of raw and frozen *Brassica* vegetables. *J Agric Food Chem* 58:4310–21.

Pérez-Conesa D, García-Alonso J, García-Valverde V, Iniesta M-D, Jacob K, Sánchez-Siles LM, Ros G, Periago MJ. 2009. Changes in bioactive compounds and antioxidant activity during homogenization and thermal processing of tomato puree. *Innov Food Sci Emerg Technol* 10:179–88.

Pérez-Gálvez A, Hornero-Méndez D, Mínguez-Mosquera MI. 2004. Changes in the carotenoid metabolism of capsicum fruits during application of modelized slow drying process for paprika production. *J Agric Food Chem* 52:518–22.

Perkins-Veazie P, Collins JK. 2004. Flesh quality and lycopene stability of fresh-cut watermelon. *Postharvest Biol Technol* 31:159–66.

Plaza L, Colina C, de Ancos B, Sánchez-Moreno C, Cano MP. 2012. Influence of ripening and astringency on carotenoid content of high-pressure treated persimmon fruit (*Diospyros kaki* L.). *Food Chem* 130:591–7.

Plaza L, Crespo I, de Pascual-Teresa S, de Ancos B, Sánchez-Moreno C, Muñoz M, Cano MP. 2011a. Impact of minimal processing on orange bioactive compounds during refrigerated storage. *Food Chem* 124:646–51.

Plaza L, Sánchez-Moreno C, de Ancos B, Elez-Martínez P, Martín-Belloso O, Cano M P. 2011b. Carotenoid and flavanone content during refrigerated storage of orange juice processed by high-pressure, pulsed electric fields and low pasteurization. LWT—Food *Sci Technol* 44:834–9.

Polyakov NE, Leshina TV, Konovalova TA, Hand EO, Kispert LD. 2004. Inclusion complexes of carotenoids with cyclodextrins: ^{1}H NMR, EPR, and optical studies. *Free Radic Biol Med* 36:872–80.

Pott I, Marx M, Neidhart S, Mühlbauer W, Carle R. 2003. Quantitative determination of β-carotene stereoisomers in fresh, dried, and solar-dried mangoes (*Mangifera indica* L.). *J Agric Food Chem* 51:4527–31.

Provesi JG, Dias CO, Amante ER. 2011. Changes in carotenoids during processing and storage of pumpkin puree. *Food Chem* 128:195–202.

Puupponen-Pimiä R, Häkkinen ST, Aarni M, Suortti T, Lampi A-M, Eurola M, Piironen V, Nuutila AM, Oksman-Caldentey K-M. 2003. Blanching and long-term freezing affect vaious bioactive compounds of vegetables in different ways. *J Sci Food Agric* 83:1389–402.

Qian C, Decker EA, Xiao H, McClements DJ. 2012a. Inhibition of β-carotene degradation in oil-in-water nanoemulsions: influence of oil-soluble and water-soluble antioxidants. *Food Chem* 135:1036–43.

Qian C, Decker EA, Xiao H, McClements DJ. 2012b. Physical and chemical stability of β-carotene-enriched nanoemulsions: influence of pH, ionic strength, temperature and emulsifier type. *Food Chem* 132:1221–9.

Qian C, Decker EA, Xiao H, McClements DJ. 2013. Impact of lipid nanoparticle physical state on particle aggregation and β-carotene degradation: potential limitations of solid lipid nanoparticles. *Food Res Int* 52:342–9.

Qiu W, Jiang H, Wang H, Gao Y. 2006. Effect of hydrostatic pressure on lycopene stability. *Food Chem* 97:516–23.

Raffo A, Baiamonte I, Paoletti F. 2008. Changes in antioxidants and taste-related compounds content during cold storage of fresh-cut red sweet pepper. *Eur Food Res Technol* 226:1167–74.

Rascón MP, Beristain CI, García HS, Salgado MA. 2011. Carotenoid retention and storage stability of spray-dried encapsulated paprika oleoresin using gum arabic and soy protein isolate as wall materials. LWT—Food *Sci Technol* 44:549–57.

Ravi H, Baskaran V. 2015. Biodegradable chitosan-glycolipid hybrid nanogels: a novel approach to encapsulate fucoxanthin for improved stability and bioavailability. *Food Hydrocoll* 43:717–25.

Reboul E, Borel P, Mikail C, Abou L, Charbonnier M, Caris-Veyrat C, Goupy P, Portugal H, Lairon D, Amiot M-J. 2005. Enrichment of tomato paste with 6% tomato peel increases lycopene and β-carotene bioavailability in men. *J Nutr* 135:790–4.

Regier M, Mayer-Miebach E, Behsnilian D, Neff E, Schuchmann HP. 2005. Influences of drying and storage of lycopene-rich carrots on the carotenoid content. *Dry Technol* 23:989–98.

Rivera-López J, Vásquez-Ortiz FA, Ayala-Zavala JF, Sotelo-Mundo RR, González-Aguilar GA. 2005. Cutting shape and storage temperature affect overall quality of fresh-cut papaya cv. 'Maradol'. *J Food Sci* 70:S482–9.

Rivera-Pastrana DM, Yahia EM, González-Aguilar GA. 2010. Phenolic and carotenoid profiles of papaya fruit (*Carica papaya* L.) and their contents under low temperature storage. *J Sci Food Agric* 90:2358–65.

Robert P, Carlsson RM, Romero N, Masson L. 2003. Stability of spray-dried encapsulated carotenoid pigments from rosa mosqueta (*Rosa rubiginosa*) oleoresin. *J Am Oil Chem Soc* 80:1115–20.

Rocha GA, Fávaro-Trindade CS, Grosso CRF. 2011. Microencapsulation of lycopene by spray drying: characterization, stability and application of microcapsules. *Food Bioprod Process* 90:37–42.

Rocha-Selmi GA, Favaro-Trindade CS, Grosso CRF. 2013. Morphology, stability, and application of lycopene microcapsules produced by complex coacervation. *J Chem 2013, Article ID* 982603, 7 p.

Rodrigues E, Mariutti LRB, Faria AF, Mercadante AZ. 2012. Microcapsules containing antioxidant molecules as scavengers of reactive oxygen and nitrogen species. *Food Chem* 134:704–11.

Rodriguez-Amaya DB. 1997. *Carotenoids and food preparation: The retention of provitamin A carotenoids in prepared, processed, and stored foods*. Arlington: Opportunities for Micronutrient Intervention.

Rodriguez-Amaya DB. 1999. Changes in carotenoids during processing and storage of foods. *Arch Latinoamer Nutr* 49:S38–47.

Rodriguez-Amaya DB. 2002. Effects of processing and storage on food carotenoids. Sight Life Newslett 3(Spec Iss):25–35.

Rodríguez-Huezo ME, Pedroza-Islas R, Prado-Barragán LA, Beristain CI, Vernon-Carter EJ. 2004. Microencapsulation by spray drying of multiple emulsions containing carotenoids. *J Food Sci* 69:E351–9.

Rozzi NL, Singh RK, Vierling RA, Watkins BA. 2002. Supercritical fluid extraction of lycopene from tomato processing byproducts. *J Agric Food Chem* 50:2638–43.

Rubio-Diaz DE, Santos A, Francis DM, Rodriguez-Saona LE. 2010. Carotenoid stability during production and storage of tomato juice made from tomatoes with diverse pigment profiles measured by infrared spectroscopy. *J Agric Food Chem* 58:8692–8.

Ruiz-Rodriguez A, Marín FR, Ocaña A, Soler-Rivas C. 2008. Effect of domestic processing on bioactive compounds. *Phytochem Rev* 7:345–84.

Rutz JK, Zambiazi RC, Borges CD, Krumreich FD, da Luz SR, Hartwig N, da Rosa CG. 2013. Microencapsulation of purple Brazilian juice in xanthan, tara gums and xanthan-tara hydrogel matrixes. *Carbohydr Polym* 98:1256–65.

Sá MC de, Rodriguez-Amaya DB. 2004. Optimization of HPLC quantification of carotenoids in cooked green vegetables: comparison of analytical and calculated data. *J Food Compos Anal* 17:37–51.

Sabio E, Lozano M, de Espinosa VM, Mendes RL, Pereira AP, Palavra AF, Coelho JA. 2003. Lycopene and β-carotene extraction from tomato processing waste using supercritical CO_2. *Ind Eng Chem Res* 42:6641–6.

Sachindra NM, Mahendrakar NS. 2005. Process optimization for extraction of carotenoids from shrimp waste with vegetable oils. *Bioresour Technol* 96:1195–200.

Sahlin E, Savage GP, Lister CE. 2004. Investigation of the antioxidant properties of tomatoes after processing. *J Food Compos Anal* 17:635–47.

Sáiz-Abajo M-J, González-Ferrero C, Moreno-Ruiz A, Romo-Hualde A, González-Navarro CJ. 2013. Thermal protection of β-carotene in re-assembled casein micelles during different processing technologies applied in food industry. *Food Chem* 138:1581–7.

Sanal IS, Bayraktar E, Mehmetoglu Ü, Çalimli A. 2005. Determination of optimum consitions for SC-(CO_2 + ethanol) extraction of β-carotene from apricot pomace using response surface methodology. *J Supercrit Fluid* 34:331–8.

Sanal IS, Güvenç A, Salgin U, Mehmetoglu Ü, Çalimli A. 2004. Recycling of apricot pomace by supercritical CO_2 extraction. *J Supercrit Fluid* 32:221–30.

Sánchez C, Baranda AB, de Marañon IM. 2014. The effect of high pressure and high temperature processing on carotenoids and chlorophylls content in some vegetables. *Food Chem* 163:37–45.

Sánchez-Moreno C, Plaza L, de Ancos B, Cano MP. 2003. Vitamin C, provitamin A carotenoids, and other carotenoids in high-pressurized orange juice during refrigerated storage. *J Agric Food Chem* 51:647–53.

Sánchez-Moreno C, Plaza L, de Ancos B, Cano MP. 2006. Impact of high-pressure and traditional thermal processing of tomato purée on carotenoids, vitamin C and antioxidant activity. *J Sci Food Agric* 86:171–9.

Sánchez-Moreno C, Plaza L, Elez-Martínez P, de Ancos B, Martín-Belloso O, Cano MP. 2005. Impact of high pressure and pulsed electric fields on bioactive compounds and antioxidant activity of orange juice in comparison with traditional thermal processing. *J Agric Food Chem* 53:4403–9.

Santana AA, Kurozawa LE, de Oliveira RA, Park KJ. 2013. Influence of process conditions on the physicochemical properties of pequi powder produced by spray drying. *Dry Technol* 31:825–36.

Schweiggert U, Kurz C, Schieber A, Carle R. 2007. Effecs of processing and storage on the stability of free and esterified carotenoids of red peppers (*Capsicum annuum* L) and hot chili peppers (*Capsicum frutescens* L.). *Eur Food Res Technol* 225:261–70.

Selim K, Tsimidou M, Biliaderis CG. 2000. Kinetics studies of degradation of saffron carotenoids encapsulated in amorphous polymer matrices. *Food Chem* 71:199–206.

Seybold C, Fröhlich K, Bitsch R, Otto K, Böhm V. 2004. Changes in contents of carotenoids and vitamin E during tomato processing. *J Agric Food Chem* 52:7005–10.

Shahidi F, Han X-Q. 1993. Encapsulation of food ingredients. *Crit Rev Food Sci Nutr* 33:501–47.

Shi I, Le Maguer M. 2000. Lycopene in tomato: Chemical and physical properties affected by food processing. *Crit Rev Biotechnol* 42:293–334.

Shi J, Le Maguer M, Bryan M, Kakuda Y. 2003. Kinetics of lycopene degradation in tomato puree by heat and light irradiation. *J Food Process Eng* 25:485–98.

Shi J, Le Maguer M, Kakuda Y, Albert Liptay A, Niekamp F. 1999. Lycopene degradation and isomerization in tomato dehydration. *Food Res Int* 32:15–21.

Shi J, Yi C, Xue SJ, Jiang Y, Ma Y, Li D. 2009. Effects of modifiers on the profile of lycopene extracted from tomato skins by supercritical CO_2. *J Food Eng* 93:431–6.

Shu B, Yu W, Zhao Y, Liu X. 2006. Study on microencapsulation of lycopene by spray-drying. *J Food Eng* 76:664–9.

Simões ADN, Allende A, Tudela JA, Puschmann R, Gil MI. 2011. Optimum controlled atmospheres minimise respiration rate and quality losses while increase phenolic compounds of baby carrots. *LWT—Food Sci Technol* 44:277–83.

Sommano S, Caffin N, McDonald J, Cocksedge R. 2013. The impact of thermal processing on bioactive compounds in Australian native food products (bush tomato and Kakadu plum). *Food Res Int* 50:557–61.

Sousdaleff M, Baesso ML, Neto AM, Nogueira AC, Marcolino VA, Matioli G. 2013. Microencapsulation by freeze-drying of potassium norbixinate and curcumin with maltodextrin: Stability, solubility, and food application. *J Agric Food Chem* 61:955–65.

Spada JC, Noreña CPZ, Marczak LDF, Tessaro IC. 2012. Study on the stability of β-carotene microencapsulated with *pinhão* (*Araucaria angustifolia* seeds) starch. *Carbohydr Polym* 89:1166–73.

Sungpuag P, Tangchitpianvit S, Chittchang U, Wasantwisut E. 1999. Retinol and beta carotene content of indigenous raw and home-prepared foods in Northeast Thailand. *Food Chem* 64:163–7.

Tai CY, Chen BH. 2000. Analysis and stability of carotenoids in the flowers of daylily (*Hemerocallis distichia*) as affected by various treatments. *J Agric Food Chem* 48:5962–8.

Takeoka GR, Dao L, Flessa S, Gillespie DM, Jewell WT, Huebner B, Bertow D, Ebeler SE. 2001. Processing effects on lycopene content and antioxidant activity of tomatoes. *J Agric Food Chem* 49:3713–7.

Toor RK, Savage GP. 2005. Antioxidant activity in different fractions of tomatoes. *Food Res Int* 38:487–94.

Toor RK, Savage GP. 2006. Changes in major antioxidant components of tomatoes during post-harvest storage. *Food Chem* 99:724–7.

Topal U, Sasaki M, Goto M, Hayakawa K. 2006. Extraction of lycopene from tomato skin with supercritical carbon dioxide: effect of operating conditions and solubility analysis. *J Agric Food Chem* 54:5604–10.

Topuz A, Ozdemir F. 2003. Influences of γ-irradiation and storage on the carotenoids of sun-dried and dehydrated paprika. *J Agric Food Chem* 51:4972–7.

Torregrosa F, Cortés C, Esteve MJ, Frígola A. 2005. Effect of high-intensity pulsed electric fields processing and conventional heat treatment on orange-carrot juice carotenoids. *J Agric Food Chem* 53:9519–25.

Uckoo RM, Jayaprakasha GK, Somerville JA, Balasubramaniam VM, Pinarte M, Patil, BS. 2013. High pressure processing controls microbial growth and minimally alters the levels of health promoting compounds in grapefruit (*Citrus paradiisi* Macfad) juice. *Innov Food Sci Emerg Technol* 18:7–14.

Updike AA, Schwartz SJ. 2003. Thermal processing of vegetables increases cis isomers of lutein and zeaxanthin. *J Agric Food Chem* 51:6184–90.

Vági E, Simándi B, Vásárhelyiné KP, Daood H, Kéry Á, Doleschall F, Nagy B. 2007. Supercritical carbon dioxide extraction of carotenoids, tocopherols and sitosterols from industrial tomato by-products *J Supercrit Fluid* 40:218–26.

Vega PJ, Balaban MO, Sims CA, O'Keefe SF, Cornell JA. 1996. Supercritical carbon dioxide extraction efficiency for carotenes from carrots by RSM. *J Food Sci* 61:757–9.

Velázquez-Estrada RM, Hernández-Herrero MM, Rüfer CE, Guamis-López B, Roig-Sagués AX. 2013. Influence of ultra high pressure homogenization processing on bioactive compounds and antioxidant activity of orange juice. *Innov Food Sci Emerg Technol* 18:89–94.

Vallverdú-Queralt A, Arranz S, Casals-Ribes I, Lamuela-Raventós RM. 2012. Stability of the phenolic and carotenoid profile of gazpachos during storage. *J Agric Food Chem* 60:1981–8.

Vallverdú-Queralt A, Odriozola-Serrano I, Oms-Oliu G, Lamuela-Raventós RM, Elez-Martínez P, Martín-Belloso O. 2013. Impact of high-intensity pulsed electric fields on carotenoids profile of tomato juice made of moderate-intensity pulsed electric field-treated tomatoes. *Food Chem* 141:3131–8.

Vanamala J, Cobb G, Turner ND, Lupton JR, Yoo KS, Pike LM, Patil BS. 2005. Bioactive compounds of grapefruit (*Citrus paradisi* cv. Rio Red) respond differently to postharvest irradiation, storage, and freeze drying. *J Agric Food Chem* 53:3980–5.

van Jaarsveld PJ, Marais DW, Harmse E, Nestel P, Rodriguez-Amaya DB. 2006. Retention of β-carotene in boiled, mashed orange-fleshed sweetpotato. *J Food Compos Anal* 19:321–9.

Vásquez-Caicedo AL, Shilling S, Carle R, Neidhart S. 2007. Effects of thermal processing and fruit matrix on β-carotene stability and enzyme inactivation during transformation of mangoes into purée and nectar. *Food Chem* 102:1172–86.

Vásquez-Caicedo AL, Sruamsiri P, Carle R, Neidhart S. 2005. Accumulation of all-*trans*-β-carotene and 9-*cis* and 13-*cis* stereoisomers during postharvest ripening of nine Thai mango cultivars. *J Agric Food Chem* 53:4827–35.

Vervoort L, van der Plancken I, Grauwet T, Verlinde P, Matser A, Hendrickx M, van Loey A. 2012. Thermal versus high pressure processing of carrots: a comparative pilot-scale study on equivalent basis. *Innov Food Sci Emerg Technol* 15:1–13.

Wenzel M, Seuss-Baum I, Schlich E. 2010. Influence of pasteurization, spray- and freeze-drying, and storage on the carotenoid content in egg yolk. *J Agric Food Chem* 58:1726–31.

Wright KP, Kader AA. 1997. Effect of controlled-atmosphere storage on the quality and carotenoid content of sliced persimmons and peaches. *Postharvest Biol Technol* 10:89–97.

Wu X, Sun C, Yang L, Zeng G, Liu Z, Li Y. 2008. β-carotene content in sweet potato varieties from China and the effect of preparation on β-carotene retention in the Yanshu No. 5. *Innov Food Sci Emerg Technol* 9:581–6.

Zhang C, Trierweiler B, Li W, Butz P, Xu Y, Rüfer CE, Ma Y, Zhao X. 2011. Comparison of thermal, ultraviolet-c, and high pressure treatments on quality parameters of watermelon juice. *Food Chem* 126:254–60.

Zhang D, Hamauzu Y. 2004. Phenolics, ascorbic acid, carotenoids and antioxidant activity of broccoli and their changes during conventional and microwave cooking. *Food Chem* 88:503–9.

Zhang Y, Zhong Q. 2013. Encapsulation of bixin in sodium caseinate to deliver the colorant in transparent dispersions. *Food Hydrocoll* 33:1–9.

Zulueta A, Barba FJ, Esteve MJ, Frígola A. 2010. Effects on the carotenoid pattern and vitamin A of a pulsed electric field-treated orange juice-milk beverage and behavior during storage. *Eur Food Res Technol* 231:525–34.

7 Isomerization and oxidation

7.1 INTRODUCTION

The highly unsaturated carotenoid molecules are prone to oxidative degradation, and losses of carotenoids during the processing and storage of foods have been reported in numerous papers, as discussed in Chapter 6. However, better understanding of the reactions and the underlying mechanisms is lacking. For lipid oxidation, there is a wealth of information on the different reactions that constitute the process, the nonvolatile and volatile products formed, and the different promoting and inhibiting factors. For carotenoid oxidation, many more investigations are needed to augment the limited and fragmentary knowledge currently available.

Since loss of color has been a serious problem in the food industry, there were attempts to elucidate the mechanisms of carotenoid degradation in the 1980s, but such efforts practically ceased when attention was directed primarily to the health effects of these pigments. In recent years, there has been renewed interest on this topic, stimulated by the finding that the degradation products can have marked effects on human health.

As for lipid oxidation, insights into the mechanisms of carotenoid oxidation can be derived from model systems, which are more easily controlled than foods, and the formation of initial, intermediate, and final products can be more easily monitored (Rodriguez and Rodriguez-Amaya, 2007, 2009). The initial amounts of the carotenoids of interest can be adjusted, and isolated effects or a combination of effects can be more clearly observed, facilitating the elucidation of mechanisms and the perception of influencing factors. Extrapolation to foods, however, has to be done with caution, considering that simple model systems may not reflect the nature and complexity of the multicomponent food matrices, in which numerous reactions and interactions occur simultaneously. Model systems should mimic foods as much as possible. This chapter focuses on this type of model systems, not those involving carotenoids dissolved in organic solvents or under conditions that do not reflect those of foods.

Epoxy carotenoids and apocarotenals, the initial products of the oxidation process, are turned over very rapidly that they do not accumulate and are found in minute amounts, making their detection and identification difficult. Epoxidation by *m*-perclorobenzoic

Food Carotenoids: Chemistry, Biology, and Technology, First Edition. Delia B. Rodriguez-Amaya.

acid (Khachik et al., 1998a,b; Rodriguez and Rodriguez-Amaya, 2007, 2009) and oxidative cleavage by $KMnO_4$ (Caris-Veyrat et al., 2003; Rodriguez and Rodriguez-Amaya, 2007, 2009) have been very useful in producing epoxides and apocarotenals that can serve as qualitative standards in the identification of the products of carotenoid oxidation in model systems and in foods.

7.2 OVERALL DEGRADATION SCHEME

The major alterations undergone by carotenoids during processing and storage of foods are geometric isomerization and oxidation (Figure 7.1). Initially, part of the all-*E*-carotenoids, the usual configuration in nature, is isomerized to the *Z*-forms. Both the *Z*- and *E*-isomers are then oxidized (Rodriguez and Rodriguez-Amaya, 2007, 2009). Shi et al. (2003) reported that the main pathway appeared to be the oxidation of the all-*E*-isomers. The rate of *Z*-isomer formation was approximately half that of direct all-*E*-isomer oxidation by heat treatment, and only 1/50 when there was exposure to light at 25°C.

Oxidation commences with epoxidation and cleavage to apocarotenals. The detection of epoxycarotenoids and apocarotenals with hydroxyl groups (Marty and Berset, 1988, 1990; Rodriguez and Rodriguez-Amaya, 2007) indicates that hydroxylation is also involved.

Subsequent fragmentations result in a series of compounds of low molecular masses, similar to those produced in fatty acid oxidation. Cleavages at different sites of the polyene chain can also directly produce short volatile fragments. The volatile compounds are mostly aldehydes, ketones, alcohols, and hydrocarbons. Now devoid of

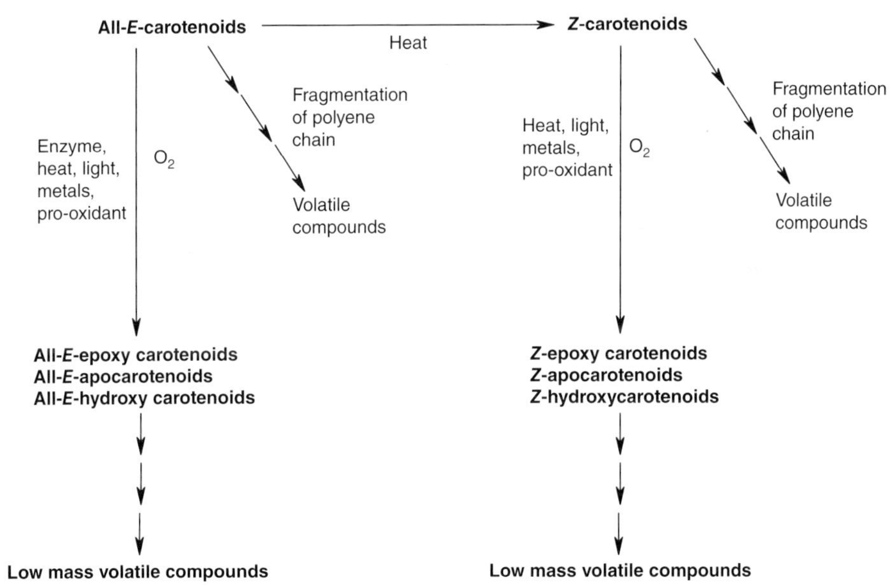

Figure 7.1 Possible overall scheme for the degradation of carotenoids in foods.

color, they contribute to the desirable flavor of foods and beverages, as in wine and tea, but also to off-flavor, as in dehydrated carrot.

Probably because studies on the various aspects of carotenoid oxidation have been for the most part carried out separately (i.e., isomerization, epoxidation, cleavage to apocarotenals, nonvolatile oxidation products, and volatile oxidation products studied separately), schemes have been proposed that show the reactions occurring separately. For example, Schwartz et al. (2008) proposed a scheme in which the oxidation of carotenoids to epoxycarotenoids, *E-Z* isomerization, and high-temperature fragmentation to volatiles occur separately. In Gregory (2008), degradation begins with epoxidation, which leads to the production of low mass products. However, *E-Z* isomerization is separate and so it is with high-temperature fragmentation. Our results and those of others taken as whole indicate that the reactions are somewhat integrated, as shown in Figure 7.1.

7.3 KINETICS

Oxidative degradation of an all-*E*-carotenoid, monitored by measuring its decreasing concentration, has been generally shown to fit first-order kinetics. Evaluating isomerization to the *Z*-form, by measuring the increasing *Z*-isomer level, is not as straightforward because, as the *Z*-carotenoid is formed, it undergoes oxidation. *Z*-carotenoids do not accumulate and their concentrations do not appear to be a good index of the occurrence of isomerization.

Carotenoid degradation (measured as total carotenoid content) and visual color followed first-order kinetics in papaya puree subjected to thermal treatment at 70°C, 80°C, 90°C, and 105°C for 0 to 3 h. (Ahmed et al., 2002). In lyophilized guava stored at ambient temperature (28°C to 32°C) for 20 days, both β-carotene and lycopene degradation followed first-order kinetics in the absence and presence of light (Ferreira and Rodriguez-Amaya, 2008). The degradation of β-carotene and color loss also followed a first-order kinetics in dehydrated blanched and unblanched carrot slices during storage at 27°C, 37°C, 47°C, and 57°C (Koca et al., 2007), and in blanched pumpkin puree at 60°C –70°C for a time period between 0 and 2 h (Dutta et al., 2006). Likewise, all-*E*-β-carotene degradation during storage of dried sweet potato chips followed first-order kinetics (Bechoff et al., 2010). α-Carotene, β-carotene, and lutein degradation followed pseudo-first-order kinetics in blanched and unblanched freeze-dried carrots (Lavelli et al., 2007).

Lycopene decreased in untreated, HIPEF-processed, and heat-treated tomato juices during storage at 4°C in darkness, following a first-order kinetics (Odriozola- Serrano et al., 2008). First-order model also explained the degradation behavior of total carotenoid, lycopene, and Hunter "a × b" value (R^2 higher than 0.93) of watermelon juice studied at 50°C–90°C for 0–5 h (Sharma et al., 2008). The kinetic data for loss of lycopene in watermelon stored at −20°C and −80°C as small chunks or puree were best fitted by application of two simultaneous first-order decay processes (Fish and Davis, 2003).

Thermal degradation kinetics of the major xanthophylls of blood orange juice were investigated at 45°C, 60°C, 75°C, and 90°C (Hadjal et al., 2013). A second-order kinetics best fitted the degradation curves of the xanthophylls. β-cryptoxanthin and lutein had similar low rates from 45°C to 90°C. The epoxy carotenoid *Z*-antheraxanthin presented the highest degradation rates at all temperatures, followed by *Z*-violaxanthin. After 200 min heat treatment at 45°C, *Z*-violaxanthin, lutein, zeaxanthin, and β-cryptoxanthin losses were 30%, 15%, 20%, and 10%, respectively. A similar trend was found by Dhuique-Mayer et al. (2007) with losses of 100%, 66%, 70%, and 5% for the same xanthophylls, although the degradation difference between β-cryptoxanthin and the other xanthophylls was more marked.

In virgin olive oil, on the other hand, first-order kinetics was found appropriate for describing the thermal degradation of epoxy xanthophylls (neoxanthin, violaxanthin, and antheraxanthin) (Aparicio-Ruiz and Gandul-Rojas, 2012).

In diluted juice of paprika heated at 80°C, 90°C, and 100°C with holding times of 0, 2, 4, 8, and 16 min, the degradation kinetics of capsanthin was studied by two groups of reaction models, including elementary reaction rate models and those of modified square root–based pseudo (MRBP-) (Shin et al., 2001). Through successive calculations, the MRBP-first-order reaction rate model was chosen as an appropriate model in view of high R^2 selection (above 0.95) and simplication of model fit.

7.4 ISOMERIZATION

Isomerization of all-*E*-carotenoids to the *Z*-isomers is well documented. It is promoted by acids, heat, and light. The release of organic acids during slicing, pulping, or juicing of fruits can be sufficient to provoke *E*-*Z* isomerization, but it occurs to a greater extent during thermal treatment.

As explained in Chapter 1, steric hindrance limits *E*-*Z* isomerization to the formation of the 9-*Z*-, 13-*Z*-, and 15-*Z*-isomers of β-carotene and zeaxanthin. Being symmetrical molecules, the 9′-*Z*- and the 13′-*Z*-isomers of these carotenoids are equivalent to the 9-*Z*- and 13-*Z*-isomers. Since the 5,6-double bond of cyclic carotenoids are involved in ring formation, 5-*Z*-isomers are not formed. However, in the acyclic lycopene, this double bond is not hindered and 5-*Z*-lycopene is a major *Z*-carotenoid in tomato and tomato products. The unsymmetrical α-carotene, β-cryptoxanthin, and lutein isomerize to 13′-*Z*- and 9′-*Z*-isomers in addition to 13-*Z*-, 9-*Z*-, and 15- *Z*-isomers.

Occurrence of *E*-*Z*-isomerization as a consequence of thermal processing has been shown by many authors. Lessin et al. (1997) reported a 10%–39% increase in the percentage of total *Z*-isomer of provitamin A carotenoids in several fruits and vegetables. The principal *Z*-isomers in processed red, yellow, and orange fruits and vegetables were 13-*Z*-, although 9-*Z*- and 15-*Z*-isomers were also detected. In processed green vegetables, 9-*Z*-β-carotene predominated, followed by 13-*Z*-β-carotene, an unidentified *Z*-isomer, and 15-*Z*-β-carotene. While the 13-*Z*-isomer increased appreciably in the tray-dried Kent mango slices, considerable formation of 9-*Z*-β-carotene occurred in the solar-dried mangos (Pott et al., 2003).

Significant isomerization was observed during sterilization of tomato puree containing oil; all-*E*-lycopene was converted mainly to 9-*Z*- and 13-*Z*-lycopene (Knockaert et al., 2012). High-pressure sterilization limited the overall lycopene isomerization, when compared to the equivalent thermal sterilization processes. The formation of 5-*Z*-lycopene seemed to be favored by high pressure. In a previous paper, while β-carotene isomerization clearly occurred during thermal sterilization of carrot, almost no isomers were formed during high-pressure sterilization (Knockaert et al., 2011).

On the other hand, Nguyen et al. (2001) reported no influence of the presence of oil on the extent or likelihood of isomerization of lycopene and other carotenoids in the all-*E*-configuration during typical cooking of tomatoes. Upon thermal treatment, β-carotene and lutein isomerized to a greater extent than δ-carotene, γ-carotene, and lycopene.

In processing tangerine tomatoes into sauce, a large decrease in tetra-*Z*-lycopene occurred, accompanied by increases in all-*E*- and other *Z*-isomers (Ishida eta l., 2007). Likewise, canning of tomato juice promoted the drastic reduction of tetra-*Z*-lycopene and its isomerization to other geometric isomers, including all-*E*-lycopene (Rubio-Diaz et al., 2010).

During dark storage of tomato juice, 15-*Z*-lycopene was the major isomer formed at 4°C, while 9-*Z*- and 13-*Z*-lycopene were favored at 25°C. 5-*Z*- and 13-*Z*-lycopene predominated at 35°C (Lin and Chen, 2005). Under lighted storage, 9-*Z*- and di-*Z*-lycopene were the main isomers generated at 35°C, while 13-*Z*- and 15-*Z*-lycopene were the most abundant at 4°C and 25°C. In carrot juice under lighted storage, photodegradation of β-carotene predominated over isomerization (Pesek and Warthesen, 1990). The 13-*Z* isomer was formed in greater amount under dark storage while accumulation of the 9-*Z* isomer was favored under lighted storage.

Pasteurization and sterilization of carrot juice at 121°C caused only minor isomerization. Sterilization at 130°C and blanching resulted in increased levels of *Z*-isomers (Marx et al., 2003). In carrot homogenate, isomerization was enhanced at short heat treatment times when sunflower oil was added prior to heating (Mayer-Miebach et al., 2005). Vacuum drying and low-pressure superheated steam drying led to more conversion of all-*E*-β-carotene to 13-*Z*-β-carotene in carrots (Hiranvarachat et al., 2008).

Cooking significantly increased the levels of 13-*Z*-β-carotene and 9-*Z*-β-carotene and resulted in the production of 15-*Z*-β-carotene, which was not detected in raw carrots (Imsic et al., 2010). During heating of carrot juice, 13-*Z*-β-carotene was formed in the largest amount, followed by 13-*Z*-lutein, and 15-*Z*-α-carotene (B.H. Chen et al., 1995). In another study on carrot juice, the formation of 9-*Z*-isomers appeared to be favored under lighted storage and 13-*Z*-isomers in the dark (H.E. Chen et al., 1996). Similarly, in carotenoid powder from carrot pulp waste stored at various temperatures, the major *Z*-isomers formed in the dark were 13-*Z*-α-carotene and 13-*Z*-β-carotene, whereas 9-*Z*-isomers of both α- and β-carotene predominated under light (B.H. Chen and Tang, 1998).

In fried sweet potato, 13-*Z*-β-carotene was the major *Z*-isomer of β-carotene; only minor amounts of 15-*Z*-β-carotene and 9-*Z*-β-carotene were formed (Kidmose et al., 2006). The total amount of *Z*-isomers generated during frying depended on the frying time and size. In leafy vegetables, only 13-*Z*-β-carotene was detected during frying.

Isomerization of β-carotene occurred in boiled spinach and, to a lesser extent, in boiled savoy cabbage (O'Sullivan et al., 2010). Canning of vegetables (broccoli, corn, kale, green peas, and spinach) increased the *Z*-isomers of lutein and zeaxanthin up to 22% and 17%, respectively (Updike and Schwartz, 2003).

Sterilization of sweet corn resulted in 26% and 29% reductions in total lutein and total zeaxanthin contents, while the *Z*-isomers of lutein and zeaxanthin increased from 12% to 30% and 7% to 25%, respectively (Aman et al., 2005). The largest increments occurred in 13-*Z*-lutein, 13′-*Z*-lutein, and 13-*Z*-zeaxanthin. Blanching of spinach caused a 17% decrease in total lutein; surprisingly, there was a decrease of the *Z*-isomers of lutein from 21% to 14%.

In the commercial frying oils palm olein and Vegetaline (hydrogenated copra-based fat), subjected to 120°C–180°C, the isomers formed were 13-*Z*- and 9-*Z*-β-carotene, and 13-*Z*, 9-*Z*-, 13′-*Z*-, 9′-*Z*-lutein (Achir et al., 2010). Although lutein had a higher number of *Z*-isomers, their total amount was lower than that of β-carotene *Z*-isomer.

7.5 OXIDATION

Loss of carotenoids during processing and storage of foods is due mainly to enzymatic and nonenzymatic oxidation, which depends on the availability of oxygen and the carotenoid structure. It is stimulated by light, heat, metals, enzymes, and peroxides, and is inhibited by antioxidants.

Enzyme-catalyzed oxidation takes place in the steps prior to heat treatment, during peeling, slicing, pulping, or juicing. It can also occur in minimally processed food and in unblanched frozen foods during thawing. Typically, carotenoid loss happens rapidly, immediately after tissue disruption, after which the carotenoid concentrations stabilize.

Nonenzymatic oxidation occurs during thermal processing and storage of processed foods. Oxidation during storage of processed foods is usually characterized by a lag phase, followed by rapid decrease of the carotenoid content, coherent with a free radical mechanism. In thermally processed guava juice (Padula and Rodriguez Amaya, 1987), mango puree and slices (Godoy and Rodriguez-Amaya, 1987), and papaya puree (Godoy and Rodriguez-Amaya, 1991), nonenzymatic oxidative degradation began only after 10 months of storage at room temperature.

7.5.1 Epoxidation

Oxidation of β-carotene at ambient temperature with atmospheric oxygen, often called autoxidation, was studied in a low-moisture system consisting of β-carotene adsorbed on starch, simulating dehydrated foods (Rodriguez and Rodriguez-Amaya, 2007). In the dark, β-carotene-5,6-epoxide, β-carotene-5,8-epoxide, β-carotene-5,6,5′′,8′-diepoxide and β-carotene-5,8,5′,8′-diepoxide, all in the all-*E*-form, were detected. Under light, only β-carotene-5,6-epoxide and β-carotene-5,8-epoxide were found in the low-moisture model and in an aqueous model system prepared by dispersing β-carotene in water with Tween 40, simulating juices or purees.

Isocryptoxanthin (β,β-caroten-4-ol) and 5,8-epoxy-β,β-caroten-4-ol were formed in both low-moisture (with or without light exposure) and aqueous model systems, indicating that hydroxylation also occurred. β-caroten-4-one was also detected under the three conditions. Semi-β-carotenone was encountered only in the aqueous model system. Isomerization also took place with the marked appearance of 13-*Z*-β-carotene under the three conditions, especially in the aqueous model system, which also had 9-*Z*-β-carotene. Formation of *Z*-isomers and *Z*-isomers with epoxy group indicated that isomerization accompanied oxidation, and *Z*-isomers, along with the all-*E*-isomers, underwent oxidation.

The occurrence of the epoxy carotenoids in commercially processed fruit products was also investigated. All-*E*-β-carotene-5,8-epoxide, all-*E*-dihydroxy-β-carotene-5,8,5′,8′-diepoxide, all-*E*-monohydroxy-β-carotene-5,8-epoxide, 9-*Z*-dihydroxy-carotene-5,8-epoxide, 9-*Z*-β-carotene-5,6-epoxide, β-carotene-5,8,5′,8′-diepoxide and 9-*Z*-β-carotene-5,6-epoxide were encountered in mango juice (Rodriguez and Rodriguez-Amaya, 2007). Except for the last two epoxides, these compounds were also detected in acerola juice. On the other hand, acerola juice had all-*E*-β-carotene-5,6-epoxide. In dried apricot, only all-*E*-5,6-epoxide and the all-*E*-5,8-epoxide were found. The three products had 9-*Z*-β-carotene and 13-*Z*-β-carotene.

In Henry et al. (2000), β-carotene was adsorbed on a C_{18} solid phase and exposed to continuous flow of water saturated with oxygen at 30°C. β-Carotene-5,6-epoxide, β-carotene-5,8-epoxide, carotene-5,8-endoperoxide, *Z*-β-carotene-5,6,5′,6′-diepoxide, and β-carotene-5,8,5′,8′-diepoxide were detected. 13-*Z*, 9-*Z*, and a di-*Z*-isomers were also found.

The other papers investigating nonenzymatic carotenoid oxidation were carried out under elevated temperature, thus representing thermal degradation. Marty and Berset (1986, 1988, 1990) simulated extrusion of β-carotene dispersed in corn starch at 180°C for 2 h. Kanasawud and Crouzet (1990a) suspended β-carotene in water by sonication and subjected it to 97°C for 3 h.

On extrusion, β-carotene-5,6-epoxide decreased while β-carotene-5,8-epoxide increased and β-carotene-5,6,5′,8′-diepoxide was formed (Marty and Berset, 1986). In subsequent papers (Marty and Berset, 1988, 1990), β-caroten-4-one, isocryptoxanthin-5,8,5′,8′-diepoxide and isozeaxanthin (β,β-caroten-4,4′-diol) were also detected. Aside from the oxidized products, 13,13′-diZ-β-carotene, 9,13′-diZ-β-carotene, 9,9′-diZ-β-carotene, 15-Z-β-carotene, 13-Z-β-carotene, and 9-Z-β-carotene were also reported in the last paper.

Kanasawud and Crouzet (1990a) identified β-carotene-5,6-epoxide, β-carotene-5,8-epoxide, *Z*-β-carotene-5,6,5′,6′-diepoxide, and β-carotene-5,8,5′,8′-diepoxide as products of β-carotene sonicated in water.

The results of these studies involving both ambient and thermal oxidation confirmed that epoxidation occurs as shown in Figure 7.2. The site of initial oxygen attack is the terminal double bond of the conjugated double bond system on one side of the molecule, and then on the other side of the molecule (Figure 7.2), forming in the case of β-carotene, β-carotene-5,6-epoxide and β-carotene-5,6,5′,6′-diepoxide, respectively. Rearrangement of the 5,6- to the 5,8-epoxide yields β-carotene-5,8-epoxide and β-carotene-5,8,5′,8′-diepoxide, respectively. Notably, β-carotene-5,6,5′,6′-diepoxide was not detected in the model systems and the processed foods investigated. This does not necessarily mean, however, that it was not formed. It might have a fast turnover that it did not accumulate at a level that could allow detection. Rearrangement of the 5,6- to the 5,8-epoxide is known to occur easily. Hydroxylation of β-carotene accompanies epoxidation, the hydroxyl group entering at the allylic carbon (position 4) situated in the β-rings.

Epoxidation of lycopene occurs both at the terminal conjugated double bonds and at the isolated double bonds, resulting in a greater number of products (Figure 7.3) and a more complicated epoxidation scheme (Figure 7.4), with the formation of lycopene 1,2-epoxide and lycopene 1,2,1′,2′-diepoxide, along with lycopene-5,6-epoxide and

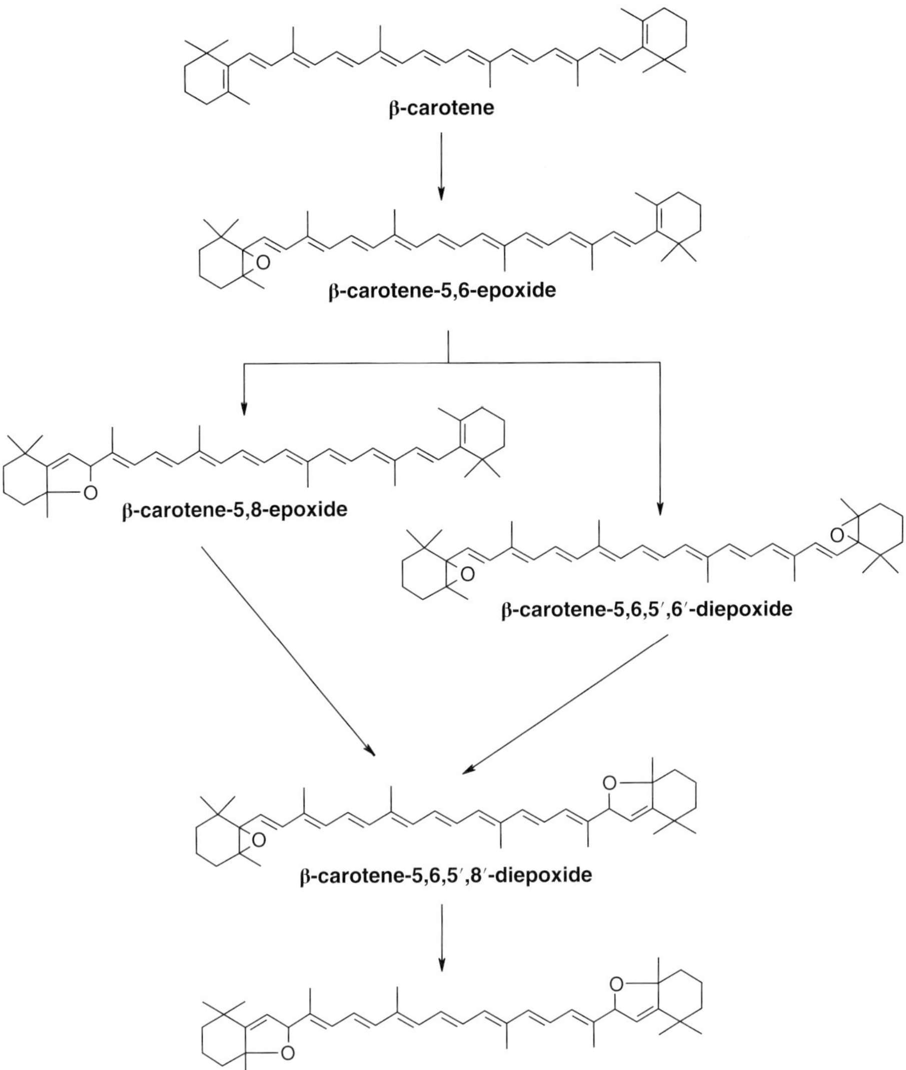

Figure 7.2 Formation of epoxy carotenoids from β-carotene. Rodriguez and Rodriguez-Amaya (2007). Reproduced with permission of Elsevier.

lycopene-5,6,5′,6′-diepoxide. Combinations of these epoxides and cyclization increase the complexity.

Khachik et al. (1998a,b) encountered lycopene-1,2-epoxide, lycopene-1,2,1′,2′-diepoxide, 2,6-cyclolycopene-1,5-diol, 2,6-cyclolycopene-1,5-epoxide, and 2,6 cyclolycopene-1,5-diol in processed tomato juice and paste. Rodriguez and Rodriguez-Amaya (2009) detected lycopene-1,2-epoxide, 2,6-cyclolycopene-1,5-diol, lycopene-1,2,5,6-diepoxide, lycopene-1,2,5′,6′-diepoxide, 2,6-cyclolycopene-1,5-epoxide, and *Z*-2,6-cyclolycopene-1,5-epoxide in both a low-moisture (lycopene isolated from tomato or watermelon, adsorbed on starch) and an aqueous model system and tomato paste.

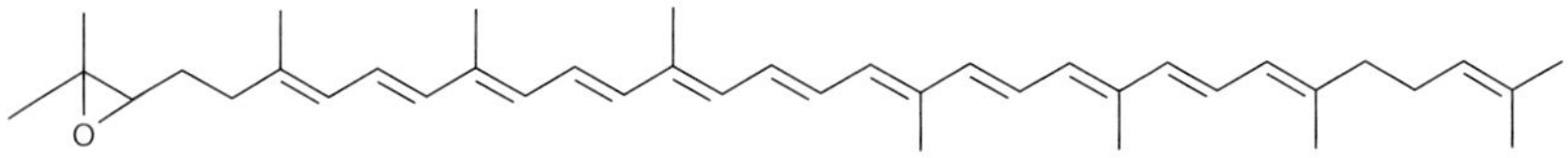

Lycopene 1,2-epoxide

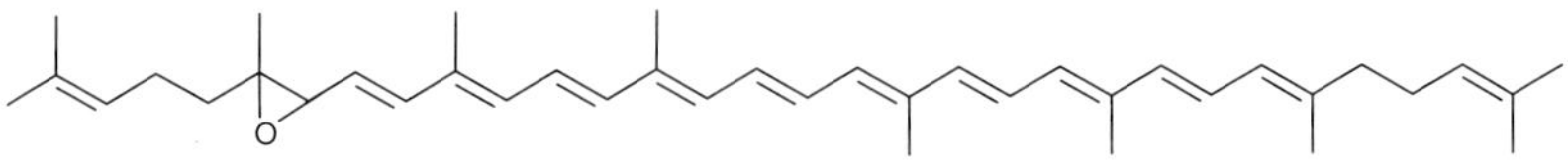

Lycopene 5,6-epoxide

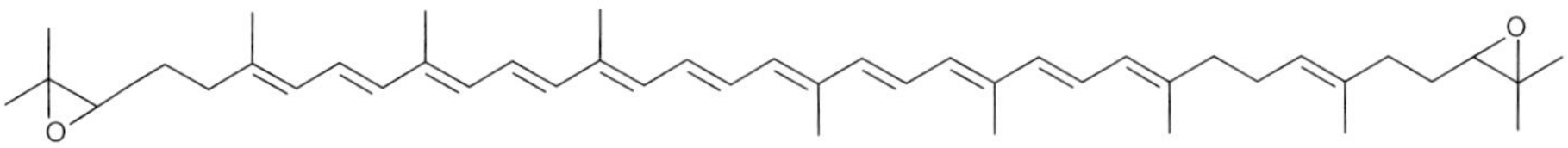

Lycopene 1,2,1′,2′-diepoxide

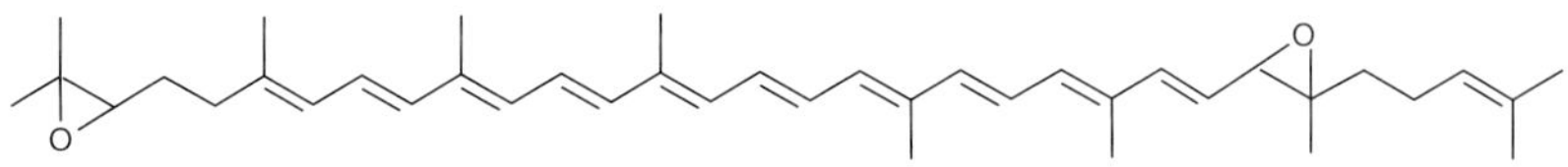

Lycopene 1,2,5′,6′-diepoxide

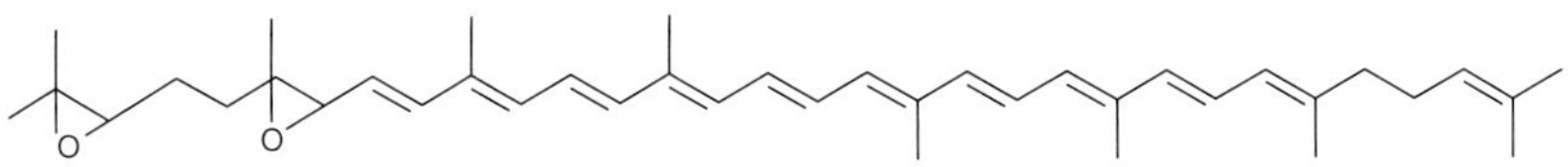

Lycopene 1,2,5,6-diepoxide

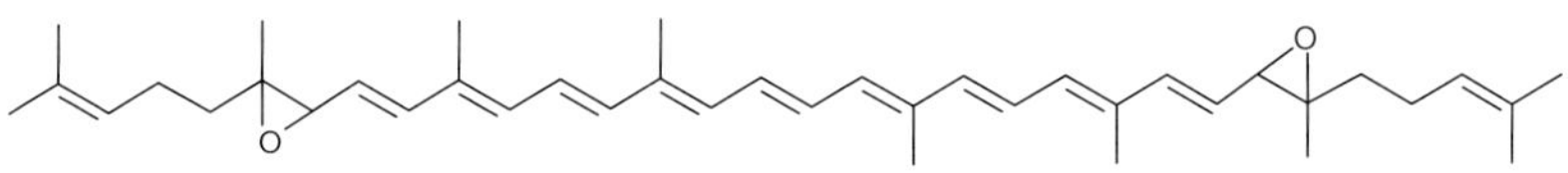

Lycopene 5,6,5′,6′-diepoxide

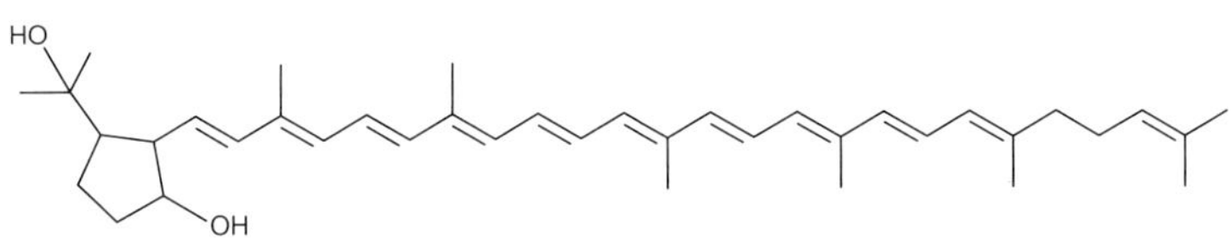

2,6-Cyclolycopene-1,5-diol

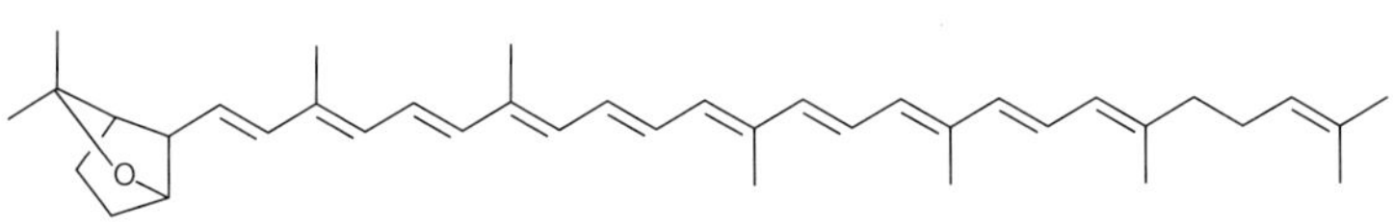

2,6-Cyclolycopene-1,5-epoxide

Figure 7.3 Epoxidation products of lycopene (Khachik et al., 1998a,b; Rodriguez and Rodriguez-Amaya, 2009).

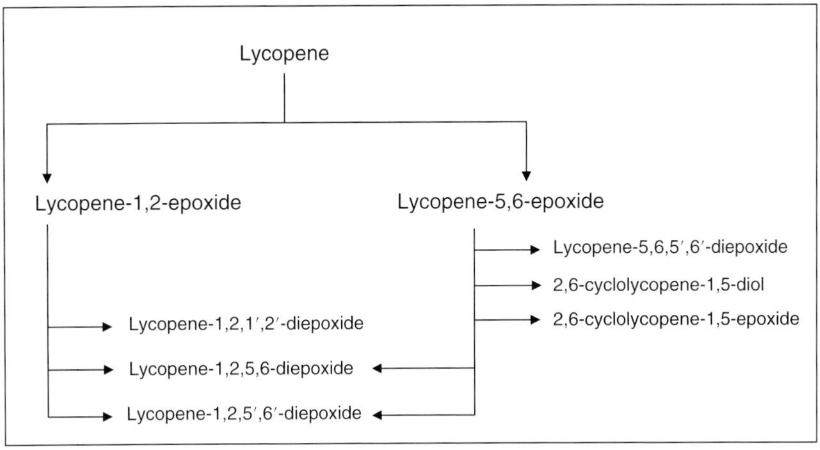

Figure 7.4 Possible pathways for the formation of oxidation products from lycopene. Taken from Rodriguez and Rodriguez-Amaya (2009).

Except for lycopene-1,2,5′,6′-diepoxide, these epoxides were found in tomato juice, and except for lycopene-1,2,5,6-diepoxide, in tomato puree. Lycopene-1,2-epoxide, 2,6-cyclolycopene-1,5-diol, 2,6-cyclolycopene-1,5-epoxide, and *Z*-2,6-cyclolycopene-1,5-epoxide were detected in guava juice. Lycopene-5,6-epoxide, lycopene-5,6,5′,6′-diepoxide, and lycopene-1,2,1′,2′-diepoxide were not detected in the model systems and in the foods analyzed. This could be due to their fast turn-over (transformation) to the subsequent products, not allowing them to accumulate at levels sufficient for detection. 9-*Z*-lycopene and 13-*Z*-lycopene were formed in the model systems and were found in the commercially processed foods (tomato juice, tomato paste, tomato puree, and guava juice).

Introduction of the 5,6-epoxide moiety and transformation of this group to the 5,8-furanoid is a common reaction in foods. A good example is the transformation of the labile violaxanthin to auroxanthin (Figure 7.5), changing the composition of fruits where violaxanthin is the major pigment. In three brands of bottled mango juice, violaxanthin, the principal carotenoid of the fresh fruits, was not detected (Mercadante and Rodriguez-Amaya, 1998). Instead, appreciable amounts of auroxanthin, which was not found in the fresh fruits, appeared. With the disappearance of violaxanthin in mango juice and canned mango slices (Cano and de Ancos, 1994), β-carotene became the predominant carotenoid.

Rearrangement of the 5,6- to the 5,8-epoxide is a common reaction for several xanthophylls in citrus juice (Dhuique-Mayer et al., 2007). In pasteurized Valencia orange juice, with the loss of violaxanthin and antheraxanthin, lutein became the major carotenoid, followed by zeaxanthin (Lee and Coates, 2003).

7.5.2 Cleavage to apocarotenals

β-apo-15-carotenal, β-apo-14′-carotenal, β-apo-12′-carotenal, and β-apo-10′-carotenal in the all-*E*-form were all found in the low-moisture model system, both in the presence and absence of light, and in the aqueous model system exposed to light (Rodriguez and Rodriguez-Amaya, 2007). β-apo-8′-carotenal and semi-β-carotenone were encountered

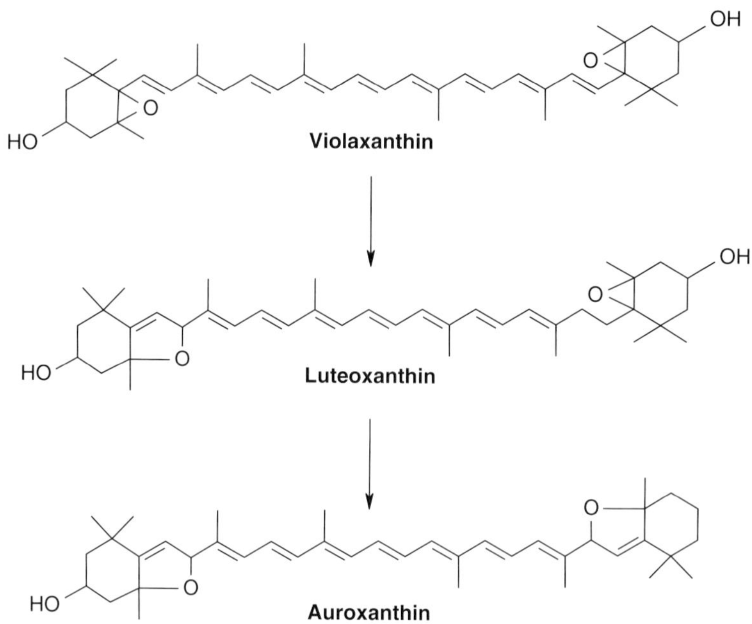

Figure 7.5 Transformation of violaxanthin during processing and storage of foods.

in the aqueous model system but not in the low-moisture system. β-apo-15-carotenal and β-apo-12-carotenal were detected in commercial mango juice.

Marty and Berset (1988, 1990) identified β-apo-15-carotenal, β-apo-14′-carotenal, β-apo-12′-carotenal, β-apo-10′-carotenal, and β-apo-8′-carotenal in a model system that simulated extrusion. Simulating commercial desodorization of bleached red palm oil to which 1% β-carotene was added at 210°C for 4 h, Ouyang et al. (1980) detected β-apo-15-carotenal, β-apo-14′-carotenal, and β-apo-13-carotenone.

Corn oil containing β-carotene was oxidized in Rancimat at 110°C from 1 to 14 h (Zeb and Murkovic, 2013). Eight products of the accelerated thermal oxidation were identified: β-apo-6′-carotenal, β-apo-8′-carotenal, 5,6-epoxy-β-apo-8′-carotenal, β-carotene-2,2′-dione, 13-*Z*-β-carotene-5,6,5′6′-diepoxide, all-*E*-β-carotene-5,8-epoxide, all-*E*-β-carotene-5,6-epoxide, and 15-*Z*-β-carotene-5,6-epoxide.

The results of the studies discussed above at ambient condition and at higher temperatures support the scheme presented in Figure 7.6 for the cleavage of β-carotene, forming β-apo-carotenals.

A similar scheme is presented in Figure 7.7 for lycopene. Apo-12′-lycopenal was formed in both the low-moisture and aqueous model systems and all the commercial food products analyzed (tomato juice, tomato paste, tomato puree, and guava juice) (Rodriguez and Rodriguez-Amaya, 2009). Apo-8′- and apo-6′-lycopenal were detected in both model systems and the tomato products. Apo-15′-lycopenal was found in the low-moisture model system while apo-10′-lycopenal was encountered in the aqueous model system and tomato puree. Apo-6′-, apo-8′-, apo-10′-, apo-12′-, and apo-14′-lycopenals were all detected and quantified in tomato products by Kopec et al. (2010). The sum of apo-lycopenals was 6.5 μg/100 g in raw tomato, 73.4 μg/100 g in tomato paste.

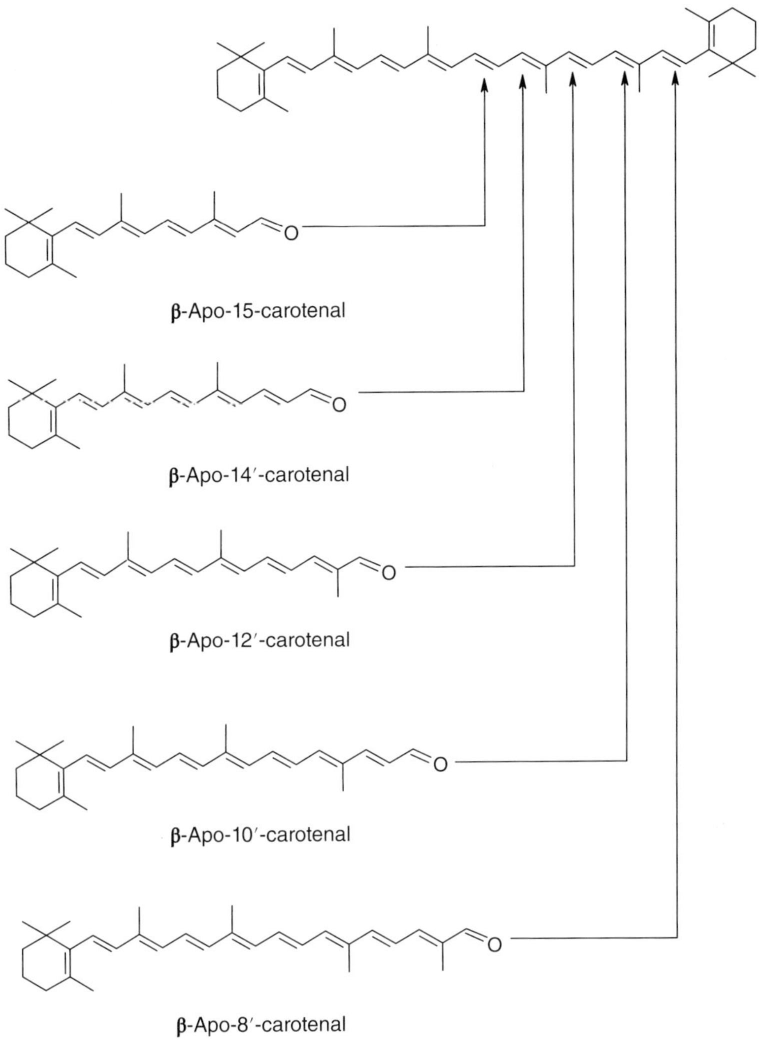

Figure 7.6 Formation of apocarotenals from β-carotene. Rodriguez and Rodriguez-Amaya (2007). Reproduced with permission of Elsevier.

Heating synthetic β-cryptoxanthin in an acidified or nonacidified aqueous system at 90°C for 1 or 2 h yielded 9-*Z*-β-cryptoxanthin, 9′-*Z*-β-cryptoxanthin, 13-Z-β-cryptoxanthin, 13′-*Z*-β-cryptoxanthin, 15-*Z*-β-cryptoxanthin, 5,6-epoxy-β-cryptoxanthin, and β-apo-12′-carotenal (Zepka and Mercadante, 2009). Heating of a cashew apple extract in the same system at 60°C and 90°C produced *Z*-lutein, 15-*Z*-β-carotene, auroxanthin, mutatoxanthin, 5,6-epoxy-β-cryptoxanthin, and 5,8-epoxy-β-carotene. Luteoxanthin and β-apo-12′-carotenal were formed only at 90°C.

It is likely that enzymatic oxidation of carotenoids occurs through the same routes as nonenzymatic oxidation. β-Apo-14′-carotenal, β-apo-12′-carotenal, β-apo-10′-carotenal, β-apo-8′-carotenal, and β-apo-13-carotenone were found in orange-fleshed melon (Fleshman et al., 2011). Ben-Aziz et al. (1973) identified lycopene-1,2-epoxide,

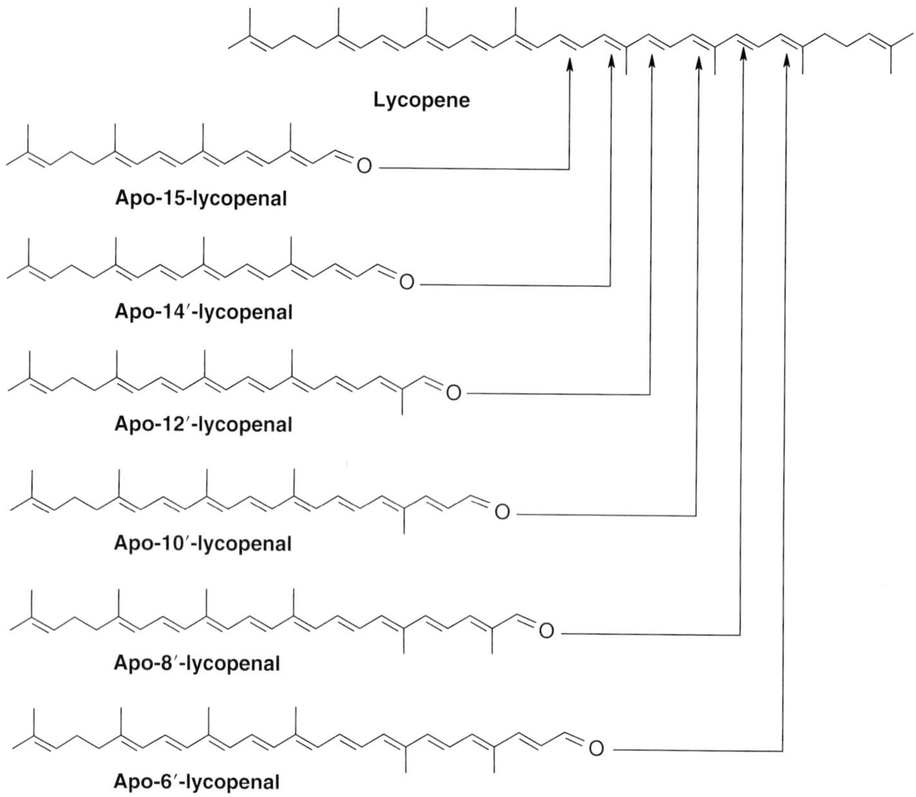

Figure 7.7 Formation of lycopenals from lycopene. Taken from Rodriguez and Rodriguez-Amaya (2009).

lycopene-5,6-epoxide, β-carotene-5,8-epoxide, phytoene -1,2-epoxide, phytofluene -1,2-epoxide and ζ-carotene -1,2-epoxide in raw tomato. Apo-6′-, apo-8′-, apo-10′-, apo-12′-, and apo-14′-lycopenals were detected and quantified in raw tomato, red grapefruit, and watermelon (Kopec et al., 2010).

7.5.3 Formation of low-mass compounds

The volatile compounds formed by carotenoid oxidation fall into three types: short acyclic compounds, which apparently come from the polyene chain; cleaved acyclic (e.g., from lycopene) and cyclic end groups (e.g., from β-carotene); and secondary products formed from the primary cleavage products, including cyclic compounds from cyclic end groups or from acyclic fragments of the polyene chain. It appears that generation of volatile compounds proceeds by direct cleavage of the carotenoid, sequential cleavage, and transformation of the initial volatile compounds.

Work done in our laboratory (Padula and Rodriguez-Amaya, unpublished results), in which nonvolatile oxidation products were identified by HPLC-MS and the volatile compounds by GC-MS, suggests that stepwise sequential cleavage may occur, from one end of the molecule to the center. In Figure 7.8, the possible formation of β-apo-8′-carotenal and β-cyclocitral from β-carotene is shown, both compounds being detected in our study involving β-carotene adsorbed in microcrystalline cellulose stored at

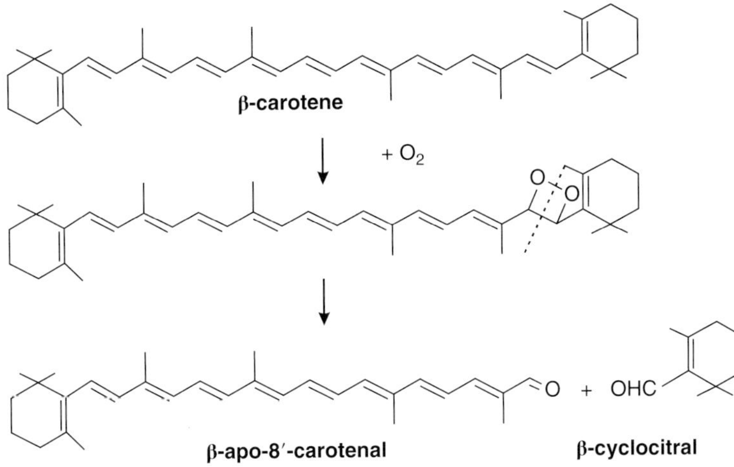

Figure 7.8 Possible mechanism for the formation of β-apo-8′-carotenal and β-cyclocitral from β-carotene.

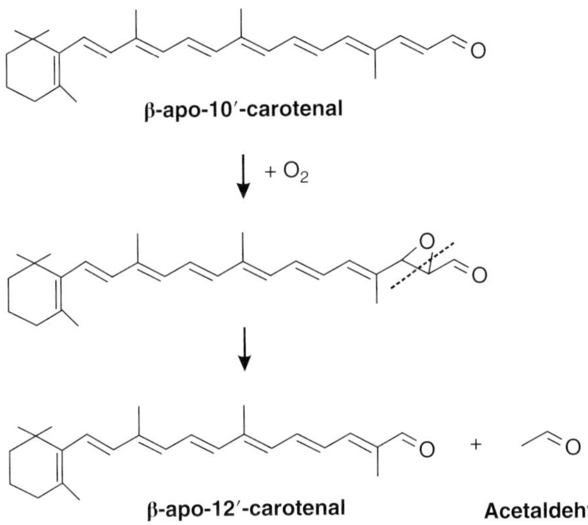

Figure 7.9 Possible mechanism for the formation of β-apo-12′-carotenal and acetaldehyde from β-apo-10′-carotenal.

ambient condition. The introduction of oxygen and cleavage at the double bond C7=C8 can occur by the dioxetane mechanism, suggested for apocarotenal formation by Ouyang et al. (1980), based solely on the identification of β-apo-14′-carotenal as a decomposition product in a simulated commercial deodorization of palm oil. A reaction pathway via a dioxetane intermediate was also proposed by Ukai et al. (1994) for the formation of 2-methyl-2-hepten-6-one and apo-6′-lycopenal by the irradiation of lycopene in an atmosphere of oxygen and in the presence of a sensitizer (methylene blue).

The identification of acetaldehyde among the volatile compounds in our unpublished work is another indication of the sequential cleavage of β-carotene. Figure 7.9 shows the possible cleavage of β-apo-10′-carotenal to β-apo-12′-carotenal and acetaldehyde.

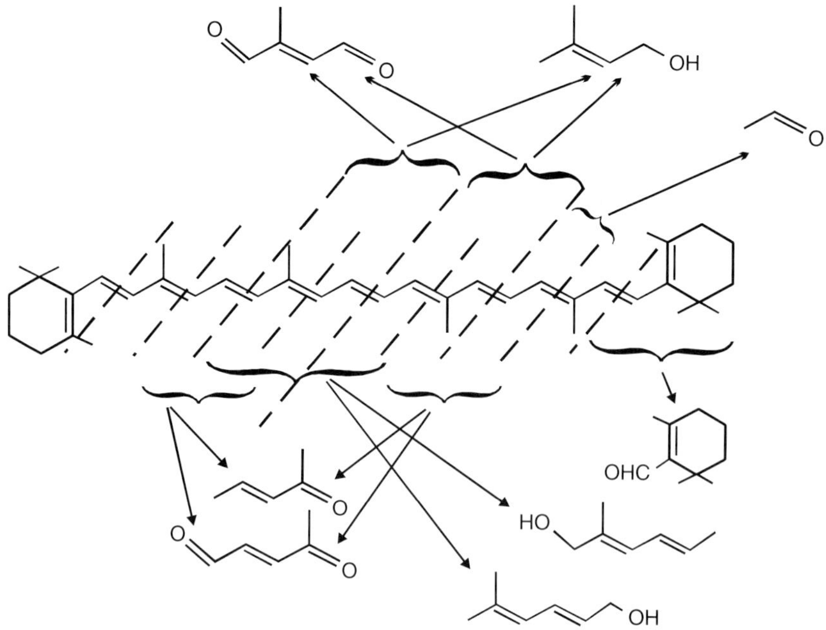

Figure 7.10 Possible formation of volatile compounds through the fragmentation of the β-carotene polyene chain.

Aside from β-cyclocitral and acetaldehyde, 3-penten-2-one, 3-methyl-2-butenol, 4-oxo-2-pentenal, 2-methyl-2-buten-1,4-dial, 2-methyl-hex-2,4-dien-1-ol, and 5-methyl-hex-2,4-dien-1-ol were also identified. These are short acyclic compounds, the possible origin of which from the β-carotene molecule can be easily be located, indicating that fragmentation can also occur by direct cleavage of the polyene chain at various sites (Figure 7.10).

The volatile compounds β-ionone, 5,6-epoxy-β-ionone, dihydroactinidiolide, and β-cyclocitral were identified in dried sweet potato chips during storage, the formation of which was attributed to degradation of all-*E*-β-carotene (Bechoff et al., 2010). Using multiresponse modeling, two isomers (9-*Z*- and 13-*Z*-β-carotene), two β-carotene epoxides (β-carotene-5,6- and β-carotene-5,8-epoxide), and four volatile compounds (β-cyclocitral, β-ionone, 5,6-epoxy-β-ionone, and dihydroactinidiolide) were investigated (Achir et al., 2014). It was concluded that (a) the formation of *Z*-isomers from β-carotene preceded oxidation, (b) β-cyclocitral arose directly from scission of β-carotene whereas the other volatiles resulted from degradation of β-carotene epoxide, and (c) *Z*-isomers were highly reactive compounds.

Kanasawud and Crouzet (1990a) identified 21 volatile thermal (3 h at 97°C) degradation products of β-carotene suspended in water by sonication and saturated with oxygen. It was postulated that 5,6-epoxy-β-ionone, formed from β-carotene-5,6,5′,6′-diepoxide, could be transformed to dihydroactinidiolide, which could also be derived from β-carotene-5,8,5′,8′-diepoxide. 5,6-Epoxy-β-ionone could also form β-ionone or be converted to 2-hydroxy-2,6,6-trimethylcyclohexane-1-carboxaldehyde, which in turn could form β-cyclocitral. 5,6-Epoxy-β-ionone could also be transformed to

2-hydroxy-2,6,6-trimethycyclohexanone, which in turn could form 2,6,6-trimethyl-2-cyclohexen-1-one. With the same model system, only dihydroactinidiolide was formed at 30°C.

As with enzymatic oxidation discussed in Chapter 8, it is more likely that 5,6-epoxy-β-ionone is formed by cleavage of β-carotene-5,6-epoxide, and dihydroactinidiolide is derived from β-carotene-5,8-epoxide. Alternatively, cleavage of β-carotene can produce β-ionone, which is epoxidized to 5,6-β-ionone, the latter in turn transformed to dihydroactinidiolide.

In a model system simulating dehydrated foods, consisting of lycopene isolated from watermelon and adsorbed on microcrystalline cellulose, ten volatile compounds (aldehydes, ketones, alcohol, furan, and pyran) were identified as oxidation products at ambient temperature, the main volatiles formed being 6-methyl-5-hepten-2-one, citral or geranial, and neral (Kobori et al., 2014). Possible routes for the formation of five of these compounds are shown in Figure 7.11. The volatiles 6-methyl-5-hepten-2-one, geranial, and neral had been previously reported as degradation products of lycopene (Caris-Veyrat et al., 2003; Kanasawud and Crouzet, 1990b). The formation of geranial and its transformation to neral was previously proposed by Kanasawud and Crouzet (1990b).

Kanasawud and Crouzet (1990b) investigated the degradation of lycopene in an aqueous model system at a temperature of 30°C to 97°C in the presence of air or oxygen for 3 h. Neral was formed only at temperatures above 50°C. Under mild conditions (temperature below 50°C), only 6-methyl-5-hepten-2-one, geranial, and pseudoionone were found. Aside from neral, 5-hexe-2-one, hexane-2,5-dione, 6-methyl-3,5-heptadien-2-one, and geranyl acetate were generated at higher temperatures. Rios et al. (2008) reported, aside from 6-methyl-5-hepten-2-one, toluene, *m*-xylene, 6-methyl-3,5-heptadien-2-one,

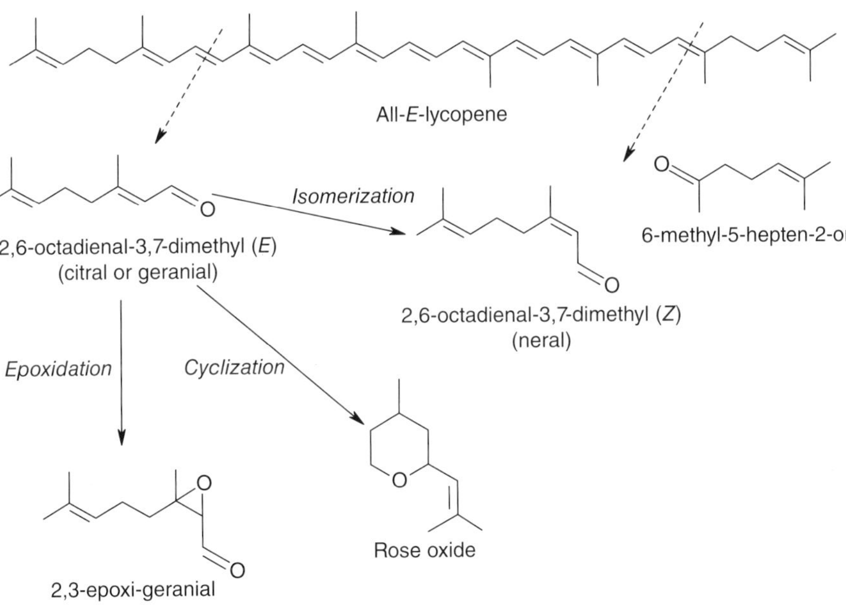

Figure 7.11 Possible routes for the formation of volatile compounds from lycopene. Kobori et al. (2014). Reproduced with permission of Elsevier.

ethanone, and β-citronellol in tomato oleoresin after thermal degradation at 50°C, 100°C, and 150°C.

Complex volatile compound profiles were obtained from the thermal degradation of carotenoids in oleoresins of paprika, tomato, and marigold (Rios et al., 2008). Intramolecular cyclization was proposed as the main reaction mechanism in the formation of the volatile compounds detected, followed by a reaction of elimination in the chain or a heterolytic fragmentation reaction. The formation of various methyl benzaldehydes or isophorone (1,1,3-trimethyl-3-cyclohexene-5-one) was taken to indicate the concurrence of reactions that affect either the central polyene chain or the end-groups.

Of the 10 volatile compounds identified by Kobori et al. (2014), 7 (1-pentanol, hexanal, 6-methyl-5-hepten-2-one, (*E*)2-octen-1-al, nonanal, neral, and geranial) were also found by Beaulieu and Lea (2006) in five varieties of watermelon, indicating similarity of enzymatic biodegradation and nonenzymatic autoxidation of carotenoids.

Hexanal, 6-methyl-5-hepten-2-one, and nonanal were detected in fresh-cut watermelon slices (Saftner et al., 2007) and, together with nonenal and geranylacetone, in watermelon juice processed by high-intensity pulsed electric field or heat (Aguiló-Aguayo et al., 2010). Geranial, neral, 6-methyl-5-hepten-2-one, and 2,3-epoxy-geranial were identified by Lewinsohn et al. (2005) in both watermelon and tomato fruits. Tandom et al. (2000) encountered hexanal, 6-methyl-5-hepten-2-one, geranylacetone, and β-ionone in fresh tomatoes. 6-Methyl-5-hepten-2-one, hexanal, and nonanal were among the volatiles identified in red-fleshed papaya fruit (Pino, 2014).

Volatile compounds generated by enzymatic oxidation of carotenoids have been more extensively studied than those derived from nonenzymatic oxidation and are discussed in detail in Chapter 8. Further discussion of aroma compounds produced by nonenzymatic oxidation of carotenoids is also provided.

7.5.4 Influencing factors

Many factors have been shown to influence the oxidative degradation of carotenoids in foods: the carotenoid involved, nature of the matrix, available oxygen, exposure to light, water content/activity, temperature, atmosphere, activity of oxidizing enzymes, presence of antioxidants, presence of metal catalysts and prooxidants, and free radical initiators and inhibitors (Rodriguez-Amaya, 1993, 2002; Xianquan et al., 2005; Pénicaud et al., 2011).

Carotenoid degradation is known to increase with the destruction of the food cellular structure, increase of surface area or porosity, duration and severity of processing conditions, duration and inadequate conditions of storage, permeability of the packaging material to O_2, and exposure to light. Carotenoids in dehydrated foods are especially prone to autoxidation because of the greater superficial area (greater exposure to oxygen).

There is ample evidence that carotenoids have varying susceptibility to oxidation, as can be noted in Chapter 6, although research results on the relative susceptibilities are somewhat inconsistent. The effects of light and heat are also well demonstrated. Only some examples will be given below.

In blanched and unblanched freeze-dried carrots, α-carotene and β-carotene had similar rate constants, whereas lutein degraded faster (Lavelli et al., 2007). β-Carotene was more stable than lycopene in watermelon chunks and puree during storage at −20°C (Fish and Davis, 2003). The yellow xanthophylls and β-carotene in pepper had the highest rates of oxidation (Pérez-Gálvez and Minguez-Mosquera, 2001). The ketocarotenoids and violaxanthin degraded at lower rates.

In both palm olein and Vegetaline, initial all-*E*-β-carotene and all-*E*-lutein degradation rates increased with temperature (Achir et al., 2010). All-*E*-lutein degraded at a slower rate than all-*E*-β-carotene. Degradation rates were lower in Vegetaline than in palm olein, explained by the initial composition of the two oils, especially their peroxide and vitamin E content.

In low-moisture model systems, consisting of β-carotene or lycopene isolated from guava, tomato, or watermelon adsorbed on cornstarch, potato starch, or microcrystalline cellulose and in an aqueous model system, greater losses were observed with lycopene from tomato (Ferreira and Rodriguez-Amaya, 2008). Since thc models were identical, the results indicated that other compounds from the food sources, coextracted with lycopene, might have influenced the oxidation. Light consistently and strongly promoted degradation under all conditions studied. Lycopene degraded much faster than β-carotene in all the model systems, but its susceptibility to degradation was much less in lyophilized guava than in the model systems, showing the marked protective influence of the food matrix.

The effect of water activity on oxidation is known to be complex (Gloria et al., 1995). Increasing water in dry matrices may raise the rate of oxidation by enhancing the mobility of reactants and bringing catalysts into solution. As the solid matrix swells, new surfaces for catalysts are exposed. On the other hand, water may also slow down the oxidation process by hydrating or diluting heavy metal catalysts or precipitating them as hydroxides. Water may also prevent peroxide decomposition by hydrogen bonding with the hydroperoxides, and by promoting radical recombination, which could interrupt the oxidation reaction. The net result is that, in many foods, the rate of oxidation reaches a minimum in the a_w corresponding to the monolayer moisture content. Dehydrated foods should therefore be stored at the monolayer a_w to decrease oxidative degradations and thus extend their shelf life.

In both blanched and unblanched freeze-dried carrots, the rate of carotenoid degradation was at a minimum over the a_w range 0.31–0.54 (Lavelli et al., 2007). In potato chips dried using an open-air sun dryer, over the range studied (0%–21% oxygen), oxygen had a more marked effect on β-carotene degradation than water activity (0.13–0.76) (Bechoff et al., 2010).

7.6 IMPLICATIONS ON FOOD QUALITY

During storage of carotenogenic foods, fading of color and development of typical flavor or off-flavor may occur, these changes being related to carotenoid decomposition.

When *E*-*Z* isomerization occurs, there is only a slight spectral shift; thus, the color of the product may not be affected or only slightly lightened. However, when oxidation takes place, the chromophore is progressively shortened until the number of conjugated double bonds falls below seven, at which point the carotenoid molecule turns colorless.

The volatile products of carotenoid degradation can be desirable, as in black tea (Ravichandran, 2002) and wine (Mendes-Pinto, 2009), where they become part of the pleasing characteristic aroma. In some processed foods, however, degradation/cleavage of carotenoids is responsible for the appearance of off-flavor, as in dehydrated carrot (Falconer et al., 1964) and in certain types of wine (Rapp and Marais, 1993).

Carotenoids, as natural antioxidants, may also contribute to the extension of the food's shelf life. Processing and storage conditions that provide optimum retention of these compounds are thus desirable.

Thermal degradation products of β-carotene acted as a prooxidant during autoxidation of soybean oil held in the dark (Steenson and Min, 2000). It was therefore recommended that food processors take the necessary measures to minimize degradation of this carotenoid to prevent the possible formation of prooxidant compounds. Thermally degraded lycopene, on the other hand, displayed antioxidant activity.

7.7 IMPLICATIONS FOR HUMAN HEALTH

For a long time the major concern about carotenoids in food processing was minimizing their degradation. Studies have shown, however, that processing (i.e., mechanical matrix disruption and/or heat treatment) can increase the bioavailability of carotenoids. The cellular structure that protects carotenoids in nature limits their bioavailability. Processing softens or breaks membranes and cell walls and denatures proteins complexed with carotenoids, facilitating the release of carotenoids from the food matrices during digestion, thereby increasing their bioavailability. Processing conditions should therefore be optimized to increase bioavailability without much degradation of the carotenoids.

Moreover, processing leads to the formation of *Z*-carotenoids, which have different biological properties from *E*-carotenoids, such as decreased vitamin A activity and altered bioavailability and antioxidant capacity (Schieber and Carle, 2005). *Z*-isomers of β-carotene have been demonstrated to be less effective in quenching singlet oxygen than all-*E*-β-carotene (Stahl and Sies, 1993). Processing effects on bioavailability, including isomerization effects, are discussed in Chapter 9.

It is generally believed that introduction of an epoxide group at one of the β-rings reduces the vitamin A activity by about half, while the epoxidation of both rings eliminates this activity.

It is now recognized that oxidation products or metabolites are involved in the biological activities attributed to carotenoids (Zhang et al., 2003; Carail and Caris-Veyrat, 2006; Khachik, 2006; Harrison et al., 2012; Wang, 2012). The studies on the health effects of these compounds, which have been carried out in human and rat cells, however, have given mixed results.

In vitro studies have shown beneficial effects such as inhibition of cell growth and cholesterol synthesis in breast cancer (MCF-7) cells by a β-carotene oxidation product identified as 5,8-endoperoxy-2,3-dihydro-β-apocarotene-13-one (Hu et al., 1998). β-apo-carotenoic acids (β-apo-14′-, β-apo-12′-, β-apo-10′- and β-apo-8′-) inhibited the proliferation of human breast cancer cells MCF-7 and Hs578T in a dose-dependent manner (Tibaduiza et al., 2002), β-apo-14′- and β-apo-12′-carotenoic acid significantly inhibited MCF-7 growth, whereas only β-apo-14′-carotenoic acid inhibited Hs578T growth.

Products of the autoxidation of lycopene induced apoptosis of HL-60 human promyelocytic leukemia cells (Nara et al., 2001; Zhang et al., 2003), suggesting that carotenoids inhibit cell growth through apoptosis induction and carotenoid oxidation products participate in the growth inhibition (Nara et al., 2001). The lycopene metabolite 2,6-cyclolycopene-1,5-diol increased connexin 43 gene expression in human HaCaT cells (King et al., 1997). Another lycopene oxidation product, identified as 2,7,11-trimethyl-tetradecahexaene-1,14-dial, showed a stimulatory effect on gap junctional communication in rat liver epithelial WB-F344 cells (Aust et al., 2003).

On the other hand, oxidized β-carotene at 5 μM inhibited, whereas β-carotene at the same concentration markedly increased gap junction intercellular communication in the human lung adenocarcinoma cell line A549 (Yeh and Hu, 2003). These results were considered suggestive that in vivo inhibition of gap junction intercellular communication by a high dose of β-carotene would be, at least in part, attributable to the effect of oxidized products of β-carotene. Cleavage products of β-carotene generated in vitro under oxidative conditions (with hypochlorous acid at room temperature) increased oxidative stress in isolated rat liver mitochondria by imparing mitochondrial respiration (Siems et al., 2002, 2005). β-apo-8′-carotenal, not β-carotene, strongly induced liver cytochromes P4501A1 and 1A2 in rat (Gradelet et al., 1996). In cultured human cells, degradation products of β-carotene autoxidation were found to be cytotoxic, and mitochondrial function was decreased in both K562 and RPE cells (Hurst et al., 2005).

Treatment of primary rat hepatocyte cultures with β-carotene did not induce any cyto- or genotoxic effects, but exposure to a mixture of β-carotene breakdown products and β-apo-8′-carotenal induced genotoxic effects (Alija et al., 2004). The mixture was obtained by degradation of β-carotene mediated by hypochlorous acid and consisted of 5,6-epoxy-β-ionone, β-ionone, ionene, β-cyclocitral, dihydroactinidiolide, and 4-oxo-β-ionone (Sommerburg et al., 2003). Cyto- and genotoxic effects on primary rat hepatocytes after supplementation of the medium with increasing concentrations of the mixture of β-carotene breakdown products during exposure to oxidative stress was subsequently investigated (Ajila et al., 2006). The results obtained demonstrated that the mixture enhanced the genotoxic effects of oxidative stress exposure, whereas it had no effect on the endpoints of cytotoxicity studied. These results were taken as further support of the hypothesis that β-carotene degradation products might be responsible for the reported carcinogenic response in the β-carotene and Retinol Efficacy Trial (CARET) and Alpha-Tocopherol Beta-carotene Cancer prevention (ATBC) chemoprevention trials, discussed in Chapter 11.

Harrison et al. (2012) suggested that a possible biological function of β-apocarotenoids is their ability to interfere with nuclear receptor signaling. This hypothesis was based on competitive radioligand binding assays, confirmed by molecular modeling studies, that showed that β-apo-13-carotenone competed directly with 9-*Z*-retinoic acid for binding to purified receptor. In their review, Salerno et al. (2005) found the data suggesting that carotenoid oxidation products may affect neutrophil viability and function by exerting proapoptotic activity and interfering with superoxide production by activated cells. They hypothesized that the prooxidant and proapoptotic activities of carotenoid oxidation products could account, at least in some cases, for the procancerogenic properties of a carotenoid-rich diet.

Autoxidation of lycopene solubilized in aqueous 5% Tween 40, which can be taken as a model system simulating food, and in liposomal suspension, representing the human body, was carried out by incubating under atmospheric oxygen at 37°C (Kim et al., 2001). 3,7,11-Trimethyl-2,4,6,10-dodecatetraen-1-al, 6,10,14-trimethy-3,5,7,9,13-pentadecapentaen-2-one, acycloretinal, apo-14′-lycopenal, apo-12′-lycopenal, apo-10′-lycopenal, and apo-8′-lycopenal were identified in both systems. Formation of apo-6′-lycopenal was observed only in the liposomal suspension.

Apo-6′-, apo-8′-, apo-10′-, apo-12′-, and apo-14′-lycopenals were detected in the plasma of individuals who had consumed tomato juice for 8 weeks (Kopec et al., 2010). 2,6-Cyclolycopene-1,5-diol was also detected in human serum (Khachick et al., 1998a). It is not clear if the metabolites of lycopene and other carotenoids in human serum are due to in vivo oxidation or if these compounds may be of dietary origin or both. More investigations are evidently needed.

References

Achir N, Pénicaud C, Bechoff A, Boulanger R, Dornier M, Dhuique-Mayer C. 2014. Use of multi-response modelling to investigate mechanisms of β-carotene degradation in dried orange-fleshed sweet potato during storage: from carotenoids to aroma compounds. *Food Bioprocess Technol* 7:1656–69.

Achir N, Randrianatoandro VA, Bohuon P, Laffargue A, Avallone S. 2010. Kinetic study of β-carotene and lutein degradation in oils during heat treatment. *Eur J Lipid Sci Technol* 112:349–61.

Aguiló-Aguayo I, Montero-Calderón M, Soliva-Fortuny R, Martín-Belloso O. 2010. Changes on flavor compounds throughout cold storage of watermelon juice processed by high-intensity pulsed electric fields or heat. *J Food Eng* 100:43–9.

Ahmed J, Shivhare US, Sandhu KS. 2002. Thermal degradation kinetics of carotenoids and visual color of papaya puree. *J Food Sci* 67:2692–5.

Alija AJ, Bresgen N, Sommerburg O, Langhans CD, Siems W, Eckl, PM. 2006. β-carotene breakdown products enhance genotoxic effects of oxidative stress in primary rat hepatocytes. *Carcinogenesis* 27:1128–33.

Alija AJ, Bresgen N, Sommerburg, O, Siems W, Eckl PM. 2004. Cytotoxic and genotoxic effects of β-carotene breakdown products on primary rat hepatocytes. *Carcinogenesis* 25:827–31.

Aman R, Biehl J, Carle R, Conrad J, Beifuss U, Schieber A. 2005. Application of HPLC coupled with DAD, APcI-MS and NMR to the analysis of lutein and zeaxanthin stereoisomers in thermally processed vegetables. *Food Chem* 92:753–63.

Aparicio-Ruiz R, Gandul-Rojas B. 2012. Thermal degradation kinetics of neoxanthin, violaxanthin, and antheraxanthin in virgin olive oils. *J Agric Food Chem* 60:5180–91.

Aust O, Ale-Agha N, Zhang L, Wollersen H, Sies H, Stahl W. 2003. Lycopene oxidation product enhances gap junctional communication. *Food Chem Toxicol* 41:1399–407.

Beaulieu JC, Lea J M. 2006. Characterization and semiquantitative analysis of volatiles in seedless watermelon varieties using solid-phase microextration. *J Agric Food Chem* 54:7789–93.

Bechoff A, Dhuique-Mayer C, Dornier M, Tomlins KI, Boulanger R, Dufour D, Westby A. 2010. Relationship between the kinetics of β-carotene degradation and formation of norisoprenoids in the storage of dried sweet potato chips. *Food Chem* 121:348–57.

Ben-Aziz A, Britton G, Goodwin TW. 1973. Carotene epoxides of *Lycopersicon esculentum*. *Phytochemistry* 12:2759–64.

Cano MP, de Ancos B. 1994. Carotenoid and carotenoid ester composition in mango fruit as influenced by processing method. *J Agric Food Chem* 42:2737–42.

Carail M, Caris-Veyrat C. 2006. Carotenoid oxidation products: from villain to savior? *Pure Appl Chem* 78:1493–503.

Caris-Veyrat C, Schmid A, Carail M, Bohm V. 2003. Cleavage products of lycopene produced by in vitro oxidations: characterization and mechanisms of formation. *J Agric Food Chem* 51:7318–25.

Chen BH, Peng HY, Chen HE. (1995). Changes of carotenoids, color, and vitamin A contents during processing of carrot juice. *J Agric Food Chem* 43:1912–8.

Chen BH, Tang YC. 1998. Processing and stability of carotenoid powder from carrot pulp waste. *J Agric Food Chem* 46:2312–8.

Chen HE, Peng HY, Chen BH. 1996. Stability of carotenoids and vitamin A during storage of carrot juice. *Food Chem* 57:497–503.

Dhuique-Mayer C, Tbatou M, Carail M, Caris-Veyrat C, Dornier M, Amiot MJ. 2007. Thermal degradation of antioxidant micronutrients in citrus juice: kinetics and newly formed components. *J Agric Food Chem* 55:4209–16.

Dutta D, Dutta A, Raychaudhuri U, Chakraborty R. 2006. Rheological characteristics and thermal degradation kinetics of beta-carotene in pumpkin puree. *J Food Eng* 76:538–46.

Falconer ME, Fishwick MJ, Lan DG, Sayer ER. 1964. Carotene oxidation and off-flavour development in dehydrated carrot. *J Sci Food Agric* 15:897–901.

Ferreira JEM, Rodriguez-Amaya DB. 2008. Degradation of lycopene and β-carotene in model systems and in lyophilized guava during ambient storage: kinetics, structure and matrix effects. *J Food Sci* 78:C589–94.

Fish WW, Davis AR. 2003. The effects of frozen storage conditions on lycopene stability in watermelon tissue. *J Agric Food Chem* 51:3582–5.

Fleshman MK, Lester GE, Riedl KM, Kopec RE, Narayanasamy S, Curley RW Jr, Schwartz SJ, Harrison EH. 2011. Carotene and novel apocarotenoid concentrations in orange-fleshed *Cucumis melo* melons: determinations of β-carotene bioaccessibility and bioavailability. *J Agric Food Chem* 59:4448–54.

Gloria, MBA, Vale SR, Bobbio PA. 1995. Effect of water activity, light and air on the stability of bixin in an annatto extract-microcrystalline cellulose model system. *Food Chem* 52:389–91.

Godoy HT, Rodriguez-Amaya DB. 1987. Changes in individual carotenoids on processing and storage of mango (*Mangifera indica*) slices and puree. *Int J Food Sci Technol* 22:451–60.

Godoy HT, Rodriguez-Amaya DB. 1991. Comportamento dos carotenóides de purê de mamão (*Carica papaya*) sob processamento e estocagem. *Ciênc Tecnol Alimen* 11:210–20.

Gradelet S, Leclerc J, Siess M-H, Astorg PO. 1996. β-apo-8′-carotenal, but not β-carotene, is a strong inducer of liver cytochromes P4501A1 and 1A2 in rat. *Xenobiotica* 26:909–19.

Gregory JF III. 2008. Vitamins. In: Damodaran S, Parkin KL, Fennema OR. editors. *Fennema's Food chemistry*, fourth edition. Boca Raton: CRC Press Taylor and Francis Group, p 439–521.

Hadjal T, Dhuique-Mayer C, Madani K, Dornier M, Achir N. 2013. Thermal degradation kinetics of xanthophylls from blood orange in model and real food systems. *Food Chem* 138:2442–50.

Harrison EH, dela Sena C, Eroglu A, Fleshman MK. 2012. The formation, occurrence, and function of β-apocarotenoids: β-carotene metabolites that may modulate nuclear receptor signaling. *Am J Clin Nutr* 96:S1189–2.

Henry LK, Puspitasari-Nienabe NL, Jarén-Galán M, van Breemen RB, Castignani GL, Schwartz SJ. 2000. Effects of ozone and oxygen on the degradation of carotenoids in an aqueous system. *J Agric Food Chem* 48:5008–13.

Hiranvarachat B, Suvarnakuta P, Devahastin S. 2008. Isomerization kinetics and antioxidant activities of β-carotene in carrots undergoing different drying techniques and conditions. *Food Chem* 107:1538–46.

Hu X, White KM, Jacobsen NE, Mangelsdorf DJ, Canfield LM. 1998. Inhibition of growth and cholesterol synthesis in breast cancer cells by oxidation products of β-carotene. *J Nutr Biochem*. 9:567-74 10.1016/S0955-2863(98)00048-5.

Hurst JS, Saini MK, Jin G-F, Awasthi YC, van Kuijk FJGM. 2005. Toxicity of oxidized β-carotene to cultured human cells. *Exp Eye Res* 81:239–43.

Imsic M, Winkler S, Tomkins B, Jones R. 2010. Effect of storage and cooking on β-carotene isomers in carrots (*Daucus carota* L. cv. 'Stefano'). *J Agric Food Chem* 58:5109–13.

Ishida BK, Roberts JS, Chapman MH, Burri BJ. 2007. Processing Tangerine tomatoes: effects on lycopene-isomer concentrations and profile. *J Food Sci* 72:C307–12.

Kanasawud P, Crouzet JC. 1990a. Mechanism of formation of volatile compounds by thermal degradation of carotenoids in aqueous medium: 1. β-Carotene degradation. *J Agric Food Chem* 38:237–43.

Kanasawud P, Crouzet JC. 1990b. Mechanism of formation of volatile compounds by thermal degradation of carotenoids in aqueous medium: 2. Lycopene degradation. *J Agric Food Chem* 38:1238–42.

Khachik F. 2006. Distribution and metabolism of dietary carotenoids in humans as a criterion for development of nutritional supplements. *Pure Appl Chem* 78:1551–7.

Khachik F, Pfander H, Traber B. 1998a. Proposed mechanisms for the formation of synthetic and naturally occurring metabolites of lycopene in tomato products and human serum. *J Agric Food Chem* 46:4885–90.

Khachik F, Steck A, Niggli UA, Pfander H. 1998b. Partial synthesis and structural elucidation of the oxidative metabolites of lycopene identified in tomato paste, tomato juice, and human serum. *J Agric Food Chem* 46:4874–84.

Kidmose U, Yang R-Y, Thilsted SH, Christensen LP, Brandt K. 2006. Contents of carotenoids in commonly consumed Asian vegetables and stability and extractability during frying. *J Food Compos Anal* 19:562–71.

Kim S-J, Nara E, Kobayashi H, Terao J, Nagao A. 2001. Formation of cleavage products by autoxidation of lycopene. *Lipids* 36:191–9.

King TJ, Khachik F, Bortkiewicz H, Fukushima LH, Morioka S, Bertram JS, 1997. Metabolites of dietary carotenoids as potential cancer preventive agents. *Pure Appl Chem* 69:2135–40.

Knockaert G, de Roeck A, Lemmens L, van Buggenhout S, Hendrickx M, van Loey A. 2011. Effect of thermal and high pressure processes on structural and health-related properties of carrots (*Daucus carota*). *Food Chem* 125:903–12.

Knockaert G, Pulissery SK, Colle I, van Buggenhout S, Hendrickx M, van Loey A. 2012. Lycopene degradation, isomerization and in vitro bioaccessibility in high pressure homogenized tomato puree containing oil: effect of additional thermal and high pressure processing. *Food Chem* 135:1290–7.

Kobori CN, Wagner R, Padula M, Rodriguez-Amaya DB. 2014. Formation of volatile compounds from lycopene by autoxidation in a model system simulating dehydrated foods. *Food Res Int* 63(Part A):49–54.

Koca N, Burdurlu HS, Karadeniz F. 2007. Kinetics of color changes in dehydrated carrots. *J Food Eng* 78:449–55.

Kopec RE, Riedl KM, Harrison EH, Curley RW Jr, Hruszkewycz DP, Clinton SK, Schwartz SJ. 2010. Identification and quantification of apo-lycopenals in fruits, vegetables, and human plasma. *J Agric Food Chem* 58:3290–6.

Lavelli V, Zanoni B, Zaniboni A. 2007. Effect of water activity on carotenoid degradation in dehydrated carrots. *Food Chem* 104:1705–11.

Lee HS, Coates GA. 2003. Effect of thermal pasteurization on Valencia orange juice color and pigments. *Lebens-Wiss u Technol* 36:153–6.

Lessin WJ, Catigani GL, Schwartz SJ. 1997. Quantification of *cis-trans* isomers of provitamin A carotenoids in fresh and processed fruits and vegetables. *J Agric Food Chem* 45:3728–32.

Lewinsohn E, Sitrit Y, Bar E, Azulay Y, Meir A, Zamir D, Tadmor Y. 2005. Carotenoid pigmentation affects the volatile composition of tomato and watermelon fruits, as revealed by comparative genetic analyses, *J Agric Food Chem* 53:3142–8.

Lin CH, Chen BH. 2005. Stability of carotenoids in tomato juice during storage. *Food Chem* 90:837–46.

Marty C, Berset C. 1986. Degradation of *trans*-β-carotene during heating in sealed glass tubes and extrusion cooking. *J Food Sci* 51:698–702.

Marty C, Berset C. 1988. Degradation products of *trans*-β-carotene produced during extrusion cooking. *J Food Sci* 53:1880–6.

Marty C, Berset C. 1990. Factors affecting the thermal degradation of all-*trans*-β-carotene. *J Agric Food Chem* 38:1063–7.

Marx M, Stuparic M, Schieber A, Carle R. 2003. Effects of thermal processing on *trans-cis*-isomerization of β-carotene in carrot juice and carotene-containing preparations. *Food Chem* 83:609–17.

Mayer-Miebach E, Behsnilian D, Regier M, Schuchmann HP. 2005. Thermal processing of carrots: Lycopene stability and isomerization with regard to antioxidant potential. *Food Res Int* 38:1103–8.

Mendes-Pinto MM. 2009. Carotenoid breakdown products the—norisoprenoids—in wine aroma. *Arch Biochem Biophys* 483:236–45.

Mercadante AZ, Rodriguez-Amaya DB. 1998. Influence of ripening, cultivar differences, and processing on the carotenoid composition of mango. *J Agric Food Chem* 46:128–30.

Nara E, Hayashi H, Kotake M, Miyashita K, Nagao A. 2001. Acyclic carotenoids and their oxidation mixtures inhibit the growth of HL-60 human promyelocytic leukemia cells. *Nutr Cancer* 39:273–83.

Nguyen M, Francis D, Schwartz S. 2001. Thermal isomerization susceptibility of carotenoids in different tomato varieties. *J Sci Food Agric* 81:910–7.

Odriozola-Serrano I, Soliva-Fortuny R, Martín-Belloso O. 2008. Changes of health-related compounds throughout cold storage of tomato juice stabilized by thermal or high intensity pulsed electric field treatments. *Innov Food Sci Emerg Technol* 9:272–9.

O'Sullivan L, Galvin K, Sherne SA, O'Brien NM. 2010. Effects of cooking on the profile and micellarization of 9-cis-, 13-cis- and all-trans-β-carotene in green vegetables. *Food Res Int* 43:1130–5.

Ouyang JM, Daun H, Chang SS, Ho CT. 1980. Formation of carbonyl compounds from β-carotene during palm oil deodorization. *J Food Sci* 45:1214–7.

Padula M, Rodriguez-Amaya DB. 1987. Changes in individual carotenoids and vitamin C on processing and storage of guava juice. *Acta Aliment* 16:209–16.

Pénicaud C, Archir N, Dhuique-Mayer C, Dornier M, Bohuon P. 2011. Degradation of β-carotene during fruit and vegetable processing or storage: reaction mechanisms and kinetic aspects: A review. *Fruits* 66:417–40.

Pérez-Gálvez A, Minguez-Mosquera MI. 2001. Structure-reactivity relationship in the oxidation of carotenoid pigments of the pepper (*Capsicum annuum* L.). *J Agric Food Chem* 49:4864–9.

Pesek CA, Warthesen JJ. 1990. Kinetic model for photoisomerization and concomitant photodegradation of β-carotenes. *J Agric Food Chem* 38:1313–5.

Pino JA. 2014. Odour-active compounds in papaya fruit cv. Red Maradol. *Food Chem* 146:120–6.

Pott I, Marx M, Neidhart S, Mühlbauer W, Carle R. 2003. Quantitative determination of β-carotene stereoisomers in fresh, dried, and solar-dried mangoes (*Mangifera indica* L.). *J Agric Food Chem* 51:4527–31.

Rapp A, Marais J. 1993. The shelf-life of wine: changes in aroma substances during storage and ageing of white wines. In: Charambous G. editor. *Shelf-life studies of food and beverages: Chemical, biological, physical and nutritional aspects*. Amsterdam: Elsevier Science Publishers, p 891–921.

Ravichandran R. 2002. Carotenoid composition, distribution and degradation to flavour volatiles during black tea manufacture and the effect of carotenoid supplementation on tea quality and aroma. *Food Chem* 78:23–8.

Rios JJ, Fernández-García E, Mínguez-Mosquera MI, Pérez-Gálvez A. 2008. Description of volatile compounds generated by the degradation of carotenoids in paprika, tomato and marigold oleoresins. *Food Chem* 106:1145–53.

Rodriguez EB, Rodriguez-Amaya DB. 2007. Formation of apocarotenals and epoxycarotenoids from β-carotene by chemical reactions and by autoxidation in model systems and processed foods. *Food Chem* 101:563–72.

Rodriguez EB, Rodríguez-Amaya DB. 2009. Lycopene epoxides and apo-lycopenals formed by chemical reactions and autoxidation in model systems and processed foods. *J Food Sci* 74:C674–82.

Rodriguez-Amaya DB. 1993. Stability of carotenoids during the storage of foods. In: Charalambous G. editor. *Shelf life studies of foods and beverages: chemical, biological, physical and nutritional aspects*. Amsterdam: Elsevier Science Publishers, p 591–628.

Rodriguez-Amaya DB. 2002. Effects of processing and storage on food carotenoids. *Sight Life Newslett* 3(Spec Iss):25–35.

Rubio-Diaz DE, Santos A, Francis DM, Rodriguez-Saona LE. 2010. Carotenoid stability during production and storage of tomato juice made from tomatoes with diverse pigment profiles measured by infrared spectroscopy. *J Agric Food Chem* 58:8692–8.

Saftner R, Luo Y, McEvoy J, Abbott JA, Vinyard B. 2007. Quality characteristics of fresh-cut watermelon slices from non-treated and 1-methylcyclopropene- and/or ethylene-treated whole fruit. *Postharvest Biol Technol* 44:71–9.

Salerno C, Crifò C, Capuozzo E, Sommerburg O, Langhans C-D, Siems W. 2005. Effect of carotenoid oxidation products on neutrophil viability and function. *Biofactors* 24:185–92.

Schieber A, Carle R. 2005. Occurrence of carotenoid *cis*-isomers in food: technological, analytical, and nutritional implications. *Trends Food Sci Technol* 16:416–22.

Schwartz AJ, von Elbe JH, Giusti MM. 2008. Colorants. In: Damodaran S, Parkin KL, Fennema OR. editors. *Fennema's food chemistry*, fourth edition, Boca Raton: CRC Press Taylor & Francis Group, p 571–638.

Sharma R, Kaur D, Oberoi DPS, Sogi DS. 2008. Thermal degradation kinetics of pigments and visual color in watermelon juice. *Int J Food Prop* 11:439–49.

Shi J, Le Maguer M, Bryan M, Kakuda Y. 2003. Kinetics of lycopene degradation in tomato puree by heat and light irradiation. *J Food Process Eng* 25:485–98.

Shin JH, Chung HL, Seo JK, Sim JH, Huh CS, Kim SK, Baek YJ. 2001. Degradation kinetics of capsanthin in paprika (*Capsicum annuum* L.) as affected by heating. *J Food Sci* 66:15–9.

Siems W, Sommerburg O, Schild L, Augustin W, Langhans C-D, Wiswedel I. 2002. β-Carotene cleavage products induce oxidative stress *in vitro* by impairing mitochondrial respiration. *FASEB J* 16:1289–91.

Siems W, Wiswedel I, Salerno C, Crifo C, Augustin W, Schild L, Langhans C-D, Sommerburg O. 2005. β-carotene breakdown products may impair mitochondrial functions: potential side effects of high-dose β-carotene supplementation. *J Nutr Biochem* 16:385–97.

Sommerburg O, Langhans CD, Arnhold J, Leichsenring M, Salerno C, Crifo C, Hoffmann GF, Debatin KM, Siem WG. 2003. β-carotene cleavage products after oxidation mediated by hypochlorous acid: a model for neutrophil-derived degradation. *Free Radic Biol Med* 35:1480–90.

Stahl W, Sies H. 1993. Physical quenching of singlet oxygen and cis-trans isomerization of carotenoids. *Ann NY Acad Sci* 691:10–19.

Steenson DF, Min DB. 2000. Effects of β-carotene and lycopene thermal degradation products on the oxidative stability of soybean oil. *J Amer Oil Chem Soc* 77:1153–60.

Tandom KS, Baldwin EA, Shewfelt RL. 2000. Aroma perception of individual volatile compounds in fresh tomatoes (*Lycopersicon esculentum*, Mill.) as affected by the medium of evaluation. *Postharvest Biol Technol* 20:261–8.

Tibaduiza EC, Fleet JC, Russell RM, Krinsky NI. 2002. Excentric cleavage products of β-carotene inhibit estrogen receptor positive and negative breast tumor cell growth in vitro and inhibit activator protein-1-mediated transcriptional activation. *J Nutr* 132:1368–75.

Ukai N, Lu Y, Etoh H, Yagi A, Ina K, Oshima S, Ojima F, Sakamoto H, Ishiguro Y. 1994. Photosensitized oxygenation of lycopene. *Biosci Biotech Biochem* 58:1718–9.

Updike AA, Schwartz SJ. 2003. Thermal processing of vegetables increases cis isomers of lutein and zeaxanthin. *J Agric Food Chem* 51:6184–90.

Wang X-D. 2012. Lycopene metabolism and its biological significance. *Am J Clin Nutr* 96:S1214–22.

Xianquan S, Shi J, Kakuda Y, Yueming J. 2005. Stability of lycopene during food processing and storage. *J Med Food* 8:413–22.

Yeh S-L, Hu M-L. 2003. Oxidized β-carotene inhibits gap junction intercellular communication in the human lung adenocarcinoma cell line A549. *Food Chem Toxicol* 41:1677–84.

Zeb A, Murkovic M. 2013. Determination of thermal oxidation and oxidation products of β-carotene in corn triacylglycerols. *Food Res Int* 50:534–44.

Zepka LQ, Mercadante AZ. 2009. Degradation compounds of carotenoids formed during heating of a simulated cashew apple juice. *Food Chem* 117:28–34.

Zhang H, Kotake-Nara E, Ono H, Nagao A. 2003. A novel cleavage product formed by autoxidation of lycopene induces apoptosis in HL-60 cells. *Free Radic Biol Med* 35:1653–63.

8 Carotenoids as food colorants and precursors of aroma compounds

8.1 INTRODUCTION

Although recent studies have been stimulated and dominated by the importance of carotenoids in human health, earlier investigations were motivated by the color they impart. As inherent food constituents, they confer the yellow, orange, or red color of many plant foods and a few animal-derived foods. They are also incorporated into food products by direct addition or indirectly through animals' feed.

Carotenoids are currently produced commercially as food and feed color additives and supplements (Jaswir et al., 2011). They are widely used by the food, cosmetic, and pharmaceutical industries. Most of commercial carotenoids (e.g., β-carotene, astaxanthin, and canthaxanthin) are products of chemical synthesis, but they are also produced by extraction from a small number of rich natural sources and by microbial fermentation.

In terms of food quality, a more recently recognized role of the multifunctional carotenoids is serving as precursors of aroma/flavor compounds. Formation of these compounds can take place enzymatically as in the ripening of fruits, or nonenzymatically during processing and storage of processed foods. For wine and tea, both enzymatic and chemical (nonenzymatic) degradation of carotenoids occur, resulting in compounds that become part of the numerous volatiles responsible for the well-appreciated aroma of these products.

8.2 CAROTENOIDS AS FOOD COLORANTS

Fruits and vegetables owe their color mainly to three groups of pigments: the green chlorophylls, the yellow-orange-red carotenoids, and the red-blue-purple anthocyanins. Exceptionally, beet is colored by the red betanin, which belongs to the pigment group of betalains.

As explained in Chapter 1, the conjugated double bond system is the chromophore responsible for the absorption of light and therefore the color of a carotenoid. The hue

Food Carotenoids: Chemistry, Biology, and Technology, First Edition. Delia B. Rodriguez-Amaya.

and intensity of carotenoid-colored foods depend on which carotenoids are present, their concentrations, and their physical state. The red-fleshed tomato and watermelon owe their color to the predominating carotenoid, the red lycopene. Orange-fleshed sweet potato and carrot have high levels of β-carotene, and mandarin orange has high concentration of β-crytoxanthin. In some animals, complexation of carotenoids with proteins extends the color to green, purple, blue, or black. A well-known example is the blue carotenoprotein crustacyanin of the lobster carapace, an astaxanthin complex. On denaturation of protein (e.g., through heating), astaxanthin is released and its vivid red color is revealed.

Colorants are added to foods for several reasons (Henry, 1996):

- To reinforce colors already present in food but less intense than the consumer would expect
- To ensure uniformity of color in food from batch to batch
- To restore the original appearance of food whose color has been affected by processing
- To give color to certain foods (e.g., sugar confectionary, soft drinks) that would otherwise be virtually colorless.

It should not be used to disguise low-quality foods.

Employing natural colors is the current marketing trend because of consumers' concern about the safety of artificial food dyes, and many natural colorants provide health benefits. The replacement of the former by the latter, however, is challenging because natural colorants are usually less stable to heat, light, and oxygen, and all the desired hues may not be obtainable (Wrolstad and Culver, 2012). Additionally, natural colors are more costly, require more material to achieve equivalent color strength, and are not as easily utilized as artificial colors (Lauro, 1991). There has been a lot of effort to improve the technical and physical properties of natural colorants, especially in making them more stable and easier to use (Downham and Collins, 2000).

Several advantages have been cited for carotenoids as food colorants: natural connotation, high tinctural potency, good stability in the pH range of most food products, provitamin A activity, and other beneficial effects on human health (Bauernfeind, 1981). Their disadvantages are limited color range, higher price compared with synthetic dyes, sensitivity to oxidative degradation, and solubility problems (Kläui, 1981; Kläui and Bauernfeind, 1981). The last two disadvantages have been dealt with in the preparation of the commercial application forms as discussed below.

8.2.1 Natural carotenoid colors

Natural carotenoid pigments have been used as additives for years to provide attractive colors to manufactured foods. There are two major concerns about plant-derived carotenoid colorants (Kläui and Bauernfeind, 1981). First, the inherent flavor and color characteristics of the plant source of the concentrate can be carried over into the product to be colored and may not be compatible with it. However, the flavor and the color of the raw material can both be desirable, and the product serves both as spice and colorant (e.g., paprika and saffron). Second, due to differences in soil, climatic conditions, age of plant, and time of harvest, the proportions of the colored and other components of the plant source may vary widely (Kläui and Bauernfeind, 1981), and there can be substantial batch-to-batch variation in coloring as well as flavor strength.

The red annatto is one of the oldest food colorants. It is derived from the resinous, thin seed coat of the capsular fruits of *Bixa orellana*, a tropical tree believed to be native to Central and South America. Although it is grown in many tropical countries, including Bolivia, Ecuador, Jamaica, the Dominican Republic, East Africa, India, and the Philippines, Peru and Brazil have been the dominant producers (Henry, 1996). It is available as oil or water solutions, suspensions, emulsions, encapsulated products, and spray-dried powders. The principal coloring agent in oil-based preparations is bixin, a monomethyl ester of a dicarboxylic *Z*-apocarotenoid having a total of 11 conjugated double bonds (Figure 1.3 in Chapter 1). It has a free carboxyl and an esterified carboxyl as the end groups. Hydrolysis (saponification) liberates the dicarboxylic, water-soluble norbixin.

Annatto is used as colorant in a wide range of foods such as butter, margarine, cheese, fats, cereals, creams, baked goods, snacks, ice cream, salad dressings, sugar, confectionaries, yogurts, drinks, and meat products. Dairy products, especially hard cheese, are the single most important application for annatto extracts.

Annatto is classified by the U.S. Food and Drug Administration (FDA) as a color additive exempt of certification (Code of Federal Regulations, 2014). In Europe, its use is more restricted, but its addition to a wide range of food commodity is permitted at a maximum level of 10 to 35 mg/kg (Scotter, 2009).

Also an old colorant and spice, paprika is a deep red, pungent powder obtained from red pepper (*Capsicum annuum*) pods. Paprika oleoresin is produced by solvent extraction of the ground powder. Paprika in edible vegetable oil and water-miscible forms of oleoresin are also available. The predominant paprika pigments are capsanthin and capsorubin (Minguez-Mosquera and Hornero-Méndez, 1993; Kim et al., 2009). Capsanthin has one end cyclized into a β-ring and the other end cyclized into a five-membered κ-ring. It has two hydroxyls attached at the 3 and 3′ position and a carbonyl substituent at the 6′ position. The carbonyl double bond brings the total number of conjugated double bonds to 11. Capsorubin has both ends cyclized into κ-rings.

Paprika is limited to those products compatible with its flavor. It is used in meat products, soups, sauces, salad dressings, processed cheese, snacks, confectionery, and baked products.

Well appreciated for its flavor-color properties and considered the world's most expensive spice, saffron is the dried stigma of *Crocus sativus* L. flowers (Giacco, 2004).

Its color comes from the carotenoid diglucoside crocin, a digentiobioside of the diapocarotenedioc acid crocetin (8,8′-diapocarotene-8,8′-dioic acid). The carboxylic and sugar portion make the molecule water soluble. Crocetin, which has a molecular formula of $C_{20}H_{24}O_4$, is a symmetrical apocarotenoid with nine double bonds, counting the carboxylic group double bonds (see Figure 1.3).

C. sativus is grown in Italy, Spain, Greece, France, Turkey, Austria, Libya, Iran, and India (Giacco, 2004). Production of saffron is labor intensive, explaining the high cost of the spice. Used for centuries, saffron is well accepted in soups, meat products, cheese, and many other foods. Both paprika and saffron are in the listing of color additives exempt from certification in the United States (Code of Federal Regulations, 2014).

More recently, tomato lycopene extract and tomato lycopene concentrate as oleoresin, powder, and water-dispersible preparation, imparting yellow to orange to red colors, have become commercially available. Several companies have obtained approval for food additives with lycopene as the key active ingredient (Sajilata and Singhal, 2006). Three products from BASF Corporation and Lyc-O-Mato product of Israel's LycoRed Ltd. have received generally recognized as safe (GRAS) certification by the FDA. Lycopene is registered as an approved food colorant in Europe and Japan. Potential applications include beverages, confectionery, bread, and cakes.

The commercial source of lutein is marigold (*Tagetes erecta* L.) flower, as fresh petals, extracts, or dried powder. Marigold lutein has been used as colorant for food and as additive in poultry feed to improve the pigmentation of the bird's fat, skin, and egg yolk. Originally cultivated in Mexico and other warmer areas of America, marigold is now naturalized in other tropical and subtropical regions (Khalil et al., 2012).

In the United States, Tagetes meal and extract are permitted for chicken feed only (Code of Federal Regulations, 2014). Marigold extracts with lutein concentrations as high as 20% are approved for use as dietary supplements but not for use as a food colorant (Wrolstad and Culver, 2012). In the European Union, lutein preparations are an approved food additive.

8.2.2 Nature-identical synthetic carotenoids

Technological advances have made possible the synthesis of carotenoids at reasonable prices with the advantage of having well-controlled, reproducible colors, without the disadvantage of fluctuations in price and quality often problematic with natural extracts. Chemical synthesis accounts for most of commercial carotenoids. However, the synthesis of certain carotenoids is very complex, and the synthesis of a new carotenoid often requires the development of a new chemical route (Ausich, 1997). Industrial synthesis of carotenoids has been comprehensively reviewed (Kläui and Bauernfeind, 1981; Paust, 1991; Ernst, 2002).

Pure carotenoid crystals have characteristics that render their commercialization in this form impractical: instability, insolubility in water, and limited solubility in fats and oils (Kläui, 1981; Kläui and Bauernfeind, 1981). To make them suitable for industrial applications, special formulations have been developed through physicochemical operations. Micronized oil suspensions are the major marketable forms for coloring fat-based foods. Because of its large surface area, microcrystalline carotenoid is extremely sensitive to oxidation in air, but suspending the microcrystals in oil considerably retards the process (Kläui, 1981, Kläui and Bauernfeind, 1981). A microcrystalline dispersion of β-carotene in an edible fat is used for margarine.

Using pure crystalline carotenoids, water-dispersable market forms can be prepared by formation of colloidal suspensions, emulsification of oily solutions, or dispersion in suitable colloids, particularly with the addition of surface-active agents (Kläui, 1981; Kläui and Bauernfeind, 1981). In these forms, the carotenoids are better protected from oxidation, but the use of food-grade antioxidants further improves stability.

Five C_{40} carotenoids, lycopene, β-carotene, zeaxanthin, canthaxanthin, and astaxanthin, have been produced synthetically on an industrial scale (Ernst, 2002). These synthetic "nature-identical" carotenoids are used as animal feed additives, particularly in poultry farming and in aquaculture. β-carotene is used for direct coloring of foods, and lycopene, β-carotene, and zeaxanthin are employed as nutritional supplements. In addition, three apocarotenoids are synthesized on an industrial scale: β-apo-8′-carotenal, which is used as food colorant, and ethyl β-apo-8′-carotenoate and citranaxanthin, employed as feed additives in poultry (Ernst, 2002). The two major industrial producers are Hoffman-La Roche and BASF.

β-carotene, the first carotenoid prepared by chemical synthesis, was introduced in 1954. It was followed by β-apo-8′-carotenal in 1960, β-apo-8′-carotenoic acid ethyl ester in 1962, and canthaxanthin in 1964. In 1968 BASF introduced citanaxanthin, and in 1984 Roche launched astaxanthin as feed additives. Astaxanthin, β-carotene (natural and synthetic), β-apo-8′-carotenal, and canthaxanthin are in the FDA's list of color additives exempt from certification (Code of Federal Regulations, 2014). However, while the use of β-carotene is according to good manufacturing practices, canthaxanthin and β-apo-8′-carotenal have restrictions on the amount that can be used in foods. Astaxanthin can only be used as salmonid fish feed.

β-carotene finds application in dairy products, cakes, soups, margarine, and confectionery. It has a long history of safe use with an acceptable daily intake of 0–5 mg/kg body weight/day (Sajilata and Singhal, 2006).

Synthetic nature-identical canthaxanthin is approved as food color worldwide (ILSI North America, 1999). There was some concern about the safety of canthaxanthin when crystalloid particles were found in human retina after prolonged and high-dose ingestion (e.g., for tanning purposes), but no ophthalmological findings have been described other than the presence of the deposits. Minor changes attributed to the presence of canthaxanthin deposits were reported to be reversible.

Astaxanthin is considered a high-value carotenoid with applications in nutraceuticals, cosmetics, food, and feed industries (Guerin et al., 2003). Astaxanthin and canthaxanthin are added to the ration of aquaculture-grown salmon, trout, and shrimp to provide the characteristic reddish pink color that these animals acquire in the wild from their diet of marine bacteria and microalgae. Aside from pigmentation and consumer appeal, astaxanthin is important in aquaculture as an essential nutritional component for adequate growth and reproduction (Higuera-Ciapara et al., 2006).

In marine organisms including salmonid fishes, astaxanthin occurs as a mixture of three different optical isomers, 3S,3′S, 3R,3′S (meso), and 3R,3′R in varying proportions (Liaaen-Jensen, 2004). Synthetic astaxanthin mimics this mixture in a 1:2:1 fixed ratio. Microbial sources contain only one of the three isomers, for example, 3S,3′S-astaxanthin in *Haematococcus* sp. or 3R,3′R-astaxanthin in *Xanthophyllomyces dendrorhous* (formerly called *Phaffia rhodozyma*).

Dufossé et al. (2005) cited the following advantages of astaxanthin over other carotenoids: (a) more stable compared to other carotenoids, (b) high antioxidant potential, (c) can easily cross the blood-brain barrier, and (d) high tinctorial property.

The Joint FAO/WHO Expert Committee on Food Additives established a group Acceptable Daily Intake for lutein and zeaxanthin of 0 to 2 mg/kg body weight (Sajilata et al., 2008). Lutein and zeaxanthin are used to enhance the yellow pigmentation of eggs. Zeaxanthin is preferred over other carotenoids for poultry and fish because it deposits evenly in the flesh and eggs (Sajilata et al., 2008).

8.2.3 Carotenoids produced by biotechnology

Intensive research has been carried out on the biosynthesis of carotenoids by appropriate microorganisms with the view of scaling it up to commercial production, especially for carotenoids that cannot be easily or economically produced by chemical synthesis (Ausich, 1997). However, these efforts have met only limited success. There are only three carotenoids actually produced commercially in this manner: β-carotene by the alga *Dunaliella* sp., astaxanthin by the alga *Haematococcus pluvialis*, and β-carotene by the fungus *Blakeslea trispora*.

Large-scale production of β-carotene by the alga *Dunaliella* sp. is a well-established technology. Commonly cultivated species are *Dunaliella salina* and *D. bardawil*. Commercial productions are in operation in Australia, China, Israel, Japan, and the United States (Ausich, 1997; Dufossé et al., 2005). Small plants are also located in Chile, Mexico, Cuba, Iran, and Taiwan. It takes advantage of the fact that this unicellular alga lacks a cell wall and produces high levels of β-carotene (3.0%–5.0% dry weight basis). Its halotolerant nature allows it to be cultivated in open saline mass culture, relatively free of competing microorganisms and predators. For high β-carotene levels, nutrient limitation, intense light, and low water activity are employed. It is suited for cultivation in coastal areas where sea water is rich in salt and nutrients.

Dunaliella β-carotene is utilized today in three forms: β-carotene extracts, *Dunaliella* powder for human use, and dried *Dunaliella* for feed use (Dufossé et al., 2005). The biomass has been shown to be safe and can be used directly for food formulation. For various formulations and applications, β-carotene can be extracted in edible oils or food-grade organic solvents.

Although greater than 95% of the market uses synthetic astaxanthin, increasing consumer demand for natural products provides an opportunity for the production of natural astaxanthin by *Haematococcus* (Lorenz and Cysewski, 2000). The cost and complexity of synthesizing optically active astaxanthin made the feasibility of producing *Haematococcus* astaxanthin worth exploring. The major producers of *Haematococcus* astaxanthin are the United States (Kona, Hawaii), Japan, and India.

Before astaxanthin production by the single-celled alga *H. pluvialis* became commercial, natural sources of astaxanthin included krill oil and meal, crayfish oil, and *Xanthophyllomyces dendrorhous*. These sources, however, have low astaxanthin concentrations, ranging from 0.15% in oils to 0.40% in *Xanthophyllomyces* yeast, compared to 1.5%–3.0% (dry weight basis) in *Haematococcus*.

The yeast *X. dendrorhous* has desirable properties as a biological source of pigment, including rapid heterotrophic metabolism and production of high cell densities in fermenters, but its content of astaxanthin in wild strains is low. Mutants have been isolated that produce >3000 μg total carotenoid per gram of yeast (>0.30%). High producers, however, are often unstable and further strain development is required.

Although *Haematococcus* has a high concentration of astaxanthin, industrial application is limited by the lengthy autotrophic cultivation in open freshwater ponds and the requirement for disruption of the tough cell wall to liberate the carotenoid (Johnson and An, 1991).

The production of astaxanthin by *H. pluvialis* is not as advantageous as the production of β-carotene by *Dunaliella*. Since *Haematococcus* is a freshwater alga, it is susceptible to competition and contamination by other organisms, making open-air culture extremely difficult (Dufossé et al., 2005). Indoor location, though more expensive, has the advantage of environmental control (Johnson and An, 1991).

Modified techniques have been developed for the production of astaxanthin by *Haematococcus* (Lorenz and Cysewski, 2000). In Sweden, completely enclosed photobioreactors (with artificial light) are utilized. In Hawaii, a combination of closed reactors and open culture ponds are being used.

In large-scale, outdoor systems, a two-step process is employed. First, vegetative cells are produced under near-optimal growth conditions with careful control of pH, temperature, and nutrient levels. When a sufficient volume of vegetative cells is produced, the culture is subjected to environmental and nutrient stress. Commercial systems induce astaxanthin production by deprivation of nitrate and phosphate, increasing temperature and light, or by the addition of sodium chloride to the culture medium (Fábregas et al., 2001; Lorenz and Cysewski, 2000).

Haematococcus algae meal has been approved in Japan as a natural red food color and as a pigment for fish feed. The alga has been approved for use as pigment in salmonid feed in Canada and the United States. It has also been cleared in the United States as a dietary supplement ingredient and approved in several European countries for human consumption.

β-carotene from the fungus *Blakeslea trispora*, marketed as a natural food color, is produced by fermentation in a reactor in the Netherlands (Downham and Collins, 2000).

8.2.4 Potential production from other microorganisms

Despite the enormous potential and the wide research interest on microbial carotenoids, few microorganisms have reached commercial production. Research on potential carotenoid-producing microorganisms, however, continues with marked intensity. The studies have focused on the search for microbial sources of potentially high-value carotenoids or carotenoids not easily obtained by chemical synthesis, as well as optimization of the medium and culture conditions to enhance carotenoid production. Lowering of productions costs, principally by using low-value industrial by-products as nutrient sources, has also been pursued. Utilization of agro-industrial by-products has the added advantage of minimizing environmental problems related to waste disposal, in line with green technology.

Reaching commercial microbial production of carotenoids is a big hurdle. Numerous papers were published about the yeast *Xanthophyllomyces dendrorhous,* but in the end, it was *H. pluviales* that was adopted for commercial production. Two examples of microorganisms currently investigated as potential commercial sources of carotenoids are discussed below.

Yeasts of the genus *Rhodotorula* have been intensely studied as possible commercial producers of carotenoids (e.g., Frengova et al., 1994; Shih and Hang, 1996; Buzzini and Martini, 1999; Buzzini, 2000, 2001; Bhosale and Gadre, 2001a,b; Aksu and Tuğba Eren, 2005; Buzzini et al., 2005; Tinoi et al., 2005; Maldonade et al., 2007, 2008, 2012; Marova et al., 2012; Ungureanu et al., 2013). The principal carotenoids of these yeasts are torulene (3′,4′-didehydro-β,ψ-carotene), torularhodin (3′,4′-didehydro-β, ψ-caroten-16′-oic acid), and β-carotene. Torulene, which is not a food constituent, is an interesting carotenoid for commercialization as food colorant. Because of its 13 conjugated double bonds, it has a nice reddish color and should be an efficient antioxidant, the antioxidant efficiency being directly associated with the length of the conjugated double bond system. Having an unsubstituted β-ring, it fulfills the requirement for a provitamin A carotenoid.

There has also been interest in the microbial production of zeaxanthin (Ruther et al., 1997; Jin et al., 2003), currently produced commercially only by chemical synthesis. Few microbes synthesize zeaxanthin as the predominant carotenoid. *Flavobacterium multivorum,* a nonfastidious and nonpathogenic bacterium that accumulates almost exclusively zeaxanthin, appears to be an important potential microbial source of this carotenoid (Johnson and Schroeder, 1996; Pasamontes et al., 1997; Alcantara and Sanchez 1999; Masetto et al., 2001; Bhosale and Bernstein, 2005). However, low carotenoid yield and a lack of information about media optimization for carotenoid production restrict the possibility of its use (Nelis and DeLeenheer, 1991). Optimization of zeaxanthin production by *F. multivorum* is being carried out (Bhosale et al., 2004; Chávez-Parga et al., 2012).

Another topic of great interest is carotenoid production in noncarotenogenic microbes (e.g., *Escherichia coli, Saccharomyces cerevisiae, Candida utilis, and Zymonas mobilis*) by the introduction of carotenoid genes from carotenogenic microbes (Misawa and Shimada, 1998). Das et al. (2007) reviewed progress in metabolic engineering of noncarotenogenic microorganisms, with particular focus on the potential of *Escherichia coli.* Many new carotenoid synthesis genes have been isolated from microorganisms, which may be utilized in the synthesis of novel and desirable carotenoids by genetic engineering (Cheng, 2006). Existing biosynthetic pathways can be modified or novel pathways established by the introduction of foreign genes into the host organisms (Sandmann, 2002). Structures not found in nature can be tailored by combining appropriate genes from organisms with different carotenogenic pathways. The application of combinatorial and evolutionary strategies to carotenoid pathway engineering can broaden the diversity of carotenoid structures synthesized in recombinant hosts.

For high-yield carotenoid production, optimization of metabolic engineering should focus on several aspects (Sandmann et al., 1999):

- Sufficient substrates (i.e., precursors) for the reactions should be available.
- A balanced level of carotenogenic enzymes should be expressed to enable efficient precursor conversion without the formation of intermediate metabolite pools.
- The correct plasmid combination is important to minimize the accumulation of intermediates and to increase the yield of end products.
- The host organism should exhibit an active central terpenoid pathway and possess a high storage capacity for carotenoids.

The success of the pathway engineering effort depends on the host metabolism, specific enzymes used, the enzyme expression levels, and the strategies employed (Ye and Bhatia, 2012). Microbial systems, especially industrial strains, have the advantages of easy genetic manipulation, a better understanding of cell metabolism, fast growth, and existing fermentation technologies for large-scale production.

Although recognizing accomplishments in metabolic engineering for increased carotenoid production, Lee and Schmidt-Dannert (2002) cited bottlenecks of microbial carotenoid biosynthesis. Carotenoid production in noncarotenogenic microorganisms might perturb other, as yet unknown metabolic pathways. Additionally, the limited carotenoid storage capability in current hosts is a major obstacle for achieving commercially relevant carotenoid production levels. While acknowledging the combination of genetic manipulation and fermentation as a giant leap forward in color production, Mortensen (2006) was mindful of the hurdle colorants made in this manner would face in terms of approval, especially in Europe.

8.3 CAROTENOIDS AS PRECURSORS OF AROMA COMPOUNDS

Perception of flavor is an integrated response to nonvolatile compounds perceived by taste receptors in the tongue and to volatile aroma compounds perceived by olfactory receptors in the nose. Some foods have one or two compounds (called character-impact compounds) that dominate or are reminiscent of the typical aroma/flavor. The aroma of many foods, however, is due to unique combinations of a large number of volatile compounds derived from different precursors.

8.3.1 Enzymatic generation of aroma compounds from carotenoids

Enzymatic cleavage of carotenoids leads to the formation of bioactive derivatives such as vitamin A (discussed in Chapter 10) and the plant hormone abscisic acid (discussed in Chapter 2), apocarotenoid pigments such as bixin and crocetin (also discussed in Chapter 2), and volatile compounds (widely called norisoprenoids) that contribute to the typical aroma of foods.

The biodegradation of carotenoids has long been recognized as an important route to aroma compounds, but studies have focused on tobacco (Enzell, 1985) rather than foods. Recent years have witnessed greater interest in carotenoid-derived food flavor compounds.

8.3.1.1 Characterization of the enzymes

Three enzymes have been associated with nonspecific cleavage of carotenoids to yield aroma compounds: lipoxygenase, xanthine oxidase, and peroxidase. Lipoxygenase catalyzes cooxidation of carotenoids in the presence of unsaturated fatty acids such as linoleic acid (Wu et al., 1999). Lipoxygenase first catalyzes the oxidation of the fatty acids to produce peroxyl radicals, which then cleave the carotenoid molecule by random attack of the polyene chain. This results in primary products, including apocarotenal, epoxycarotenal, apocarotenone, and epoxycarotenone, that can then serve as substrates for further free radical propagated reactions, resulting in the volatile compounds.

Lipoxygenase isolated from tomato fruit was used to catalyze the cooxidation of β-carotene in the presence of linoleic acid (Allen and Gramshaw, 1996). The volatiles produced were β-ionone, β-cyclocitral, and 5,6-epoxy-β-ionone.

Two pathways have been suggested for the formation of epoxy-β-ionone. In the first pathway, suggested by Enzell (1985), Bosser et al. (1995), and Wu et al. (1999), β-carotene is first oxidized to 5,6-epoxy-β-carotene, which rearranges to 5,8-epoxy-β-carotene. These epoxy carotenoids are cleaved to 5,6-epoxy-β-ionone and dihydroactinidiolide, respectively. The second pathway, noted by Bosser et al. (1995), involves the cleavage of β-carotene to β-ionone, which is converted to 5,6-β-ionone, then lactonized to dihydroactinidiolide.

Xanthine oxidase catalyzes the cooxidation of carotenoids in the presence of an aldehyde to give diverse volatile products (Bosser et al., 1994). Aldehyde oxidation generates the highly reactive superoxide anion $O_2^{\bullet -}$, which gives rise to other free radicals (Wache et al., 2002). Reproduced in vitro in aqueous solution, this cooxidation led to the formation of β-ionone, epoxy-β-ionone, dihydroactinidiolide, β-cyclocitral, pseudoionone, from β-carotene, initiated by free radical formation (Bosser and Belin, 1994). Through this process, cleavage of the 9-10 bond of neoxanthin gave rise to precursors of damascenone, including grasshopper ketone (Wache et al., 2002).

The multiplicity of the volatile compounds generated by lipoxygenases and xanthine oxidases suggests unspecific cleavage of the polyene chromophore or uncontrolled termination of the reaction (Bouvier et al., 2005).

The third enzyme is peroxidase. A peroxidase from mushroom that cleaves β-carotene into flavor compounds, including β-ionone and derivatives, has been cloned (Zorn et al., 2003).

The last decade has seen increasing attention to aroma compounds derived from oxidative cleavage of specific double bonds of the carotenoid polyene chain, catalyzed by a family of enzymes termed carotenoid cleavage dioxygenases (CCDs) (Giuliano et al., 2003; Wys, 2004; Ohmiya, 2009). The classification of CCDs as monooxygenase or dioxygenase has been the subject of debate. Monooxygenases rely on atmospheric O_2 for one oxygen atom, whereas dioxygenases incorporate both oxygen atoms into the products (Auldridge et al., 2006). For CCDs, a dioxygenase mechanism was proposed in which atmospheric O_2 is added across the double bond to form a dioxetane intermediate, which would subsequently break down to the cleavage products (Schwartz et al., 2003). Labeling experiments using $H_2{}^{18}O$ or ${}^{18}O_2$ showed that the oxygen in the keto-group of β-ionone is derived solely from molecular dioxygen, unambiguously demonstrating a dioxygenase mechanism for AtCCD1 from *Arabidopsis thaliana* (Schmidt et al., 2006).

CCD1 is the enzyme considered to be primarily involved in the formation of aroma compounds in fruits and vegetables. For dicyclic carotenoids, such as β-carotene, cleavage at the 9,10 and/or 9′,10′ double bonds is favored (Figure 8.1) (Camara and Bouvier, 2004; Walter and Strack, 2011). Cleavage at one of these bonds yields a C_{13} volatile compound (Figure 8.1) and a C_{27} apocarotenal (β-apo-10′-carotenal). The non-volatile C_{27} apocarotenoid can then undergo a second dioxygenase cleavage, generating an additional C_{13} volatile and a C_{14} fragment, coming from the central portion of the polyene chain. Cleavage at both bonds yields a C_{14} dialdehyde and two C_{13} compounds, which vary according to the carotenoid substrate (Schwartz et al., 2001). For acyclic

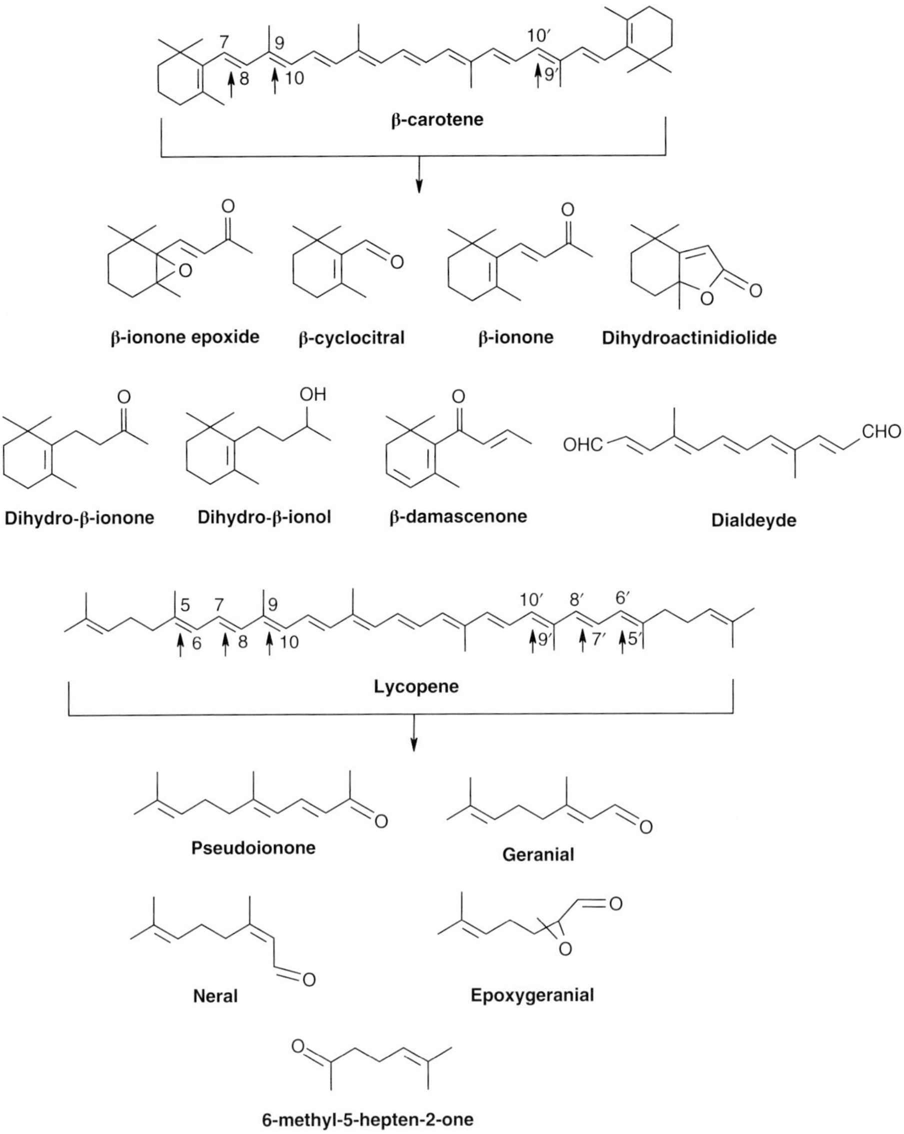

Figure 8.1 Cleavage products derived enzymatically from β-carotene and lycopene.

carotenoids, such as lycopene, CCD1 has lower regioselectivity for cleavage, targeting double bonds other than 9,10 (9′,10′) (Figure 8.1) (Walter and Strack, 2011). Maize and tomato CCD1 enzymes cleaved lycopene to generate 6-methyl-5-hepten-2-one (Figure 8.1) (Vogel et al., 2008). This volatile, an important flavor compound in tomato, is produced by cleavage at the 5,6/5′,6′ bond positions of lycopene. Ilg et al. (2009) showed that rice CCD1 converts lycopene into three volatiles, pseudoionone, 6-methyl-5-hepten-2-one, and geranial (C_{10}), suggesting that the 7,8/7′,8′ double bonds of acyclic carotenoid constitute another cleavage site for plant CCD1 (Figure 8.1). Primary products resulting from the initial cleavages may undergo modifications involving oxidation, reduction, dehydration, rearrangement, and glycosylation (Camara and Bouvier, 2004). Acid-catalyzed conversions of nonvolatile metabolites to aroma compounds occur during processing of food (Winterhalter and Rouseff, 2002).

Carotenoids accumulate predominantly inside plastids, while CCD1 is cytoplasmic (Simkin et al., 2004). Only a small portion of the carotenoids in ripening fruits is metabolized to volatile compounds, suggesting that a structural change associated with chromoplast differentiation permits limited access to the carotenoid pool (Lewinsohn et al., 2005b; Tieman et al., 2006). It has also been suggested that the cleavage to C_{13} compounds might be a sequential, differentially compartmentalized process, involving a plastidial cleavage enzyme with direct access to the C_{40} carotenoid, forming a C_{27} apocarotenoid intermediate, which is then exported from the plastid to the cytosol and cleaved further by cytosolic CCD1 to the C_{13} compound (Floss et al., 2008; Floss and Walter, 2009; Walter and Strack, 2011). This suggestion is supported by the finding that apocarotenoids rather than carotenoids are the substrates of OsCCD1 (Golden Rice CCD1) *in planta* (Ilg et al., 2010).

CCD1 is a promiscuous enzyme (wide substrate specificity) that is able to utilize phytoene, ζ-carotene, lycopene, β-carotene, δ-carotene, zeaxanthin, and violaxanthin as substrate in vitro to synthesize various products (Auldridge et al., 2006). CCD1 homologs have been identified genetically and/or biochemically, and functionally characterized in quince fruit (Fleischmann et al., 2002), crocus (Bouvier et al., 2003; Rubio et al., 2008), star fruit (Fleischmann et al., 2003), tomato (Simkin et al., 2004; Ilg et al., 2014), grape (Mathieu et al., 2005; Lashbrooke et al., 2013), citrus (Kato et al., 2006), melon (Ibdah et al., 2006), nectarine (Baldermann et al., 2005), and carrot (Yahyaa, 2013).

The grape VvCCD1 cleaved zeaxanthin symmetrically, yielding 3-hydroxy-β-ionone (a C_{13}-compound) and a C_{14}-dialdehyde (Mathieu et al., 2005). Recombinant citrus CitCCD1 cleaved β-cryptoxanthin, zeaxanthin, and all-E-violaxanthin at the 9-10 and 9′,10′ positions, and cleaved 9-Z-violaxanthin at the 9′,10′ position (Kato et al., 2006). Gene expression of *CitCCD1* increased in the flavedos and juice sacs of satsuma mandarin, Valencia orange, and Lisbon lemon during maturation. CCD1 from melon (CmCCD1) was shown to cleave carotenoids at positions 9,10 (9′,10′), generating geranylacetone from phytoene, pseudoionone from lycopene, β-ionone from β-carotene, and α-ionone and pseudoionone from δ-carotene (Ibdah et al., 2006). The carrot DcCCD1 was observed to cleave cyclic carotenoids, such as β-carotene and the cyclic part of δ-carotene, but not acyclic carotenoids, such as phytoene, lycopene, and the acyclic moiety of δ-carotene (Yahyaa et al., 2013).

The tomato genome contains two closely related genes potentially encoding carotenoid cleavage dioxygenases, *LeCCD1A* and *LeCCD1B* (Simkin et al., 2004). *LeCCD1B* is highly expressed in ripening fruit. LeCCD1 is not plastid-localized. They were shown to symmetrically cleave multiple carotenoid substrates at the 9,10 (9′,10′) positions to produce a C_{14} dialdehyde and two C_{13} cyclohexones that vary depending on the substrate. A recent paper reported wide specifity, both in terms of substrate and of cleavage site, for tomato CCD1A and, to a larger extent, CCD1B, mediating the oxidative cleavage of *Z*- and all-*E*-carotenoids as well as different apocarotenoids at many more double bonds than previously reported (Ilg et al., 2014). A plenitude of volatiles, monoapocarotenoids, and dialdehyde products, such as *Z*-pseudoionone, neral, geranial, and farnesylacetone, are produced.

Not much is known about CCD subclass 4, which is also involved in the formation of carotenoid-derived aroma compounds in fruits and flowers. MdCCD4 from *MdCCD4* gene isolated from apple and expressed in *Escherichia coli* cleaved β-carotene to yield β-ionone (Huang et al., 2009). It has also been reported that the saffron CsCCD4 could cleave β-carotene at the 9,10 (9′,10′) positions to yield β-ionone (Rubio et al., 2008). However, while CCD1 is cytosolic, CsCCD4 (from *C. sativus*) were found localized in plastids, specifically in plastoglobules (Rubio et al., 2008). Identification and functional characterization of the grape VvCCD4a and VvCCD4b suggested that these enzymes are primarily responsible for catalyzing the cleavage of plastidial carotenoids (Lashbrooke et al., 2013). Based on their work on yellow- and white-fleshed peaches, Brandi et al. (2011) concluded that differential expression of CCD4 could be the major determinant in the accumulation of carotenoid and carotenoid-derived volatiles in peach fruit flesh.

VvCCD1 expression was constitutive, whereas *VvCCD4a* expression was predominant in leaves and *VvCCD4b* in the fruits. VvCCD1, VvCCD4a, and VvCCD4b were capable of catalyzing cleavage of C_{40} carotenoid substrates at the 9,10 (9′,10′) (ζ-carotene, β-carotene and/or ε-carotene) and lycopene at the 5,6 (5′,6′) double bond positions, confirming cleavage of both cyclic and acyclic substrates. This is contrary to Huang et al.'s (2009) conclusion, after analyzing five different plant species (including apple but not grape), that CCDs catalyze the cleavage of cyclic apolar carotenoids (e.g., β-carotene), not acyclic carotenoids (e.g., lycopene and ζ-carotene), and carotenoids containing a hydroxyl group (e.g., zeaxanthin and lutein).

8.3.1.2 Carotenoid-derived aroma compounds of fruits and vegetables

Among the most prominent changes during maturation of vegetables or ripening of fruits are enhanced biosynthesis of the vividly colored carotenoids and their oxidative cleavage to volatile compounds that contribute to the typical aroma/flavor of ripe fruits. Important fruit aroma compounds include mono- and sequiterpenes, phenolic derivatives, and compounds derived from lipids, amino acids, and carotenoids.

The quince (*Cydonia oblonga*) fruit and starfruit (*Averrhoa carambola*) were among the first fruits for which it was recognized that the flavor was strongly influenced by carotenoid-derived volatile compounds (Ishihara et al., 1986; Winterhalter and Schreier, 1988; Lutz and Winterhalter, 1992). A considerable number of C_{13} compounds has been reported, with β-ionone derivatives predominating (Güldner and Winterhalter, 1991; Winterhalter et al., 1991). C_{10} and C_{12} compounds, termed marmelo lactones, marmelo oxides, and quince oxepine, have also been found (Näf and Velluz, 1991), apparently derived from the central part of the carotenoid polyene chain, left after the cleavage of the end groups (Lutz and Winterhalter, 1992).

A large number of carotenoid degradation products have been detected in starfruit, including β-damascenone, megastigma-4,6,8-trienes, megastigma-4,6,8-triene-3-ones, megastigma-5,8-dien-4-one, 4-hydroxy-β-ionol, 3-hydroxy-β-ionol, 4-oxo-β-ionol, 3-hydroxy-β-ionone, 3-oxo-α-ionol, 3-oxo-*retro*-α-ionol, 3-oxo-4,5-dihydro-α-ionol, 3-oxo-7,8-dihydro-α-ionol, 3-hydroxy-β-damascone, 3,5-dihydroxy-megastigma-6,7-diene-9-one ('grasshopper ketone'), 3-hydroxy-5,6-epoxy-β-ionone, 3-hydroxy-5,6-epoxy-β-ionol, 3,4-dihydro-3-hydroxyactinidol, vomifoliol, 4,5-dihydrovomifoliol, and 7,8-dihydrovomifoliol (Macleod and Ames, 1990; Herderich et al., 1992). The majority of starfruit carotenoid-derived volatiles are formed from degradation of glycosidically bound precursors (Winterhalter and Schreier, 1995). Some C_{13} compounds resulting from cleavage at the 9,10 double bond of the carotenoid precursor have also been found.

Labeling experiments are lacking, but a structural relation between the precursor carotenoid and the resulting volatile compound can be easily perceived. The major carotenoid-derived volatile compounds found in lycopene-containing tomatoes and watermelon are acyclic, such as geranial, neral, 6-methyl-5-hepten-2-one, 2,6-dimethyl-hept-5-1-al, 2,3-epoxygeranial, (*E,E*)-pseudoionone, geranyl acetone, and farnesyl acetone, presumably derived from lycopene (Figure 8.1) and other acyclic carotenoids (Lewinsohn et al., 2005b). β-Ionone, dihydroactinodiolide, and β-cyclocitral are predominant in tomato and watermelon containing β-carotene; α-ionone was detected only in an orange-fleshed δ-carotene accumulating tomato mutant.

Geraniol, neral, geranial, 6-methyl-5-hepten-2-one, β-ionone, β-ionone epoxide, and farnesyl acetone were among the 71 volatiles identified in watermelon by Yajima et al. (1985). 6-Methyl-5-hepten-2-one was detected in fresh-cut watermelon slices (Saftner et al., 2007) and in red-fleshed papaya fruit (Pino, 2014). 6-Methyl-5-hepten-2-one and geranylacetone were found in untreated and treated (high-intensity pulsed electric field or heat) watermelon juices (Aguiló-Aguayo et al., 2010).

α-Ionone, β-ionone, β-cyclocitral, and β-damascenone were found in orange juice (Mahattanatawee et al., 2005). The putative precursors were identified as α- and β-carotene, α- and β-cryptoxanthin, and neoxanthin.

In tomato 'Sunny' and 'Solar Set', analyzed at five ripening stages, 6-methyl-5-hepten-2-one and geranylacetone were among the eight volatile compounds that increased in concentration during ripening, peaking in the turning, pink, or red stage of maturity (Baldwin et al., 1991).

Some carotenoid-derived volatiles possess extremely potent odor thresholds. For example, β-ionone and β-damascenone have thresholds of 0.007 and 0.002 ppb, respectively (Winterhalter and Rouseff, 2002), and have strong effects on the overall human appreciation of the aromas. Although generally present at relatively low levels in fruits, β-ionone, 5,6-epoxy-β-ionone and dihydroactinidiolide are often associated with fruity, floral and woody notes. 6-Methyl-5-hepten-2-one can be described as mushroom, earthy, vinyl, and rubber (Jordán et al., 2002). On the other hand, geranial and neral are frequently associated with a floral/lemon and citrus/musty note, respectively (Pherobase, 2013).

Having an agreeable scent reminiscent of lemon, citral is actually a mixture of the *Z*- and *E*-acyclic monoterpene aldehyde isomers neral and geranial, respectively (Lewinsohn et al., 2005a). In many plants, citral is believed to be biosynthesized directly from geranyl diphosphate, but it does not appear to be the case in tomato and watermelon (Lewinsohn et al., 2005a). In these two fruits, geranial and neral are probably derived from lycopene because citral is not found in tomatoes or canary yellow watermelons, which are devoid of lycopene.

8.3.1.3 Carotenoid-derived aroma compounds of saffron

Interestingly, Figure 8.2 shows that the three major metabolites responsible for saffron quality comes from the same C_{40} carotenoid zeaxanthin, which serves as precursor of the apocarotenoid pigment crocetin, and an aroma compound, safranal. Crocetin,

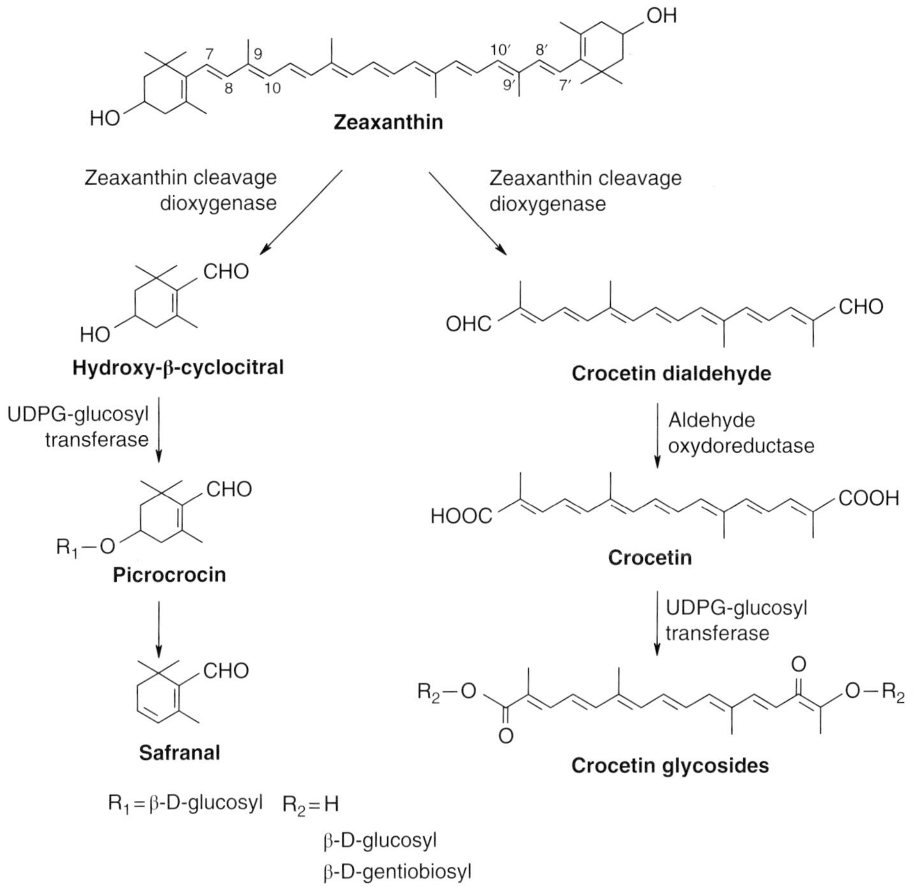

Figure 8.2 Proposed pathway for the formation of crocetin and safranal. Matthews and Wurtzel (2008). Reproduced by permission of Taylor and Francis Group, LLC, a division of Informa plc.

picrocrocin, and safranal are largely responsible for the much appreciated color, pleasant bitter taste, and aroma, respectively, of saffron.

Safranal composes 70% of the volatile fraction of saffron (Curro et al., 1986, cited by Giaccio, 2004). There is no smell in the fresh stigmas of *C. sativus*. The distinctive smell appears during drying and storage of saffron. Bouvier et al. (2003) cloned the Crocus zeaxanthin 7,8 (7′,8′)-cleavage dioxygenase gene (*CsZCD*) and Crocus carotenoid 9,10 (9′,10′)-cleavage dioxygenase gene (*CsCCD*). *CsZCD* expression is restricted to the style branch tissues, whereas *CsCCD* is expressed in flower and leaf tissues. The CsCCD enzyme acts on a broader range of precursors.

The proposed pathway (Figure 8.2) commences with the symmetric cleavage at both ends of zeaxanthin at the 7,8 (7′,8′) positions, yielding 3-hydroxy-β-cyclocitral and crocetin dialdehyde, which are glycosylated and dehydrogenated to picrocrocin (4-(β-D-glucopyranosyloxy)-2,6,6-trimethyl-1-cyclohexene-1-carboxaldehyde) and crocetin, respectively. Picrocrocin is then transformed to safranal (2,6,6-trimethyl-1,3-cyclohexadiene-1-carboxaldehyde) by thermal treatment or alkaline-acid hydrolysis.

As discussed above, the enzyme that catalyzes the cleavage has been thought to be CsZCD (Bouvier et al., 2003). A recent paper, however, reported that the enzyme responsible would actually be cytoplasmic CCD2 (Frusciante et al., 2014). Frusciante et al., used deep transcriptome sequencing of six stigma stages to identify all CCDs expressed during saffron stigma development. Seven different *CCD* transcripts were identified, including *CCD1*, three *CCD4* isoforms, *ZCD*, *CCD7*, and *CCD2*. CCD2 cleaved the 7,8 and 7′,8′ double bonds, converting zeaxanthin to crocetin dialdehyde via 3-OH-β-apo-8′-carotenal. ZCD did not cleave zeaxanthin or 3-OH-β-apo-8′-carotenal in the test systems used. Sequence comparison and structure prediction suggested that ZCD was an N-truncated CCD4 form.

Carmona et al. (2006) conceded that in saffron dehydrating at room temperature, which would last for many hours or even days, picrocrocin would certainly be the precursor of safranal, provided enzyme activity would be viable. However, reported results obtained with thermal dehydration were no longer in accordance with the proposed pathway, and Carmona et al., suggested mechanisms for safranal generation from crocetin.

Although safranal is the principal volatile compound of saffron, other carotenoid-derived aroma compounds have been identified in the fresh stigmas of *C. sativus*. Rubio et al. (2008) reported that before and at anthesis, the aromatic compound β-ionone becomes the principal volatile in the stigma. In this study, four carotenoid cleavage dioxygenase (CCD) genes, *CsCCD1a*, *CsCCD1b*, *CsCCD4a*, and *CsCCD4b*, were isolated from *C. sativus*. *CsCCD1a* was constitutively expressed, *CsCCD1b* was unique to the stigma tissue, but only *CsCCD4a* and *CsCCDb* had expression patterns consistent with the highest levels of β-carotene and emission of β-ionone during stigma development. CsCCD1a, CsCCD1b, and CsCCD4 could all cleave β-carotene at the 9,10 (9′,10′) positions to yield β-ionone.

8.3.2 Nonenzymatic generation of aroma compounds from carotenoids

Much less work has been dedicated to nonenzymatic formation of aroma compounds from carotenoids, which occurs during autoxidation at ambient temperature, photodegradation, and thermal degradation. Similar to the enzymatic process, nonvolatile compounds are initially formed, and subsequent fragmentations give rise to low-mass volatile compounds. More attention has been given to the characterization and identification of the nonvolatile apocarotenals and epoxycarotenoids, the initial products of nonenzymatic oxidative degradation of carotenoids. This topic is discussed in detail in Chapter 7.

In a model system simulating dehydrated foods, with β-carotene adsorbed on microcrystalline cellulose, exposed to a flow of synthetic air, at ambient temperature (30°C), β-cyclocitral, acetaldehyde, 3-penten-2-one, 3-methyl-2-butenol, 4-oxo-2-pentenal, 2-methyl-2-buten-1,4-dial, 2-methyl-hex-2,4-dien-1-ol, and 5-methyl-hex-2,4-dien-1-ol were identified (Padula and Rodriguez-Amaya, unpublished results). With the exception of β-cyclocitral, these are short acyclic compounds, the possible origin of which from the β-carotene molecule can be easily be located, indicating that the volatile compounds resulted from the cleavage of the end groups, as well as direct cleavage of the polyene chain at various sites (see Figure 7.10).

Kanasawud and Crouzet (1990a) identified 21 volatile compounds resulting from thermal (3 h at 97°C) degradation of β-carotene suspended in water by sonication and saturated with oxygen. The most abundant were 5,6-epoxy-β-ionone and dihydroactinidiolide, which were apparently produced at the beginning of the degradation process. It was postulated that 5,6-epoxy-β-ionone was formed from cleavage of the β-carotene-5,6,5′,6′-diepoxide, and it could be transformed to dihydroactinidiolide, which could also be derived directly from β-carotene-5,8,5′,8′-diepoxide. 5,6-Epoxy-β-ionone could also form β-ionone or be converted to 2-hydroxy-2,6,6-trimethylcyclohexane-1-carboxaldehyde, which in turn could form β-cyclocitral. 5,6-Epoxy-β-ionone could also be transformed to 2-hydroxy-2,6,6-trimethylcyclohexanone, which in turn could form 2,6,6-trimethyl-2-cyclohexen-1-one. With the same model system, only dihydroactinidiolide was formed at 30°C.

In a model system simulating dehydrated foods, consisting of lycopene isolated from watermelon or synthetic lycopene adsorbed on microcrystalline cellulose, ten volatile compounds were identified as oxidation products at ambient temperature, the main volatiles generated being 6-methyl-5-hepten-2-one, citral or geranial, and neral (Kobori et al., 2014). Seven of these compounds (1-pentanol, hexanal, 6-methyl-5-hepten-2-one, (E)2-octen-1-al, nonanal, neral, geranial) were also found by Beaulieu and Lea (2006) in five varieties of fresh watermelon, indicating similarity of products formed by enzymatic biodegradation and nonenzymatic autoxidation of carotenoids.

Kanasawud and Crouzet (1990b) investigated the degradation of lycopene in an aqueous model system at a temperature of 30°C to 97°C in the presence of air or oxygen for 3 h. Neral was formed only at temperatures above 50°C. Under mild conditions (temperature below 50°C), only 6-methyl-5-hepten-2-one, geranial, and pseudoionone were found. Aside from neral, 5-hexe-2-one, hexane-2,5-dione, 6-methyl-3,5-heptadien-2-one, and geranyl acetate were generated at higher temperatures.

The possible scheme for the formation of volatile compounds during thermal degradation of lycopene is shown in Figure 8.3 (Crouzet et al., 2002). 2-Methyl-2-hepten-6-one (the same as 6-methyl-5-hepten-2-one), pseudoionone, and geranial are generated by direct cleavage of lycopene. Pseudoionone can then be transformed to geranyl acetone or 3,5-heptadien-2-one. Geranial can be converted to neral, and 2-methyl-2-hepten-6-one to hexane-2,5-dione and 5-hexene-2-one.

Rios et al. (2008) studied thermal degradation (100°C, and 150°C) of carotenoids in oleoresins of marigold, tomato, and paprika. Some of the volatile compounds detected were identical to those reported for biodegradation. However, others were derived exclusively from the thermal degradation process, such *m*-xylene, toluene, and 2,6-dimethylnapthalene). Toluene and *m*-xylene were found in all three oleoresins, whereas methylbenzaldehyde was detected in paprika and marigold oleoresins but not in tomato oleoresin. 6-Methyl-3,5-heptadien-2-one, 6-methyl-5-hepten-2-one, and ethanone were identified in both paprika and tomato oleoresins. Isophorone, ketoisophorone, 2,6-dimethylnapththalene, and loliolide were encountered only in the marigold oleoresin, and β-ionone only in the paprika oleoresin.

The similarity of the products formed by ambient temperature autoxidation, photo-oxidation, and thermal degradation indicate that these processes might involve the same

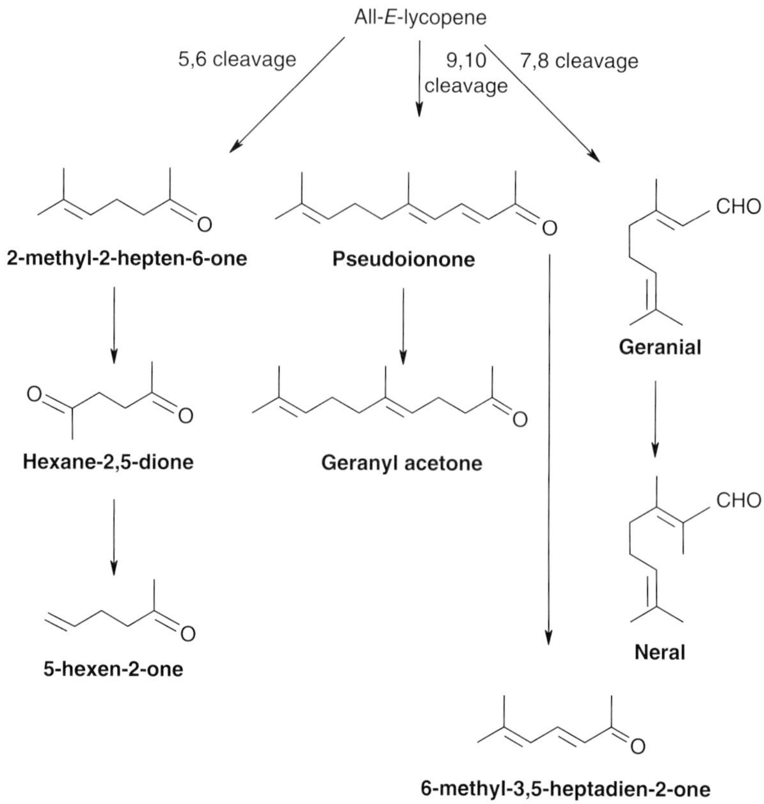

Figure 8.3 Proposed mechanism for the formation of main volatile compounds during thermal degradation of lycopene. Crouzet et al. (2002). Reproduced by permission of Oxford University Press, USA.

reactions, with further reactions taking place in thermal degradation after those that occur under autoxidation at ambient temperature. A lot more work is needed on carotenoid oxidative degradation in different foods and food simulating systems, under different conditions, before the mechanisms can be satisfactorily elucidated.

In tomato juice treated by different technological methods, neral and geranial were encountered (Schreier et al., 1979). Of 44 major aroma components of tomato paste, β-damascenone, β-ionone, and 6-methyl-5-heptane-2-one were among the 11 considered to be most important to tomato paste (Buttery et al., 1990).

Bechoff et al. (2010) studied the formation of volatile compounds during storage of dried sweet potato chips. The presence of the volatile compounds β-ionone, 5,6-epoxy-β-ionone, dihydroactinidiolide, and β-cyclocitral was related to the degradation of all-*E*-β-carotene, and it was suggested that carotenoid degradation in dried sweet potato was by autoxidation.

The volatile products of the degradation of carotenoids are desirable, as in tea and wine, where they become part of the characteristic aroma. In some processed foods, however, degradation/cleavage of carotenoids is undesirable because it is responsible for the development of off flavor, as in dehydrated carrot (Ayer et al., 1964; Falconer et al., 1964) and in certain types of wine (Winterhalter, 1991; Rapp and Marais, 1993).

8.3.4 Carotenoid-derived aroma compounds of tea and wine

Most of the aroma compounds in tea are formed during processing and are derived from carotenoids, amino acids, and unsaturated fatty acids (Ravichandran and Parthiban, 1998). Carotenoid decomposition occurs mainly by oxidative enzymatic reaction that occurs during withering and fermentation and a pyrolytic reaction during firing (Sanderson and Graham, 1973). Carotenoids also undergo photo- and auto-oxidative reactions. During drying and processing, carotenoids of the green tea leaves give rise to smaller oxygenated compounds that contribute to tea flavor and aroma (Sanderson and Graham, 1973; Weeks, 1986). Carotenoid derivatives found in tea are β-ionone, α-ionone, 3-hydroxy-5,6-epoxy-ionone, 5-dihydroxy-4,5-dihydro-6,7-didehydro-α-ionone, linalool, and other terpenoid aldehydes and ketones, with β-ionone as the major degradation product (Ravichandran, 2002). Dihydroactinidiolide, theaspirone, 2,2,6-trimethylcyclohexanone, and 2,2, 6-trimethyl-6-hydroxycyclohexanone are probably formed from the primary oxidation product (i.e., β-ionone). Dehydro-β-ionone, β-ionol, and β-ionone epoxide are also found in black tea (Weeks, 1986). Geraniol, dihydroactinidiolide, geranyl acetone, and 5,6-epoxy-β-ionone were among the volatiles that highly contributed to the quality of green tea and could be possible markers for overall quality evaluation (Jumtee et al., 2011).

In a comparison of carotenoid-derived aroma compounds in brewed extracts of different teas, only theaspirone and dihydroactinidiolide were found in black tea (Kawakami and Kobayashi, 2002). Aside from these two volatiles, 2,6,6-trimethyl-2-hydroxycyclohexanone, 3,3-dimethyl-2,7-octanedione, and 5,6-epoxy-β-ionone were also detected in both green and oolong teas. Green tea also had 6-methyl-(*E*)-3,5-heptadien-2-one, 2,6,6,trimethylcyclohex-2-en-1,4-dione, and β-ionone, whereas 6-methyl-5-hepten-2-one, α-farnesene, and nerolidol were also detected in oolong tea. Following changes during manufacturing of Toyama-kurocha tea, the composition and amount of carotenoid-derived compounds at each manufacturing stage were extremely varied.

β-damascenone (honeylike) is one of the most important aroma components of Japanese green tea (Kumazawa and Masuda, 1999). Heat processing of black tea infusion increased its concentration, and 3-hydroxy-7,8-didehydro-β-ionol was determined to be one of its precursors (Kumazawa and Masuda, 2001).

Major glycosidic precursors of damascenone were isolated and identified in green tea infusions (9-O-β-D-glucopyranosyl –megastigma-6,7-dien-3,5,9-triol, 9-O-β-D-glucopyranosyl -3-hydroxy-7,8-didehydro-β-ionol, 3-O-β-D-glucopyranosyl -3-hydroxy-7,8-didehydro-β-ionol, 3-O-β-D-glucopyranosyl –megastigma-6,7-dien-3,5,9-triol) (Kinoshita et al., 2010). The glycosidic precursors were not hydrolyzed to give damascenone under slightly acidic conditions but could be transformed to damascenone in the presence of green tea infusions even under equal conditions.

Carotenoid-derived aroma compounds have been identified in both white and red wines, such as port, Madeira, Rioja, Grenache, merlot, Fiano, Riesling, chardonnay, chenin blanc, Shiraz, Semillon, cabernet sauvignon, sauvignon blanc, and pinot noir (Leino et al., 1993; Guth, 1997a,b; Aznar et al., 2001; Baumes et al., 2002; Sabon et al., 2002; Winterhalter and Rouseff, 2002; Mendes-Pinto et al., 2005; Lee et al., 2007; Petrozziello et al., 2012). The compounds considered important to the aroma of wines are 2,2,6-trimethylcyclohexanone, β-damascenone, β-ionone, vitispirane, actinidiol,

1,1,6-trimethyl-1,2-dihydronaphthalene (TDN), and Riesling acetal. With the exception of 2,2,6-trimethylcyclohexanone (TCH), which is a C_9 compound and is found only in ports, the other compounds are C_{13}. The determinant factors for the aroma of wine are the grape carotenoid profile, the fermentation process, and the wine storage conditions (Mendes-Pinto, 2009). The most important carotenoid-derived aroma compounds in wine are formed by complex chemical transformations from multiple odorless precursors that happen during winemaking and storage (Winterhalter et al., 1990, 1991; Skouroumounis and Sefton, 2000).

Carotenoid-derived compounds, including β-damascenone, TCH, TDN, and vitispirane, were determined in 14-year young and 15-year old port wines. In a high oxygen environment, as in the case of port wine, the levels of these compounds decreased while oxygen was being consumed. However, during barrel ageing, TDN, vitispirane, and TCH increased significantly while β-ionone and β-damascenone decreased (Pinho et al., 2013).

As with tea, aroma compounds in wine can be formed by direct degradation of carotenoids (e.g., β-carotene and neoxanthin) or they can be stored as glycoconjugates, which can release their volatile aglycones during fermentation via enzymatic and acid hydrolysis (Mendes-Pinto, 2009). In chardonnay juice, used for winemaking in Australia, 70% of the total concentration of volatile secondary metabolites consisted of C_{13} compounds, which were mainly observed in the acid- and the glycosidase enzyme-released fractions (Sefton et al., 1993).

Three C_{13} compounds, 3,6,9-trihydroxymegastigma-4,7-diene, 3,4,9-trihydroxymegastigma-5,7-diene, and the actinidols, have all been synthesized and subjected to acid hydrolysis. All three were shown to generate (*E*)-1-(2,3,6-trimethylphenyl) buta-1,3-diene under wine conservation conditions (Cox et al., 2005).

Glycoconjugation of geraniol in grapes reduced the flavor impact of this compound in wine and the rate of formation of other flavor compounds from it during bottle aging (Skouroumounis and Sefton, 2000).

References

Aguiló-Aguayo I, Montero-Calderón M, Soliva-Fortuny R, Martín-Belloso O. 2010. Changes on flavor compounds throughout cold storage of watermelon juice processed by high-intensity pulsed electric fields or heat. *J Food Eng* 100:43–9.

Aksu Z, Tuğba Eren A. 2005. Carotenoids production by the yeast *Rhodotorula mucilaginosa*: use of agricultural wastes as a carbon source. *Process Biochem* 40:2985–91.

Alcantara S, Sanchez S. 1999. Influence of carbon and nitrogen sources on *Flavobacterium* growth and zeaxanthin biosynthesis. *J Ind Microbiol Biotechnol* 23:697–700.

Allen CL, Gramshaw JW. 1996. The co-oxidation of carotenoids by lipoxygenase in tomatoes. In: Taylor AJ, Mottram DS. editors. *Flavour science: recent developments*. Reading: The Royal Society of Chemistry, p 32–7.

Auldridge ME, McCarty DR, Klee HJ. 2006. Plant carotenoid cleavage oxygenases and their apocarotenoid products. *Curr Opin Plant Biol* 9:315–21.

Ausich RL. 1997. Commercial opportunities for carotenoid production by biotechnology. *Pure Appl Chem* 69:2169–73.

Ayer JE, Fishwick MJ, Land DG, Swain T. 1964. Off-flavour of dehydrated carrot stored in oxygen. *Nature* 203:81–2.

Aznar M, López R, Cacho JF, Ferreira V. 2001. Identification and quantification of impact odorants of aged red wines from Rioja: GC-olfactometry, quantitative GC-MS, and odor evaluation of HPLC fractions. *J Agric Food Chem* 49:2924–9.

Baldermann S, Naim M, Fleischmann P. 2005. Enzymatic carotenoid degradation and aroma formation in nectarines (*Prunus persica*). *Food Res Int* 38:833–6.
Baldwin EA, Nisperos-Carriedo MO, Moshonas MG. 1991. Quantitative analysis of flavor and other volatiles and for certain constituents of two tomato cultivars during ripening. *J Am Soc Hort Sci* 116:265–9.
Bauernfeind JC. 1981. Natural food colors. In: Bauernfeind JC. editor. *Carotenoids as colorants and vitamin A precursors*. New York and London: Academic Press, p 1–45.
Baumes R, Wirth J, Bureau S, Gunata Y, Razungles A. 2002. Biogeneration of C13-norisoprenoid compounds: experiments supportive for an apo-carotenoid pathway in grapevines. *Anal Chim Acta* 458:3–14.
Beaulieu JC, Lea JM. 2006. Characterization and semiquantitative analysis of volatiles in seedless watermelon varieties using solid-phase microextration. *J Agric Food Chem* 54:7789–93.
Bechoff A, Dhuique-Mayer C, Dornier, M, Tomlins KI, Boulanger R, Dufour D, Westby A. 2010. Relationship between the kinetics of β-carotene degradation and formation of norisoprenoids in the storage of dried sweet potato chips. *Food Chem* 121:348–57.
Bhosale P, Bernstein PS. 2005. Microbial xanthophylls. *Appl Microbiol Biotechnol* 68:445–55.
Bhosale P, Gadre RV. 2001a. Optimization of carotenoid production from hyper-producing *Rhodotorula glutinis* mutant 32 by a factorial design. *Lett Appl Microbiol* 33:12–6.
Bhosale P, Gadre RV. 2001b. β-Carotene production in sugarcane molasses by a *Rhodotorula glutinis* mutant. *J Ind Microbiol Biotechnol* 26:327–32.
Bhosale P, Larson AJ, Bernstein PS. 2004. Factorial analysis of tricarboxylic acid cycle intermediates for optimization of zeaxanthin production from *Flavobacterium multivorum*. *J Appl Microbiol* 96:623–9.
Bosser A, Belin JM. 1994. Synthesis of β-ionone in an aldehyde/xanthine/β-carotene system involving free radical formation. *Biotechnol Prog* 10:129–33.
Bosser A, Paplorey E, Belin J-M. 1995. A simple way to (+/−)-dihydroactinidiolide from β-ionone related to the enzymic co-oxidation of β-carotene in aqueous solution. *Biotechnol Prog* 11:689–92.
Bouvier F, Isner J-C, Dogbo O, Camara B. 2005. Oxidative tailoring of carotenoids: a prospect towards novel functions in plants. *Trends Plant Sci* 10:187–94.
Bouvier F, Suire C, Mutterer J, Camara B. 2003. Oxidative remodeling of chromoplast carotenoids: identification of the carotenoid dioxygenase *CsCCD* and *CsZCD* genes involved in *Crocus* secondary metabolite biogenesis. *Plant Cell* 15:47–62.
Brandi F, Bar E, Mourgues F, Horváth G, Turcsi E, Giuliano G, Liverani A, Tartarini S, Lewinsohn E, Rosati C. 2011. Study of 'Redhaven' peach and its white-fleshed mutant suggests a key role of CCD4 carotenoid dioxygenase in carotenoid and norisoprenoid volatile metabolsim. *BMC Plant Biol* 11:24.
Buttery RG, Teranishi R, Ling LC, Turnbaugh JG. 1990. Quantitative and sensory studies on tomato paste volatiles. *J Agric Food Chem* 38:336–40.
Buzzini P. 2000. An optimization study of carotenoid production by *Rhodotorula glutinis* DBVPG 3853 from substrates containing concentrated rectified grape must as the sole carbohydrate source. *J Ind Microbiol Biotechnol* 24:41–5.
Buzzini P. 2001. Batch and fed-batch carotenoid production by *Rhodotorula glutinis-Debaryomyces castellii* co-cultures in corn syrup. *J App Microbiol* 90:843–7.
Buzzini P, Martini A. 1999. Production of carotenoids by strains of *Rhodotorula glutinis* cultured in raw materials of agro-industrial origin. *Bioresour Technol* 71:41–4.
Buzzini P, Martini A, Gaetani M, Turchetti B, Pagnoni UM, Davoli, P. 2005. Optimization of carotenoid production by *Rhodotorula graminis* DBVPG 7021 as a function of trace element concentration by means of response surface analysis. *Enzyme Microb Technol* 36:687–92.
Camara B, Bouvier F. 2004. Oxidative remodeling of plastid carotenoids. *Arch Biochem Biophys* 430:16–21.
Carmona M, Zalacain A, Salinas R, Alonso GL. 2006. Generation of saffron volatiles by thermal carotenoid degradation. *J Agric Food Chem* 54:6825–34.
Chávez-Parga MDC, Munguía-Franco A, Aguilar-Torres M, Escamilla-Silva EM. 2012. Optimization of zeaxanthin production by immobilized *Flavobacterium* sp. cells in fluidized bed bioreactor. *Adv Microbiol* 2:598–604.
Cheng Q. 2006. Structural diversity and functional novelty of new carotenoid biosynthesis genes. *J Ind Microbiol Biotechnol* 33:552–9.
Code of Federal Regulations. 2014. 21 CFR Part 73—Listing of color additives exempt from certification. Washington DC: US Food Drug Admin. Available at: http://www.fda.gov/ForIndustry/ColorAdditives/default.htm.

Cox A, Skouroumounis GK, Elsey GM, Perkins MV, Sefton MA. 2005. Generation of (*E*)-1-(2,3,6-trimethylphenyl)buta-1,3-diene from C13-norisoprenoid precursors. *J Agric Food Chem* 53:6777–83.

Crouzet J, Kanasawud P, Sakho M. 2002. Thermal generation of carotenoid-derived compounds. In: Winterhalter P, Rouseff RI. editors. *Carotenoid-derived aroma compounds*. Washington DC: ACS Symposium Series 802, American Chemical Society, p 115–29.

Das A, Yoon S-H, Lee S-H, Kim J-Y, Oh D-K, Kim S-W. 2007. An update on microbial carotenoid production: application of recent metabolic engineering tools. *Appl Microbiol Biotechnol* 77:505–12.

Downham A, Collins. 2000. Colouring our foods in the last and next millennium. *Int J Food Sci Technol* 35:5–22.

Dufossé L, Galaup P, Yaron A, Arad SM, Blanc P, Murthy KNC, Ravishankar GA. 2005. Microorganisms and microalgae as sources of pigments for food use: a scientific oddity or an industrial reality? *Trends Food Sci Technol* 16:389–406.

Enzell C. 1985. Biodegradation of carotenoids: an important route to aroma compounds. *Pure Appl Chem* 57:693–700.

Ernst H. 2002. Recent advances in industrial carotenoid synthesis. *Pure Appl Chem* 74:1369–82.

Fábregas J, Otero A, Maseda A, Domínguez A. 2001. Two-stage cultures for the production of astaxanthin from *Haematococcus pluvialis*. *J Biotechnol* 89:65–71.

Falconer ME, Fishwick MJ, Lan DG, Sayer ER. 1964. Carotene oxidation and off-flavour development in dehydrated carrot. *J Sci Food Agric* 15:897–901.

Fleischmann P, Studer K, Winterhalter P. 2002. Partial purification and kinetic characterization of a carotenoid cleavage enzyme from quince fruit (*Cydonia oblonga*). *J Agric Food Chem* 50:1677–80.

Fleischmann P, Watanabe N, Winterhalter P. 2003. Enzymatic carotenoid cleavage in star fruit (*Averrhoa carambola*). *Phytochem* 63:131–7.

Floss DS, Schliemann W, Schmidt J, Strack D, Walter MH. 2008. RNA interference-mediated repression of MtCCD1 in mycorrhizal roots of *Medicago truncatula* causes accumulation of C27 apocarotenoids, shedding light on the functional role of CCD1. *Plant Physiol* 148:1267–82.

Floss DS, Walter MH. 2009. Role of carotenoid cleavage dioxygenase 1 (CCD1) in apocarotenoid biogenesis revisited. *Plant Signal Behav* 4:3172–5.

Frengova G, Simova E, Pavlova K, Beshkova D, Grigorova D. 1994. Formation of carotenoids by *Rhodotorula glutinis* in whey ultrafiltrate. *Biotechnol Bioeng* 44:888–94.

Frusciante S, Diretto G, Bruno M, Ferrante P, Pietrella M, Prado-Cabrero A, Rubio-Moraga A, Beyer P, Gomez-Gomez L, Al-Babili S, Giuliano G. 2014. Novel carotenoid cleavage dioxygenase catalyzes the first dedicated step in saffron crocin biosynthesis. *Proc Natl Acad Sci* 111:12246–51.

Giacco M. 2004. Crocetin from saffron: an active component of an ancient spice. *Crit Rev Food Sci Nutr* 44:155–72.

Giuliano G, Al-Babili S, von Lintig J. 2003. Carotenoid oxygenases: cleave it or leave it. *Trends Plant Sci* 8:145–9.

Guerin M, Huntley ME, Olaizola M. 2003. Haematococcus astaxanthin: applications for human health and nutrition. *Trends Biotechnol* 21:210–6.

Güldner A, Winterhalter P. 1991. Structures of two new ionone glycosides from quince fruit (*Cydonia oblonga* Mill.). *J Agric Food Chem* 39:2142–6.

Guth H. 1997a. Identification of character impact odorants of different white wine varieties. *J Agric Food Chem* 45:3022–6.

Guth H. 1997b. Quantitation and sensory studies of character impact odorants of different white wine varieties. *J Agric Food Chem* 45:3027–32.

Henry BS. 1996. Natural food colours. In: Hendrey GAF, Houghton, JD. editors. *Natural food colorants*. London: Blackie Academic & Professional, p 40–79.

Herderich M, Neubert C, Winterhalter P, Schreier P, Skouroumounis GK. 1992. Identification of C13-norisoprenoid flavour precursors in starfruit (*Averrhoa carambola* L.). *Flavour Frag J* 7:179–85.

Higuera-Ciapara I, Félix-Valenzuela L, Goycoolea FM. 2006. Astaxanthin: a review of its chemistry and applications. *Crit Rev Food Sci Nutr* 46:185–96.

Huang F-C, Molnár P, Schwab W. 2009. Cloning and functional characterization of carotenoid cleavage dioxygenase 4 genes. *J Exp Bot* 60:3011–22.

Ibdah M, Azulay Y, Portnoy V, Wasserman B, Bar E, Meir A, Burger Y, Hirschberg J, Schaffer AA, Katzir N, Tadmor Y, Lewinsohn E.2006. Functional characterization of CmCCD1, a carotenoid cleavage dioxygenase from melon. *Phytochem* 67:1579–89.

Ilg A, Beyer P, Al-Babili S. 2009. Characterization of the rice carotenoid cleavage dioxygenase 1 reveals a novel route for geranial biosynthesis. *FEBS* J 276:736–47.

Ilg A, Bruno M, Beyer P, Al-Babili S. 2014. Tomato carotenoid cleavage dioxygenases 1A and 1B: relaxed double bond specificity leads to a plenitude of dialdehydes, mono-apocarotenoids and isoprenoid volatiles. *FEBS Open Bio* 4:584–93.

Ilg A, Yu Q, Schaub P, Beyer P, Al-Babili S. 2010. Overexpression of the *rice carotenoid cleavage dioxygenase 1* gene in Golden Rice endosperm suggests apocarotenoids as substrates *in planta. Planta* 232:691–9.

ILSI (1999). ILSI North America food component reports: canthaxanthin. *Crit Rev Food Sci Nutr* 39:297–316.

Ishihara M, Tsuneya T, Shiota H, Shiga M, Nakatsu K. 1986. Identification of new constituents of quince fruit flavor (*Cydonia oblonga* Mill. = *C. vulgaris* Pers.). *J Org Chem* 51:491–5.

Jaswir I, Noviendri D, Hasrini RF, Octavianti F. 2011. Carotenoids: sources, medicinal properties and their application in food and nutraceutical industry. *J Med Plants Res* 5:7119–31.

Jin ES, Feth B, Melis A. 2003. A mutant of the green alga *Dunaliella salina* constitutively accumulates zeaxanthin under all growth conditions. *Biotechnol Bioeng* 81:115–24.

Johnson EA, An G-H. 1991. Astaxanthin from microbial sources. *Crit Rev Biotechnol* 11:297–326.

Johnson EA, Schroeder WA. 1996. Microbial carotenoids. *Adv Biochem Eng Biotechnol* 53:119–78.

Jordán MJ, Margaría CA, Shaw PE, Goodner KL. 2002. Aroma active components in aqueous kiwi fruit essence and kiwi fruit puree by GC-MS and multidimensional GC/GC-O. *J Agric Food Chem* 50:5386–90.

Jumtee K, Komura H, Bamba T, Fukusaki E. 2011. Prediction of Japanese green tea (Sen-cha) ranking by volatile profiling using gas chromatography mass spectrometry and multivariate analysis. *J Biosci Bioeng* 112:252–5.

Kanasawud P, Crouzet JC. 1990a. Mechanism of formation of volatile compounds by thermal degradation of carotenoids in aqueous medium. 1: β-carotene degradation. *J Agric Food Chem* 38:237–43.

Kanasawud P, Crouzet JC. 1990b. Mechanism of formation of volatile compounds by thermal degradation of carotenoids in aqueous medium. 2: Lycopene degradation. *J Agric Food Chem* 38:1238–42.

Kato M, Matsumoto H, Ikoma Y, Okuda H, Yano M. 2006. The role of carotenoid cleavage dioxygenases in the regulation of carotenoid profiles during maturation in citrus fruit. *J Exp Bot* 57:2153–64.

Kawakami M, Kobayashi A. 2002. Carotenoid-derived aroma compounds in tea. In: Winterhalter P, Rouseff RI. editors. *Carotenoid-derived aroma compounds*. Washington DC: ACS Symposium Series 802, American Chemical Society, p 145–59.

Khalil M, Raila J, Ali M, Islam KMS, Schenk R. 2012. Stability and bioavailability of lutein ester supplements from *Tagetes* flower prepared under processing conditions. *J Funct Foods* 4:602–10.

Kim S, Ha TY, Hwang IK. (2009). Analysis, bioavailability and potential healthy effects of capsanthin, natural red pigment from *Capsicum* spp. *Food Rev Int* 25:198–213.

Kinoshita T, Hirata S, Yang Z, Baldermann S, Kitayama E, Matsumoto S, Suzuki M, Fleischmann P, Winterhalter P, Watanabe N. 2010. Formation of damascenone derived from glycosidically bound precursors in green tea infusions. *Food Chem* 123:601–6.

Kläui H. 1981. Carotenoids and their applications. In: Counsell JN. editor. *Natural colours for food and other uses*. Barking, Essex: Applied Science Publishers Ltd.

Kläui H, Bauernfeind JC. 1981. Carotenoids as food colors. In: Bauernfeind JC. editor. *Carotenoids as colorants and vitamin A precursors*. New York and London: Academic Press, p 47–317.

Kobori CN, Wagner R, Padula M, Rodriguez-Amaya DB. 2014. Formation of volatile compounds from lycopene by autoxidation in a model system simulating dehydrated foods. *Food Res Int* 63(Part A):49–54.

Kumazawa K, Masuda H. 1999. Identification of potent odorants in Japanese green tea (Sen-cha). *J Agric Food Chem* 47:5169–72.

Kumazawa KI, Masuda H. 2001. Change in the flavor of black tea drink during heat processing. *J Agric Food Chem* 49:3304–9.

Lashbrooke JG, Young PR, Dockrall SJ, Vasanth K, Vivier MA. 2013. Functional characterization of three members of the *Vitis vinifera* L. carotenoid cleavage dioxygenase gene family. *BMC Plant Biol* 13:156.

Lauro GJ. 1991. A primer on natural colors. *Cereal Foods World* 36:949–53.

Lee PC, Schmidt-Dannert C. 2002. Metabolic engineering towards biotechnological production of carotenoids in microorganisms. *Appl Microbiol Biotechnol* 60:1–11.

Lee S-H, Seo M-J, Riu M, Cotta JP, Block DE, Dokoozlian NK, Ebeler SE. 2007. Vine microclimate and norisoprenoid concentration in Cabernet Sauvignon grapes and wines. *Am J Enol Vitic* 58:291–301.

Leino M, Francis LI, Kallio H, Williams PJ. 1993. Gas chromatographic headspace analysis of Chardonnay and Semillon wines after thermal processing. Z. *Lebensm Unters Forsch* 197:29–33.

Lewinsohn E, Sitrit Y, Bar E, Azulay Y, Ibdah M, Meir A, Yosef E, Zamir D, Tadmor Y. 2005a. Not just colors: carotenoid degradation as a link between pigmentation and aroma in tomato and watermelon fruit. *Trends Food Sci Technol* 16:407–15.

Lewinsohn E, Sitrit Y, Bar E, Azulay Y, Meir A, Zamir D, Tadmor Y. 2005b. Carotenoid pigmentation affects the volatile composition of tomato and watermelon fruits, as revealed by comparative genetic analyses. *J Agric Food Chem* 53:3142–8.

Liaaen-Jensen S. 2004. Basic carotenoid chemistry. In: Krinsky NI, Mayne ST, Sies H. editors. *Carotenoids in health and disease*. New York: Marcel Dekker, p 1–30.

Lorenz RT, Cysewski GR. 2000. Commercial potential of *Haematococcus* microalgae as a natural source of astaxanthin. *Trends Biotech* 18:160–7.

Lutz A, Winterhalter P. 1992. Isolation of additional carotenoid metabolites from quince fruit (*Cydonia oblonga* Mill.). *J Agric Food Chem* 40:1116–20.

MacLeod G, Ames JM. 1990. Volatile components of starfruit. *Phytochem* 29:165–72.

Mahattanatawee K, Rouseff R, Valim MF, Naim M. 2005. Identification and aroma impact of norisoprenoids in orange juice. *J Agric Food Chem* 53:393–7.

Maldonade IR, Rodriguez-Amaya DB, Scamparini ARP. 2008. Carotenoids of yeasts isolated from the Brazilian ecosystem. *Food Chem* 107:145–50.

Maldonade IR, Rodriguez-Amaya DB, Scamparini ARP. 2012. Statistical optimisation of cell growth and carotenoid production by *Rhodotorula mucilaginosa*. *Braz J Microbiol* 43:109–15.

Maldonade IR, Scamparini ARP, Rodriguez-Amaya DB. 2007. Selection and characterization of carotenoid-producing yeasts from Campinas region, Brazil. *Braz J Microbiol* 38:65–70.

Marova I, Carnecka M, Halienova A, Certik M, Dvorakova T, Haronikova A. 2012. Use of several waste substrates for carotenoid-rich yeast biomass production. *J Environ Manage* 95:S338–42.

Masetto A, Flores-Cotera LB, Diaz C, Langley E, Sanchez S. 2001. Application of a complete factorial design for the production of zeaxanthin by *Flavobacterium* sp. *J Biosci Bioeng* 92:55–8.

Mathieu S, Terrier N, Procureur J, Bigey F, Günata Z. 2005. A carotenoid cleavage dioxygenase from *Vitis vinifera* L.: functional characterization and expression during grape berry development in relation to C_{13}-norispoprenoid accumulation. *J Exp Bot* 56:2721–31.

Matthews PD, Wurtzel ET. 2008. Biotechnology of food colorant production. In: Socaciu C. editor. *Food colorants: chemical and functional properties*. Boca Raton: CRC Press. Taylor and Francis, p 347–398.

Mendes-Pinto MM. 2009. Carotenoid breakdown products—the norisoprenoids—in wine aroma. *Arch Biochem Biophys* 483:236–45.

Mendes-Pinto MM, Ferreira ACS, Caris-Veyrat C, de Pinho PG. 2005. Carotenoid, chlorophyll, and chlorophyll-derived compounds in grapes and Port wines. *J Agric Food Chem* 53:10034–41.

Minguez-Mosquera MI, Hornero-Méndez D. 1993. Separation and quantification of the carotenoid pigments in red peppers (*Capsicum annuum* L.), paprika, and oleoresin by reversed-phase HPLC. *J Agric Food Chem* 41:1616–20.

Misawa N, Shimada H. 1998. Metabolic engineering for the production of carotenoids in non-carotenogenic bacteria and yeasts. *J Biotechnol* 59:169–81.

Mortensen A. 2006. Carotenoids and other pigments as natural colorants. *Pure Appl Chem* 78:1477–91.

Näf R, Velluz A. 1991. Isolation of acyclic precursors of the marmelo oxides, the marmelo lactones and the quince oxepine from quince fruit (*Cydonia oblonga* mil.). *Tetrahedron Lett* 32:4487–90.

Nelis HJ, De Leenheer AP. 1991. Microbial sources of carotenoid pigments used in foods and feeds. *J Appl Bacteriol* 70:181–91.

Ohmiya A. 2009. Carotenoid cleavage dioxygenases and their apocarotenoid products in plants. *Plant Biotechnol* 26:351–8.

Pasamontes L, Hug D, Tessier M, Hohmann HP, Schierle J, van Loon AP. 1997. Isolation and characterization of the carotenoid biosynthesis genes of *Flavobacterium* sp. strain R1534. *Gene* 185:35–41.

Paust J. 1991. Recent progress in commercial retinoids and carotenoids. *Pure Appl Chem* 63:45–58.

Petrozziello M, Borsa D, Guaita M, Gerbi V, Bosso A. 2012. Quantification by solid phase micro extraction and stable isotope dilution assay of norisoprenoid compounds in red wines obtained from Piedmont rare varieties. *Food Chem* 135:2483–9.

Pherobase. 2013. Database of insect pheromones and semiochemicals. Available at: http://www.pherobase.com.

Pinho PG de, Martins RC, Vivier MA, Young PR, Oliveira CM, Silva AC. 2013. Monitoring carotenoids and derived compounds in grapes and Port wines: impact on quality. In: Winterhalter P, Ebeler SE. editors.

Carotenoid cleavage products. Washington DC: ACS Symposium Series 1134, American Chemical Society, p 139–54.

Pino JA. 2014. Odour-active compounds in papaya cv. Red Maradol. *Food Chem* 146:120–6.

Rapp A, Marais J. 1993. The shelf-life of wine: changes in aroma substances during storage and ageing of white wines. In: Charambous G. editor. *Shelf-life studies of food and beverages: chemical, biological, physical and nutritional aspects*. Amsterdam: Elsevier Science Publishers, p 891–921.

Ravichandran R. 2002. Carotenoid composition, distribution and degradation to flavour volatiles during black tea manufacture and the effect of carotenoid supplementation on tea quality and aroma. *Food Chem* 78:23–8.

Ravichandran R, Parthiban R. 1998. The impact of processing techniques on tea volatiles. *Food Chem* 62:347–53.

Rios JJ, Fernández-García E, Mínguez-Mosquera MI, Pérez-Gálvez A. 2008. Description of volatile compounds generated by the degradation of carotenoids in paprika, tomato and marigold oleoresins. *Food Chem* 106:1145–53.

Rubio A, Rambla JL, Santaella M, Gómez MD, Orzaez D, Granell A, Gómez-Gómez L. 2008. Cytosolic and plastoglobule-targeted carotenoid dioxygenases from *Crocus sativus* are both involved in β-ionone release. *J Biol Chem* 283:24816–25.

Ruther A, Misawa N, Boger P, Sandmann G. 1997. Production of zeaxanthin in *Escherichia coli* transformed with different carotenogenic plasmids. *Applied Microbiol Biotechnol* 48:162–7.

Sabon I, de Revel G, Kotseridis Y, Bertrand A. 2002. Determination of volatile compounds in Grenache wines in relation with different terroirs in the Rhone Valley. *J Agric Food Chem* 50:6341–5.

Saftner R, Luo Y, McEvoy J, Abbott JA, Vinyard B. 2007. Quality characteristics of fresh-cut watermelon slices from non-treated and 1-methylcyclopropene- and/or ethylene-treated whole fruit. *Postharvest Biol Technol* 44:71–9.

Sajilata MG, Singhal RS. 2006. Isolation and stabilisation of natural pigments for food application. *Stewart Postharvest Rev* 5:11.

Sajilata MG, Singhal RS, Kamat MY. 2008. The carotenoid pigment zeaxanthin: a review. *Compr Rev Food Sci Food Safety* 7:29–49.

Sanderson GW, Graham HN. 1973. On the formation of black tea aroma. *J Agric Food Chem* 21:576–85.

Sandmann, G. 2002. Combinatorial biosynthesis of carotenoids in a heterologous host: a powerful approach for the biosynthesis of novel structures. *ChemBioChem* 3:629–35.

Sandmann G, Albrecht M, Schnurr G, Knörzer O, Böger P. 1999. The biotechnological potential and design of novel carotenoids by gene combination in *Escherichia coli*. *TIBTECH* 17:233–7.

Schmidt H, Kurtzer R, Eisenreich W, Schwab W. 2006. The carotenase AtCCD1 from *Arabidopsis thaliana* is a dioxygenase. *J Biol Chem* 281:9845–51.

Schreier P, Drawert F, Junker A. 1979. The quantitative composition of natural and technologically changed aroma of plants. IV: Enzymic and thermal reaction products formed during the processing of tomatoes. *Z Lebensm-Unters Forsch* 165:23–7.

Schwartz SH, Qin X, Zeevaart JAD. 2001. Characterization of a novel carotenoid cleavage dioxygenase from plants. *J Biol Chem* 276:25208–11.

Schwartz SH, Tan BC, McCarty DR, Welch W, Zeevaart JAD. 2003. Substrate specificity and kinetics for VP14, a carotenoid cleavage dioxygenase in the ABA biosynthetic pathway. *Biochim Biophys Acta* 1619:9–14.

Scotter M. 2009. The chemistry and analysis of annatto food colouring: a review. *Food Addit Contam* 26:1123–45.

Sefton MA, Francis IL, Williams PJ. 1993. The volatile composition of Chardonnay juices: a study by flavor precursor analysis. *Am J Enol Vitic* 44:359–70.

Shih CT, Hang YD. 1996. Production of carotenoids by *Rhodotorula rubra* from sauerkraut brine. *Lebensm Wiss Technol* 29:570–2.

Simkin AJ, Schwartz SH, Auldridge M, Taylor MG, Klee HJ. 2004. The tomato carotenoid cleavage dioxygenase 1 genes contribute to the formation of the fruit volatiles beta-ionone, pseudoionone, and geranylacetone. *Plant J* 40:882–92.

Skouroumounis GK, Sefton MA. 2000. Acid-catalyzed hydrolysis of alcohols and their β-D-glucopyranosides. *J Agric Food Chem* 48:2033–9.

Tieman DM, Zeigler M, Schmeiz EA, Taylor MG, Bliss P, Kirst M, Klee HJ. 2006. Identification of loci affecting flavor volatile emissions in tomato fruit. *J Exp Biol* 57:887–96.

Tinoi J, Rakariyathan N, Deming RL. 2005. Simplex optimization of carotenoid production by *Rhodotorula glutinis* using hydrolyzed mung bean waste flour as substrate. *Process Biochem* 40:2551–7.

Ungureanu C, Marchal L, Chirvase AA, Foucault A. 2013. Centrifugal partition extraction, a new method for direct metabolites recovery from culture broth: case study of torularhodin recovery from *Rhodotorula rubra*. *Bioresour Technol* 132:406–9.

Vogel JT, Tan B-C, McCarty DR, Klee HJ. 2008. The carotenoid cleavage dioxygenase 1 enzyme has broad substrate specificity, cleaving multiple carotenoids at two different bond positions. *J Biol Chem* 283:11364–73.

Wache Y, Bosser-DeRatuld A, Belin J-M. 2002. Production of aroma compounds by enzymatic cooxidation of carotenoids. In: Winterhalter P, Rouseff RI. editors. *Carotenoid-derived aroma compounds*. Washington DC: ACS Symposium Series 802, American Chemical Society, p 102–113.

Walter MH, Strack D. 2011. Carotenoids and their cleavage products: biosynthesis and functions. *Nat Prod Rep* 28:663–92.

Weeks WW. 1986. Carotenoids: a source of flavor and aroma. In: Parliament TH, Croteau R. editors. *Biogeneration of aromas*. Washington DC: American Chemical Society, p 157–66.

Winterhalter P. 1991. 1,1,6-Trimethyl-1,2-dihydronaphthalene (TDN) formation in wine. 1: Studies on the hydrolysis of 2,6,10,10-tetramethyl-1-oxaspiro[4.5]dec-6-ene-2,8-diol rationalizing the origin of TDN and related C13 norisoprenoids in Riesling wine. *J Agric Food Chem* 39:1825–9.

Winterhalter P, Harmsen S, Trani F. 1991. A C13-norisoprenoid gentiobioside from quince fruit. *Phytochem* 30:3021–5.

Winterhalter P, Rouseff RI. 2002. Carotenoid-derived aroma, an introduction. In: Winterhalter P, Rouseff RI. editors. *Carotenoid-derived aroma compounds*. Washington DC: ACS Symposium Series 802, American Chemical Society, p 1–17.

Winterhalter P, Schreier P. 1988. Free and bound C13 norisoprenoids in quince (*Cydonia oblonga*, Mill.) fruit. *J Agric Food Chem* 36:1251–6.

Winterhalter P, Schreier P. 1995. The generation of norisoprenoid volatiles in starfruit (*Averrhoa carambola* L.): a review. *Food Rev Int* 11:237–54.

Winterhalter P, Sefton MA, Williams PJ. 1990. Volatile C_{13}-norisoprenoid compounds in Riesling wine are generated from multiple precursors. *Am J Enol Vitic* 41:277–83.

Wrolstad RE, Culver CA. 2012. Alternatives to those artificial FD&C food colorants. *Annu Rev Food Sci Technol* 3:59–77.

Wu Z, Robinson DS, Hughes RK, Casey R, Hardy D, West SI. 1999. Co-oxidation of β-carotene catalyzed by soybean and recombinant pea lipoxygenases. *J Agric Food Chem* 47:4899–906.

Wys, A. (2004). Carotene oxygenases: a new family of double bond cleavage enzymes. *J Nutr* 134:S246–50.

Yahyaa M, Bar E, Dubey NK, Meir A, Davidovich-Rikanati R, Hirschberg J, Aly R, Tholl D, Simon PW, Tadmor Y, Lewinsohn E, Ibdah M. 2013. Formation of norisoprenoid flavor compounds in carrot (*Daucus carota* L.) roots: characterization of a cyclic-specific carotenoid cleavage dioxygenase 1 gene. *J Agric Food Chem* 61:12244–52.

Yajima I, Sakakibara H, Ide J, Yanai T, Hayashi K. 1985. Volatile flavor components of watermelon (*Citrullus vulgaris*). *Agric Biol Chem* 49:3145–50.

Ye VM, Bhatia SK. 2012. Pathway engineering strategies for production of beneficial carotenoids in microbial hosts. *Biotechnol Lett* 34:1405–14.

Zorn H, Langhoff S, Scheibner M, Nimtz M, Berger RG. 2003. A peroxidase from *Lepista irina* cleaves β,β-carotene to flavor compounds. *Biol Chem* 384:1049–56.

9 Bioaccessibility and bioavailability

9.1 INTRODUCTION

Before carotenoids can perform their health-promoting functions, they have to reach their sites of action. They must be absorbed from the intestine, transported in the circulation, and delivered to target tissues. These complicated processes are subject to many influencing factors.

Carotenoid bioavailability refers to the fraction of the ingested carotenoid that is absorbed and becomes available for utilization in normal physiological functions or for storage in the human body (Castenmiller and West, 1998). A component of bioavailability, bioaccessibility (release and micellarization) is used to designate the fraction of ingested carotenoid that is released from the food matrix during digestion and made available for absorption. Bioavailability is best determined through human studies; bioaccessibility has been widely evaluated in vitro. It is in this context that these two terms will be used in this chapter. Unless otherwise stated, quoted bioavailability data were obtained from human studies and bioaccessibility values were acquired by in vitro assays as described in Chapter 4.

9.2 ABSORPTION, METABOLISM, AND TRANSPORT

Carotenoids undergo the following steps in the human body: (1) breakdown of the food matrix and release of the carotenoids, (2) dispersion in gastric lipid emulsion particles, (3) incorporation in micelles stabilized by biliary salts in the intestinal lumen, (4) uptake by intestinal mucosal cells, (5) intracellular metabolism (of provitamin A carotenoids), and (6) incorporation into chylomicrons and secretion into the lymphatic system (Figure 9.1) (Furr and Clark, 1997; Deming and Erdman, 1999; Yonekura and Nagao, 2007; During, 2008).

Carotenoids are released from the food by mastication, gastric action (grinding and gastric churning), and digestive enzymes (enzymatic hydrolysis of lipids and proteins). The extent of release from the food matrix is highly variable, depending on the food

Food Carotenoids: Chemistry, Biology, and Technology, First Edition. Delia B. Rodriguez-Amaya.

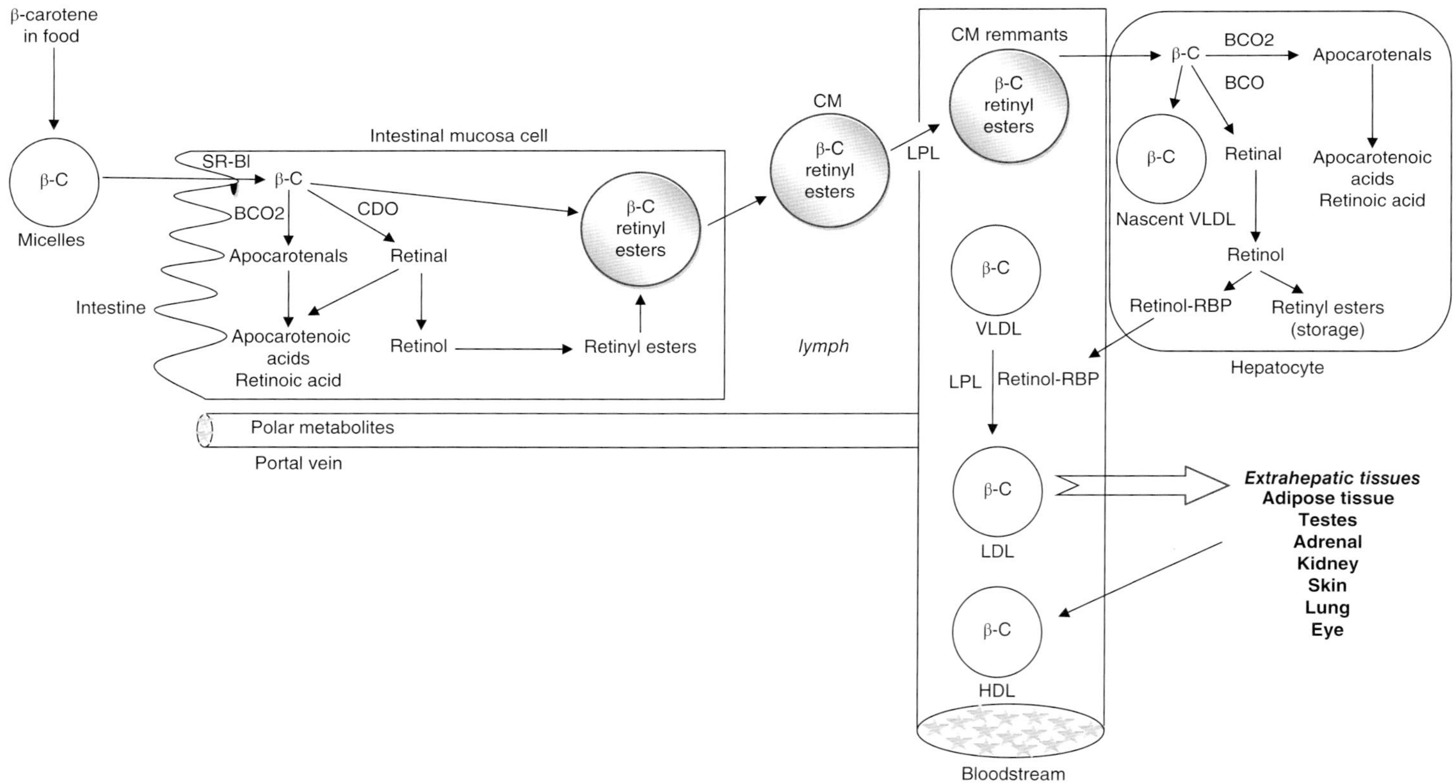

Figure 9.1 Absorption, metabolism, and transport of β-carotene. CM = chylomicrons, VLDL = very-low-density lipoprotein, LDL = low-density lipoprotein, HDL = high-density lipoprotein, BCO = β-carotene 15,15′-oxygenase, BCO_2 = β-carotene 9′,10′-oxygenase, LPL = lipoprotein lipase, RBP = retinol binding protein, SR-BI = scavenger receptor class B, type I. During (2008). Reproduced by permission of Taylor and Francis Group, LLC, a division of Informa plc.

consumed, whether the carotenoids are complexed with other components (e.g., protein), or are in the crystallized form as in the carrot root or dissolved in dietary oils as in corn or palm oils. It also depends on whether the food is finely chopped or puréed, raw or cooked, and if fat is consumed simultaneously or not.

The carotenoids liberated from the food matrix solubilize into lipid globules in the stomach, generating lipid emulsion particles in the otherwise aqueous environment of the gastric chyme. Solubilization of individual carotenoids into lipid emulsions differs according to polarity, the apolar carotenes migrating to the triacylglycerol-rich core of the particles and the more polar xanthophylls orienting at the surface along with proteins, phospholipids, and partially ionized fatty acids (Borel et al., 1996; Furr and Clark, 1997; Tyssandier et al., 2001). This localization explains, at least in part, the now well-documented greater bioaccessibility of xanthophylls in comparison with the carotenes. The surface components can more easily transfer from the lipid droplets to mixed micelles, whereas components associated with the emulsion core require digestion of the triacylglycerols before transfer.

Carotenoids solubilized in lipid emulsion particles are transported to the duodenum of the small intestine. Dietary fat in the duodenum triggers the release of bile acids from the gall bladder. These acids aid in the reduction of lipid particle size and stabilization into mixed micelles. Carotenoids are solubilized into mixed micelles along with dietary triacylglycerols, their hydrolysis products, phospholipids, cholesterol esters, and bile acids. Mixed micelle formation is necessary to move apolar lipids and lipid-soluble compounds such as carotenoids across the unstirred water layer prior to uptake by intestinal epithelial cells.

Intestinal uptake of carotenoids had been thought of as a simple passive diffusion through gut cells. According to this mechanism, the micelles migrate through the unstirred water layer to the brush border membrane; the carotenoid then leaves the micellar structure, diffusing through the membrane into the cytoplasm of enterocytes (Yonekura and Nagao, 2007). Recent studies indicate that absorption actually consists of complex mechanisms involving receptor-mediated transport of carotenoids. The participation of transporters, such as the scavenger receptor class B type I (SR-BI), is strongly indicated (Reboul et al., 2005; van Bennekum et al., 2005; During et al., 2005; Borel et al., 2013). Studies with Caco-2 monolayers have shown cellular uptake and secretion to be curvilinear, time-dependent, saturable, and concentration-dependent processes, characteristics more consistent with the participation of a specific epithelial transporter than with passive diffusion. In addition to the kinetics of cellular uptake and secretion, inhibition of intestinal absorption of one carotenoid by another and cellular isomer discrimination all suggest that carotenoid uptake by intestinal cells is a facilitated process (During et al., 2002).

In the intestinal mucosa, provitamin A carotenoids are partly metabolized by one or two routes to form retinal, retinoic acid, and small amounts of β-apocarotenoids. Conversion of the provitamins A to vitamin A is discussed in detail in Chapter 10.

Both carotenoids and vitamin A, mainly retinyl ester, are incorporated into chylomicrons and secreted into the lymphatic system. In the blood circulation, the chylomicrons undergo lipolysis, catalyzed by a lipoprotein lipase, forming chylomicron remnants. These remnants containing carotenoids and retinyl ester are taken up by the liver, where retinyl esters are hydrolyzed, reesterified, and stored mainly in hepatic stellate cells

(Nayak et al., 2001). Depending on the need and physiological conditions, retinyl esters are hydrolzyed, and free retinol is resecreted into the bloodstream in very-low-density lipoprotein (VLDL) (Johnson and Russell, 1992).

Nonprovitamin A carotenoids, unesterified carotenols, and part of the provitamin A carotenoids are absorbed intact. Fatty acid esters of xanthophylls are cleaved in the lumen of the small intestine prior to uptake by the mucosa, as reported for β-cryptoxanthin esters (Wingerath et al., 1995; Breithaupt et al., 2002, 2003). The enzyme responsible for the hydrolysis of xanthophyll esters is most likely carboxyl ester hydrolase secreted by the pancreas. In an in vitro study, human pancreatic lipase accepted only retinyl palmitate as substrate; carotenoid mono- and diesters were not hydrolyzed (Breithaupt et al., 2002). Granado-Lorencio et al. (2007a) also observed that xanthophyll esters were cleaved by cholesterol esterase but not by human pancreatic lipase. In a later study (Breithaupt et al., 2007), recombinant pancreatic lipase did hydrolyze esters of xanthophylls (β-cryptoxanthin, lutein, zeaxanthin), but the conversion rates were extremely low, hardly explaining the high amounts of free xanthophylls found in human serum after ingestion of carotenoid ester–containing diets (Bowen et al., 2002) or the increasing amounts of free β-cryptoxanthin and absence of β-cryptoxanthin esters in the chylomicrons and serum after ingestion of tangerine juice (rich in β-cryptoxanthin esters) (Wingerath et al., 1995). On the other hand, cholesterol esterase cleaved both retinyl palmitate and β-cryptoxanthin esters with high yields. This enzyme is responsible for the hydrolysis of dietary cholesterol esters, esters of fat-soluble vitamins, phospholipids, lysophospholipids, ceramide, and mono-, di-, and triacylglycerols.

In the liver, the chylomicron remnant-associated carotenoid can be metabolized into vitamin A and other metabolites and stored, or repackaged and released in the bloodstream. Transported exclusively by lipoproteins, the carotenoids are finally distributed to extrahepatic tissues. The liver secretes carotenoids associated with hepatic VLDL, but in the fasted state, hydrocarbon carotenoids are carried predominantly by low-density lipoprotein (LDL). The xanthophylls are carried by both high-density lipoprotein (HDL) and LDL and, to a lesser extent, by VLDL (Johnson and Russell, 1992; Traber et al., 1994; Parker 1996). Hydrocarbon carotenoids are mainly located in the hydrophobic core of the particles, whereas the xanthophylls reside on the surface (Parker, 1996).

In humans, carotenoids accumulate in many tissues including the liver, adipose, serum, breast milk, adrenal gland, prostate, macula, kidney, lung, brain, and skin. Tissue-specific accumulation (e.g., lycopene in the prostate, lutein and zeaxanthin in the macula) could suggest a biological effect.

9.3 METHODS FOR DETERMINING BIOAVAILABILITY

In vitro methods for determining bioaccessibility are discussed in Chapter 4. Methods for studying the bioavailability of carotenoids from dietary sources or supplements in humans fall under four major approaches: (a) serum/plasma response after carotenoid ingestion, (b) oral-fecal balance technique, (c) chylomicron response after carotenoid ingestion, and (d) stable isotope studies (Parker, 1997; Parker et al., 1999; Yeum and Russell, 2002; During, 2008).

Carotenoid bioavailability has been widely assessed by following changes in the plasma carotenoid concentrations after single or long-term ingestion of supplements or food sources. Usually, a plasma concentration-versus-time plot is generated, from which the area under the curve is determined and used as indicator of the absorption of the carotenoid. Serum response curves to determine bioavailability are limited by several factors: (a) The serum response to a single oral dose of carotenoid is highly variable. (b) The concentration of carotenoids in the serum represents a balance between intestinal absorption, breakdown, tissue uptake, and release from body stores. (c) Human serum contains substantial endogenous concentrations of carotenoids such as α-carotene, β-carotene, lycopene, β-cryptoxanthin, and lutein. (d) Relatively large doses, usually exceeding the typical daily intake by at least fivefold, are needed for a significant increase in carotenoid concentration over baseline levels. (e) The intestinal metabolism (into retinol and retinyl esters) of the provitamin A carotenoids during passage through the intestinal mucosa is often not accounted for. A major problem of this method is the wide variation in plasma carotenoid response between individuals.

The traditional oral-fecal balance method gives only rough estimates because (a) it does not account for carotenoid degradation in the upper (chemical oxidation) or lower (microbial degradation or alteration) regions of the gastrointestinal tract; (b) in the fecal sample, it does not differentiate between exogenous carotenoids from foods or supplements and endogenously secreted carotenoids; and (c) it does not account for the loss of carotenoids via the skin (During, 2008).

Chylomicron-associated carotenoids are used as indicators of their absorption. Advantages of the chylomicron response over the serum response curve method are as follows: (a) The method accounts for intestinal conversion to retinyl ester. (b) It improves the distinguishability of newly absorbed carotenoids from endogenous pools. (c) It allows for the use of smaller doses (Yeum and Russell, 2002). However, this method is not able to separate the liver-derived VLDL from the intestine-derived chylomicrons, and isolation of the chylomicron fraction is not easy. Intra- and interindividual variation can be another problem.

The development of stable isotope labeled carotenoids has made it possible to (a) distinguish between dosed and endogenous carotenoids, (b) assess the extent of intestinal conversion of vitamin A, (c) estimate absolute and postabsorptive metabolism for subsequent empirical or compartmental modeling, and (d) use doses that are low enough to avoid influencing endogenous pools (Yeum and Russell, 2002).

Lieshout et al. (2003) reviewed in detail various aspects of isotopic tracer techniques, including study design, choice of isotopic tracers, dosing regimen, collection of samples, chemical analysis of samples, and data analysis. It was concluded that these techniques could meet the need for accurate and precise estimates of the bioavailability, bioconversion, and bioefficacy of dietary carotenoids in humans.

9.4 DIETARY FACTORS AFFECTING BIOAVAILABILITY

The bioavailability of carotenoids is extremely variable, influenced by many diet-related factors (e.g., food matrix, dose and type of carotenoids, food processing techniques, amount of dietary fat, fiber, and other food components), as well as by host-related factors (e.g., vitamin A status, nutrient deficiencies, gut integrity, and genetic polymorphism associated with provitamin A carotenoid metabolism) (Furr and Clark, 1997; Castenmiller and West, 1998; van het Hof et al., 2000b; Yeum and Russell, 2002; Zaripheh and Erdman, 2002; Yonekura and Nagao, 2007). This section will highlight food-related factors, which have been investigated intensely in recent years through in vitro bioaccessibility studies, the findings of which are generally coherent with those of human studies on bioavailability. In vitro bioaccessibility differs widely among carotenoids in a given food as well as for a specific carotenoid in different foods (Granado-Lorencio et al., 2007b).

For each of the factors cited below, in vitro bioaccessibility will be discussed first, followed by bioavailability results from human studies.

9.4.1 Nature of the food matrix

More than the chemical form (i.e., structure) of the different carotenoids found in foods, their subcellular location and the nature of the food matrix are important determinants of bioavailability. Carotenoids in plant foods are located in chloroplasts as part of the photosynthetic apparatus (in green leafy and nonleafy vegetables) or in chromoplast, dissolved in oil droplets (in fruits) or as semi-crystalline membrane-bound solids (in carrot).

The low bioavailability of carotenoids from plant sources has been attributed primarily to the food matrix (Yeum and Russell, 2002). Carotenoids in foods are often bound within plant matrices of indigestible polysaccharides, fibers, and phenolic compounds, which reduce the bioavailability. Bioaccessibility has been shown to be highly dependent on the physical and chemical properties of the food matrix and the way these change during digestion (Cilla et al., 2012). The intracellular localization of nutrients and bioactive compounds implies that their bioaccessibility can be hindered by several structural elements.

Some studies suggested that ingestion of purified carotenoids is needed to achieve major increase in plasma carotenoid concentrations (E.D. Brown et al., 1989; Micozzi et al., 1992; Bulux et al., 1994). However, in a randomized crossover study with healthy volunteers, lycopene appeared to be equally bioavailable from tomato juice and the supplement (lycopene beadlet) used (Paetau et al., 1998). Moreover, the study of Yeum et al. (1996) indicated that most of the carotenoids (lutein, β-cryptoxanthin, α-carotene, 13-*Z*-β-carotene, all-*E*-β-carotene, all-*E*-lycopene, and *Z*-lycopenes) that exist in human plasma can be increased in a relatively short time by dietary intake of fruits and vegetables. Similarly, results of Riso et al. (2003) suggest that the intake of one single dose of lutein from different sources is able to bring about a significant plasma response in the short term.

Mango (10%) had higher bioaccessibility of β-carotene, followed by papaya (5.3%), tomato (3.1%), and carrot (3.1%) (Schweiggert et al., 2012). The bioaccessibility of lycopene from papaya and tomato did not differ significantly. The physical form of carotenoid deposition in plant chromoplasts is believed to have major impact on their liberation efficiency from the food matrices. Chromoplasts from carrot and tomato contain large crystalloid β-carotene and lycopene aggregates, respectively (Vásquez-Caicedo et al., 2006; Schweiggert et al., 2011). On the other hand, β-carotene and other provitamin A carotenoids in papaya accumulate in numerous but much smaller globular and tubular structures, in a lipid-dissolved or liquid-crystalline form. For carrots, cell walls and chromoplast substructure were important barriers for carotenoid bioaccessibility, whereas in tomatoes, the chromoplast substructure represented the most important barrier (Palmero et al., 2013). The highest increase in bioaccessibility, for all matrices, was obtained when carotenoids were transferred into the oil phase, a system lacking cell walls and chromoplast substructures that could hamper carotenoid release.

Bioaccessibility varied markedly among the nine raw whole fruits and vegetables evaluated by Jeffrey et al. (2012b), with values of 1%–39% for lycopene, 18%–20% for α-carotene, 7%–49% for β-carotene, 9%–59% for lutein, 4%–22% for violaxanthin, and 47%–96% for phytoene. Per 100 g of food, grapefruit and watermelon had the most accessible lycopene (69 and 64 μg, respectively); carrot the most accessible α-carotene (559 μg), β-carotene (1078 μg), lutein (91 μg), and phytoene (23 mg); and mango the most accessible violaxanthin (177 μg). Digestive stability averaged 80%, except for the xanthophylls, which exhibited a wider and lower range of stabilities.

Watermelon and melon cells were shown to be the largest cells concomitant with thin, nonfibrous cell walls (Jeffery et al., 2012a). Carrot, hypodermal grapefruit, and sweet potato cells were the smallest with fibrous or dense cell walls. Mango fruit showed the highest proportion of globules to other substructures. Carrot, papaya, and tomato contained many crystalline structures, while watermelon, mango, and butternut squash had a high proportion of membranous structures.

The xanthophyll carotenoids (lutein, zeaxanthin, and β-cryptoxanthin), when present, were highly bioaccessible from fruits (orange, kiwi, red grapefruit and honeydew melon), ranging from 50% to 100% (O'Connell et al., 2007). Lutein bioaccessibility was lower (19%–38%) in dark green vegetables (spinach and broccoli) than in fruits (100%–109%).

The β-carotene bioaccessibility of field-grown orange-fleshed honeydew melons was 3.3%, uptake in Caco-2 cells was about 11%, and chromoplast structure was globular not crystalline (Fleshman et al., 2011). The bioaccessibility of β-carotene from orange-fleshed honeydew melons was comparable to that of carrot.

The extent of micellarization of both lycopene and β-carotene in gac fruit was considerably greater than those reported for these carotenoids in other fruits and vegetables subjected to the same in vitro procedure (Failla et al., 2008). This difference may be due to the localization of the carotenoids in the lipid-rich matrix of gac aril, which contains as much as 22% fatty acids by weight, with palmitate, oleate, and linoleate comprising ~30% each of total fatty acyl pool.

The structural quality of carrots, represented by the texture, and β-carotene bioaccessibility were observed to be inversely related, that is, carrots with firm texture have low β-carotene bioaccessibility (Lemmens et al., 2009). In this vegetable, β-carotene is located in the chromoplasts (surrounded by a cell membrane and a cell wall), where it is associated with proteins and/or residual membranes (Hornero-Méndez and Mínguez-Mosquera, 2007). Several physical barriers have to be broken before β-carotene can be released from the matrix.

In carrot- and tomato-derived suspensions, only particles smaller than an individual cell resulted in high bioaccessibility values, pointing to the importance of the cell wall as the main barrier for carotenoid uptake (Moelants et al., 2012). However, predictions based on the relation between particle size and bioaccessibility indicated that bioaccessibility is determined not only by the cell wall integrity but also by interactions between structural compounds of the complex food matrix.

In 20 varieties of sun-dried chili peppers, red peppers had higher carotenoid content and bioaccessibility than either the orange peppers or yellow peppers (Pugliese et al., 2014b).

For various cassava cultivars, the efficiency of micellarization of total β-carotene (30% with no significant difference between isomers) was linearly proportional to the concentration in cooked cassava, and accumulation of all-*E*-β-carotene by Caco-2 cells was proportional to the quantity present in micelles (Thakkar et al., 2007). Bioaccessibility and Caco-2 cell uptake of β-carotene in cooked transgenic cassava were significantly greater than those for identically processed wild roots (Failla et al., 2008).

Daly et al. (2010) found that the bioaccessibility of carotenoids from eight herbs varied from 0% to 43%, with lutein (+zeaxanthin) and β-cryptoxanthin being more bioaccessible than β-carotene. Carotenoid bioaccessibility from spinach was highest with milk (4% fat) and lowest when skimmed milk or more complex food matrices such as sausage were added to the meal (Biehler et al., 2011).

The stability of carotenoids under digestion conditions was >75%, regardless of the food analyzed; micellarization ranged from 5% to 100%, depending on the carotenoid and the food analyzed (Granado-Lorencio et al., 2007b). Xanthophyll ester hydrolysis was incomplete (<40%); both free and esterified forms were incorporated into micelles, regardless of the xanthophyll involved and the food assessed.

Carotenoid bioaccessibility was shown to be generally higher from sorghum (63%–81%) compared to maize (45%–47%) (Kean et al., 2011). Micellarization of xanthophylls (75%) was more efficient than carotenes (52%) in sorghum, but was similar in maize (40%–49%). The bioaccesibility of carotenoids from durum wheat pasta was also high (71%) (Werner and Böhm, 2011).

Using a dynamic gastric model of digestion, almost 100% bioaccessibility of lutein was found after duodenal digestion, with no difference between three samples (raw pistachios, roasted and salted pistachios, and muffins made with raw pistachios) (Mandalari et al., 2013).

In a randomized crossover study, the bioavailability of β-carotene from papaya was approximately three times higher than that from carrot and tomato (Schweiggert et al., 2014). The difference between carrot and tomato was not significant. Lycopene was approximately 2.6 times more available from papaya than from tomato. Papaya β-cryptoxanthin was 2.9 and 2.3 times more bioavailable than papaya β-carotene and lycopene, respectively. The differences in bioavailability were hypothesized to be mainly due to the morphology of the chromoplast and physical deposition form of the carotenoids.

As cited by van het Hof et al. (2000b), the relative bioavailability of β-carotene from vegetables compared with purified β-carotene ranged from 3% to 6% for green leafy vegetables, from 19% to 34% for carrots, and from 22% to 24% for broccoli (Micozzi et al., 1992; Pee et al., 1995; Törrönen et al., 1996; Castenmiller et al., 1999; van het Hof et al., 1999b). Broccoli and green peas induced a greater β-carotene response in the plasma than whole-leaf and chopped spinach, in spite of a 10 times lower β-carotene content in the former vegetables (van het Hof et al., 1999a). β-carotene from orange fruit was found to be more effective in increasing plasma concentrations of retinol and β-carotene than were green leafy vegetables (Pee et al., 1998). Thürmann et al. (2002) reported superior bioavailability of β-carotene from a water-dispersible powder in a commercially available drink when compared with a carrot juice drink.

Bioavailability of lutein from lutein-enriched eggs was higher than that of lutein, lutein ester supplements, and spinach, the bioavailability not differing significantly in these other sources (Chung et al., 2004). Lutein from yellow carrots was found to be highly bioavailable and did not decrease the β-carotene concentration that would accompany administration of lutein supplements (Molldrem et al., 2004).

A randomized, double-blind, crossover, comparative, single-dose study in healthy subjects confirmed that the bioavailability of lutein and zeaxanthin was critically dependent on the formulation used (Evans et al., 2012). The superiority of a starch-based over an alginate-based product was documented.

Human trials showed that the serum transfer efficiency of β-cryptoxanthin was statistically higher in emulsified formulation than in fresh mandarin juice (Takaishi et al., 2012). Caco-2 cell permeability studies indicated that emulsifiers preferentially accelerated the absorption of the nonesterified form of β-cryptoxanthin.

Based on a review of the literature, Boileau et al. (1999) presented a bioavailability ranking, with raw green leafy vegetables having the lowest bioavailability and synthetic carotenoids in oil having the highest bioavailability: raw green leafy vegetables < raw yellow or orange vegetables < raw juice without fat < mildly cooked yellow or orange vegetables < processed juice with fat containing meal < tubers < fruits < natural or synthetic carotenoids in oil. Pure β-carotene in an oily solution or supplement is absorbed more efficiently than an equivalent amount of β-carotene in fruits and vegetables. Although the absorption of carotenoids from fruits is generally more efficient than that from fibrous vegetables, it is still low compared with β-carotene in oil.

On the other hand, in a fully randomized crossover study, in which lycopene was provided in the form of ketchup and oleoresin capsules at low levels (5, 10, 20 mg), the serum lycopene levels increased significantly at all levels of intake, but there was no significant difference between the two treatments (Rao and Shen, 2002).

9.4.2 Carotenoid species

Bioaccessibility in raw and canned carrot, raw tomato and sauce, watermelon, cooked spinach, lettuce, and canned green beans was dependent on the carotenoid species: lutein > β-carotene and α-carotene > lycopene (Reboul et al., 2006).

Although it varies depending on the type of product, processing conditions, and method of assessment, it is widely accepted that the bioaccessibility of lycopene is generally low (Garrett et al., 1999a, 2000; Reboul et al., 2006; Goñi et al., 2006; Huo et al., 2007; Colle et al., 2010a).

Assessing the bioaccessibility of provitamin A carotenoids from boiled bananas and derived dishes, the bioaccessibility of all-*E*-β-carotene ranged from 10% to 32%, depending on the food recipes, modified particularly by the addition of provitamin A–rich ingredients (palm oil/amaranth) (Ekesa et al., 2012). Efficiency of micellarization of all-*E*-β-carotene was similar to that of all-*E*-α-carotene and dependent on the cultivar (Musilongo, plantain type, 16%; Vulambya, East African cooking type, 28%); that of

13-*Z*-isomer was higher (21%–34%). From a blended fruit juice (orange, kiwi, and pineapple), bioaccessibility of α- and β-carotene was 9.3% and 10%, respectively (Rodríguez-Roque et al., 2013).

Many studies have demonstrated the greater bioaccesibility of xanthophylls compared to carotenes. Micellarization of lutein (25%–40%) from a meal (prepared with baby food carrots, spinach, meat, and tomato sauce) exceeded that of α- and β-carotene (12%–18%) and lycopene (<0.5%) (Garret et al., 1999a). From a stir-fried meal, the percentages of lutein, lycopene, α-carotene, and β-carotene transferred from the meal to the micellar fraction were 29, 3.2, 15, and 16, respectively (Garret et al., 2000). In another study, micellarization of lutein and zeaxanthin from meals exceeded that of β-carotene and was greater for xanthophylls in oil-based supplements than in spinach (Chitchumroonchokchai et al., 2004). The efficiency of micellarization of lutein from drumstick leaves (Pullakhandam and Failla, 2007) and of xanthophylls (lutein, zeaxanthin, and β-cryptoxanthin) from loquat, orange, and broccoli (Granado-Lorencio et al., 2007a) also exceeded that of β-carotene.

From different chili peppers, the xanthophyll carotenoids were more efficiently transferred to micelles (Pugliese et al., 2013). In a subsequent work, capsanthin and zeaxanthin had the highest bioaccessibility at an average value of 36% to 40%, followed by antheraxanthin (26%) (Pugliese et al., 2014a). β-cryptoxanthin, violaxanthin, and β-carotene had much lower bioaccessibility, averaging 6.1%, 4.8%, and 4.0%, respectively. Neoxanthin and lutein were not detected in the micelles.

Employing a bioaccessibility model that included enzymatic digestion and colonic fermentation, Goñi et al. (2006) evaluated the bioaccessibilities of major carotenoids of common fruits and vegetables in the Spanish diet. Lutein was found to have greater small intestine bioaccessiblity (79%) than β-carotene (27%) and lycopene (40%) In the large intestine, however, similar and greater amounts of lycopene and β-carotene were released from the matrix (57%) than lutein (17%). Results of this study suggested that 91% of β-carotene, lutein, and lycopene contained in fruits and vegetables was available in the gut during the entire digestion process. In an earlier study involving green leafy vegetables (Serrano et al., 2005), the amount of β-carotene and lutein released from the food matrix by digestive enzymes ranged from 22% to 67% and 27% to 77%, respectively. The carotenoids released by the vitro colonic fermentation ranged from 2% to 11%.

Digestive stability of xanthophylls was also shown to surpass that of carotenes. As studied with a dynamic in vitro gastrointestinal system, zeaxanthin and lutein were stable throughout digestion, whereas β-carotene and all-*E*-lycopene were degraded (~30% and 20% loss at the end of digestion, respectively) in the jejunal and ileal compartments (Blanquet-Diot et al., 2009). The recovery of β-carotene in the digesta of a red tomato meal was significantly lower than that of a yellow tomato meal. Isomeric configuration also influenced the stability, 5-*Z*-lycopene being the most stable followed by all-*E*- and 9-*Z*-lycopene. No *E*-*Z* isomerization of lycopene took place in the intestinal tract model.

In contrast to micellarization, Caco-2 cellular uptake of β-carotene exceeded that of lutein (Garrett et al., 1999b; Liu et al., 2004). Caco-2 cellular uptake of β-carotene, free β-cryptoxanthin, and β-cryptoxanthin esters was 14%, 3.9%, and 0.7%, respectively (Dhuique-Mayer et al., 2007). In another study with Caco-2 cells, absorption of α-carotene, lutein, and lycopene was 10%, 7%, and 2.5%, respectively (During et al., 2002).

Chitchumroonchokchai and Failla (2006) reported the presence of zeaxanthin monoester in the Caco-2 cells but indicated that free zeaxanthin was taken up by the cells more efficiently than zeaxanthin esters.

The relative bioavailability of lutein from a diet supplemented with a variety of leafy vegetables was much greater than that of β-carotene (67% and 14%, respectively) (van het Hof et al., 1999a). The same trend was reported for lutein and β-carotene from spinach (45% and 5.1%, respectively) (Castenmiller et al., 1999). Enzymatic disruption of the matrix enhanced the bioavailability of β-carotene from whole-leaf and minced spinach but had no effect on lutein bioavailability. In the presence of high amounts of β-carotene, there was preferential uptake of lutein as compared to all-*E*-β-carotene from the intestinal lumen into chylomicrons (Gärtner et al., 1996). The greater serum lutein response compared to that of β-carotene was also shown in other human studies with green vegetables (van het Hof et al., 1999c; Novotny et al., 2005). During 4 weeks of supplementation, serum lutein response from unesterified lutein exceeded that from esterified lutein (Norkus et al., 2010).

Disruption of the food matrix and increasing the amount of fat appear to enhance absorption of carotenes to a greater extent than xanthophylls (Yonekura and Nagao, 2007). Xanthophylls seem to be more easily released from the food matrix and more efficiently micellarized than the carotenes. The bioavailability of hydrocarbon carotenoids is relatively lower than oxygenated carotenoids because the latter are incorporated in the outer portions of lipid micelles and can be more easily taken up by enterocyte membranes and eventually by the chylomicrons (Yeum and Russell, 2002).

The bioavailability of epoxy carotenoids appears to be very low. In humans supplemented for 1 week with spinach and wakame (edible brown alga), the plasma concentration of neoxanthin and fucoxanthin remained very low, whereas those of β-carotene and lutein increased markedly (Asai et al., 2008).

9.4.3 Geometric configuration

In blended foods containing orange-fleshed sweet potato flour (chapati, mandazi, and porridge), the incorporation into micelles of 13-Z-β-carotene was significantly higher than all-*E*-β-carotene (Bechoff et al., 2011). Efficiency of micellarization of *Z*-β-carotene isomers from water-soluble beadlets or *Dunaliella salina* also exceeded that of all-*E*-β-carotene (Ferruzzi et al., 2006). Caco-2 cell uptake, however, was not isomer specific at the concentrations utilized in the study.

In contrast, preferential transport of all-*E*-β-carotene versus either 9-Z- or 13-Z-β-carotene through the Caco-2 cell monolayers was observed by During et al. (2002). Under linear concentration conditions at 16 h incubation, the extent of absorption with Caco-2 cells of all-*E*-β-carotene was 11%, whereas absorption of 9-*Z*- and 13-*Z*-β-carotene was significantly lower (2%–3%). For α-carotene, lutein, and lycopene, absorption was 10%, 7%, and 3%, respectively.

All-*E*-β-carotene has been found to preferentially accumulate in human chylomicrons, very-low-density lipoproteins (Stahl et al., 1995), and human serum (Stahl et al.,1993; Gaziano et al., 1995; Ben-Amotz and Levy, 1996) compared to 9-*Z*-β-carotene. Two possibilities have been raised to explain this difference in plasma response between the geometric isomers: selective intestinal transport of all-*E*-β-carotene or isomerization of all-*E*- to the *Z*-isomer. The second possibility is supported by the finding of You et al. (1996) that [^{13}C]-all-*E*-β-carotene accumulated significantly in the plasma of subjects who ingested a dose of [^{13}C]-9-*Z*-β-carotene. The first possibility is in agreement with the results of During et al. (2002) discussed above that the *Z*-isomers of β-carotene were taken up by the Caco-2 cells to only one-fifth of the extent of all-*E*- β-carotene.

The greater in vitro micellarization of *Z*-β-carotene, compared to all-*E*-β-carotene, appears at first glance to be incoherent with the greater bioavailability of all-*E*-β-carotene in human studies. The in vitro micellarization trend can, however, be compensated for by the preferential transport of all-*E*-β-carotene versus Z-β-carotenes through the Caco-2 cells.

The situation is different with lycopene. With rice cooked with the lycopene-rich gac aril or oil, micellarization and the subsequent uptake by Caco-2 cells were both more efficient with *Z*-lycopenes than with all-*E*-lycopene (Failla et al., 2008). The human serum has been found to contain high levels of *Z*-lycopene isomers (Sakamoto et al., 1994; Schierle et al., 1997), accounting for more than 50% of total lycopene (Stahl et al., 1992), in spite of the absolute predominance of all-*E*-lycopene in foods.

The different isomeric profile of lycopene in foods and plasma has been attributed to better absorption of the Z-isomers of lycopene compared to the all-*E* form because of the shorter length of the bent Z-isomer molecule, making it easier to fit into the micelle (Boileau et al., 2002). Z-lycopene also has greater solubility in mixed micelles and lower tendency to aggregate, thus increasing micellar uptake. It also is possible that Z-lycopene binds more favorably to membrane transporters responsible for the uptake of carotenoids across the brush border membrane of absorptive intestinal cells (During et al., 2005; Reboul et al., 2005).

Isomerization of all-*E* to the *Z*-configuration within the mixed micelles or following incorporation into enterocytes is another possibility. Conversion of all-*E*- to *Z*-isomers of lycopene was reported when lycopene and tomato puree were added to simulated and human gastric fluids (Re et al., 2001) and in a tributyrin model system at gastric pH (Moraru and Lee, 2005), the isomerization being attributed to the acidic condition in the gastric milieu.

A significant increase in the absorption of lycopene, measured in the plasma triacylglycerol-rich lipoprotein fractions, was observed when tomato sauce was enriched in Z-isomers by heat treatment (Unlu et al., 2007b). This was considered in agreement with preferential absorption of Z-lycopene in man. However, the considerable increase in the proportion of lycopene Z-isomers in biological samples could not be explained by this observation alone, probably reflecting an additional in vivo isomerization of the all-*E*- to *Z*-isomers.

Unlu et al. (2007a) reported that absorption of lycopene from tangerine tomato sauce, containing 97% tetra-*Z*- and other *Z*-isomers, was about 2.5 times greater than lycopene absorption from a high β-carotene variety of tomato that contained all-*E*-lycopene as the predominant isomer. The percentage distribution of lycopene Z-isomers in the tangerine tomato sauce was reflected in a similar triacylglycerol-rich lipoprotein response pattern from the human subjects, suggesting minimal isomerization during digestion and absorption. Burri et al. (2009) also conducted a crossover human study with sauces made from tangerine or red tomatoes. Tangerine tomato sauce caused a greater increase of serum lycopene, suggesting that Z-isomers of lycopene might facilitate lycopene absorption.

9.4.4 Carotenoid-carotenoid interaction

It is widely recognized that interactions between carotenoids occur during absorption and postabsorptive metabolism. The most likely explanations for these interactions appeared to be competition for incorporation into micelles, carotenoid exchange between lipoproteins in the postprandial state, and inhibition of provitamin A cleavage (van den Berg, 1999). As already noted by van den Berg in his review of earlier papers, however, much of the evidence continues to be equivocal, with discrepant findings between studies, in magnitude, and/or in the direction of the interactions observed.

Tyssandier et al. (2001) studied specifically the transfer of carotenoids to mixed micelles from emulsion lipid droplets, mimicking dietary lipid emulsions in the human gastrointestinal tract during digestion. The transfer was inversely related to carotenoid hydrophobicity, and maximum between pH 6 and 7 and from 2 mmol/L bile salts. Both carotenes and xanthophylls could impair the transfer of carotenes, but they apparently had no effect on the transfer of lutein.

β-Carotene incorporation into mixed micelles was slightly increased during simulated small intestinal digestion of carotenoid-enriched oil (concentration of lutein sixfold or more greater than β-carotene), or of white maize porridge supplemented with oil (ninefold molar excess of lutein to β-carotene) (Thakkar and Failla, 2008). Mean micellarization efficiencies of β-carotene, β-cryptoxanthin, lutein, and zeaxanthin were 17%, 28%, 30%, and 28%, respectively, during simulated digestion of maize porridge prepared from flours containing 0.4–11.3 μg/g endogenous provitamin A carotenoids. Lutein, however, attenuated uptake of β-carotene by Caco-2 cells from micelles in a dose-dependent manner with inhibition reaching 35% when the molar ratio of lutein to β-cryptoxanthin was 13.

In a Caco-2 cell system, the main carotenoid interactions occurred only between the apolar carotenes (β-carotene with α-carotene and β-carotene with lycopene), suggesting that these hydrocarbon carotenoids with similar structural characteristics could follow similar pathways for their cellular uptake and/or incorporation into chylomicrons. (During et al., 2002; During and Harrison, 2004).

In summarizing earlier work, Castenmiller and West (1998) noted that β-carotene supplementation increased concentrations of α-carotene in a dose-dependent but non-linear manner, and appeared to decrease serum concentrations of lutein, lycopene, and canthaxanthin. Fotouhi et al. (1996), however, found that long-term β-carotene supplementation in men resulted in higher β-carotene concentration in the plasma, without lowering concentrations of other carotenoids (α-carotene, β-cryptoxanthin, lycopene, and lutein).

When combined in the same dose, β-carotene significantly reduced the serum AUC (area under the curve) values for lutein (54%–61% of control values), whereas lutein reduced the AUC value for β-carotene in five subjects but enhanced it in three subjects (Kostic et al., 1995). On the other hand, the ingestion of a combined dose of β-carotene and lycopene did not affect the AUC for β-carotene, but the AUC for lycopene was significantly greater (Johnson et al., 1997). This behavioral difference was attributed to the fact that β-carotene and lycopene are both hydrocarbons, while lutein, as a hydroxylated carotenoid, might have a different absorption mechanism. Van den Berg and Van Vliet (1998) showed in male subjects that lutein, but not lycopene, negatively affected β-carotene absorption when given simultaneously with β-carotene but apparently had no effect on β-carotene cleavage.

In the presence of high amounts of β-carotene, there was preferential uptake of lutein and zeaxanthin from the intestinal lumen into chylomicrons, compared to all-*E*-β-carotene (Gärtner et al., 1996). Gaziano et al. (1995) found that β-carotene supplementation significantly reduced the lycopene concentrations in low-density lipoproteins.

The mean serum total lycopene response to synthetic (Lycovit, BASF, Germany) and tomato-derived lycopene (Lyc-O-Mato, LycoRed Natural Products, Israel) was not significantly different (Hoppe et al., 2003). Neither lycopene source interacted with other serum carotenoids (α-carotene, β-carotene, β-cryptoxanthin, lutein, and zeaxanthin). Supplementation with natural palm oil carotenoids, added to a mixed meal, resulted in significant increases in plasma levels of the supplied carotenoids as compared to the consumption of a low-carotenoid meal (van het Hof et al., 1999b). The relative plasma response was similar to that of synthetic β-carotene, suggesting that the presence of α-carotene did not affect the bioavailability of β-carotene from palm oil.

Ingestion of concurrent doses of β-carotene and canthaxanthin reduced peak serum canthaxanthin, but canthaxanthin did not inhibit the appearance of β-carotene in the serum (White et al., 1994). In another study, a combined dose of β-carotene and canthaxanthin inhibited the appearance of canthaxanthin in plasma, chylomicrons, and VLDL subfractions but did not affect the rapid accumulation of canthaxanthin in LDL within 10 h (Paetau et al., 1997). The appearance of β-carotene in plasma or plasma lipoproteins was not significantly affected.

Adding a second carotenoid to a meal that provided a first carotenoid diminished the chylomicron response to the first carotenoid (Tyssandier et al., 2002). However, this cosupplementation did not diminish the medium-term plasma response to the first carotenoid.

9.4.5 Amount and type of fat

Dietary fat has multiple roles that impact carotenoid bioaccessibility/bioavailability (Furr and Clark, 1997; Yeum and Russell, 2002). It facilitates carotenoid extraction from the food matrix and maintains carotenoid solubility in emulsions during the transfer of gastric chyme to the small intestine. It stimulates the secretion of pancreatic enzymes and bile salts and facilitates the formation of micelles, including serving as structural components of the mixed micelles. It also promotes vitamin A and carotenoid absorption by providing the lipid components for intestinal chylomicron assembly.

Lycopene bioaccessibility clearly depends on the type and the quantity of lipids. Adding 5% lipid to raw tomato pulp improved lycopene bioaccessibility for all the lipids tested (Colle et al., 2012). The largest increase in lycopene bioaccessibility was observed with the addition of 5% sunflower oil, followed by olive oil and cocoa butter. In another study, the addition of olive oil (2%) during digestion, especially as an oil-in-water emulsion, resulted in substantial increase in all-*E*-β-carotene and all-*E*-lycopene bioaccessibility in carrot- and tomato-derived particles, respectively (Moelants et al., 2012).

From sun-dried Tanzanian green leaves (amaranth, cow pea, sweet potato, pumpkin, and cassava) cooked without oil, 8%–29% of the β-carotene content became accessible after in vitro digestion (Hedrén et al., 2002b). Accessibility increased to 39%–94% when the leaves were cooked with sunflower or red palm oil. Adding red palm oil instead of sunflower oil resulted in about twice as much accessible β-carotene. In a subsequent study, the amount of in vitro accessible all-*E*-β-carotene in green leafy vegetables cooked without oil by traditional and an improved method ranged from 5% to 12% and 4% to 15%, respectively (Mulokozi et al., 2004). The same vegetables cooked with the improved method with oil had 2–5 times higher amount of accessible all-*E*-β-carotene. Chandrika et al. (2006) also demonstrated the importance of the addition of fat during cooking of Sri Lankan green leafy vegetables. Addition of peanut oil (5%) increased micellarization of both β-carotene and lutein from drumstick leaves (Pullakhandam and Failla, 2007).

In vitro transfer of α-carotene, β-carotene, and lycopene from chyme to mixed micelles during digestion requires minimal (0.5%–1%) lipid content in the meal and is affected by the length of fatty acyl chains but not the degree of unsaturation in the triacylglycerol (Huo et al., 2007). Relatively low amounts of triolein and canola oil (0.5%–1%) were required for maximum micellarization of carotenes, but more oil (~2.5%) was required when triacylglycerol with medium chain saturated fatty acyl groups (e.g., trioctanoin and coconut oil) was added to the test salad. In contrast, fatty acyl chain length had limited or no impact on carotenoid uptake by Caco-2 cells.

Lutein and zeaxanthin provided by sweet corn and spinach in a test meal had greater bioaccessibility (about 20%–30%) with butter and palm oil than with olive and fish oils (Gleize et al., 2013). The results suggested that saturated fatty acids improved the bioaccessibility of these carotenoids. There was no significant effect of the type of triacylglycerol fatty acid on xanthophyll uptake by Caco-2 cells.

The percentage of accessible all-*E*-β-carotene in the micellar phase (fraction of carotenoids transferred from the food matrix to a micellar phase obtained by microfiltration) varied from 0.5% to 1.1% in heat-processed orange-fleshed sweet potato without fat and between 11% and 22% with the addition of 2.5% cooking oil (Bengtsson et al., 2009). The percentage of accessible all-*E*-β-carotene in the supernatant phase (obtained after low-speed centrifugation) was significantly higher: 24% to 41% without fat and 28% to 46% with fat.

Adding lipids prior to processing clearly enhanced the lycopene bioaccessibility. The type of lipid added was of minor importance compared to the process conditions applied (Colle et al., 2013). High-pressure homogenization (HPH) or microwave heating of tomato pulp in the presence of lipids for 20 min at 70°C and 90°C did not improve the lycopene bioaccessibility significantly. When HPH was applied prior to the heat treatment, microwave heating at 90°C could improve the lycopene bioaccessibility. It is hypothesised that HPH damages the cellular barriers for lycopene bioaccessibility, which can be further disrupted by thermal processing, improving lycopene release during digestion. Finally, heating for 20 min at 120°C as such facilitated the lycopene bioaccessibility remarkably. HPH preceding this thermal treatment was of no extra value in terms of lycopene bioaccessibility.

The importance of dietary fat in the absorption of β-carotene and its bioconversion to vitamin A is well established (Prince and Frisoli, 1993; Jalal et al., 1998; Takyi, 1999;

Ribaya-Mercado, 2002). An increase in dietary fat content resulted in higher serum β-carotene concentration in young subjects within 8 and 24 hours post-β-carotene administration (Shiau et al., 1994).

Both the amount and type of fat affect the bioavailability of some (i.e., lutein) but not all carotenoids (Borel et al., 1998; Roodenburg et al., 2000). Borel (1998) showed that incorporation of β-carotene into chylomicrons was markedly low when men ingested β-carotene with medium-chain rather than long-chain triacylglycerols. Carotenoid absorption from raw vegetable salads with a moderate amount of dietary fat is likely to be greatest when consumed in one meal rather than smaller doses over multiple meals (Goltz et al., 2013).

Essentially no absorption of carotenoids was observed when salads with fat-free salad dressing were consumed (M.J. Brown et al., 2004). A substantially greater absorption of carotenoids was observed when salads were consumed with full-fat than reduced-fat salad dressings. The addition of avocado to salsa enhanced lycopene and β-carotene absorption, resulting in 4.4 and 2.6 times the mean AUC after intake of avocado-free salsa, respectively (Unlu et al., 2005). Likewise, addition of 150 g avocado or 24 g avocado oil to salad enhanced the absorption of α-carotene, β-carotene, and lutein, resulting in 7.2, 15.3, and 5.1 times the mean AUC after intake of avocado-free salad, respectively. This enhancement of the carotenoid absorption was attributed primarily to the lipids in avocado. The appearance of β-carotene in chylomicrons and in VLDL subfractions was lower after ingestion of a meal containing sunflower oil than after ingestion of a meal containing beef tallow (Hu et al., 2000).

Only a small amount of fat in the diet is needed to improve the bioavailability of provitamin A carotenoids from plant foods. Jalal et al. (1998) indicated that the cutoff point is between 3 and 5 g of fat. A larger amount of fat was required for a comparable amount of lutein esters (Roodenburg et al., 2000).

9.4.6 Amount and type of dietary fiber

The low bioavailability of carotenoids in plant foods is often explained, at least in part, by the presence of dietary fiber. Studies verifying this effect, however, are lacking.

Several explanations have been raised for this role (Palafox-Carlos et al., 2011): (a) Dietary fiber may impede the release of carotenoids from the food matrix. (b) It may entrap lipids and bile salts, thereby avoiding micelle formation with carotenoids. (c) It increases the viscosity of the intestinal content, resulting in reduced absorption because of the slowing down of enzymatic activity in the pancreas and increased difficulty in contacting intestinal enterocytes.

The amount of β-carotene transferred to the micelle fraction during simulated digestion increased significantly as the fruit ripened (Ornelas-Paz et al., 2008). Qualitative and quantitative changes that occur in pectin of the mango pulp during ripening influenced the efficiency of micellarization of β-carotene.

In another in vitro study, there was a significant correlation between small intestine availability of lutein and β-carotene and the content of Klason lignin, nonstarch polysaccharide, and resistant protein of green vegetables (Serrano et al., 2005). According to the authors, the nondigestible compounds might directly affect the intestinal carotenoid availability because they could act as a barrier to the action of digestive enzymes and to the release of carotenoids from the food matrix.

Citrus pectin reduced β-carotene absorption and plasma β-carotene levels significantly in humans (Rock and Swendseid, 1992). Oat β-glucan, a different type of soluble fiber, did not have the same effect as citrus pectin (Deming and Erdman, 1999).

The mean AUC over 24 h of β-carotene was significantly reduced by the water-soluble fibers pectin, guar, and alginate with a mean decrease of 33%–43% (Riedl et al., 1999). All tested fibers also significantly reduced the AUC of lycopene and lutein by 40%–74%; the effect on canthaxanthin was almost significant.

In a three-week intervention trial, no effect on the serum β-carotene or lutein responses could be observed from the addition of dietary fiber (prepared from sugar beet) to enzymatically liquefied spinach (Castenmiller et al., 1999). This suggested that once the cell wall components are broken down, addition of dietary fiber in amounts previously found in the food has no effect on carotenoid bioavailability.

9.4.7 Other food constituents

The addition of grapefruit juice significantly decreased the bioaccessibility (up to 30%) but not the Caco-2 cellular uptake of β-carotene from boiled orange-fleshed sweet potato (Poulaert et al., 2012). Lycopene, but more probably naringin, of the grapefruit juice was suspected to be responsible for this inhibitory effect, apparently due in part to competition for incorporation between β-carotene and naringin into mixed micelles during in vitro digestion.

Studying the influence of antioxidant spices (turmeric and onion) and food acidulants (amchur, lime, tamarind, kokum), Veda et al. (2008) observed that turmeric significantly enhanced the bioaccessibility of β-carotene from all of the vegetables tested, especially when heat processed. Onion enhanced β-carotene bioaccessibility from pressure-cooked carrot and amaranth and from open-pan-boiled pumpkin and fenugreek leaf.

Both plant-free sterols and sterol esters reduced the bioavailability of β-carotene by ~50% in normocholesterolemic men (Richelle et al., 2004). The reduction was significantly less with free sterols than with sterol esters.

Lutein response in the chylomicron-rich fraction in men was weakest after ingestion of a meal containing the antioxidants vitamin C, vitamin E, and polyphenols (Reboul et al., 2007). When the effect of each class of antioxidants and potential interactions was evaluated, a mixture of carotenoids (lycopene plus β-carotene) significantly impaired lutein uptake, while vitamins C and E (at physiological concentrations) had no significant effect. Subsequent experiments showed that the aglycone flavanone naringenin was the only polyphenol responsible for the effect of the polyphenol mixture.

The presence of milk or milk-derived peptides (i.e., casein phosphopeptides) and milk plus iron in fruit juices (orange, peach, grape juice) did not influence the bioavailability of carotenoids from the juices in women (Granado-Lorencio et al., 2009).

The addition of tomato puree to spinach did not decrease lutein plasma concentration (Riso et al., 2004).

9.4.8 Processing

Although processing, especially thermal processing, can substantially decrease the carotenoid content, an increasing number of in vitro and human studies have shown that it can increase the carotenoid bioaccessibility/bioavailability. The magnitude of such increase depends on the cooking/processing conditions.

9.4.8.1 Home cooking

Food processing such as grinding, fermentation, and mild heating may increase bioavailability, most likely as a result of disruption of the cell walls of plant tissues, dissociation of the nutrient or bioactive compound-matrix complexes, or transformation into more active molecular structures (Parada and Aguilera, 2007).

Investigating β-carotene, lycopene, β-cryptoxanthin, and lutein in zucchini, red pepper, and tomato, micellarization varied from 1.7% to 100% depending on the food, carotenoid, and cooking method (boiling, steaming, grilling, or microwave-cooking) (Ryan et al., 2008).

Crushing or homogenization of tomatoes in itself was not enough to increase the in vitro accessibility of lycopene (Tibäck et al., 2009). However, when intense crushing was followed by heat treatment, in the form of either a heat shock or boiling, the lycopene accessibility increased significantly.

Bioaccessibility strongly depended on the particle size in raw (cut and blended) and gently cooked (boiling for 3 min) carrots (Lemmens et al., 2010). Intense cooking (boiling for 25 min) released a considerable amount of all-*E*-β-carotene from cell fragments (smaller than a cell) as well as from small and large cell clusters. In another study, cooked carrot puree (consisting primarily of single plant cell particles) had the highest release of carotenes and Caco-2 cell uptake, followed by blanched carrots (consisting primarily of plant cell clusters) and raw carrot puree (consisting of larger plant cell clusters) (Netzel et al., 2011).

Bioaccessibility varied substantially from the raw to the cooked/processed vegetables: α-carotene from 1.6% to 14% and β-carotene from 2.6% to14% for carrot juice; β-carotene from 2.4% to 17% and lutein from 38% to 48% for boiled spinach; lycopene from <0.1% to 6.0% in processed tomato (Reboul et al., 2006). Even in the same food, bioaccessibility percentages varied in different studies, although the trend is the same (i.e., greater bioaccesibility of cooked food compared to the raw food). According to Hedrén et al. (2002a), homogenization released 21% of the total β-carotene content of carrot. Cooking the pulp increased the accessibility to 27%. Addition of cooking oil to the cooked pulp increased the released amount to 39%. The trend is similar for α-carotene. In Hornero-Méndez and Mínguez-Mosquera (2007), micellarization was 52% from cooked carrots and 29% from raw carrots. Addition of olive oil resulted in higher amounts of micellarized carotenes (80%). These differences can be attributed mainly to differing conditions during processing and during the in vitro assay of bioaccessibility. Boiling spinach for 20 min at 98°C decreased the carotenoid contents, but this was compensated by significantly better micellarization from 15-fold for β-carotene to 72-fold for lutein (Courraud et al., 2013).

Conventional boiling (10 min at 100°C) decreased the carotenoid content in some samples of chili peppers; however, the micellar content was generally not lower for processed peppers, indicating that bioaccessibility of carotenoids from processed peppers is enhanced in relation to unprocessed peppers (Pugliese et al., 2013). Freezing increased the bioaccessiblity of β-cryptoxanthin in all of 13 cultivars of red chili peppers (Pugliese et al., 2014a). It also increased the bioaccessibility of capsanthin, β-carotene, zeaxanthin, antheraxanthin, and violaxanthin in most cultivars. Boiling increased the bioaccessibility of β-cryptoxanthin, but for the other carotenoids, bioaccessibility was increased in some cultivars and decreased in others. Red peppers had higher carotenoid content and bioaccessibility than either orange or yellow peppers (Pugliese et al., 2014b). Xanthophylls showed greater bioaccessibility than carotenes.

Percentage bioaccessibility of β-carotene ranged from 6.7 in fenugreek leaves to 20 in carrot (Veda et al., 2006). Pressure-cooking increased the β-carotene bioaccessibility by 100%, 48%, and 19% from fenugreek leaves, amaranth leaves, and carrots, respectively. Stir-frying in the presence of a small amount of oil led to an enormous increase in the β-carotene bioaccessibility: 263% for fenugreek leaves, 192% for amaranth leaves, 63% for carrot, and 53% for pumpkin.

The efficiency of micellarization of all-*E*- and *Z*-isomers of β-carotene was 25%–30% for boiled cassava and gari (roasted cassava granules), independent of the cultivar (Thakkar et al., 2009). Micellarization of β-carotene from fermented and cooked fufu cassava paste was only 12%–15%. Gari and fufu are traditional African foods. Fried cassava roots showed higher micellarization efficiency for total carotenoid and all-*E*-β-carotene (14% for both), compared with boiled samples (Gomes et al., 2013).

The efficiency of micellarization of all-*E*-β-carotene was 50% for sweet potato with oil added after homogenization and boiling, 48% for porridge with oil added to the milled flour from freeze-dried roots before cooking, 31% for porridge with oil added after cooking of flour, and 16% for sweet potato that was pureed and oil was added after boiling (Bengtsson et al., 2010).

Notably, cellular transport (cellular uptake plus secretion by Caco-2 cells) of lutein was reported to be generally greater from uncooked spinach rather than cooked spinach, irrespective of whether it was fresh, frozen, or canned (O'Sullivan et al., 2008). There was no significant difference in the micellarization of lutein between the cooking (boiling or microwave cooking) and processing methods (freezing, canning).

Microwave thawing of ultrafrozen orange juice caused a significant decrease in the provitamin A carotenoids, lutein, and zeaxanthin but increased their bioaccessibility (Stinco et al., 2013).

For yellow corn meal, micellarization efficiency of xanthophylls was similar from extruded puff (63%) and bread (69%), lower from porridge (48%) (Kean et al., 2008). For whole yellow cornmeal products, xanthophyll micellarization was highest in bread (85%) and similar in extruded puff (46%) and porridge (47%). β-carotene micellarization for extruded puffs and breads was 10%–23% but higher in porridge (40%–43%).

In humans, the bioavailability of lycopene was shown to be greater from cooked or processed tomato then from fresh tomato. Uptake of lycopene and its geometric isomers was greater from boiled tomato juice (1 h with 1% corn oil) than from unprocessed tomato juice (Stahl and Sies, 1992).

In a three-week dietary intervention, the enzymatic disruption of cell walls in liquefied spinach significantly increased the serum β-carotene response, compared to that of whole and minced spinach preparations (Castenmiller et al., 1999). Serum lutein responses were higher than those of β-carotene and were not influenced by the changes in the vegetable matrix. The lower plasma appearance of β-carotene could be due to its cleavage to retinol. With intrinsically labeled carotenoids in kale, however, it was shown that the bioavailability of β-carotene was lower than that of lutein, even when the conversion to retinol is considered (Novotny et al., 2005). [^{13}C]lutein AUC was three times greater than [^{13}C]β-carotene AUC and 1.6 times greater than [^{13}C]β-carotene plus [^{13}C]retinol AUC.

9.4.8.2 Industrial processing

Industrial extraction of orange juice reduced the particle size (volume and surface area mean diameter) and increased the bioaccessibility of carotenoids (Stinco et al., 2013). The carotenoid bioaccessibility was greater from the industrially extracted than from the homemade juice.

Page et al. (2012) reported that lycopene accessibility from tomato puree was not strictly related to tissue disruption. It was linked to the kinetics of the heat treatment: rapid temperature rise in hot-break treatment led to greater bioaccessibility than did slow temperature rise. In another study, thermal processing improved the bioaccessibility of lycopene in tomato pulp, but the improvement was significant only at temperatures of 130°C and 140°C (Colle et al., 2010a).

Tomato juice subjected to high-pressure processing (500-700 MPa, 30°C), pressure-assisted thermal processing (500–700 MPa, 100°C), and thermal processing (0.1 MPa, 100°C) showed significantly higher all-*E*-β-carotene micellarization as compared to the raw unprocessed juice, the amount of micellarized all-*E*-β-carotene not differing significantly among the treatments (Gupta et al., 2011). Lycopene micellarization was limited regardless of the processing method used (below 0.5%). Microscopic evaluation revealed that the treatments were not severe enough to solubilize the lycopene crystals and facilitate its micellarization.

An inverse relationship between the homogenization pressure, and thus the tomato network strength, and the lycopene bioaccessibility was observed in tomato pulp (Colle et al., 2010b). Thermal processing (90°C, 30 min), subsequent to high-pressure homogenization, was not able to sufficiently decrease the strength of the fiber network in order to improve lycopene bioaccessibility. High-pressure homogenization (HPH) (100 bar) or microwave heating of tomato pulp in the presence of lipids during 20 min at 70°C and 90°C did not improve lycopene bioaccessibility significantly (Colle et al., 2013). HPH applied prior to microwave heating at 90°C could improve lycopene bioaccessibility. The authors hypothesized that HPH damaged the cellular barriers for lycopene bioaccessiblity, which could be further disrupted by thermal processing, thereby improving lycopene release during digestion. Microwave heating at 120°C for 20 min as such facilitated lycopene bioaccessibility remarkably.

In another recent paper, HPH decreased the particle size due to matrix disruption and increased product consistency due to the formation of a fiber network (Panozzo et al., 2013). It also resulted in a decrease of in vitro bioaccessibility of lycopene, ζ-carotene, and lutein, which was attributed to a structuring effect of HPH.

HPH of carrot puree could improve β-carotene bioaccessibility by disrupting cells, but only at a pressure higher than 50 MPa (Knockaert et al., 2012a). A subsequent thermal pasteurization resulted in further increase in β-carotene bioaccessibility by softening of the cell walls. The high temperature also induced formation of *Z*-isomers. In high-pressure homogenized tomato puree containing oil, lycopene bioaccessibility decreased during subsequent thermal or high-pressure processing (Knockaert et al., 2012b).

In contrast to the thermally treated samples, almost no β-carotene isomerization was observed in the high-pressure processed carrot (Knockaert et al., 2011). However, the effect of high pressure on β-carotene bioaccessibility was dependent on the intensity of the process. Going from mild to strong pasteurization then to sterilization, the β-carotene bioaccessibility of the high-pressure-treated samples changed from 1.2 times higher, to over 1.2 times lower, then to 2.5 times lower than that of the thermally treated samples.

Extrusion cooking reduced the lycopene content of extruded snacks enriched with tomato derivatives, but the proportion of bioaccessible lycopene increased (Dehghan-Shoar et al., 2011). Lycopene uptake by Caco-2 cells from the extruded snacks exceeded by 5% that of the control in which lycopene was not extruded.

Ultrasound treatment at 24 kHz and 100 μm caused loss of tomato cell integrity, a decrease in the degree of pectin esterification, and a marked decrease in lycopene bioaccessibility (Anese et al., 2013). It was inferred that the decrease in bioaccessibility was due to the formation of a new network through hydrogen bonding and hydrophobic interactions among the de-esterified pectin molecules, entrapping lycopene in the matrix and making it less accessible for digestion.

Both high-pressure processing (400 MPa, 40°C, 5 min) and thermal treatment (90°C, 30 sec) resulted in significant decrease of carotenoid bioaccessibility from milk- (whole and skimmed milk) and soy-based fruit (orange, kiwi, pineapple, and mango juices) beverages (Cilla et al., 2012). High-pressure-processed samples showed higher carotenoid bioaccesibility than thermally treated samples.

Caco-2 cell studies indicated that emulsifiers preferentially accelerated the absorption of the nonesterified form of β-cryptoxanthin (Takaishi et al., 2012). In human trials, emulsified β-cryptoxanthin maintained higher serum β-cryptoxanthin levels than that from satsuma mandarin juice or satsuma mandarin fruit. The AUC of emulsified β-cryptoxanthin was 1.6 and 1.8 times higher than those of the satsuma mandarin juice and fruit, respectively.

In canned tomatoes, mechanical homogenization enhanced the lycopene and β-carotene responses significantly, both in triacylglycerol-rich lipoproteins and plasma (van het Hof et al., 2000a). Additional heating also tended to enhance the responses. It was concluded that the intactness of the cellular matrix of tomatoes determined the bioavailability of carotenoids and that matrix disruption by mechanical homogenization and/or heat treatment enhances the bioavailability. Ingestion of tomato paste yielded 2.5-fold higher total and all-*E*-lycopene peak concentrations and 3.8-fold higher AUC responses than ingestion of fresh tomatoes (Gärtner et al., 1997).

Carotenoid mass-balanced calculations after ingestion of a single meal by ileostomy volunteers indicated a higher absorption and plasma response of beta-carotene from cooked pureed carrot meals (65%) than from raw chopped carrots (41%) (Livny et al.,

2003). Daily consumption of processed carrots and spinach over a 4-week period resulted in an increase in plasma β-carotene concentration that averaged three times that obtained with the consumption of the same amount of β-carotene from these vegetables in the raw form (Rock et al., 1998).

Using an extrinsic stable isotope reference method, absorption of β-carotene and α-carotene was found to be approximately twofold greater in commercial carrot puree (baby food) than in boiled mashed carrot (Edwards et al., 2002). Retinol yield was only marginally affected by the different treatment. Carotene and retinol ester absorption from raw grated carrot was intermediate and not significantly different from the processed/cooked preparations.

Modified atmosphere packaging did not affect significantly the bioavailability of carotenoids and tocopherols from broccoli in humans (Granado-Lorencio et al., 2008).

References

Anese M, Mirolo G, Beraldo P, Lippe G. 2013. Effect of ultrasound treatments of tomato pulp on microstructure and lycopene in vitro bioaccessibility. *Food Chem* 136:458–63.

Asai A, Yonekura L, Nagao A. 2008. Low bioavailability of dietary epoxyxanthophylls in humans. *Brit J Nutr* 100:273–7.

Bechoff A, Poulaert M, Tomlins KI, Westby A, Menya G, Young S, Dhuique-Mayer C. 2011. Retention and bioaccessibility of β-carotene in blended foods containing orange-fleshed sweet potato flour. *J Agric Food Chem* 59:10373–80.

Ben-Amotz A, Levy Y. 1996. Bioavailability of a natural mixture compared with synthetic all-trans β-carotene in human serum. *Am J Clin Nutr* 63:729–34.

Bengtsson A, Alminger ML, Svanberg U. 2009. In vitro bioaccessibility of β-carotene from heat-processed orange-fleshed sweet potato. *J Agric Food Chem* 57:9693–8.

Bengtsson A, Brackmann C, Enejder A, Alminger ML, Svanberg U. 2010. Effects of thermal processing on the in vitro bioaccessibility and microstructure of β-carotene in orange-fleshed sweet potato. *J Agric Food Chem* 58:11090–6.

Biehler E, Kaulmann A, Hoffmann L, Krause E, Bohn T. 2011. Dietary and host-related factors influencing carotenoid bioaccessibility from spinach (*Spinacia oleracea*). *Food Chem* 125:1328–34.

Blanquet-Diot S, Soufi M, Rambeau M, Rock E, Alric M. 2009. Digestive stability of xanthophylls exceeds that of carotenes as studied in a dynamic in vitro gastrointestinal system. *J Nutr* 139:876–83.

Boileau TW-M, Boileau AC, Erdman JW Jr. 2002. Bioavailability of all-trans and cis-isomers of lycopene. *Exp Biol Med* 227:914–9.

Boileau TWM, Moore AC, Erdman JW Jr. 1999. Carotenoids and vitamin A. In: Papas AM. editor. *Antioxidant status, diet, nutrition, and health*. Washington DC: CRC Press, p 133–58.

Borel P, Grolier P, Armand M, Partier A, Lafont H, Lairon D, Azais Braesco V. 1996. Carotenoids in biological emulsions: solubility, surface-to-core distribution, and release from lipid droplets. *J Lipid Res* 37:250–61.

Borel P, Lietz G, Goncalves A, de Edelenyi FS, Lecompte S, Curtis P, Goumidi L, Caslake MJ, Miles EA, Packard C, Calder PC, Mathers JC, Minihane AM, Tourniaire F, Kesse-Guyot E, Galan P, Hercberg S, Breidenassel C, Gross MG, Moussa M, Meirhaeghe A, Reboul E. 2013. CD36 and SR-BI are involved in cellular uptake of provitamin A carotenoids by Caco-2 and HEK cells, and some of their genetic variants are associated with plasma concentrations of these micronutrients in humans. *J. Nutr.* 143:448–56.

Borel P, Tyssandier V, Mekki N, Grolier P, Rochette Y, Alexander-Gouabau MC, Lairon D, Azaïs-Braesco V. 1998. Chylomicron β-carotene and retinyl palmitate responses are dramatically diminished when men ingest β-carotene with medium rather than long-chain triglycerides. *J Nutr* 128:1361–7.

Bowen PE, Herbst-Espinosa SM, Hussain EA, Stacewicz-Sapuntzakis M. 2002. Esterification does not impair lutein bioavailability in humans. *J Nutr* 132:3668–73.

Breithaupt DE, Alpmann A, Carrière F. 2007. Xanthophyll esters are hydrolyzed in the presence of recombinant human pancreatic lipase. *Food Chem* 103:651–6.

Breithaupt DE, Bamedi A, Wirt U. 2002. Carotenol fatty acid esters: easy substrates for digestive enzymes? *Comp Biochem Physiol B* 132:721–8.

Breithaupt DE, Weller P, Wolters M, Hahn A. 2003. Plasma response to a single dose of dietary β-cryptoxanthin esters from papaya (*Carica papaya* L.) or non-esterified β-cryptoxanthin in adult human subjects: a comparative study. *Br J Nutr* 90:795–801.

Brown ED, Micozzi MS, Craft NE, Bieri JG, Beecher G, Edwards BK, Rose A, Taylor PR, Smith JC Jr. 1989. Plasma carotenoids in normal men after a single ingestion of vegetables or purified beta-carotene. *Am J Clin Nutr* 49:1258–65.

Brown MJ, Ferruzi MG, Nguyen ML, Cooper DA, Eldridge A. L. Schwartz SJ, White WS. 2004. Carotenoid bioavailability is higher from salads ingested with full-fat than with fat-reduced salad dressings as measured with electrochemical detection. *Am J Clin Nutr* 80:396–403.

Bulux J, Serrano JQ, Giuliano AR, Perez CYL, Rivera C, Solomons NW, Canfield LM. 1994. Plasma response of children to short-term chronic β-carotene supplementation. *Am J Clin Nutr* 59:1369–75.

Burri BJ, Chapman MH, Neidlinger TR, Seo JS, Ishida BK. 2009. Tangerine tomatoes increase total and tetra-cis-lycopene isomer concentrations more than red tomatoes in healthy adult humans. *Int J Food Sci Nutr* 60(s1):1–16.

Castenmiller JJM, West CE. 1998. Bioavailability and bioconversion of carotenoids. *Annu Rev Nutr* 18:19–38.

Castenmiller JJM, West CE, Linssen JPH, van het Hof KH, Voragen AGJ. 1999. The food matrix of spinach is a limiting factor in determining the bioavailability of β-carotene and to a lesser extent of lutein in humans. *J Nutr* 129:349–55.

Chandrika UG, Svanberg U, Jansz ER. 2006. In vitro accessibility of β-carotene from cooked Sri Lankan green leafy vegetables and their estimated contribution to vitamin A requirement. *J Sci Food Agric* 86:54–61.

Chitchumroonchokchai C, Failla ML. 2006. Hydrolysis of zeaxanthin esters by carboxyl ester lipase during digestion facilitates micellarization and uptake of the xanthophyll by Caco-2 human intestinal cells. *J Nutr* 136:588–94.

Chitchumroonchokchai C, Schwartz SJ, Failla ML. 2004. Assessment of lutein bioavailability from meals and a supplement using simulated digestion and Caco-2 human intestinal cells. *J Nutr* 134:2280–6.

Chung H-Y, Rasmussen HM, Johnson EJ. 2004. Lutein bioavailability is higher from lutein-enriched eggs than from supplements and spinach in men. *J Nutr* 134:1887–93.

Cilla A, Alegría A, de Ancos B, Sánchez-Moreno C, Cano MP, Plaza L, Clemente G, Lagarda MJ, Barberá R. 2012. Bioaccessibility of tocopherols, carotenoids, and ascorbic acid from milk- and soy-based fruit beverages: influence of food matrix and processing. *J Agric Food Chem* 60:7282–90.

Colle IJP, Lemmens L, van Buggenhout S, Met K, van Loey AM, Hendrickx ME. 2013. Processing tomato pulp in the presence of lipids: the impact on lycopene bioaccessibility. *Food Res Int* 51:32–8.

Colle I, Lemmens L, van Buggenhout S, van Loey A, Hendrickx M. 2010a. Effect of thermal processing on degradation, isomerization, and bioaccessibility of lycopene in tomato pulp. *J Food Sci* 75:C753–59.

Colle IJP, van Buggenhout S, Lemmens L, van Loey AM, Hendrickx ME. 2012. The type and quantity of lipids present during digestion influence the in vitro bioaccessibility of lycopene from raw tomato pulp. *Food Res Int* 45:250–5.

Colle I, van Buggenhout S, van Loey A, Hendrickx M. 2010b. High pressure homogenization followed by thermal processing of tomato pulp: influence on microstructure and lycopene in vitro bioaccessibility. *Food Res Int* 43:2193–200.

Courraud J, Berger J, Cristol J-P, Avallone S. 2013. Stability and bioaccessibility of different forms of carotenoids and vitamin A during in vitro digestion. *Food Chem* 136:871–7.

Daly T, Jiwan MA, O'Brien NM, Aherne SA. 2010. Carotenoid content of commonly consumed herbs and assessment of their bioaccessibility using an in vitro digestion model. *Plant Foods Hum Nutr* 65:164–9.

Dehghan-Shoar Z, Mandimika T, Hardacre AK, Reynolds GW, Brennan CS. 2011. Lycopene bioaccessibility and starch digestibility for extruded snacks enriched with tomato derivatives. *J Agric Food Chem* 59:12047–53.

Deming, D M, Erdman, J W Jr. (1999). Mammalian carotenoid absorption and metabolism. *Pure Appl Chem* 71:2213–23.

Dhuique-Mayer C, Borel P, Reboul E, Caporiccio B, Besancon P, Amiot M-J. 2007. β-Cryptoxanthin from *Citrus* juices: assessment of bioaccessibility using an in vitro digestion/Caco-2 cell culture model. *Brit J Nutr* 97:883–90.

During A. 2008. Bioavailability of natural pigments. In: Socaciu C. editor. *Food colorants. chemical and functional properties*. Boca Raton: Taylor and Francis Goup, p 147–75.
During A, Dawson HD, Harrison EH. 2005. Carotenoid transport is decreased and expression of the lipid transporters SR-BI, NPC1L1, and ABCA1 is down-regulated in Caco-2 cells treated with ezetimibe. *J Nutr* 135:2305–12.
During A, Harrison EH. 2004. Intestinal absorption and metabolism of carotenoids: insights from cell culture. *Arch Biochem Biophys* 430:77–88.
During A, Hussain MM, Morel DW, Harrison EH. 2002. Carotenoid uptake and secretion by Caco-2 cells: β-carotene isomer selectivity and carotenoid interactions. *J Lipid Res* 43:1086–95.
Edwards AJ, Nguyen CH, You C-S, Swanson JE, Emenhiser C, Parker RS. 2002. α- and β-carotene from a commercial carrot puree are more bioavailable to humans than from boiled-mashed carrots, as determined using an extrinsic stable isotope reference method. *J Nutr* 132:159–167.
Ekesa B, Poulaert M, Davey MW, Kimiywe J, van den Bergh I, Blomme G, Dhuique-Mayer C. 2012. Bioiaccessibility of provitamin A carotenoids in banana (*Musa* spp.) and derived dishes in African countries. *Food Chem* 133:1471–7.
Evans M, Beck M, Elliott J, Etheve S, Roberts R, Schalch W. 2012. Effects of formulation on the bioavailability of lutein and zeaxanthin: a randomized, double-blind, cross-over, comparative, single-dose study in healthy subjects. Eur J Nutr. Epub 2012 Sep 30.
Failla ML, Chitchumroonchokchai C, Ishida BK. 2008. In vitro micellarization and intestinal cell uptake of *cis* isomers of lycopene exceed those of all-*trans* lycopene. *J Nutr* 138:482–6.
Ferruzzi MG, Lumpkin JL, Schwartz SJ, Failla M. 2006. Digestive stability, micellarization, and uptake of β-carotene isomers by Caco-2 human intestinal cells. *J Agric Food Chem* 54:2780–5.
Fleshman MK, Lester GE, Riedl KM, Kopec RE, Narayanasamy S, Curley RW Jr, Schwartz SJ, Harrison EH. 2011. Carotene and novel apocarotenoid concentrations in orange-fleshed *Cucumis melo* melons: determinations of β-carotene bioaccessibility and bioavailability. *J Agric Food Chem* 59:4448–54.
Fotouhi N, Meydani M, Santos MS, Meydani SN, Hennekens CH, Gaziano JM. 1996. Carotenoid and tocopherol concentrations in plasma, peripheral blood mononuclear cells, and red blood cells after long-term beta-carotene supplementation in men. *Am J Clin Nutr* 63:553–8.
Furr HC, Clark RM. 1997. Intestinal absorption and tissue distribution of carotenoids. *J Nutr Biochem* 8:364–77.
Garrett DA, Failla ML, Sarama RJ. 1999a. Development of an in vitro digestion method to assess carotenoid bioavailability from meals. *J Agric Food Chem* 47:4301–9.
Garrett DA, Failla ML, Sarama RJ. 2000. Estimation of carotenoid bioavailability from fresh stir-fried vegetables using an in vitro digestion/Caco-2 cell culture model. *J Nutr Biochem* 11:547–80.
Garrett DA, Failla ML, Sarama RJ, Craft N. 1999b. Accumulation and retention of micellar β-carotene and lutein by Caco-2 human intestinal cells. *J Nutr Biochem* 10:573–81.
Gärtner C, Stahl W, Sies H. 1996. Preferential increase in chylomicron levels of the xanthophylls lutein and zeaxanthin compared to β-carotene in the human. *Int J Vit Nutr Res* 66:119–25.
Gärtner C, Stahl W, Sies H. 1997. Lycopene is more bioavailable from tomato paste than from fresh tomatoes. *Am J Clin Nutr* 66:116–22.
Gaziano JM, Johnson EJ, Russell RM, Manson JE, Stampfer MJ, Ridker PM, Frei B, Hennekens CH, Krinsky NI. 1995. Discrimination in absorption or transport of beta-carotene isomers after oral supplementation with either all-trans- or 9-cis-beta-carotene. *Am J Clin Nutr* 61:1248–52.
Gleize B, Tourniaire F, Depezay L, Bott R, Nowicki M, Albino L, Lairon D, Kesse-Guyot E, Galan P, Hercberg S, Borel P. 2013. Effect of type of TAG fatty acids on lutein and zeaxanthin bioavailability. *Brit J Nutr* 110:1–10.
Goltz SR, Sapper TN, Failla ML, Campbell WW, Ferruzzi MG. 2013. Carotenoid bioavailability from raw vegetables and a moderate amount of oil in human subjects is greatest when the majority of daily vegetables are consumed at one meal. *Nutr Res* 33:358–66.
Gomes S, Torres AG, Godoy R, Pacheco S, Carvalho J, Nutti M. 2013. Effects of boiling and frying on the bioaccessibility of β-carotene in yellow-fleshed cassava roots (*Manihot esculenta* Crantz cv. BRS Jari). *Food Nutr Bull* 34:65–74.
Goñi I, Serrano J, Saura-Calixto F. 2006. Bioaccessibility of β-carotene, lutein, and lycopene from fruits and vegetables. *J Agric Food Chem* 54:5382–7.
Granado-Lorencio F, Herrero-Barbudo C, Blanco-Navarro I, Pérez-Sacristán B, Olmedilla-Alonso B. 2009. Bioavailability of carotenoids and α-tocopherol from fruit juices in the presence of absorption modifiers: in vitro and in vivo assessment. *Brit J Nutr* 101:576–82.

Granado-Lorencio F, Olmedilla-Alonso B, Herrero-Barbudo C, Blanco-Navarro I, Pérez-Sacristán B, Blázquez-García S. 2007a. In vitro bioaccessibility of carotenoids and tocopherols from fruits and vegetables. *Food Chem* 102:641–8.

Granado-Lorencio F, Olmedilla-Alonso B, Herrero-Barbudo C, Pérez-Sacristán B, Blanco-Navarro I, Blázquez-García S. 2007b. Comparative in vitro bioaccessibility of carotenoids from relevant contributors to carotenoid intake. *J Agric Food Chem* 55:6387–94.

Granado-Lorencio F, Olmedilla-Alonso B, Herrero-Barbudo C, Sánchez-Moreno C, de Ancos B, Martínez JA, Pérez-Sacristán B, Blanco-Navarro I. 2008. Modified- atmosphere packaging (MAP) does not affect the bioavailability of tocopherols and carotenoids from broccoli in humans: a cross-over study. *Food Chem* 106:1070–6.

Gupta R, Kopec RE, Schwartz SJ, Balasubramanian VM. 2011. Combined pressure-temperature effects on carotenoid retention and bioaccessibility in tomato juice. *J Agric Food Chem* 59:7808–17.

Hedrén E, Diaz V, Svanberg U. 2002a. Estimation of carotenoid accessibility from carrots determined by in vitro digestion method. *Eur J Clin Nutr* 56:425–30.

Hedrén E, Mulokozi G, Svanberg U. 2002b. In vitro accessibility of carotenes from green leafy vegetables cooked with sunflower oil or red palm oil. *Int J Food Sci Nutr* 53:445–53.

Hoppe PP, Krämer K, van den Berg H, Steenge G, van Vliet T. 2003. Synthetic and tomato-based lycopene have identical bioavailability in humans. *Eur J Nutr* 42:272–8.

Hornero-Méndez D, Mínguez-Mosquera MI. 2007. Bioaccessibility of carotenes from carrots: effect of cooking and addition of oil. *Innov Food Sci Emerg Technol* 8:407–12.

Hu X, Jandacek RJ, White WS. 2000. Intestinal absorption of β-carotene ingested with a meal rich in sunflower oil or beef tallow: postprandial appearance in triacylglycerol-rich lipoproteins in women. *Am J Clin Nutr* 71:1170–80.

Huo T, Ferruzzi MG, Schwartz SJ, Failla ML. 2007. Impact of fatty acyl composition and quantity of triglycerides on bioaccessibility of dietary carotenoids. *J Agric Food Chem* 55:8950–7.

Jalal, Nesheim MC, Agus Z, Sanjur D, Habicht JP. 1998. Serum retinol concentrations in children are affected by food sources of beta-carotene, fat intake, and anthelmintic drug treatment. *Am J Clin Nutr* 68:623–9.

Jeffery J, Holzenburg A, King S. 2012a. Physical barriers to carotenoid bioaccessibility. Ultrastructure survey of chromoplast and cell wall morphology in nine carotenoid-containing fruits and vegetables. *J Sci Food Agric* 92:2594–602.

Jeffery JL, Turner ND, King SR. 2012b. Carotenoid bioaccessibility from nine raw carotenoid-storing fruits and vegetables using an in vitro model. *J Sci Food Agric* 92:2603–10.

Johnson EJ, Qin J, Krinsky NI, Russell RM. 1997. Ingestion by men of a combined dose of β-carotene and lycopene does not affect the absorption of β-carotene but improves that of lycopene. *J Nutr* 127:1833–7.

Johnson EJ, Russell RM. 1992. Distribution of orally administered beta-carotene among lipoproteins in healthy men. *Am J Clin Nutr* 56:128–35.

Kean EG, Bordenave N, Ejeta G, Hamaker BR, Ferruzi MG. 2011. Carotenoid bioaccessibility from whole grain and decorticated yellow endosperm sorghum porridge. *J Cereal Sci* 54:450–9.

Kean EG, Hamaker BR, Ferruzi MG. 2008. Carotenoid bioaccessibility from whole grain and degermed maize meal products. *J Agric Food Chem* 56:9918–26.

Knockaert G, de Roeck A, Lemmens L, van Buggenhout S, Hendrickx M, van Loey A. 2011. Effect of thermal and high pressure processes on structural and health-related properties of carrots (*Daucus carota*). *Food Chem* 125:903–12.

Knockaert G, Lemmens L, van Buggenhout S, Hendrickx M, van Loey A. 2012a. Changes in β-carotene bioaccessibility and concentration during processing of carrot puree. *Food Chem* 133:60–7.

Knockaert G, Pulissery SK, Colle I, van Buggenhout S, Hendrickx M, van Loey A. 2012b. Lycopene degradation, isomerization and in vitro bioaccessibility in high pressure homogenized tomato puree containing oil: effect of additional thermal and high pressure processing. *Food Chem* 135: 1290–7.

Kostic D, White WS, Olson JA. 1995. Intestinal absorption, serum clearance, and interactions between lutein and β-carotene when administered to human adults in separate or combined oral doses. *Am J Clin Nutr* 62:604–10.

Lemmens L, van Buggenhout S, Oey I. van Loey A, Hendrickx M. 2009. Towards a better understanding of the relationship between the β-carotene in vitro bio-accessibility and pectin structural changes: a case study on carrots. *Food Res Int* 42:1323–30.

Lemmens L, van Buggenhout S, van Loey AM, Hendrickx ME. 2010. Particle size reduction leading to cell wall rupture is more important for the β-carotene bioaccessibility of raw compared to thermally processed carrots. *J Agric Food Chem* 58:12769–76.

Liu C-S, Glahn RP, Liu RH. 2004. Assessment of carotenoid bioavailability of whole foods using a Caco-2 cell culture model coupled with an in vitro digestion. *J Agric Food Chem* 52:4330–7.

Livny O, Reifen R, Levy I, Madar Z, Faulks R, Southon S, Schwartz B. 2003. β-carotene bioavailability from differently processed carrot meals in human ileostomy volunteers. *Eur J Nutr* 42:338–45.

Mandalari G, Bisignano C, Filocamo A, Chessa S, Sarò M, Torre G, Faulks RM, Dugo P. 2013. Bioaccessibility of pistachio polyphenols, xanthophylls, and tocopherols during simulated human digestion. *Nutrition* 29:338–44.

Micozzi MS, Brown ED, Edwards BK, Bieri JG, Taylor PR, Khachik F, Beecher GR, Smith JC Jr. 1992. Plasma carotenoid response to chronic intake of selected foods and β-carotene supplements in men. *Am J Clin Nutr* 55:1120–5.

Moelants KRN, Lemmens L, Vandebroeck M, van Buggenhout S, van Loey AM, Hendrickx ME. 2012. Relation between particle size and carotenoid bioaccessibility in carrot- and tomato-derived suspensions. *J Agric Food Chem* 60:11995–2003.

Molldrem KL, Li J, Simon PW, Tanumihardjo SA. 2004. Lutein and β-carotene from lutein-containing yellow carrots are bioavailable in humans. *Am J Clin Nutr* 80:131–6.

Moraru C, Lee T-C. 2005. Kinetic studies of lycopene isomerization in a tributyrin model system at gastric pH. *J Agric Food Chem* 53:8997–9004.

Mulokozi G, Hedrén E, Svanberg U. 2004. In vitro accessibility and intake of β-carotene from cooked green leafy vegetables and their estimated contribution to vitamin A requirements. *Plant Foods Hum Nutr* 59:1–9.

Nayak N, Harrison EH, Hussain MM. 2001. Retinyl ester secretion by intestinal cells: a specific and regulated process dependent on assembly and secretion of chylomicrons. *J Lipid Res* 42:272–80.

Netzel M, Netzel G, Zabaras D, Lundin L, Day L, Addepalli R, Osborne SA, Seymour R. 2011. Release and absorption of carotenes from processed carrots (*Daucus carota*) using in vitro digestion coupled with a Caco-2 cell trans-well culture model. *Food Res Int* 44:868–74.

Norkus EP, Norkus KL, Dharmarajan TS, Schierle J, Schalch W. 2010. Serum lutein response is greater from free lutein than from esterified lutein during 4 weeks of supplementation in healthy adults. *J Am Coll Nutr* 29:575–85.

Novotny JA, Kurilic AC, Britz SJ, Clevidence BA. 2005. Plasma appearance of labeled β-carotene, lutein and retinol in humans after consumption of isotopically labeled kale. *J Lipid Res* 46:1896–903.

O'Connell OF, Ryan L, O'Brien NM. 2007. Xanthophyll carotenoids are more bioaccessible from fruits than dark green vegetables. *Nutr Res* 27:258–64.

Ornelas-Paz JJ, Failla ML, Yahia EM, Gardea-Bejar A. 2008. Impact of the stage of ripening and dietary fat on in vitro bioaccesibility of β-carotene in 'Ataulfo' mango. *Agric Food Chem* 56:1511–6.

O'Sullivan L, Ryan L, Aherne SA, O'Brien NM. 2008. Cellular transport of lutein is greater from uncooked rather than cooked spinach irrespective of whether it is fresh, frozen, or canned. *Nutr Res* 28:532–8.

Paetau I, Chen H, Goh NM-Y, White WS. 1997. Interactions in the postprandial appearance of β-carotene and canthaxanthin in plasma triacylglycerol-rich lipoproteins in humans. *Am J Clin Nutr* 66:1133–43.

Paetau I, Khachik F, Brown ED, Beecher GR, Kramer TR, Chittams J, Clevidence BA. 1998. Chronic ingestion of lycopene-rich tomato juice or lycopene supplements significantly increases plasma concentrations of lycopene and related tomato carotenoids in humans. *Am J Clin Nutr* 68:1187–95.

Page D, van Stratum E, Degrou A, Renard CMGC. 2012. Kinetics of temperature increase during tomato processing modulate the bioaccessibility of lycopene. *Food Chem* 135:2462–9.

Palafox-Carlos H, Ayala-Zavala JF, González-Aguilar GA. 2011. The role dietary fiber in the bioaccessibility and bioavailability of fruit and vegetable antioxidants. *J Food Sci* 76:R6–15.

Palmero P, Lemmens L, Ribas-Agustí A, Sosa C, Met K, Umutonmi JD, Hendrickx M, van Loey A. 2013. Novel targeted approach to better understand how natural structural barriers govern carotenoid in vitro bioaccessibility in vegetable-based systems. *Food Chem* 141:2036–43.

Panozzo A, Lemmens L, van Loey A, Manzocco L, Nicoli MC, Hendrickx M. 2013. Microstructure and bioaccessibility of different carotenoid species as affected by high pressure homogenisation: a case study on differently coloured tomato. *Food Chem* 141:4094–100.

Parada J, Aguilera JM. 2007. Food microstructure affects the bioavailability of several nutrients. *J Food Sci* 72:R21–32.

Parker RS. 1996. Absorption, metabolism, and transport of carotenoids. *FASEB J* 10:542–51.
Parker RS. 1997. Bioavailability of carotenoids. *Eur J Clin Nutr* 51(Suppl. 1):S86–90.
Parker RS, Swanson JE, You C-S, Edwards AJ, Huang T. 1999. Bioavailability of carotenoids in human subjects. *Proc Nutr Soc* 58:155–62.
Pee S de, West CE, Muhilal, Daryadi D, Hautvast JGAJ. 1995. Lack of improvement in vitamin A status with increased consumption of dark-green leafy vegetables. *Lancet* 346:75–81.
Pee S de, West CE, Permaesih D, Martuti S, Muhilal, Hautvast JGAJ. 1998. Orange fruit is more effective than are dark-green, leafy vegetables in increasing serum concentrations of retinol and β-carotene in school-children in Indonesia. *Am J Clin Nutr* 68:1058–67.
Poulaert M, Borel P, Caporiccio B, Gunata Z, Dhuique-Mayer C. 2012. Grapefruit juices impair the bioaccessibility of β-carotene from orange-fleshed sweet potato but not its intestinal uptake by Caco-2 cells. *J Agric Food Chem* 60:685–91.
Prince MR, Frisoli JK. 1993. Beta-carotene accumulation in serum and skin. *Am J Clin Nutr* 57:175–81.
Pugliese A, Loizzo MR, Tundis R, O'Callaghan Y, Galvin K, Menichini F, O'Brien N. 2013. The effect of domestic processing on the content and bioaccessibility of carotenoids from chili peppers (*Capsicum* species). *Food Chem* 141:2606–13.
Pugliese A, O'Callaghan Y, Tundis, R, Galvin K, Menichini F, O'Brien N, Loizzo MR. 2014a. In vitro investigation of the bioaccessibility of carotenoids from raw, frozen and boiled red chili peppers (*Capsicum annuum*). *Eur J Nutr* 53:501–10.
Pugliese A, O'Callaghan Y, Tundis, R, Galvin K, Menichini F, O'Brien N, Loizzo MR. 2014b. In vitro assessment of the bioaccessibility of carotenoids from sun-dried chili peppers. *Plant Foods Hum Nutr.* 69:8–17.
Pullakhandam R, Failla ML. 2007. Micellarization and intestinal cell uptake of β-carotene and lutein from drumstick (*Moringa oleifera*) leaves. *J Med Food* 10:252–7.
Rao AV, Shen H. 2002. Effect of low dose lycopene intake on lycopene bioavailability and oxidative stress. *Nutr Res* 22:1125–31.
Re R, Fraser PD, Long M, Bramley PM, Rice-Evans C. 2001. Isomerization of lycopene in the gastric milieu. *Biochem Biophys Res Commun* 281:576–81.
Reboul E, Abou L, Mikail C, Ghiringhelli O, Andre M, Portugal H, Jourdheuil-Rahmani D, Amiot MJ, Lairon D, Borel P. 2005. Lutein transport by Caco-2 TC-7 cells occurs partly by a facilitated process involving the scavenger receptor class B type I (SR-BI). *Biochem J* 387:455–61.
Reboul E, Richelle M, Perrot E, Desmoulins-Mazelet C, Pirisi V, Borel P. 2006. Bioaccessibility of carotenoids and vitamin E from their main dietary sources. *J Agric Food Chem* 54:8749–55.
Reboul E, Thap S, Tourniaire F, André M, Juhel C, Morange S, Amiot M-J, Lairon D, Borel P, 2007. Differential effect of dietary antioxidant classes (carotenoids, polyphenols, vitamins C and E) on lutein absorption. *Br J Nutr* 97:440–6.
Ribaya-Mercado JD. 2002. Influence of dietary fat on β-carotene absorption and bioconversion into vitamin A. *Nutr Rev* 60:104–10.
Richelle M, Enslen M, Hager C, Groux M, Tavazzi I, Godin J-P, Berger A, Métairon S, Quaile S, Piquet-Welsch C, Sagalowicz L, Green H, Fay LB. 2004. Both free and esterified plant sterols reduce cholesterol absorption and the bioavailability of β-carotene and α-tocopherol in normocholesterolemic humans. *Am J Clin Nutr* 80:171–7.
Riedl J, Linseisen J, Hoffman J, Wolfram G. 1999. Some dietary fibers reduce the absorption of carotenoids in women. *J Nutr* 129:2170–6.
Riso P, Brusamolino A, Ciappellano S, Porrini M. 2003. Comparison of lutein bioavailability from vegetables and supplement. *Int J Vitam Nutr Res* 73:201–5.
Riso P, Brusamolino A, Scalfi L, Porrini, M. 2004. Bioavailability of carotenoids from spinach and tomatoes. *Nutr Metab Cardiovasc Dis* 14:150–6.
Rock CL, Lovalvo JL, Emenhiser C, Ruffin MT, Flatt SW, Schwartz SJ. 1998. Bioavailability of β-carotene is lower in raw than in processed carrots and spinach in women. *J Nutr* 128:913–6.
Rock CL, Swendseid ME. 1992. Plasma beta-carotene response in humans after meals supplemented with dietary pectin. *Am J Clin Nutr* 55:96–9.
Rodríguez-Roque MJ, Rojas-Graü MA, Elez-Martínez P, Martín-Belloso O. 2013. Changes in vitamin C, phenolic, and carotenoid profiles throughout in vitro gastrointestinal digestion of blended fruit juice. *J Agric Food Chem* 61:1859–67.
Roodenburg AJC, Leenen R, van het Hof KH, Weststrate JA, Tijburg LBM. 2000. Amount of fat in the diet affects bioavailability of lutein esters but not of α-carotene, β-carotene, and vitamin E in humans. *Am J Clin Nutr* 71:1187–93.

Ryan L, O'Connell O, O'Sullivan L, Aherne SA, O'Brien NM. 2008. Micellarization of carotenoids from raw and cooked vegetables. *Plant Foods Hum Nutr* 63:127–33.

Sakamoto H, Mori H, Ojima F, Ishiguro Y, Arimoto A, Imae Y, Nanba T, Ogawa M, Fukuba H. 1994. Elevation of serum carotenoids after continual ingestion of tomato juice. *Nippon Eiyo Shokuryo Gakkai-shi* 47:93–9.

Schierle J, Bretzel W, Bühler I, Faccin N, Hess D, Steiner K, Schüep W. 1997. Content and isomeric ratio of lycopene in food and human blood plasma. *Food Chem* 59:459–65.

Schweiggert RM, Kopec RE, Villalobos-Gutierrez MG, Högel J, Quesada S, Esquivel P, Schwartz SJ, Carle R. 2014. Carotenoids are more bioavailable from papaya than from tomato and carrot in humans: a randomized cross-over study. *Brit J Nutr* 111:490–8.

Schweiggert RM, Mezger D, Schimpf F, Steingass CB, Carle R. 2012. Influence of the chromoplast morphology on carotenoid bioaccessibility of carrot, mango, papaya, and tomato. *Food Chem* 135:2736–42.

Schweiggert RM, Steingass CB, Heller A, Esquivel P, Carle R. 2011. Characterization of chromoplasts and carotenoids of chromoplasts and carotenoids of red and yellow fleshed papaya (*Carica papaya* L.). Food Res. *Int* 44:1373–80.

Shiau A, Mobarhan S, Stacewicz-Sapuntzakis M, Benya R, Liao Y, Ford C, Bowen P, Friedman H, Frommel TO. 1994. Assessment of the intestinal retention of beta-carotene in humans. *J Am Coll Nutr* 13:369–75.

Serrano J, Goñi I, Saura-Calixto F. 2005. Determination of β-carotene and lutein available from green leafy vegetables by an in vitro digestion and colonic fermentation method. *J Agric Food Chem* 53: 2936–40.

Stahl W, Schwarz W, Sies H.1993. Human serum concentrations of all-*trans* β- and α-carotene but not 9-*cis* β-carotene increase upon ingestion of a natural isomer mixture obtained from *Dunaliella salina* (Betatene). *J Nutr* 123:847–51.

Stahl W, Schwarz W, Sundquist AR, Sies H. 1992. *Cis-trans* isomers of lycopene and β-carotene in human serum and tissues. *Arch Biochem Biophys* 294:173–7.

Stahl W, Schwarz W, von Laar J, Sies H. 1995. All-trans β-carotene preferentially accumulates in human chylomicrons and very low density lipoproteins compared with 9-cis geometrical isomer. *J Nutr* 125:2128–33.

Stahl W, Sies H. 1992. Uptake of lycopene and its geometrical isomers is greater from heat-processed than from unprocessed tomato juice in humans. *J Nutr* 122:2161–6.

Stinco CM, Fernández-Vásquez R, Heredia FJ, Meléndez-Martínez AJ, Vicario IM. 2013. Bioaccessibility, antioxidant activity and colour of carotenoids in ultrafrozen orange juices: influence of thawing conditions. LWT—Food *Sci Technol* 53:458–63.

Takaishi N, Satsu H, Takayanagi K, Mukai K, Shimizu M. 2012. *In vivo* and in vitro studies on the absorption characteristics of β-cryptoxanthin in the intestine. *Biosci Biotechnol Bioche*.76:2124–8.

Takyi EEK. 1999. Children's consumption of dark green leafy vegetables with added fat enhances serum retinol. *Am J Clin Nutr* 129:1549–54.

Thakkar SK, Failla ML. 2008. Bioaccessibility of pro-vitamin A carotenoid is minimally affected by non-provitamin A xanthophylls in maize (*Zea mays* sp). *J Agric Food Chem* 56:11441–6.

Thakkar SK, Huo TH, Maziya-Dixon B, Failla ML. 2009. Impact of style of processing on retention and bioaccessibility of β-carotene in cassava (*Manihot esculanta*, Crantz). *J Agric Food Chem* 57: 1344–8.

Thakkar SK, Maziya-Dixon B, Dixon AGO, Failla ML. 2007. β-carotene micellarization during in vitro digestion and uptake by Caco-2 cells is directly proportional to β-carotene content in different genotypes of cassava. *J Nutr* 137:2229–33.

Thürmann PA, Steffen J, Zwernemann C, Aebischer C-P, Cohn W, Wendt G, Schalch W. 2002. Plasma concentration response to drinks containing β-carotene as carrot juice or formulated as a water dispersible powder. *Eur J Nutr* 41:228–35.

Tibäck EA, Svelander CA, Colle IJP, Altskär AI, Alminger MAG, Hendrickx MEG, Ahrné LM, Langton MIBC. 2009. Mechanical and thermal pretreatments of crushed tomatoes: effects on consistency and in vitro accessibility of lycopene. *J Food Sci* 74:E386–95.

Törrönen R, Lehmusaho M, Häkkinen S, Hänninen O, Mykkänen H. 1996. Serum β-carotene response to supplementation with raw carrots, carrot juice or purified β-carotene in healthy non-smoking women. *Nutr Res* 16:565–75.

Traber MG, Diamond SR, Lane JC, Brody RI, Kayden HJ. 1994. β-carotene transport in human lipoproteins: comparison with alpha-tocopherol. *Lipids* 29:665–9.

Tyssandier V, Cardinault N, Caris-Veyrat C, Amiot M-J, Grolier P, Bouteloup C, Azais-Braesco V, Borel P. 2002. Vegetable-borne lutein, lycopene, and β-carotene compete for incorporation into chylomicrons, with no adverse effect on the medium-term (3-wk) plasma status of carotenoids in humans. *Am J Clin Nutr* 75:526–34.

Tyssandier V, Lyan B, Borel P. 2001. Main factors governing the transfer of carotenoids from emulsion lipid droplets to micelles. *Biochim Biophys Acta* 1533:285–92.

Unlu NZ, Bohn T, Clinton SK, Schwartz SJ. 2005. Carotenoid absorption from salad and salsa by humans is enhanced by the addition of avocado or avocado oil. *J Nutr* 135:431–6.

Unlu NZ, Bohn T, Francis DM, Clinton SK, Schwartz SJ. 2007a. Carotenoid absorption in humans consuming tomato paste sauces obtained from tangerine or high-β-carotene varieties of tomatoes. *J Agric Food Chem* 55:1597–603.

Unlu NZ, Bohn T, Francis DM, Nagaraja HN, Clinton SK, Schwartz SJ. 2007b. Lycopene from heat-induced *cis*-isomer-rich tomato sauce is more bioavailable than from all-*trans*-rich tomato sauce in human subjects. *Brit J Nutr* 98:140–6.

van Bennekum A, Werder M, Thuahnai ST Han C-H, Duong P, Williams DL, Wettstein P, Schulthess G, Phillips MC, Hauser H. 2005. Class B scavenger receptor-mediated intestinal absorption of dietary β-carotene and cholesterol. *Biochem* 44:4517–25.

van den Berg H. 1999. Carotenoid interactions. *Nutr Rev* 57:1–10.

van den Berg H, van Vliet T. 1998. Effect of simultaneous, single oral doses of beta-carotene with lutein or lycopene on the beta-carotene and retinyl ester responses in the triacylglycerol-rich lipoprotein fraction of men. *Am J Clin Nutr* 68:82–9.

van het Hof KH, Brouwer IA, West CE, Haddeman E, Steegers-Theunissen RP, van Dusseldorp M, Weststrate JA, Eskes TK, Haustvast JG. 1999a. Bioavailability of lutein from vegetables is 5 times higher than that of β-carotene. *Am J Clin Nutr* 70:261–8.

van het Hof KH, Gärtner C, Wiersma A, Tijburg LBM, Weststrate JA. 1999b. Comparison of the bioavailability of natural palm oil carotenoids and synthetic β-carotene in humans. *J Agric Food Chem* 47:1582–6.

van het Hof KH, Tijburg LBM, Pietrzik K, Weststrate JA. 1999c. Influence of feeding different vegetables on plasma level of carotenoids, folate and vitamin C. Effect of disruption of the vegetable matrix. *Br J Nutr* 82:203–12.

van het Hof KH, de Boer BCJ, Tijburg LBM, Lucius BRHM, Zijp I, West CE, Hautvast JGAF, Weststrate JA. 2000a. Carotenoid bioavailability in humans from tomatoes processed in different ways determined from the carotenoid response in the triglyceride-rich lipoprotein fraction of plasma after a single consumption and in the plasma after four days of consumption. *J Nutr* 130:1189–96.

van hetHof KH, West CE, Weststrate JA, Haustvast JGAJ. 2000b. Dietary factors that affect the bioavailability of carotenoids. *J Nutr* 130:503–6.

van Lieshout M, West CE, van Breemen RB. 2003. Isotopic tracer techniques for studying the bioavailability and bioefficacy of dietary carotenoids, particularly β-carotene, in humans: a review. *Am J Clin Nutr* 77:12–28.

Vásquez-Caicedo AL, Heller A, Neidhart S, Carle R. 2006. Chromoplast morphology and β-carotene accumulation during postharvest ripening of mango cv. ‘Tommy Atkins’. *J Agric Food Chem* 54:5769–76.

Veda S, Kamath A, Platel K, Begum K, Srinivasan K. 2006. Determination of bioaccessibility of β-carotene in vegetables by in vitro methods. *Mol Nutr Food Res* 50:1047–52.

Veda S, Platel K, Srinivasan K. 2008. Influence of food acidulants and antioxidant spices on the bioaccessibility of β-carotene from selected vegetables. *J Agric Food Chem* 56:8714–9.

Werner S, Böhm V. 2011. Bioaccessibility of carotenoids and vitamin E from pasta: evaluation of an in vitro digestion model. *J Agric Food Chem* 59:1163–1170.

White WS, Stacewicz-Sapuntzakis M, Erdman JW Jr, Bowen PE. 1994. Pharmacokinetics of beta-carotene and canthaxanthin after ingestion of individual and combined doses by human subjects. *J Am Coll Nutr* 13:665–71.

Wingerath T, Sies H, Stahl W. 1995. β-Cryptoxanthin selectively increases in human chylomicrons upon ingestion of tangerine concentrate rich in β-cryptoxanthin esters. *Arch Biochem Biophys* 324:385–90.

Yeum K-J, Booth SL, Sadowski JA, Liu C, Tang G, Krinsky NI, Russell RM. 1996. Human plasma carotenoid response to the ingestion of controlled diets high in fruits and vegetables. *Am J Clin Nutr* 64:594–602.

Yeum K-J, Russell RM. 2002. Carotenoid bioavailability and bioconversion. *Annu Rev Nutr* 22:483–504.

Yonekura L, Nagao A. 2007. Intestinal absorption of dietary carotenoids. *Mol Nutr Food Res* 51:107–115.

You CS, Parker RS, Goodman KJ, Swanson JE, Corso TN. 1996. Evidence of *cis-trans*-isomerization of 9-*cis*-β-carotene during absorption in human. *Am J Clin Nutr* 64:177–83.

Zaripheh S, Erdman JW JR. 2002. Factors that influence the bioavailability of xanthophylls. *J Nutr* 132:S531–4.

10 Provitamin A activity

10.1 INTRODUCTION

The best established function of carotenoids in terms of human health is the provitamin A activity. Vitamin A can be obtained from foods in two forms: preformed vitamin A (retinyl esters and retinol) and provitamin A carotenoids (mainly β-carotene). Preformed vitamin A comes from foods of animal origin, mainly liver, egg, milk, and dairy products. Provitamin A carotenoids are provided by green and yellow or orange vegetables and fruits. Provitamin A carotenoids provide about 20% to 35% of the habitual intake of vitamin A in the Western diet (FAO/WHO, 1988; IOM, 2001; Weber and Grune, 2012). In contrast, because of the high cost or unavailability of animal foods, about 80% of dietary vitamin A originates from provitamin A carotenoids in developing countries (WHO, 2009).

Structurally, vitamin A (retinol) is essentially one-half of the molecule of β-carotene with an added molecule of water at the end of the lateral polyene chain. Thus, β-carotene is a potent provitamin A to which 100% activity is assigned. An unsubstituted β ring with an 11-carbon polyene chain is the minimum requirement for vitamin A activity. γ-Carotene, α-carotene, β-cryptoxanthin, and β-carotene-5,6-epoxide, all of which have one unsubstituted ring, would have about half the bioactivity of β-carotene. The acyclic carotenoids, which are devoid of β-rings, and the xanthophylls other than those mentioned above, in which the β-rings have hydroxy, epoxy, and carbonyl substituents, are not provitamins A.

Vitamin A is necessary for normal vision, embryonic development, normal growth, reproduction, gene expression, cell and tissue differentiation, and immune function. Chronic shortage of dietary vitamin A results in vitamin A deficiency (VAD), the most specific clinical effect of which is xerophthalmia and its various stages, including night blindness, conjunctival xerosis, Bitot's spot, corneal xerosis, corneal ulceration, and scarring (McLaren and Friggs, 2001; IOM, 2006). The leading cause of preventable childhood blindness, VAD is also associated with reduced immunity toward infections, which results in increased mortality from childhood diseases (e.g., gastrointestinal disease, measles) (Beaton et al., 1993; Maida et al., 2008).

Food Carotenoids: Chemistry, Biology, and Technology, First Edition. Delia B. Rodriguez-Amaya.

VAD is defined as liver stores below 20 μg (0.07 μmol) of retinol per gram (Sommer and Davidson, 2002). VAD disorders are defined as health and physiologic consequences attributable to VAD, whether clinically evident (xerophthalmia, anemia, growth retardation, increased infectious morbidity, and mortality) or not (impaired iron mobilization, disturbed cellular differentiation, and depressed immune response).

VAD remains a public health problem (i.e., 15% or more of children sampled have serum retinol levels of <20 μg/dL (0.7 μmol/L) in developing countries. In 2009, it was estimated that about 190 million preschool-age children and 19.1 million pregnant women had low serum retinol levels; about 5.2 million preschool-age children and 9.8 million pregnant women were night blind (WHO, 2009). In 2010, the United Nations System Standing Committee on Nutrition reported that VAD affected some 160 million preschool children in low-income countries, with prevalence estimated at about 30%. South-central Asia (which includes India) has the highest prevalence, having two-thirds of the affected children. Along with central and west Africa, it had a prevalence of more than 40%. South and Central America and the Caribbean had the lowest prevalences, near 10%. The situation had improved but only at somewhat less than 0.5 percentage points per year. At this rate, these low-income countries would take more than 50 years to get to the levels typical of industrialized countries.

10.2 BIOCONVERSION OF PROVITAMIN A CAROTENOIDS

Bioconversion refers to the proportion of absorbed provitamin A that is converted to retinol. Bioefficacy is the combination of absorption and bioconversion; it is defined as the efficiency with which ingested dietary provitamin A carotenoid is absorbed and converted to active retinol (van Lieshout et al., 2001).

Within the intestinal absorptive cells, carotenoids undergo oxidative cleavage to form vitamin A, or may pass unmetabolized across the intestine. There are two pathways for the cleavage of provitamin A carotenoids to vitamin A: central and eccentric (Figure 10.1) (Wyss, 2004; Harrison, 2012). The predominant pathway for β-carotene cleavage, central cleavage yields two molecules of retinal in the intestinal cell and liver cytosol (Goodman and Olson, 1969). Retinal can be reversibly reduced to retinol by retinal reductase or irreversibly oxidized to retinoic acid by retinal dehydrogenase (Olson and Lakshman, 1990; Parker, 1996).

Although the enzyme has been known for a long time (Goodman and Huang, 1965; Olson and Hayaishi, 1965), it was successfully cloned and characterized only in the 2000s in different species, including humans (Yan et al., 2001). The mechanism of reaction of β-carotene 15,15′-oxygenase (BCO1), however, has been controversial. It was initially thought to be a dioxygenase. Incubation of the substrate analogue α-carotene in the presence of highly enriched $^{17}O_2$ and $H_2{}^{18}O$ incorporated oxygen from both O_2 and H_2O in the cleavage product, indicating a monooxygenase mechanism (Leuenberger et al., 2001). The enzyme has thus been referred to as β-carotene 15,15′-monooxygenase (BCMO1). Arguing that this study used conditions that favored oxygen exchange with water, Dela Seña et al. (2014) incubated BCO1 and β-carotene in $H_2{}^{18}O$-$^{16}O_2$ and $H_2{}^{16}O$-$^{18}O_2$ with minimal reaction and processing times to minimize oxygen exchange

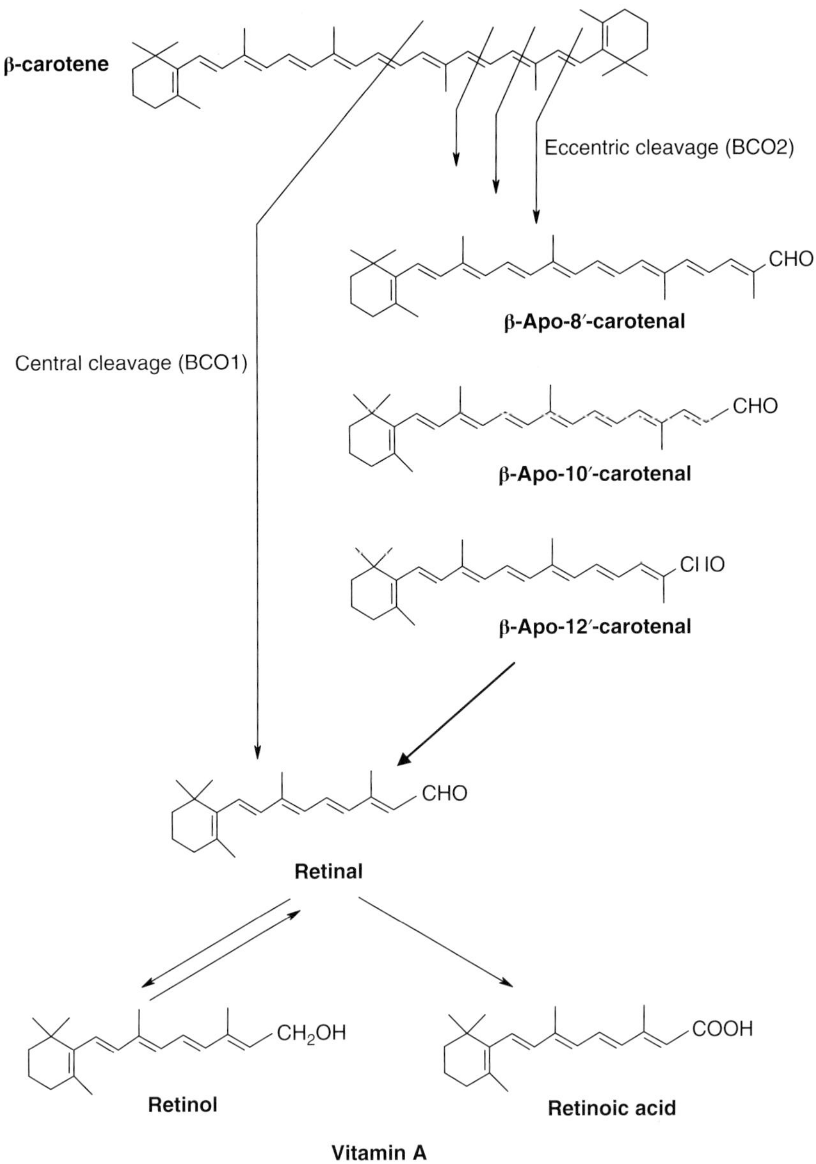

Figure 10.1 Central and eccentric cleavages of β-carotene. Adapted from Harrison (2012).

between retinal and water. Retinals were formed that contained oxygen atoms originating solely from O_2, demonstrating a dioxygenase mechanism.

Purified recombinant human BCO1 enzyme had been characterized and found to be highly expressed in the digestive tissues and the liver (Lindqvist and Andersson, 2002). It is also expressed in nondigestive tissues where it may convert provitamin A carotenoids obtained from the plasma into retinal locally.

An alternative route involves eccentric or assymetric cleavage (Figure 10.1), catalyzed primarily by dioxygenase 2 (BCDO2) (von Lintig, 2012). It was first proposed by

Glover and Redfearn (1954), who observed cleavage at several double bonds in the polyene chain of β-carotene aside from the central 15,15′-double bond to produce β-apo-carotenals with different chain lengths, which can be subsequently converted to retinal (Figure 10.1). X.-D.Wang et al. (1991) demonstrated the formation of significant amounts of β-apo-12′-, β-apo-10′-, and β-apo-8′-carotenals, retinal, and retinoic acid in vitro during incubation of intestinal homogenates prepared from human, monkey, ferret, and rat tissues. Evidence for this pathway was provided by the identification of β-carotene-9′,10′-oxygenase (BCDO2), which acts specifically at the 9′,10′ double bond of β-carotene to produce β-apo-10'-carotenal and β-ionone (Kiefer et al., 2001).

BCO1 has high specificity toward the double bond at the 15,15′-position, and at least one unsubstituted β-ionone ring is required (Lindqvist and Andersson, 2002). BCDO2 exhibits a broad substrate specificity, converting both carotenes and xanthophylls by oxidative cleavage at 9,10 and 9′,10′ double bonds. These enzymes are located at different sites within the cell; BCO1 is cytoplasmic (Lindqvist and Andersson, 2002) while BCDO2 is located in the mitochondria (Amengual et al., 2011).

While there is general agreement that the key enzyme for the production of vitamin A is BCO1, the physiological role of BCDO2 is less known. It has been linked with regulation. Oxidative stress led to increased eccentric cleavage of β-carotene, and the mixture of cleavage products led to disruption of retinoid signaling via indirect mechanisms (Eroglu et al., 2012). Specific β-apocarotenoids exerted anti–vitamin A activity by directly interacting with retinoid acid receptors as high-affinity antagonists. Carotenoids can accumulate in the mitochondria and impair respiration, causing oxidative stress. With its mitochondrial localization, BCDO2 can prevent this accumulation (Lobo et al., 2012).

Lobo et al.'s study (2010) revealed a diet-responsive regulatory network that controls β-carotene absorption and vitamin A production by negative feedback mechanism. Retinoic acid via retinoic acid receptors induced expression of the intestinal transcription factor ISX, which repressed the expression of SR-B1 and BCO1.

10.3 BIOEFFICACY AND VITAMIN A EQUIVALENCY OF PROVITAMIN A CAROTENOIDS

Reviewing earlier publications, Nestel and Trumbo (1999) noted that the efficiency of the bioconversion of β-carotene to vitamin A may vary depending on vitamin A status: (a) more efficient when the status is lower, and (b) less efficient the more β-carotene is consumed. These observations have been amply confirmed by later studies.

High dietary doses of β-carotene limits its absorption and conversion to vitamin A (Lin et al., 2000; Tang et al., 2000; Hickenbottom et al., 2002a,b; Novotny et al., 2010), indicating that possible vitamin A toxicity is avoided and β-carotene is a safer source to provide vitamin A. Bioconversion of plant carotenoids to vitamin A in school-aged children varied inversely with vitamin A status (Ribaya-Mercado et al., 2000). Discussing the factors that influence BCO1 activity, Lietz (2010) considered vitamin A status as possibly the most important factor.

In 1967 WHO established that 6 μg of β-carotene is equivalent to 1 μg of retinol (FAO/WHO, 1967). This was based on two assumptions: (a) the mass ratio of the maximum conversion of β-carotene in oil, its most bioavailable form, to vitamin A in vivo was 2:1, and (b) the bioavailability of β-carotene from foods on average was one-third that of β-carotene in oil (Olson, 1999). Thus, one retinol equivalent is equivalent to 6 μg (2 × 3 μg) of dietary β-carotene. Other carotenoids, such as α-carotene and β-cryptoxanthin, were considered half as active as β-carotene. *Z*-isomers were later considered half as active as their all-*E* counterparts as well.

Based on later studies (van Het Hof et al., 1999) that suggested that the relative vitamin A activity of β-carotene was 50% less than previously thought, the retinol activity equivalent (RAE) for dietary β-carotene was established to be 12 μg (2 × 6 μg) and is equal to 1 μg retinol (IOM, 2001; Trumbo et al., 2003). Considering that the vitamin A activity of α-carotene and β-cryptoxanthin would be approximately half that of β-carotene, one RAE would be 24 μg of either of these two provitamins A. Given possible future changes in equivalency, it is recommended that the actual weights of carotenoids found in specific foods be listed in food tables to allow future adjustments when more data are available (Trumbo et al., 2001).

In the 2004 report of WHO/FAO, the committee retained the vitamin A equivalence of β-carotene of 6:1, originally derived on the basis of balance studies, until there is firm confirmation of more precise methodologies from ongoing studies.

Thurnham (2007) reexamined the data that were used to support the RAE ratio, including bioequivalence studies done in developing and developed countries, depletion and repletion studies, feeding with vegetable sources of β-carotene or pure supplements, influence of helminths, carotenoid interactions and matrix effects, and studies using stable isotopes. Stable isotope studies showed that the bioefficacy of β-carotene conversion to retinol is generally poor even for pure β-carotene unless the dose is small and fed regularly until equilibration is reached. Retinol formation appeared to be inversely influenced by previous vitamin A intake, the amount of material given, and current vitamin A status. The author called for more stable isotope studies where liver reserves of vitamin A are determined pre- and postintervention to evaluate β-carotene bioefficacy of different vegetable sources.

From compilations of Haskell (2012) and van Loo-Bouwman (2014), the mean vitamin A equivalency of β-carotene (defined as the amount of ingested β-carotene in micrograms that is absorbed and converted into 1 μg retinol) in oil in studies with more than one subject ranged from 2:1 to 9:1 by weight (van Lieshout et al., 2001; You et al., 2002; Tang et al., 2003, 2012; Haskell et al., 2004; Z. Wang et al., 2004; van Loo-Bouwman et al., 2009, 2010; Li et al., 2010; Liu et al., 2010). Notably, in Z. Wang et al. (2004) and Tang et al. (2003), the within-study variability was very high, the equivalency ratios ranging from 3.8:1 to 22.8:1 for rural Chinese adults and from 2.4:1 to 20:2 in U.S. adults, respectively, suggesting that there were genetic differences in β-carotene metabolism among the study participants (Haskell, 2012). Haskell attributed the variability of the vitamin A equivalency of β-carotene in oil to differences in the size of the oral dose of β-carotene administered, genetic polymorphisms related to β-carotene metabolism, and vitamin A status.

The vitamin A equivalencies for plant β-carotene estimated in populations in developed and developing countries were highly variable, the mean ratios ranging from 3.6:1 to 28:1 (Tang 2010; Haskell, 2012; van Loo-Bouwman et al., 2014). As pointed out by Haskell (2012), part of the variation might have come from the studies' experimental designs, assessing various response indicators for β-carotene and vitamin A of either single meals (Edwards, 2001; You et al., 2002; Tang, 2005, 2009, 2012; J. Wang et al., 2008; Li et al., 2010; Liu et al., 2010; Muzhingi et al., 2011; Ghavami et al., 2012; La Frano, 2013) or longer term provisions (~50–60 d) (Pee et al., 1998; Tang et al., 1999; Haskell et al., 2004; Khan et al., 2007, van Loo-Bouwman, 2009, 2010) of β-carotene-containing foods. The equivalence ratio would also be dependent on characteristics of the target population, such as differences in vitamin A status, nutrient deficiencies, gut integrity, and genetic polymorphisms associated with β-carotene metabolism, aside from the food-related factors that affect bioavailability discussed in Chapter 9. The vitamin A equivalency ratio was very high (26.1 or 28:1) when cooked green leafy vegetables were consumed by anemic Indonesian school children or by anemic lactating Vietnamese women with marginal vitamin A status and a high prevalence of intestinal helminths (≥48% and ≥62%, respectively) (Pee et al., 1998; Khan et al., 2007). The iron status of the school children was inadequate; that of the women was not reported. Retinol homeostasis can be disrupted in iron deficiency, resulting in low serum retinol concentration. The ratio was lower (10:1) when cooked pureed spinach was consumed by Bangladeshi men with marginal vitamin A status who were treated for intestinal helminths (Haskell et al., 2004).

In their review, van Loo-Bouwman et al. (2014) proposed a vitamin A equivalence for β-carotene in a mixed diet of 9:1–16:1 for a Western diet under Western conditions. For a non-Western diet including a variety of commonly consumed vegetables, an equivalence of 9:1 to 28:1 in a mixed diet was considered prudent. These authors also cited genetic polymorphisms in the *BCO1* gene and the degree of regulation of the expression of *BCO1* in response to vitamin A status as possible cause of the interindividual variations in reported equivalence ratios.

Considering the numerous factors that impact bioefficacy, manifested in the highly variable equivalency ratios obtained in the different studies, it is an oversimplication to establish a single conversion factor for β-carotene and another single factor for the other provitamin A carotenoids, as pointed out by Rodriguez-Amaya (1989, 1996). It is more realistic to establish ratios for different food groups (e.g., raw leafy vegetables, cooked leafy vegetables, raw fruits, processed fruits, roots), preferably with different sets of ratios for developed and developing countries.

10.4 STRATEGIES TO COMBAT VITAMIN A DEFICIENCY

There is no single solution to combat micronutrient malnutrition. Countries should choose the strategy that best fits their particular needs and conditions, and often, simultaneous implementation of interventions is needed. Global efforts to control vitamin A deficiency date back to the 1970s when three strategies were proposed: (a) periodic supplementation with high-dose vitamin A capsules, (b) food fortification, and (c) dietary diversification. More recently, biofortication and conservation of biodiversity for food and nutrition have been advocated.

In the December 1992 UN International Conference on Nutrition Declaration and Plan of Action (FAO/WHO, 1992), the recommendation for vitamin A was as follows: "Implement the most appropriate combination of the following measures: improved food availability, food preservation, food and nutrition education and training, dietary diversification, food fortification, supplementation, and pertinent public-health measures such as primary health care, promotion of breast-feeding, and safe drinking water." It was further stated that food-based strategies be given first priority, favoring locally available foods and taking into account local food habits, and that supplementation should be progressively phased out as soon as micronutrient-rich food-based strategies enable adequate consumption of micronutrients.

10.4.1 Vitamin A supplementation

Supplementation is an immediate and cost-effective strategy to improve the vitamin A status of populations in which there is acute vitamin A deficiency (Ross 2002). It has been widely implemented (e.g., Pedro et al., 2004; Aguayo et al., 2005; Donnen et al., 2007; Idindili et al., 2007). It is, however, a short-term, temporary approach that must be employed until food-based strategies provide sufficient vitamin A intake. Under these programs, children aged 6 months to 5 years receive a high dose of vitamin A (100,000 international units for children 6–11 months and 200,000 international units for children 1–5 years), usually in the form of a capsule, at 6-month intervals.

The periodic vitamin A supplementation of preschool children has been reported not only to reduce clinical signs of vitamin A deficiency but also to reduce the mortality rate in children in developing countries. A review of 43 randomized trials representing 215,633 children showed that giving vitamin A capsules to children aged 6 months to 5 years could reduce death and some diseases (Imdad et al., 2010). The results of 17 of the studies indicated that vitamin A reduced the overall risk of death by 24%. This is in accordance with the earlier report of Beaton et al. (1993), which also affirmed that vitamin A supplementation resulted in an average reduction of 23% in mortality rates of infants and children between 6 months and five years.

In general, periodic high-dose vitamin A supplementation brought benefits to malnourished children but no benefit or some adverse effects in well-nourished children. There are reports associating high-dose vitamin A with adverse effects, particularly in children with respiratory infection (Bresee et al., 1996; Donnen et al., 1998; Fawzi et al., 2000; Mahalanabis et al., 2004).

In the Philippines, a detectable impact of vitamin A capsules on serum retinol was limited to groups with the highest prevalence of vitamin A deficiency and lasted up to 4 months after supplementation (Pedro et al., 2004). It therefore appeared that distribution of high-dose capsules would be necessary every 3 or 4 months.

Supplementation (50,000 international units) is also recommended for non-breast-fed infants or breast-fed infants (less than 6 months old) whose mothers have not received supplemental vitamin A. To enhance the vitamin A status of the mother and the breast-fed infant, supplementation in lactating mothers (200,000 international units within 8 weeks of childbirth) has been recommended.

Although conceptually simple, periodic high-dose supplementation has operational problems. It is often integrated in national immunization days to take advantage of the same structure, thus lowering operational costs and insuring high coverage. Nevertheless, irregular or inadequate supplies, budget constraints at the national level, poor orientation and low motivation of health workers, and lack of supervision have been cited as causes of poor outreach of the program. Coverage varies widely and is often inadequate, with more remote areas being more difficult to reach and being often neglected due to poor infrastructure. In India, for example, weak implementation strategies were reported to have kept the vitamin A supplementation program from achieving its target coverage (Bhutia et al., 2013). The coverage for children aged 12–59 months was only 20% for one dose in 6 months. The current program suffers from an absence of clear guidelines, diminishing organizational effectiveness, and lack of community involvement and social accountability.

Although the favored approach of international agencies, vitamin A supplementation has achieved inadequate coverage and is usually not sustainable without external support. For this reason, there has been increasing emphasis on a sustainable dietary approach to the prevention of subclinical vitamin A deficiency.

10.4.2 Food fortification

In developed countries, fortification (the addition of essential nutrients to foods for prevention or correction of a dietary deficiency) is common and has contributed immensely to the reduction of micronutrient deficiency. Without it, many individuals in the United States would not meet recommended micronutrient intakes (Dwyer et al., 2014). It does not require changes in the dietary habits of the population, can be implemented relatively quickly, and can be sustainable over long periods of time (FAO/ILSI, 1997). Fortification programs require careful planning to ensure that appropriate food vehicles and fortificants are chosen.

Indiscriminate fortification of foods can result in overfortification or underfortification in the food supply and nutrient imbalances in the diets of individuals (Dwyer et al., 2014). Guidelines have been developed to avoid the indiscriminate addition of nutrients to foods. The American Medical Association, Institute of Food Technologists, Food and Nutrition Board guidelines recommend the following prerequisites to justify fortification: (a) the intake of a particular nutrient is inadequate for a substantial portion of the population, (b) the food is consumed by most individuals in the target population, (c) there is reasonable assurance that excessive intake will not occur, and (d) the cost is reasonable for the intended population (cited by Gregory, 2008).

Fortifying a widely consumed centrally processed food with critical nutrients can be a viable strategy to reduce the prevalence and severity of micronutrient deficiency in developing countries. Various aspects of fortification should be addressed: selecting an appropriate vehicle and an adequate level of fortification to meet the requirements, along with stability, quality control, and monitoring. The safety and appropriateness of fortification levels should be monitored and assured at both the production and household level. A major problem is that most poor populations cannot afford centrally processed foods.

In a forum held in the Philippines in 2000 on food fortification policy for the protection of populations from mineral and vitamin deficiencies in Asia and the Pacific, the following consensus was reached: all people in the region should have access to affordable, safe, and efficacious fortified foods as a long-term and permanent commitment to the elimination of micronutrient malnutrition; all salt intended for human consumption should be iodized; flour fortification with essential vitamins and minerals should be an integral part of all strategies to control and prevent malnutrition;

fortification of staple foods like rice, cereals, and oils as well as condiments and industrially processed complementary foods should be encouraged, particularly the fortification with iron, vitamin A, zinc, and folic acid (Solon, 2000).

Food fortification with vitamin A, especially of oil or sugar, has been launched in developing countries (Mokhtar et al., 2001; Dary and Moura 2002; Darnton-Hill and Nalubola, 2002; Klemm et al., 2010; Fiedler and Afidra, 2010). Sugar has been fortified with vitamin A in Central American countries, and biological efficacy and program effectiveness are well established (Dary and Moura, 2002). In many countries, margarine is fortified with vitamin A (Darnton-Hill and Nalubola, 2002) or β-carotene, which acts as both a coloring agent and a nutrient. Oils used in light cooking or salads can also serve as carriers. In the Philippines, the efficacy of vitamin A-fortified margarine and pandesal bread has been proven (Solon et al., 2000).

10.4.3 Dietary diversification

Investments in reducing micronutrient malnutrition have focused on supplementation and fortification programs and policies to the detriment of food-based approaches, which focus on increasing the amount of micronutrients consumed in the diet and on enhancing bioavailability. Food-based approaches are complex and require collaboration of different sectors, including agriculture, nutrition, food science and technology, education, and economics. Notwithstanding the difficulty in implementation and evaluation of efficacy, these strategies are the long-term approaches to combatting VAD and are believed to be more sustainable and culturally acceptable than supplementation or fortification. Moreover, contrary to single nutrient interventions, foods have various micronutrients and bioactive substances, and can therefore address several deficiencies as well as chronic degenerative diseases. It is now recognized that the food's beneficial effect on health is due not to single compounds or a single class of compounds but to the combined (additive or synergistic) effects of several constituents.

Underwood (2000) cited several advantages of dietary strategies:

- Multiple macro- and micronutrient deficiencies may be at least partially corrected through diversifying vitamin A sources in diets. For example, green leafy vegetables contain iron, vitamin E, vitamin K, riboflavin, folate, and frequently vitamin C.
- The natural balance of essential nutrients in foods minimizes the risk of adverse nutrient interactions and toxicity.
- Household empowerment is enhanced through dietary strategies. For example, informed household decisions facilitate self-reliant control over family well-being.
- The underlying cause of vitamin A deficiency and of malnutrition in general (i.e., inadequate intake of nutritious foods relative to need) can be eased.
- Leadership and management capacities are developed by dietary strategies that enable community participation in the identification, solving, and monitoring of problems, and as a consequence, overall community development is stimulated.
- Flexibility in diversification, modification, and food-to-food enhancement of menus based on local resources is accommodated.
- Functional components in food beyond those now recognized as beneficial for health are made available.

Additionally, dietary approaches frequently engage women and the poor, fostering culturally acceptable sustainable solutions, and in the process build self-worth, confidence, and reliance (Smitasiri et al., 1999). Food-based strategies promote self-sufficiency and food security while other approaches tend to perpetuate dependency on external donor agencies (Greiner, 2013). The rationale for and the multiple benefits of food-based strategies have been increasingly recognized (FAO/ILSI, 1997; Chakravarty, 2000; Balcha, 2001; Latham 2010; Blasbalg et al., 2011; Kennedy et al., 2011; Thompson and Amoroso, 2013; Greiner, 2013; Tang 2013). Food-based strategies can draw both direct impact on nutritional status and health by changing the production, preparation, and consumption of foods, and indirect impact by changing associated aspects such as income, expenditure, and empowerment of women (Pee et al., 2000). The combination of these impacts, each subject to confounding factors, makes evaluation of effectiveness highly complicated.

Difficulties with dietary approaches has also been pointed out (Underwood, 2000):

- A unified national approach may be difficult because of variable conditions and resources across regions and within countries.
- Local adaptations are necessary and, therefore, require local planning where management skills may be lacking.
- Homestead food-production strategies are susceptible to seasonality, environmental disasters (e.g., persistent drought), and environmental contamination.
- Among poor households, home food production is open to economic draw of markets and to pressures to produce quantity for a few marketable crops rather than quality and diversity for home consumption to provide family nutritional and health gains.

Some reviews have found little evidence for an effect of agricultural interventions on the nutritional status of children (Ruel, 2001; Berti et al., 2004; Leroy and Frongillo, 2007). Masset et al. (2012), however, attributed this result to the lack of statistical power of the studies rather than to the lack of effectiveness of the interventions.

Dietary diversification includes increased production and consumption of plant foods rich in provitamins A, better storage and preparation methods to preserve the provitamins, and small livestock and fishery projects. It involves changes in food production practices, food selection patterns, and traditional household methods for preparing and processing indigenous foods. It should include increasing women's access to food processing technologies that extend the availability of vitamin A and provitamin A–rich foods, reduce nutrient losses due to traditional processing, and improve hygienic and nutritional quality of the processed food products (Mulokozi et al., 2001). An improved solar-drying method, for example, retained more β-carotene in green leafy vegetables than traditional sun-drying.

10.4.3.1 Home gardening

Considered by many as the most effective food-based approach in most low-income settings (Marsh, 1998), home gardening programs have been practiced and evaluated in Bangladesh (Talukder et al., 2000; Bushamuka et al., 2005), India (Vijayaraghavan et al.,

1997), Nepal (Shankar et al., 1998), South Africa (Faber et al., 2001, 2002; Faber and van Jaarsveld, 2007), and the Philippines (Miura et al., 2003). In Bangladesh, a pilot study was successfully scaled up to a national homestead-gardening program (Talukder et al., 2000).

Home gardens can provide the household with direct access to important nutrients, therefore addressing multiple nutritional requirements simultaneously. Moreover, a garden can serve as a possible source of additional income for the household.

Low consumption of fruits and vegetables has been shown to be due to lack of awareness, aside from low availability of these foods at the household level. This led to projects promoting the production and consumption of carotenoids-rich foods through home and school gardening, complemented by information, education, and communication strategies. In order to be successful, gardening projects should be supported by nutrition education programs to raise awareness of the importance of micronutrients and consequences of their deficiency, assess dietary consumption, diversify food production, and improve food preparation, processing, preservation, storage, and marketing of micronutrient-rich foods. The low bioavailability of plant provitamins A has led to the promotion of home or small-scale production of fish, poultry, and small animals to increase consumption of animal-derived foods rich in preformed vitamin A and bioavailable iron.

Diet diversification programs should take advantage of the diversity of local indigenous and traditional crops and wild plant species, which are often rich in nutrients and bioactive compounds, promoting their production, marketing, and consumption. Complementary public health measures that help reduce micronutrient malnutrition should also be implemented, such as deworming, malaria prevention and control, and improved water and sanitation facilities.

10.4.3.2 Breast-feeding

An essential way to prevent deficiency of vitamin A and a range of other nutrients and protective factors in infants and young children is breast-feeding. Breast milk can supply the vitamin A that an infant needs for the first 6 months of life and can continue to be an important source through to the age of 2 years. Although vitamin A concentration in human milk depends on the mother's vitamin A status, vitamin A deficiency is rare among breast-fed infants, even in parts of the world where vitamin A deficiency is endemic. The promotion of exclusive breast-feeding for 4–6 months and continued breast-feeding with complementary foods thereafter should be a part of any dietary intervention to improve vitamin A status.

10.4.3.3 Reduction of postharvest losses

It is estimated that roughly one-third of the food produced in the world for human consumption every year—approximately 1.3 billion tons—gets lost or wasted (Gustavsson et al., 2011). In medium- and high-income countries, food is to a significant extent wasted at the consumption stage. In the low-income countries, food losses occur mostly at the production, harvest, postharvest, and processing stages.

The problems are mainly inadequate harvest techniques, poor postharvest management and logistics, lack of infrastructure, poor processing and packaging, and lack of marketing information that would allow production to match demand better.

Increased production of provitamin A–rich food will not be sufficient in ameliorating VAD if postharvest losses are not prevented or at least reduced. Fruits, vegetables, roots, and tubers, the major sources of provitamins A, are highly perishable and have the highest losses/wastage rates.

10.4.4 Conservation of biodiversity for food and nutrition

Led by the Food and Agriculture Organization of the United Nations (FAO) and Bioversity International, there is an international, multidisciplinary initiative that promotes the sustainable use of biodiversity for food security and nutrition. This represents a merging of two objectives: conservation of biodiversity and promoting food and nutritional security.

Recognizing the prolonged worldwide decline of biodiversity, the Convention on Biological Diversity (CBD) was adopted in 1992 and signed by over 150 governments at the United Nations Conference on Environment and Development in Rio de Janeiro, Brazil. Since then, 192 countries and the European Union have ratified the agreement. It has three main goals: conservation of biodiversity, sustainable use of its components, and sharing of the benefits arising from the commercial and other utilization of genetic resources in a fair and equitable way (CBD, 2014).

Sustainable development is defined as development that meets the needs of the present without compromising the ability of future generations to meet their own needs. In the CBD report, sustainable use is the "use of components of biological diversity in a way and at a rate that does not lead to the long-term decline of biological diversity, thereby maintaining its potential to meet the needs and aspirations of present and future generations" (CBD, 2014).

The first program created under CBD was Agricultural Biodiversity. Under this program, there is an initiative titled *Mainstreaming Biodiversity Conservation and Sustainable Use for Improved Nutrition and Well-Being*. This initiative aims to promote the sustainable use of biodiversity in programs contributing to food security and improved human nutrition (Toledo and Burlingame, 2006; Johns and Eyzaguirre, 2007).

Bioversity International is a center of the Consultative Group on International Agricultural Research. It is a research institute with a mandate to advance the conservation and use of genetic diversity for the well-being of present and future generations (Bioversity International, 2014). FAO leads international efforts to defeat hunger (FAO, 2014). Its mandate is to raise the levels of nutrition, improve agricultural productivity, better the lives of rural populations, and contribute to the growth of the world economy.

The framework of the Biodiversity for Food and Nutrition Initiative is built around four elements: (a) Developing and documenting knowledge; (b) Integration of biodiversity, food, and nutrition issues into research and policy instruments; (c) Conserving and promoting wider use of biodiversity for food and nutrition; (d) Public awareness and supporting activities (FAO, 2015). The initiative addresses major global health issues and trends such as micronutrient deficiencies, the decline of dietary diversity, and the concomitant rise in chronic diseases that are affecting developing countries, particularly among the poor. It promotes the use of local biodiversity, including traditional foods of indigenous and local ecosystems, with their many sources of nutritionally rich species and varieties, as readily accessible, locally empowering, and sustainable sources of quality nutrition.

The following important findings in food and nutrition are recognized:

- A diversity of foods from plants and animals remains the best means to achieve a balanced diet. Nutritional status and child growth improve with consumption of greater food diversity, and available research indicates the health benefits of varied diets, particularly in fruits and vegetables.
- Because it is difficult to identify optimal diets, eating a wide range of foods provides a safeguard against nutritional deficiencies. Diverse diets contribute to the fight against problems of malnutrition and obesity in both developing and developed countries.
- Biodiversity is important in supporting agricultural production and sustainability. Genetic diversity can provide access to seeds and planting materials better adapted to existing conditions (e.g., drought-resistant traits or resistance to pests and diseases) and is the basis of adaptation as needs and conditions change.
- The general global trend toward diet simplification has negative impacts on human food security, nutritional balance, and health.

Diets low in variety but high in energy contribute to the escalating problems of obesity and chronic diseases, which are increasingly found along with micronutrient deficiencies and undernutrition (FAO, 2015). FAO is promoting a series of activities toward "sustainable diets" linking local food products, biodiversity, nutrition, and sustainability.

Studies show that foods from native, wild, and semicultivated species have higher contents of micronutrients and other health-promoting compounds than those derived from commercially grown plants. These studies provide additional strong justification for the Biodiversity Initiative. Determination of the composition of nutrients, carotenoids, and other bioactive compounds of indigenous species is being actively pursued around the world. FAO promotes training in food composition; courses have been held in Europe, Africa, Asia, Latin America, the Near East, and Oceania.

10.4.5 Biofortification

A recent approach, complementary to existing strategies for the reduction of micronutrient deficiency in high-risk countries, is to fortify the major staple foods with micronutrients (e.g., rice and wheat with iron and zinc; sweet potato, cassava, and maize with β-carotene), using the best traditional breeding practices and modern biotechnology (Nestel et al., 2006). Called biofortification, this approach takes advantage of the fact that millions of people, mostly in poorer countries, have regular daily intake of staple foods that fill the stomach but do not have sufficient micronutrients (Bouis, 1996). No behavioral change on the part of consumers is required. The population is allowed to grow and consume the same foods they are accustomed to eating while improving their micronutrient intake. It is intended to offer a sustainable and low-cost strategy to reach people with poor access to formal markets and health care systems in developing countries at a fraction of the recurring costs of either supplementation or fortification.

Once high-yielding biofortified cultivars are developed that meet the target nutrient levels, they are widely disseminated. The farmers are expected to continue to grow the biofortified crop year after year. A challenge is to get farmers and consumers to accept the biofortified crops and increase their intake of the target nutrient.

The HarvestPlus biofortification project initially focused on six staple crops: beans, cassava, maize, rice, sweet potatoes, and wheat. The potential for nutrient enhancement is also being examined in additional crops important in diets of those suffering from micronutrient deficiencies: bananas, barley, cowpeas, groundnuts, lentils, millet, pigeon, peas, plantains, potatoes, sorghum, and yams.

In order to be considered successful, biofortification should fulfill three requirements (Bouis and Welch, 2010):

- The breeding must be successful, high-nutrient density being combined with high yields and high profitability.
- Efficacy must be demonstrated, the micronutrient status of human subjects being improved when consuming the biofortified cultivars as normally eaten.
- The biofortified crops must be adopted by farmers and consumed by those suffering from micronutrient malnutrition in significant numbers.

In terms of vitamin A, the most successful product of the biofortication program so far is orange-fleshed sweet potato (OFSP). The production and consumption of OFSP, the result of efforts of plant breeders to select varieties with enhanced levels of β-carotene using conventional methods, is being actively pursued in sub-Saharan Africa and elsewhere to address vitamin A deficiency, amply fulfilling the three requirements for successful biofortification enumerated above.

Conventionally bred OFSP with β-carotene content reaching 194 μg/g had good stability during cooking (van Jaarsveld et al., 2006). Each serving of 125 g per day for 53 school days to 5-to-10-year-old children in Durban, South Africa, showed significant improvement of vitamin A status (van Jaarsveld et al., 2005). In rural Mozambique, a study (Low et al., 2007) found that OFSP was well accepted by young children and confirmed the effectiveness of OFSP in increasing vitamin A intake and the serum retinol concentrations in the children. Introduction of OFSP to Ugandan farming households also increased vitamin A intakes among malnourished children and women and was associated with improved vitamin A status among children (Hotz et al., 2012).

It is estimated that biofortified OFSP varieties can provide 50%–100% of daily vitamin A needs. They are high yielding, virus resistant, and drought tolerant. According to the HarvestPlus 2012 Annual Report, from 2007 to 2009 OFSP was disseminated to more than 10,000 households in Uganda. More than 60% of households adopted, grew, and ate OFSP (HarvestPlus, 2013). Consequently, the intake of OFSP increased by two-thirds for older children and nearly doubled for young children and women. In 2013, HarvestPlus and its partners delivered OFSP to more than 50,000 Ugandan farming households. In total, 126,000 households—more than three-quarters of a million Ugandans—are now eating OFSP (HarvestPlus, 2014).

β-Carotene biofortified cassava was released in Nigeria in 2011 and β-carotene fortified maize in 2012 in Zambia. More than 100,000 Nigerian farmers in more than 2,000 villages planted the biofortified cassava stems for the first time in 2013

(HarvestPlus, 2013). Since its official release, biofortified maize has reached more than 10,000 Zambian households. With β-carotene content much lower than that of OFSP, it is estimated that biofortified cassava can furnish 50% and biofortified maize 25% of the daily vitamin A needs.

β-carotene of biofortified cassava and maize have been shown to have good bioavailability (La Frano et al., 2014). The vitamin A equivalence of β-carotene in β-carotene-biofortified cassava porridge, evaluated in U.S. women, was 2.8:1 (Liu et al., 2010). In a second study, also with U.S. women, vitamin A conversion was 4.2:1 and 4.5:1, with and without added oil, respectively (La Frano et al., 2013). Another study of U.S. women showed that on average, 6.48 μg β-carotene in β-carotene-biofortified maize porridge was equivalent to 1 μg retinol (Li et al., 2010). In healthy Zimbabwean men, the vitamin A equivalency of β-carotene in high β-carotene cooked yellow maize was 3.2:1 (Muzhingi et al., 2011).

10.5 POTENTIAL PROVITAMIN A SOURCES FOR ALLEVIATING VAD

Considering that animal sources, though providing highly bioavailable vitamin A, are expensive or not available, the low-cost, available, and diverse plant foods rich in provitamin A represent the viable sustainable options for overcoming vitamin A deficiency in developing countries. As shown in Chapter 5, there are numerous plant-derived foods with high levels of β-carotene and some foods with moderate amounts of β-cryptoxanthin that can be promoted as possible provitamin A sources for food-based strategies to combat VAD.

10.5.1 Red palm oil

Red palm oil (RPO) is a highly concentrated source of bioavailable β- and α-carotene. Palm oil production and yields are high. It is inexpensive and produced in great quantities. Various small-scale human feeding studies have been successful in showing that red palm oil increases or at least maintains vitamin A status, and this oil has been widely investigated and proposed for food-based intervention for VAD amelioration (e.g., Lian et al., 1967; Rao, 1994, 2001; Mahapatra and Manorama, 1997; Manorama et al., 1997; Solomons, 1998, 2003; Canfield and Kaminsky, 2000; Lietz et al., 2000, 2001, 2006; van Stuijvenberg and Benadé, 2000; van Stuijvenberg et al., 2000, 2001; Delisle et al., 2001; Sivan et al., 2001, 2002; Benadé, 2003; Radhika et al., 2003; Zagre et al., 2003; Zhang et al., 2003; Zeba et al., 2006). RPO was found to have a retinol equivalency of 5.7:1 (You et al., 2002). Four days of supplementation with palm oil carotenoids or synthetic β-carotene improved the plasma β-carotene status substantially (van het Hof et al., 1999).

In a survey of 420 children in Benin, mangoes, eggs, and various plant-based sauces were the main vitamin A–rich foods consumed by young children, although the percentage of children consuming them was low (5%–11%) (Amoussa-Hounkpatin et al., 2012). Mangoes are seasonal and are available only 2 or 3 months a year, while very few children consumed eggs, probably because of their cost. Plant-based sauces, which have generally high contents of provitamin A coming from red palm oil/palm nut juice, were among the vitamin A–rich food consumed by the largest number of children.

Noting that despite its abundance, RPO has seldom been used for VAD prevention on a national level, Burri (2012) concluded that the important barriers appear to be the following: (a) RPO requires refining, limiting its profitability and availability for small farmers. (b) The goal of most refining methods is to create a low-cost bland, odorless, and colorless fat, which requires removal of carotenoids. (c) Production cost is prohibitive, since RPO use competes with high-value vitamin A supplements, which are heavily subsidized. Refining, however, is required for the production of colorless palm oil. For RPO as a source of provitamin A, refining is not needed. Different raw materials (red palm fruits) are used separately for the oil and the provitamin A source or the carotenoid fraction is separated prior to refining to produce the oil. Moreover, in many developing countries, RPO is a traditional food, and its strong color and taste are appreciated rather than considered a drawback.

Consumption of RPO increased the concentrations of α- and β-carotene significantly in both plasma and breast milk (Lietz et al., 2001). It was concluded that breast-milk retinol might be maintained through increased intake of RPO and use of mild cooking preparation methods (such as the addition of the oil at the end of cooking and avoiding frying).

10.5.2 Green leafy vegetables

Relatively easy to produce and available practically all year round, dark green leafy vegetables are the most affordable and available sources of provitamin A in developing countries. They also provide other nutrients (vitamins and minerals) and bioactive substances (phenolic compounds, fiber). Both Rodriguez-Amaya (1997) and Reddy (2000) cited green leafy vegetables among the rich sources of β-carotene. A survey of earlier work revealed that dark green leafy vegetables are the most common rich sources of β-carotene in developing countries, such as India, Thailand, Malaysia, Bangladesh, Nepal, and Brazil (Rodriguez-Amaya, 1997).

Chapter 5 cites many examples of green leafy vegetables with substantial amounts of β-carotene, such as moringa, amaranth, spinach, sweet potato leaves, taro, kale, and numerous indigenous edible leaves. Spinach is the most studied green leafy vegetable, especially in developed countries. India, Sri Lanka, Tanzania, and Fiji have many analyzed indigenous dark green leafy vegetables with high levels of β-carotene. In Brazil, along with indigenous varieties of squash, native leafy vegetables dominate the ten richest sources of β-carotene among vegetables (Rodriguez-Amaya et al., 2008). Carrot, often referred to as the richest source of this carotenoid in the international literature, is only seventh among the Brazilian sources.

The potential role of provitamin A carotenoids from green leafy vegetables in furnishing adequate amounts of vitamin A has been challenged because of their low bioavailability (Pee et al., 1995, 1998). Later research, however, showed a substantial increase in serum β-carotene in children successfully treated for *Ascaris lumbricoides*, after feeding with a moderately high cumulative dose of dark green leafy vegetable for 6 weeks (Persson et al., 2001). Moreover, addition of oil to vegetables during cooking enhanced the in vitro accessibility of all-*E*-β-carotene several fold, and consumption of vegetables cooked with oil might make it possible to achieve the daily recommended safe intake of vitamin A within one meal (Mulokozi et al., 2004). Other studies have also indicated that it is possible to improve the in vitro accessibility (Chandrika et al., 2006) and the total body vitamin A pool size, and restore low liver vitamin A contents (Ribaya-Mercado et al., 2007) by eating sufficient amounts of carotene-rich yellow vegetables and green leafy vegetables with a minimum amount of fat. Consumption of yellow and dark green leafy vegetables produced in home gardens significantly improved the vitamin A status of 2-to-5-year-old children in a rural village in South Africa (Faber et al., 2002). Using isotope-dilution techniques, Tang et al. (1999) showed that carotenoid-rich green-yellow vegetables could provide adequate vitamin A nutrition in the diet of kindergarten children and protect them from becoming vitamin A deficient during seasons when the provitamin A food source was limited. Using intrinsically deuterated vegetables in conjunction with an isotope reference method, it was shown in women that spinach or carrot, cooked in various ways, could provide significant amounts of vitamin A (Tang et al., 2005).

10.5.3 Carrot and orange-fleshed sweet potato

Two root crops, carrot and orange-fleshed sweet potato, are available worldwide and are important sources of provitamin A carotenoids. Especially in developed countries, carrot is a major source of provitamin A carotenoids (α- and β-carotene). It is often referred to as the richest source of β-carotene in the international literature.

OFSP was promoted as part of food-based approaches to overcome VAD even before the HarvestPlus biofortification program was started. Sweet potato is a staple food in many developing countries. Unfortunately, the most consumed varieties are white-fleshed, practically devoid of carotenoids. However, indigenous varieties of orange-fleshed potatoes are available.

Evaluating orange-fleshed sweet potato as an intervention food to prevent VAD, Burri (2011) calculated that 6 to 33 g/day (0.02 to 0.13 cup/day) for a 3-year-old child with marginal vitamin A status and 68 to 381 g/day (0.27 to 1.49 cups/day) for a lactating woman with good status would be needed to meet vitamin A requirements.

Plant-based complementary foods are key sources of nutrients in addition to breast milk for infants in lower income countries. A household-level sweet potato–based infant food rich in provitamin A was developed to complement vitamin A supplementation initiatives in sub-Saharan Africa (Amagloh et al., 2012).

Cultivation of β-carotene vegetables was promoted in a crop-based intervention in South Africa (Laurie et al., 2008). Children from project households consumed carrot, butternut, spinach, and orange-fleshed sweet potato more frequently than children from control households. In an earlier study in Kenya (Hagenimana et al., 2001) children in the intervention group consumed vitamin A–rich foods almost twice as frequently as control children (93% more), especially orange-fleshed sweet potatoes, mangoes, dark-green leafy vegetables, butter, and eggs. β-Carotene values were high enough that one cup of boiled and mashed sweet potato fed daily to children of weaning age was considered sufficient to meet their vitamin A requirement, even using the higher 12:1 β-carotene to retinol conversion.

10.5.4 Tropical fruits

Unlike temperate fruits in which anthocyanin pigments predominate, many tropical and subtropical fruits are carotenogenic, as shown in Chapter 5. Provitamin A carotenoids have generally lower levels in fruits than in leafy vegetables but are more bioavailable, as discussed in Chapter 9. Among fruits, mango and papaya are often mentioned in programs aimed at combatting VAD. For example, mango has been promoted as source of vitamin A for young children in the rural areas of Burkina Faso (Nana et al., 2006).

Chapter 5 also cites other tropical fruits, especially indigenous fruits, with high levels of β-carotene. In Brazil, the palm fruit buriti has the highest β-carotene concentration among the numerous foods already analyzed (Rodriguez-Amaya et al., 2008). It also has substantial amounts of γ-carotene. The native palm fruits tucumã, umari, and bocaiúva are also rich sources of β-carotene. Moreover, through in vitro assay (Oliveira and Rodriguez-Amaya, 2010), β-carotene from buriti, tucumã, and pupunha were found to have better bioaccessibility than that from commercially produced fruits, apparently due to their lipid content. The non-palm fruits, orange-fleshed melons and vitamin C-rich acerola are also good sources of β-carotene.

In Vietnam, the gac fruit is an excellent source of β-carotene (170–350 μg/g), surpassing by a wide margin 16 other commonly consumed fruits and vegetables (Vuong, 2000; Vuong et al., 2002). Although easy to grow, it is available only 3 months a year, and there have been no efforts to educate the at-risk population about its health benefits.

10.6 CURRENT STATUS OF β-CAROTENE RESEARCH

Experts in the field of carotenoids met at the Hohenheim consensus conference in July 2009 to discuss the current status of β-carotene research. The following consensuses were drawn (Grune et al., 2010):

- When comparing food-derived all-*E*-β-carotene with synthetic all-*E*-β-carotene, there is no evidence that the latter is deleterious.
- Based on in vitro data, there is evidence that β-carotene has effects that go beyond the established provitamin A function. However, such effects have not yet been unequivocally proven in humans.
- Compared with other carotenoids, the primary role of β-carotene is its provitamin A activity.
- Dietary β-carotene intake varies widely and is not normally distributed in the population. The majority of people consume 1–2 mg/d (reported for the United States and the United Kingdom), although, in rare cases, an intake of 10 mg/d has been reported.
- The number of people at risk for poor vitamin A status depends on the intake of total vitamin A, which is defined as preformed vitamin A plus provitamin A. Based on numerous studies, it is evident that parts of the world's population do not meet the recommendations for vitamin A intake with dietary sources of preformed vitamin A.

To fill the gap between the low intake from sources containing preformed vitamin A, adequate amounts of provitamin A must additionally be supplied.

- According to the German National Nutrition Survey II, foods fortified with β-carotene often are important contributors (up to 30%) to the daily supply of vitamin A. The extent (roughly estimated as 3%–12%) differs in various countries and depends on different food sources (fortified nonalcoholic beverages, cheese, butter, etc.).
- Although fruits and vegetables contribute to the daily vitamin A supply, the recommended β-carotene intake of 2–4 mg/d is not achieved in the general population. Even based on a conversion ratio of 6:1, it is not possible to ensure that the whole population consumes the recommended intake of vitamin A (including intake of preformed vitamin A).
- The intake of preformed vitamin A in large parts of the Asian population is very low. β-Carotene is only partially able to ensure an optimal total vitamin A intake and is mostly derived from leafy vegetables and fruits.
- The bioavailability of β-carotene from natural sources depends on the food matrix and individual response.
- The following food-related factors largely influence the bioavailability of β-carotene: food matrix, food processing, fat in the meal (including avocado fat and fat replacers such as sucrose polyester), other carotenoids in the meal, and dietary fiber. Additional consumer-related factors include polymorphisms related to metabolism, vitamin A status, and gut integrity.
- In any given population, the conversion rate appears to differ substantially among individuals, resulting in a population mean with a high variance. Following early intestinal conversion, there is continuous postabsorptive conversion over time. There may be tissue-specific differences in the propensity for uptake, storage, and cleavage, but they have not yet been systematically defined.
- Conversion efficiency depends at least in part on the individual's vitamin A status, BMI, and comorbidities. Genetic factors are becoming known that influence bioavailability of β-carotene.
- There is a specific distribution of β-carotene in adipose tissue, skin, intestine, adrenal gland, liver, corpus luteum, and the macula. However, the regulation, if any, of β-carotene uptake, retention, and turnover in these tissues is largely unknown.
- Based on recent data, including food composition and data from national surveys, the intake of preformed vitamin A is inadequate in a substantial part of the general population. For many people, the gap between the RDA/recommended nutrient intake (or other reference intake) and the quantity of vitamin A consumed as preformed vitamin A cannot be closed by consumption of 2–4 mg/day of β-carotene from a regular diet.
- The basic need for β-carotene in its provitamin A function is defined by the existing gap between preformed vitamin A intake and recommendations for total vitamin A intake. In cases of poor vitamin A status due to low intake of preformed vitamin A, an intake of β-carotene in the range of 2–4 mg/d still might not sufficiently correct the individual vitamin A status. Indeed, an appropriate intake of β-carotene from food and/or supplement will safely compensate the gap of vitamin A.
- There are various groups at risk for an inadequate vitamin A supply, especially young individuals as well as pregnant and lactating women.

The conclusions are:

- Due to its unique structure and cleavage efficiency, β-carotene is the most efficient provitamin A carotenoid. As an antioxidant, the compound quenches singlet molecular oxygen and scavenges reactive oxygen species, especially peroxyl radicals. Singlet oxygen quenching is likely to be restricted to the skin as the only light-exposed tissue that contains higher levels of β-carotene; other carotenoids demonstrate similar activity. Upon radical scavenging, β-carotene decomposes and cannot be regenerated. Thus, it is suggested that the major function of β-carotene in human nutrition is that of a provitamin A.
- The provitamin A function of β-carotene is well established. Nutritional surveys from various countries consistently report β-carotene intake to be essential to meet vitamin A requirements.

References

Aguayo VM, Baker SK, Crespin X, Hamani H, Mamadoul Taïbou A. 2005. Maintaining high vitamin A supplementation coverage in children: lessons from Niger. *Food Nutr Bull* 26:26–31.

Amagloh FK, Hardacre A, Mutukumira AN, Weber JL, Brough L, Coad J. 2012. A household-level sweet potato-based infant food to complement vitamin A supplementation initiatives. *Matern Child Nutr* 8:512–21.

Amengual J, Glenn P, Lobo GP, Golczak M, Li HNM, Klimova T, Hoppel CL, Wyss A, Palczewski K, von Lintig J. 2011. A mitochondrial enzyme degrades carotenoids and protects against oxidative stress. *FASEB J* 25:948–59.

Amoaful EF. 2001. Planning a national food-based strategy for sustainable control of vitamin A deficiency in Ghana: steps toward transition from supplementation. *Food Nutr Bull* 22:361–5.

Amoussa-Hounkpatin W, Mouquet-Rivier C, Dossa RAM, Picq C, Avallone S. 2012. Contribution of plant-based sauces to the vitamin A intake of young children in Benin. *Food Chem* 131:948–55.

Balcha HM. 2001. Experience of World Vision Ethiopia Micronutrient Program in promoting the production of vitamin A-rich foods. *Food Nutr Bull* 22:366–9.

Beaton GH, Martorell R, Aronson KJ, Edmonston B, McCabe G, Ross AC, Harvey B. 1993. Effectiveness of vitamin A supplementation in the control of young child morbidity and mortality in developing countries. Nutrition policy discussion paper No. 13. Geneva: United Nations Administrative Committee Coordination/Subcommittee on Nutrition.

Benadé AJS. 2003. A place for palm fruit oil to eliminate vitamin A deficiency. *Asia Pac J Clin Nutr* 12:369–72.

Berti PR, Krasevec J, FitzGerald S. 2004. A review of the effectiveness of agriculture interventions in improving nutrition outcomes. *Public Health Nutr* 7:599–609.

Bhutia DT, de Pee S, Zwanikken PAC. 2013. Vitamin A coverage among under-five children. A critical appraisal of the vitamin A supplementation program in India. *Sight Life* 27(1):12–19.

Bioversity International. 2014. Improving lives through biodiversity research. Retrieved 1 Jun 2014 from http://www.bioversityinternational.org/.

Blasbalg TL, Wispelwey B, Deckelbaum RJ. 2011. Econutrition and utilization of food-based approaches for nutritional health. *Food Nutr Bull* 32:S4–13.

Bouis H. (1996). Enrichment of food staples through plant breeding: a new strategy for fighting micronutrient malnutrition. *Nutr. Rev.* 54:131–7.

Bouis HE, Welch RM. 2010. Biofortification: a sustainable agricultural strategy for reducing micronutrient malnutrition in the global south. *Crop Sci* 50:S20–32.

Bresee JS, Fischer M, Dowell SF, Johnston BD, Biggs VM, Levine RS, Lingappa JR, Keyserling HL, Petersen KM, Bak JR, Gary HE Jr, Sowell AL, Rubens CE, Anderson LJL. 1996. Vitamin A therapy for children with respiratory syncytial virus infection: a multicenter trial in the United States. *Pediatr Infect Dis* 15:777–82.

Burri BJ. 2011. Evaluating sweet potato as an intervention food to prevent vitamin A deficiency. *Compr Rev Food Sci Food Safety* 10:118–30.

Burri BJ. 2012. Evaluating global barriers to the use of red palm oil as an intervention food to prevent vitamin A deficiency. *Compr Rev Food Sci Food Safety* 11:221–32.

Bushamuka VN, de Pee S, Talukder A, Kiess L, Panagides D, Abu T, Bloem M. 2005. Impact of a homestead gardening program on household food security and empowerment of women in Bangladesh. *Food Nutr Bull* 26:17–25.

Canfield LM, Kaminsky RG. 2000. Red palm oil in the maternal diet improves the vitamin A status of lactating mothers and their infants. *Food Nutr Bull* 21:144–8.

CDB. 2014. The Convention on Biological Diversity. Retrieved Dec 2014 from https://www.cdbint/convention/.

Chakravarty I. 2000. Food-based strategies to control vitamin A deficiency. *Food Nutr Bull* 21:135–43.

Chandrika UG, Svanberg U, Jansz ER. 2006. *In vitro* accessibility of β-carotene from cooked Sri Lankan green leafy vegetables and their estimated contribution to vitamin A requirement. *J Sci Food Agric* 86:54–61.

Darnton-Hill I, Nalubola R. 2002. Fortification strategies to meet micronutrient needs: successes and failures. *Proc Nutr Soc* 61:231–41.

Dary O, Mora JO. 2002. Food fortification to reduce vitamin A deficiency: International Vitamin A Consultative Group recommendations. *J Nutr* 132:S2927–33.

Dela Seña C, Riedl KM, Narayanasamy S, Curley RW Jr, Schwartz SJ, Harrison EH. 2014. The human enzyme that converts dietary provitamin A carotenoids to vitamin A is a dioxygenase. *J Biol Chem* 289:13661–6.

Delisle H, Zagré N, Ouedraogo V. 2001. Marketing of red palm oil as a food source of vitamin A in Burkina Faso: a pilot project involving women's groups. *Food Nutr Bull* 22:388–94.

Donnen P, Dramaix M, Brasseur D, Bitwe R, Vertongen F, Hennart P. 1998. Randomized placebo-controlled clinical trial of the effect of a single high dose or daily low doses of vitamin A on the morbidity of hospitalized, malnourished children. *Am J Clin Nutr* 68:1254–60.

Donnen P, Sylla A, Dramaix M, Sall G, N Kuakuvi N, Hennart P. 2007. Effect of daily low dose of vitamin A compared with single high dose on morbidity and mortality of hospitalized mainly malnourished children in Senegal: a randomized controlled clinical trial. *Eur J Clin Nutr* 61:1393–9.

Dwyer JT, Woteki C, Bailey R, Britten P, Carriquiry A, Gaine PC, Miller D, Moshfegh A, Murphy MM, Edge MS. 2014. Fortification: new findings and implications. *Nutr Rev* 72:127–41.

Edwards AJ, You C-S, Swanson JE, Parker RS. 2001. A novel extrinsic reference method for assessing the vitamin A value of plant foods. *Am J Clin Nutr* 74:348–55.

Eroglu A, Hruszkewycz DP, dela Seña C, Narayanasamy S, Riedl KM, Kopec RE, Schwartz SJ, Curley RW Jr, Harrison EH. 2012. Naturally occurring eccentric cleavage products of provitamin A β-carotene function as antagonists of retinoid acid receptors. *J Biol Chem* 287:15886–95.

Faber M, Phungula MAS, Venter SL, Dhansay MA, Benadé AJS. 2002. Home gardens focusing on the production of yellow and dark-green leafy vegetables increase the serum retinol concentrations of 2-5-y-old children in South Africa. *Am J Clin Nutr* 76:1048–54.

Faber M, van Jaarsveld PJ. 2007. The production of provitamin A-rich vegetables in home-gardens as a means of addressing vitamin A deficiency in rural African communities. *J Sci Food Agric* 87: 366–77.

Faber M, Venter S, Phungula MAS, Benadé AJS. 2001. An integrated primary health-care and provitamin A household food-production program: impact on food-consumption patterns. *Food Nutr Bull* 22:370–5.

FAO. 2014. The Food and Agriculture Organization of the United Nations. Retrieved 1 Jun 2014 from http://www.fao.org/.

FAO. 2015. Biodiversity and nutrition a common path. Retrieved 6 Jan 2015 from http://fao.org/infoods/infoods/food-biodiversity/en/.

FAO/ILSI. 1997. *Preventing micronutrient malnutrition: a guide to food-based approaches*. A manual for policy makers and programme planners. Washington DC: International Life Sciences Institute Press.

FAO/WHO. 1967. *Requirements of vitamin A, thiamine, riboflavine and niacin*. Report of a Joint FAO/WHO Expert Group. WHO technical report series 362. Geneva: World Health Organization.

FAO/WHO. 1988. *Requirements of vitamin A, iron, folate and vitamin B_{12}*. FAO/WHO Joint Expert Consultation. FAO Food and Nutrition Series no. 23. Rome: Food and Agriculture Organization of the United Nations/World Health Orgranization.

FAO/WHO. 1992. *International Conference on Nutrition. World Declaration and Plan of Action. Final statement as agreed by all UN member states*. Rome: Food and Agriculture Organization of the United Nations/World Health Organization.

Fawzi WW, Mbise R, Spiegelman D, Fataki M, Hertzmark E, Ndossi G. 2000. Vitamin A supplements and diarrheal and respiratory tract infections among children in Dar es Salaam, Tanzania. *J Pediatr* 137:660–7.

Fiedler JL, Afidra R. 2010. Vitamin A fortification in Uganda: Comparing the feasibility, coverage, costs, and cost-effectiveness of fortifying vegetable oil and sugar. *Food Nutr Bull* 31:193–205.

Ghavami AQ, Coward WA, Bluck LJC. 2012. The effect of food preparation on the bioavailability of carotenoids from carrots using intrinsic labeling. *Br J Nutr* 107:1350–66.

Glover J, Redfearn ER. 1954. The mechanism of transformation of β-carotene into vitamin A in vivo. *Biochem J* 58:xv–xvi.

Goodman DS, Huang HS. 1965. Biosynthesis of vitamin A with rat intestinal enzyme. *Science* 149:879–80.

Goodman DS, Olson JA. 1969. The conversion of all-*trans* β-carotene into retinal. *Methods Enzymol* 15:462–475.

Gregory JF III. 2008. Vitamins. In: Damodaran S, Parkin KL, Fennema OR. editors. *Fennema's food chemistry*, 4th ed. Boca Raton: CRC Press Taylor & Francis Group, p 439–521.

Greiner T. 2013. *Vitamin A: moving the food-based approach forward*. FAO and WHO.

Grune T, Lietz G, Palou A, Ross AC, Stahl W, Tang G, Thurnham D, Yin S, Biesalski HK. 2010. β-Carotene is an important vitamin A source for humans. *J Nutr* 140:S2268–85.

Gustavsson J, Cederberg C, Sonesson U, van Otterdijk R, Meybeck A. 2011. *Global food losses: extent, causes and prevention*. Rome: FAO.

Hagenimana V, Low J, Anyango M, Kurz K, Gichuki ST, Kabira J. 2001. Enhancing vitamin A intake in young children in western Kenya: orange-fleshed sweet potatoes and women farmers can serve as key entry points. *Food Nutr Bull* 22:376–87.

Harrison EH. 2012. Mechanisms involved in the intestinal absorption of dietary vitamin A and provitamin A carotenoids. *Biochim Biophys Acta* 1821:70–7.

HarvestPlus. 2013. Bridging the delta. 2012 annual report. Available at http://r4d.dfid.gov.uk/pdf/outputs/Misc_Crop/HarvestPlus-Annual-Report-2012.pdf.

HarvestPlus. 2014. Diving into delivery. 2013 annual report. Available at http://r4d.dfid.gov.uk/pdf/outputs/Misc_Crop/HarvestPlus-2013-AnnualReport.pdf.

Haskell MJ. 2012. The challenge to reach nutritional adequacy for vitamin A: β-carotene bioavailability and conversion—evidence in humans. *Am J Clin Nutr* 96(suppl):S1193–203.

Haskell MJ, Jamil KM, Hassan F, Peerson JM, Hossain MI, Fuchs GJ, Brown KH. 2004. Daily consumption of Indian spinach (*Basella alba*) or sweet potatoes has a positive impact on total body vitamin A stores in Bangladeshi men. *Am J Clin Nutr* 80:705–14.

Hickenbottom SJ, Follett JR, Lin Y, Dueker SR, Burri BJ, Neidlinger TR, Clifford AJ. 2002a. Variability in conversion of β-carotene to vitamin A in men as measured by using a double-tracer study design. *Am J Clin Nutr* 75:900–7.

Hickenbottom SJ, Lemke SL, Ducker SR, Lin Y, Follett JR, Carkeet C, Buchholz BA, Vogel JS, Clifford AJ. 2002b. Dual isotope test for assessing β-carotene cleavage to vitamin A in humans. *Eur J Nutr* 41:141–7.

Hotz C, Loechl C, Lubowa A, Tumwine JK, Ndeezi G, Masawi AN, Baingana R, Carriquiry A, de Brauw A, Meenakshi JV, Gilligan DO. 2012. Introduction of β-carotene-rich orange sweet potato in rural Uganda resulted in increased vitamin A intakes among children and women and improved vitamin A status among children. *J Nutr* 142:1871–80.

Idindili B, Masanja H, Urassa H, Bunini W, van Jaarsveld P, Aponte JJ, Kahigwa E, Mshinda H, Ross D, Schellenberg DM. 2007. Randomized controlled safety and efficacy trial of 2 vitamin A supplementation schedules in Tanzanian infants. *Am J Clin Nutr* 85:1312–9.

Imdad A, Herzer K, Mayo-Wilson E, Yakoob MY, Bhutta ZA. 2010. Vitamin A supplementation for preventing morbidity and mortality in children from 6 months to 5 years of age. Cochrane Database of Systematic Reviews 2010 Issue 12, CD008524. doi:10.1002/14651858.CD008524.pub2.

IOM (Institute of Medicine). 2001. *Dietary reference intakes for vitamin A, vitamin K, arsenic, boron, chromium, copper, iodine, iron, manganese, molybdenum, nickel, silicon, vanadium, and zinc*. Washington DC: National Academy Press.

IOM (Institute of Medicine). 2006. *Dietary reference intakes: the essential guide to nutrient requirements*. Washington DC: National Academy Press.

Johns T, Eyzaguirre PB. 2007. Biofortification, biodiversity and diet: a search for complementary applications against poverty and malnutrition. *Food Policy* 32:1–24.

Kennedy E, Webb P, Walker P, Saltzman E, Maxwell D, Nelson M, Booth S. 2011. The evolving food and nutrition agenda: policy and research priorities for the coming decade. *Food Nutr Bull* 32:60–8.

Khan NC, West CE, de Pee S, Bosch D, Phuong HD, Hulshof PJM, Khoi HH, Verhoef H, Hautvast JGAJ. 2007. The contribution of plant foods to the vitamin A supply of lactating women in Vietnam: a randomized controlled trial. *Am J Clin Nutr* 85:1112–20.

Kiefer C, Hessel S, Lampert JM, Vogt K, Lederer MO, Breithaupt DE, von Lintig J. 2001. Identification and characterization of a mammalian enzyme catalyzing the asymmetric oxidative cleavage of provitamin A. *J Biol Chem* 276:14110–6.

Klemm RDW, West KP Jr, Palmer AC, Johnson Q, Randall P, Ranum P, Northrop-Clewes C. 2010. Vitamin A fortification of wheat flour: considerations and current recommendations. *Food Nutr Bull* 31:S47–61.

La Frano MR, de Moura FF, Boy E, Lönnerdal B, Burri BJ. 2014. Bioavailability of iron, zinc, and provitamin A carotenoids in biofortified staple crops. *Nutr Rev* 72:289–307.

La Frano MR, Woodhouse LR, Burnett DJ, Burri BJ. 2013. Biofortified cassava increases β-carotene and vitamin A concentrations in the TAG-rich plasma layer of American women. *Br J Nutr* 110:310–20.

Latham M. 2010. The great vitamin A fiasco. *J World Public Health Nutr Assoc* 1:1–20.

Laurie SM, Faber M. 2008. Integrated community-based growth monitoring and vegetable gardens focusing on crops rich in β-carotene: project evaluation in a rural community in the Eastern Cape, South Africa. *J Sci Food Agric* 88:2093–101.

Leroy JL, Frongillo EA. 2007. Can interventions to promote animal production ameliorate undernutrition? *J Nutr* 137:2311–6.

Leuenberger MG, Engeloch-Jarret C, Woggon W-D. 2001. The reaction mechanism of the enzyme-catalyzed central cleavage of β-carotene to retinal. *Angew Chem Int Ed Engl* 40:2613–7.

Li S, Nugroho A, Rocheford T, White W. 2010. Vitamin A equivalence of the β-carotene in β-carotene-biofortified maize porridge consumed by women. *Am J Clin Nutr* 92:1105–12.

Lian OK, Tie LT, Rose CS, Prawiranegara DD, Gyorgy P. 1967. Red palm oil in the prevention of vitamin A deficiency: a trial of preschool children in Indonesia. *Am J Clin Nutr* 20:1267–74.

Lietz G, Henry CJK, Mulokozi G, Mugyabuso J, Ballart A, Ndossi GD, Lorri W, Tomkins A. 2000. Use of red palm oil for the promotion of maternal vitamin A status. *Food Nutr Bull* 21:215–8.

Lietz G, Henry CJK, Mulokozi G, Mugyabuso JKL, Ballart A, Ndossi GD, Lorri W, Tomkins A. 2001. Comparison of the effects of supplemental red palm oil and sunflower oil on maternal vitamin A status. *Am J Clin Nutr* 74:501–9.

Lietz G, Lange J, Rimbach G. 2010. Molecular and dietary regulation of 15,15′-monooxygenase 1 (BCMO1). *Arch Biochem Bophys* 502:8–16.

Lietz G, Mulokozi G, Henry JCK, Tomkins AM. 2006. Xanthophyll and hydrocarbon carotenoid patterns differ in plasma and breast milk of women supplemented with red palm oil during pregnancy and lactation. *J Nutr* 136:1821–7.

Lin Y, Dueker SR, Burri BJ, Neidlinger TR, Clifford AJ. 2000. Variability of the conversion of β-carotene to vitamin A in women measured by using a double-tracer study design. *Am J Clin Nutr* 71:1545–54.

Lindqvist A, Andersson S. 2002. Biochemical properties of purified recombinant human β-carotene 15,15′-monooxygenase. *J Biol Chem* 277:23942–8.

Liu W, Zhou Y, Sanchez T, Ceballos H, White WS. 2010. The vitamin A equivalence of β-carotene in β-carotene-biofortified cassava ingested by women. *FASEB J* 24 (Meeting Abstract Supplement) 92.7.

Lobo GP, Amengual J, Palczewski G, Babino D, von Lintig J. 2012. Mammalian carotenoid-oxygenases: key players for carotenoid function and homeostasis. *Biochim Biophys Acta* 1821:78–87.

Lobo GP, Hessel S, Eichinger A, Noy N, Moise AR, Wyss A, Palczewski K, von Lintig J. 2010. ISX is a retinoic acid-sensitive gatekeeper that controls intestinal β,β-carotene absorption and vitamin A production. *FASEB J* 24:1656–66.

Low JW, Arimond M, Osman N, Cunguara B, Zano F, Tschirley D. 2007. A food-based approach introducing orange-fleshed sweet potatoes increased vitamin A intake and serum retinol concentrations in young children in rural Mozambique. *J Nutr* 137:1320–7.

Mahalanabis D, Lahiri M, Paul D, Gupta S, Gupta A, Wahed MA, Khaled MA. 2004. Randomized, double-blind, placebo-controlled clinical trial of the efficacy of treatment with zinc or vitamin A in infants and young children with severe acute lower respiratory infection. *Am J Clin Nutr* 79:430–6.

Mahapatra S, Manorama R. 1997. The protective effect of red palm oil in comparison with massive vitamin A dose in combating vitamin A deficiency. *Asia Pac J Clin Nutr.* 6:246–50.

Maida JM, Mathers K, Alley CL. 2008. Pediatric ophthalmology in the developing world. *Curr Opin Ophthalmol* 19:403–8.

Manorama R, Sarita M, Kavita R, Rukmini C. 1997. Red palm oil for combating vitamin A deficiency. *Asia Pac J Clin Nutr* 6:56–9.

Marsh R. 1998. Building on traditional gardening to improve household food security. *Food Nutr Agric* 22:4–14.

Masset E, Haddad L, Cornelius A, Isaza-Castro J. 2012. Effectiveness of agricultural interventions that aim to improve nutritional status of children: systematic review. *BMJ* 344:d8222– doi:10.1136/bmj.d8222.

McLaren DS, Frigg M. 2001. *Sight and life manual on vitamin A deficiency disorders (VADD)*, 2nd ed. Basel: Task Force Sight and Life.

Miura S, Kunii O, Wakai S. 2003. Home gardening in urban poor communities of the Philippines. *Int J Food Sci Nutr* 54:77–88.

Mokhtar N, Belhadj H, Kress D, Zerrari A, Chaouki N, Aguenaou H. 2001. Food-fortification program in Morocco. *Food Nutr Bull* 22:427–30.

Mulokozi G, Hedrén E, Svanberg U. 2004. In vitro accessibility and intake of β-carotene from cooked green leafy vegetables and their estimated contribution to vitamin A requirements. *Plant Foods Hum Nutr* 59:1–9.

Mulokozi G, Mselle L, Mugyabuso J, Johnson-Welch C. 2001. Reducing subclinical vitamin A deficiency through women's adoption of appropriate technologies in Tanzania. *Food Nutr Bull* 22:400–7.

Muzhingi T, Gadaga TH, Siwela AH, Grusak MA, Russell RM, Tang G. 2011. Yellow maize with high β-carotene is an effective source of vitamin A in healthy Zimbabwean men. *Am J Clin Nutr* 94:510–9.

Nana CP, Brouwer ID, Zagré NM, Kok FJ, Traoré AS. 2006. Impact of promotion of mango and liver as sources of vitamin A for young children: a pilot study in Burkina Faso. *Public Health Nutr* 9:808–13.

Nestel P, Bouis HE, Meenakshi JV, Pfeiffer W. 2006. Biofortification of staple food crops. *J Nutr* 136:1064–7.

Nestel P, Trumbo P. 1999. The role of provitamin A carotenoids in the prevention and control of vitamin A deficiency. *Archiv Latinoamer Nutr* 49:S26–33.

Novotny JA, Harrison DJ, Pawlosky R, Flanagan VP, Harrison EH, Kurilich AC. 2010. β-Carotene conversion to vitamin A decreases as the dietary dose increases in humans. *J Nutr* 140:915–8.

Oliveira GPR de, Rodriguez-Amaya DB. 2010. In vitro bioaccessibility of the carotenoids of fresh and processed fruits. Paper presented at the 28th International Horticultural Congress, Lisbon. In: Book of Symposium Abstracts. p 762.

Olson J. 1999. Bioavailability of carotenoids. *Archiv Latinamer Nutr* 49:S21–5.

Olson JA, Hayaishi O. 1965. The enzymatic cleavage of β-carotene into vitamin A by soluble enzymes of rat liver and intestine. *Proc Nat'l Acad Sci USA* 54:1364–70.

Olson JA, Lakshman MR. 1990. Carotenoid conversions. *Methods Enzymol* 189:425–32.

Parker RS. 1996. Absorption, metabolism, and transport of carotenoids. *FASEB J* 10:542–51.

Pedro MRA, Madriaga JR, Barba CVC, Habito RCF, Gana AE, Deitchler M, Mason JB. 2004. The National Vitamin A Supplementation Program and subclinical vitamin A deficiency among preschool children in the Philippines. *Food Nutr Bull* 25:319–29.

Pee S de, Bloem MW, Kiess L. 2000. Evaluating food-based programmes for their reduction of vitamin A deficiency and its consequences. *Food Nutr Bull* 21:232–8.

Pee S de, West CE, Hautvast JGAJ, Muhilal, Karyadi D. 1995. Lack of improvement in vitamin A status with increased consumption of dark-green leafy vegetables. *Lancet* 346:75–81.

Pee S de, West CE, Permaesih D, Martuti S, Muhilal, Hautvast JG. 1998. Orange fruit is more effective than are dark-green, leafy vegetables in increasing serum concentrations of retinol and beta-carotene in schoolchildren in Indonesia. *Am J Clin Nutr* 68:1058–67.

Persson V, Ahmed F, Gebre-Medhin M, Greiner T. 2001. Increase in serum beta-carotene following dark green leafy vegetable supplementation in Mebendazole-treated school children in Bangladesh. *Eur J Clin Nutr* 55:1–9.

Radhika MS, Bhaskaram P, Balakrishna N, Ramalakshmi BA. 2003. Red palm oil supplementation: a feasible diet-based approach to improve the vitamin A status of pregnant women and their infants. *Food Nutr Bull* 24:208–17.

Rao BSN. 1994. Potential use of red palm oil in combating vitamin A deficiency in India. *Food Nutr Bull* 21:202–11.

Rao BSN. 2001. Dietary approaches to the prevention of vitamin A deficiency: Indian experience with red palm oil as a source of vitamin A. *Food Nutr Bull* 22:395–9.

Reddy V. 2000. Comments on the development of high-carotene foods with the use of biotechnology. *Food Nutr Bull* 21:247.

Ribaya-Mercado JD, Maramag CC, Tengco LW, Dolnikowski GG, Blumberg JB, Solon FS. 2007. Carotene-rich plant foods ingested with minimal dietary fat enhance the total-body vitamin A pool size in Filipino schoolchildren as assessed by stable-isotope-dilution methodology. *Am J Clin Nutr* 85:1041–9.

Ribaya-Mercado JD, Solon FS, Solon MA, Cabal-Barza MA, Perfecto CS, Tang G, Solon JAA, Fjeld CR, Russell RM. 2000. Bioconversion of plant carotenoids to vitamin A in Filipino school-aged children varies inversely with vitamin A status. *Am J Clin Nutr* 72:455–65.

Rodriguez-Amaya DB. 1989. Critical review of provitamin A determination in plant foods. *J Micronutr Anal* 5:191–225.

Rodriguez-Amaya DB. 1996. Assessment of the provitamin A contents of foods: the Brazilian experience. *J Food Compos Anal* 9:196–230.

Rodriguez-Amaya DB. 1997. *Carotenoids and food preparation: the retention of provitamin A carotenoids in prepared, processed, and stored foods*. Washington DC: John Snow Inc./OMNI Project.

Rodriguez-Amaya DB, Kimura M, Godoy HT, Amaya-Farfan J. 2008. Updated Brazilian database on food carotenoids: factors affecting carotenoid composition. *J Food Compos Anal* 21:445–63.

Ross DA. 2002. Recommendations for vitamin A supplementation. *J Nutr* 132:S2902–6.

Ruel MT. 2001. *Can food-based strategies help reduce vitamin A and iron deficiencies? A review of recent evidence*. Washington DC: International Food Policy Research Institute.

Shankar AV, Gittelsohn J, Pradhan EK, Dhungel C, West KP Jr. 1998. Home gardening and access to animals in households with xerophthalmic children in rural Nepal. *Food Nutr Bull* 19:34–41.

Sivan YS, Jayakumar YA, Arumughan C, Sundaresan A, Balachandran C, Job J, Deepa SS, Shihina SL, Damodaran M, Soman CR, Raman Kutty V, Sankara Sarma P. 2001. Impact of β-carotene supplementation through red palm. *J Trop Pediatr* 47:67–72.

Sivan YS, Jayakumar YA, Arumughan C, Sundaresan A, Jayalekshmy A, Suja KP, Soban Kumar DR, Deepa SS, Damodaran M, Soman CR, Raman Kutty V, Sankara Sarma P. 2002. Impact of vitamin A supplementation through different dosages of red palm oil and retinol palmitate on preschool children. *J Trop Pediatr* 48:24–8.

Smitasiri S, Sa-ngobwarchar K, Kongpunya P, Subsuwan C, Banjong O, Chitchumroonechokchai C, Rusami-Sopaporn W, Veeravong S, Dhanamitta S. 1999. Sustaining behavioural change to enhance micronutrient status through community- and women-based interventions in north-east Thailand: vitamin A. *Food Nutr Bull* 20:243–51.

Solomons NW. 1998. Plant sources of vitamin A and human nutrition: red palm oil does the job. *Nutr Rev* 56:309–11.

Solomons NW, Orozco M. 2003. Alleviation of vitamin A deficiency with palm fruit and its products. *Asia Pac J Clin Nutr* 12:373–84.

Solon, F. (2000). The Manila forum on food fortification policy. The potential for protecting populations from mineral and vitamin deficiencies in Asia and the Pacific. *Sight and Life Newsletter* 2:27–28.

Solon FS, Sanchez-Fermin LE, Wambangco LS. 2000. Strengths and weaknesses of the food fortification programme for the elimination of vitamin A deficiency in the Philippines. *Food Nutr Bull* 21:239–46.

Sommer A, Davidson FR. 2002. Assessment and control of vitamin A deficiency: the Annecy Accords. *J Nutr* 132:S2845–50.

Talukder A, Kiess L, Huq N, de Pee S, Darnton-Hill I, Bloem MW. 2000. Increasing the production and consumption of vitamin A-rich fruits and vegetables: lessons learned in taking the Bangladesh homestead gardening programme to a national scale. *Food Nutr Bull* 21:165–72.

Tang G. 2010. Bioconversion of dietary provitamin A carotenoids to vitamin A in humans. *Am J Clin Nutr* 91:S1468–73.

Tang G. 2013. Using plant foods rich in β-carotene to combat vitamin A deficiency. *Sight Life* 27:20–28.

Tang G, Gu X-F, Hu S-m, Xu Q-M, Qin J, Dolnikowski GG, Fjeld CR, Gao X, Russell R M, Yin S-A. 1999. Green and yellow vegetables can maintain body stores of vitamin A in Chinese children. *Am J Clin Nutr* 70:1069–76.

Tang G, Hu Y, Yin S, Wang Y, Dallal GE, Grusak MA, Russell RM. 2012. β-Carotene in Golden Rice is as good as β-carotene in oil at providing vitamin A to children. *Am J Clin Nutr* 96:658–64.

Tang G, Qin J, Dolnikowski GG, Russell RM. 2003. Short-term (intestinal) and long-term (postintestinal) conversion of β-carotene to retinol in adults as assessed by a stable-isotope reference method. *Am J Clin Nutr* 78:259–66.

Tang G, Qin J, Dolnikowski GG, Russell RM, Grusak MA. 2005. Spinach or carrots can supply significant amounts of vitamin A as assessed by feeding with intrinsically deuterated vegetables. *Am J Clin Nutr* 82:821–8.

Tang G, Qin J, Dolnikowski GG, Russell RM, Grusak MA. 2009. Golden Rice is an effective source of vitamin A. *Am J Clin Nutr* 89:1776–83.
Thompson B, Amoroso L. 2013. *Improving diets and nutrition: food-based approaches*. Oxfordshire, UK: CABI.
Thurnham DI. 2007. Bioequivalence of β-carotene and retinol. *J Sci Food Agric* 87:13–39.
Toledo A, Burlingame B. 2006. Biodiversity and nutrition: a common path toward global security and sustainable development. *J Food Compos Anal* 19:477–83.
Trumbo P, Yates AA, Schlicker S, Poos M. 2001. Dietary Reference Intakes: vitamin A, vitamin K, arsenic, boron, chromium, copper, iodine, iron, manganese, molybdenum, nickel, silicon, vanadium, and zinc. *J Am Diet Assoc* 101:294–301.
Trumbo PR, Yates AA, Schlicker-Renfro S, Suitor C. 2003. Dietary Reference Intakes: revised nutritional equivalents for folate, vitamin E and provitamin A carotenoids. *J Food Compos Anal* 16:379–82.
Underwood BA. 2000. Dietary approaches to the control of vitamin A deficiency: an introduction and overview. *Food Nutr Bull* 21:117–23.
United Nations System Standing Committee on Nutrition. 2010. *6th report on the world nutrition situation*. Geneva: United Nations System Standing Committee on Nutrition.
van het Hof KH, Gärtner C, Wiersman A, Tijburg LBM, Weststrate JA. 1999. Comparison of the bioavailability of natural palm oil carotenoids and synthetic β-carotene in humans. *J Agric Food Chem* 47:1582–6.
van Jaarsveld PJ, Faber M, Tanumihardjo SA, Nestel P, Lombard CJ, Benadé AJS. 2005. β-carotene-rich orange-fleshed sweet potato improves the vitamin A status of primary school children assessed with the modified-relative-dose response test. *Am J Clin Nutr* 81:1080–7.
van Jaarsveld PJ, Marais DW, Harmse E, Nestel P, Rodriguez-Amaya DB. 2006. Retention of β-carotene in boiled, mashed orange-fleshed sweet potato. *J Food Compos Anal* 19:321–9.
van Lieshout M, West CE, Muhilal, Permaesih D, Wang Y, Xu X, van Breemen RB, Creemers AFL, Verhoeven MA, Lugtenburg J. 2001. Bioefficacy of β-carotene dissolved in oil studied in children in Indonesia. *Am J Clin Nutr* 73:949–58.
van Loo-Bouwman CA, Naber THJ, Schaafsma G. 2014. A review of vitamin A equivalency of β-carotene in various food matrices for human consumption. *Br J Nutr* 111:2153–66.
van Loo-Bouwman CA, Naber THJ, van Breemen RB, Zhu D, Dicke H, Siebelink E, Hulshof PJM, Russel FGM, Schaafsma G, West CE. 2010. Vitamin A equivalency and apparent absorption of β-carotene in ileostomy subjects using a dual-isotope dilution technique. *Br J Nutr* 103:1836–43.
van Loo-Bouwman CA, West CE, van Breemen RB, Zhu D, Siebelink E, Versloot P, Hulshof PJM, van Lieshout M, Russel FGM, Schaafsma G, Naber THJ. 2009. Vitamin A equivalency of β-carotene in healthy adults: limitation of the extrinsic dual-isotope dilution technique to measure matrix effect. *Br J Nutr* 101:1837–45.
van Stuijvenberg ME, Benadé AJS. 2000. South African experience with the use of red palm oil to improve the vitamin A status of primary schoolchildren. *Food Nutr Bull* 21:212–4.
van Stuijvenberg ME, Dhansay MA, Lombard CJ, Faber M, Benade AJ. 2001. The effect of a biscuit with red palm oil as a source of β-carotene on the vitamin A status of primary school children: a comparison with β-carotene from a synthetic source in a randomized controlled trial. *Eur J Clin Nutr* 55:657–62.
van Stuijvenberg ME, Faber M, Dhansay MA, Lombard CJ, Vorster N, Benadé AJS. 2000. Red palm oil as a source of β-carotene in a school biscuit used to address vitamin A deficiency in primary school children. *Int J Food Sci Nutr* 51:S43–50.
Vijayaraghavan K, Nayak U, Bamji M, Ramana GNV, Reddy V. 1997. Home gardening for combating vitamin A deficiency in rural India. *Food Nutr Bull* 18:337–43.
von Lintig J. 2012. Metabolism of carotenoids and retinoids related to vision. *J Biol Chem* 287:1627–34.
Vuong LT. 2000. Underutilized β-carotene-rich crops of Vietnam. *Food Nutr Bull* 21:173–81.
Vuong LT, Dueker SR, Murphy SP. 2002. Plasma β-carotene and retinol concentrations of children increase after a 30-d supplementation with the fruit *Momordica cochinchinensis* (gac). *Am J Clin Nutr* 75:872–9.
Wang J, Wang Y, Wang Z, Li L, Qin J, Lai W, Fu Y, Suter PM, Russell RM, Grusak MA, Tang G, Yin S. 2008. Vitamin A equivalence of spirulina β-carotene in Chinese adults as assessed by using stable-isotope reference method. *Am J Clin Nutr* 87:1730–7.
Wang X-D, Tang G-W, Fox JG, Krinsky NI, Russell RM. 1991. Enzymatic conversion of β-carotene into β-apo-carotenals and retinoids by human, monkey, ferret, and rat tissues. *Arch Biochem Biophys* 285:8–16.
Wang Z, Yin S, Zhao X, Russell RM, Tang G. 2004. β-Carotene-vitamin A equivalence in Chinese adults assessed by an isotope dilution technique. *Br J Nutr* 91:121–31.

Weber D, Grune T. 2012. The contribution of β-carotene to vitamin A supply of humans. *Mol Nutr Food Res* 56:251–8.

WHO. 2009. *Global prevalence of vitamin A deficiency in populations at risk 1995–2005: WHO global database on vitamin A deficiency*. Geneva: World Health Organization.

WHO/FAO. 2004. *Vitamin and mineral requirements in human nutrition. WHO/FAO Joint Expert Consultation*, 2nd ed. Geneva: World Health Organization/Food and Agriculture Organization of the United Nations.

Wyss A. 2004. Carotene oxygenases: a new family of double bond cleavage enzymes. *J Nutr* 134:S246–50.

Yan W, Jang G-F, Haeseleer F, Esumi N, Chang J, Kerrigan M, Campochiaro M, Campochiaro P, Palczewski K, Zack DJ. 2001. Cloning and characterization of a human β,β-carotene-15,15′-dioxygenase that is highly expressed in the retinal pigment epithelium. *Genomics* 72:193–202.

You C-S, Parker RS, Swanson, JE. 2002. Bioavailability and vitamin A value of carotenes from palm oil assessed by an extrinsic isotope reference method. *Asia Pac J Clin Nutr* 11:S438–42.

Zagre NM, Delpeuch F, Traissac P, Delisle H. 2003. Red palm oil as source of vitamin A for mothers and children: impact of a pilot plant project in Burkina Faso. *Publ Health Nutr* 6:733–42.

Zeba AN, Prével YM, Somé IT, Delisle HF. 2006. The positive impact of red palm oil in school meals on vitamin A status: study in Burkina Faso. *Nutr J* 5:17.

Zhang J, Wang C-R, Xue A-N, Ge, KY. 2003. Effects of red palm oil on serum lipids and plasma carotenoids level in Chinese male adults. *Biomed Environ Sci* 16:348–54.

11 Carotenoids and chronic diseases

11.1 INTRODUCTION

Numerous studies have documented the association between the consumption of diets rich in fruits and vegetables and a lower risk for chronic degenerative diseases, especially cancer (Steinmetz and Potter, 1996; Cohen et al., 2000; van't Veer et al., 2000; Voorrips et al., 2000; Trichopoulou et al., 2003; Wright et al., 2003; Genkinger et al., 2004; Chan et al., 2005; Michels et al., 2006; Pomerleau et al., 2006; Freedman et al., 2008; Boffetta et al., 2010) and cardiovascular diseases (Liu et al., 2000, 2001; van't Veer et al., 2000; Fung et al., 2001; Joshipura et al., 2001; Bazzano et al., 2002; Trichopoulou et al., 2003; Genkinger et al., 2004; Hung et al., 2004; Dauchet et al., 2005, 2006, 2007; He et al., 2006, 2007; Pomerleau et al., 2006; Heidermann et al., 2008; Nöthlings et al., 2008; S. Wang et al., 2011). Fruit and vegetable intake has also been associated with cognitive function (Ortega et al., 1997; L. Lee et al., 2001; Morris et al., 2006).

Among the bioactive compounds (also called phytochemicals) credited with the health-promoting effects of fruits and vegetables, carotenoids are among the most cited and investigated. Independent of the provitamin A activity, carotenoids have been associated with decreased risk of cancer, cardiovascular diseases, cataract, and macular degeneration (Astorg, 1997; Olson, 1999; Tapiero et al., 2004; Krinsky and Johnson, 2005; Voutilainen et al., 2006; Rao and Rao, 2007; Tanaka et al., 2012).

11.2 EVIDENCE OF HEALTH BENEFITS/EFFICACY

As emphasized by the World Cancer Research Fund (WCRF)/American Institute for Cancer Research (AICR) (2007), no one kind of study, however careful its methods, can produce definitive results. Reliable judgment on disease causation is based on assessment of a variety of well-designed epidemiological and experimental studies.

Food Carotenoids: Chemistry, Biology, and Technology, First Edition. Delia B. Rodriguez-Amaya.

Evidence for a relationship between a food or a bioactive component of food and a disease is derived from the following methods of investigation (WCRF/AICR, 2007; Ashwell, 2002):

- Epidemiological studies (also referred to as observational human studies)
- Biochemical, tissue/cellular, or animal studies
- Intervention studies (also referred to as human clinical trials, supplementation, or experimental human trials).

Epidemiology examines the correlation of a food or a dietary constituent to an outcome. It does not establish a cause-and-effect relationship. The possibility that the beneficial effect is due to another compound or multiple compounds, including or excluding the compound of interest, cannot be ruled out. Of the different types of epidemiological studies, the most commonly used in food and health investigations are the retrospective case control studies, retrospective cohort studies, and the prospective cohort studies.

In case-control retrospective studies, individuals diagnosed with the disease (case) are compared with otherwise similar individuals without the disease (control) with regard to a possible risk factor (e.g., diet). Dietary habits before the onset of the disease are assessed retrospectively by questionnaire or interview. The major drawback is the heavy dependence on subjects' recall, which may differ in accuracy between cases and controls. Case-control studies are usually less expensive than the cohort studies and can be completed over a shorter time.

Problems with recall bias are avoided in prospective cohort studies. Dietary information is collected from a large population, free of the disease at the beginning of the study, followed through time, usually a decade or more, until a sufficient number of participants develop the disease. The relationship of specific characteristics of individual diets and the incidence of the disease is then analyzed. Cohort studies allow repeated assessments of diets at regular intervals, examination of the effects of diet on the disease in question as well as other diseases, and collection and storage of tissue samples for analysis. This type of study, however, takes a long time, requires a large number of subjects, and is very expensive.

Numerous biochemical, cellular, and animal studies have been carried out to investigate the factors that influence the carotenoid–chronic disease relationship and possible mechanisms of action. Extrapolation of the findings of these studies to humans, however, is questionable. In considering health claims for consumption of tomatoes, tomato products, and/or lycopene and risk of prostate cancer, the U.S. Food and Drug Administration stated that it "did not consider the animal and in vitro studies as providing any supportive information about the substance-disease relationship because such studies cannot mimic the normal physiology that may be involved in the risk reduction of any type of cancer, nor can the studies mimic the human body's response to the consumption of tomato lycopene, tomatoes, and tomato products, which contain lycopene" (USFDA, 2005). For conclusive evidence of efficacy, therefore, human studies, especially intervention/clinical studies, are necessary. Thus, this book focuses on human studies.

Intervention studies are considered more useful than observational studies because they are less susceptible to bias. The researcher can be more certain that the measured effect is attributable to the specific intervention, not to other bioactive compounds or factors. In these studies, subjects are allocated to different groups (normally an intervention group and a control group) and exposed to different conditions (such as different diets or bioactives). The most reliable method of assigning subjects to different groups is by random allocation, and the allocation ideally should be concealed from both investigators and subjects (the double-blind method). The double-blind, randomized intervention study (otherwise known as the double-blind randomized controlled trial or RCT) is considered an efficient way to get evidence for the effects of a bioactive compound on a target function.

In spite of the voluminous literature about bioactive compounds (e.g., carotenoids) and human health, the results are still inconsistent, inconclusive, and sometimes conflicting. A perusal of the literature reveals that there are at least three major inherent difficulties in efficacy studies:

- The effect of bioactive compounds on the human body may be very small over relatively short periods (months or a few years) but can contribute significantly throughout life as part of the daily diet. Thus, the health effect may not be observed during the study period, perhaps explaining studies reporting no significant effect. Long-term studies, although costly, laborious, and complicated, are recommended. There is also a tendency to use doses above the physiological levels in an attempt to observe the outcome better, but the findings cannot be extrapolated to actual human situations.
- Reduction of the risk of chronic degenerative diseases is not due to a single compound or a single class of compounds but to the range of bioactive compounds contained in foods. These compounds have different modes of action and act at different stages of disease development, often demonstrating synergy. Thus, while the evidence for the beneficial effects of plant foods is compelling, that for individual phytochemicals is often inconclusive or inconsistent. On the other hand, when food is used, attributing the effects to a specific bioactive compound is presumptive.
- There is considerable variation of interindividual responses to the administered bioactive compound, further masking the health effects and making it difficult to draw conclusions. Genetic variation appears to be a key factor in explaining this huge interindividual variability.

Genetic variants in genes encoding for proteins involved in carotenoid metabolism in humans may affect their expression or activity and, in turn, carotenoid metabolism and carotenoid status (Borel 2012). As reviewed by Borel, a genomewide association study and several candidate gene association studies have shown that groups of subjects bearing different alleles in single nucleotide polymorphisms located in or near several of the genes display different blood and/or tissue concentrations of carotenoids, which may in turn affect the ability of carotenoids to prevent some diseases.

Ashwell (2002) recommended the following general principles to improve the validity of studies used to substantiate health claims, applicable to both epidemiological and intervention studies:

- The subjects are representative of the target group for the claim.
- The subjects consume a reasonable amount of food or food component in question at a reasonable frequency, consistent with realistic consumption patterns.

- The study is large enough to demonstrate the proposed beneficial effect.
- The study is long enough to justify any implication of the claim that a beneficial effect is a long-term rather than a short-term effect.
- The outcomes are measured properly and according to standard procedures.
- The outcomes are identical or similar to those of the claimed effect.
- Possible confounding variables are taken into account.

11.3 MODE OF ACTION

Oxidative stress caused by reactive oxygen and nitrogen species has been widely postulated to be a causative factor in the development and progression of several degenerative chronic diseases. These reactive species can damage biologically important molecules like lipids, DNA, and proteins. The carotenoids' action against diseases has been widely attributed to their antioxidant activity, through quenching of singlet oxygen and scavenging of free radicals (Krinsky, 1989, 2001; Palozza and Krinsky, 1992; Edge et al., 1997; Palace et al., 1999; Kaur and Kapoor, 2001; Young and Lowe, 2001; Stahl and Sies, 2003, 2005; Astley et al., 2004a,b; Kiokias and Gordon, 2004; Willcox et al., 2004; Agarwal et al., 2012). The physiological significance of this activity has been questioned, or more information/evidence is considered necessary (Britton, 1995; Temple, 2000; A.R. Collins, 2001; Stanner et al., 2003; Kaliora et al., 2006; Voutilainen et al., 2006; Chong et al., 2007). Astley et al. (2004a) cited two overlapping but distinct effects: antioxidant protection by scavenging DNA-damaging free radicals and modulation of DNA repair mechanisms.

Several human studies have been carried out to demonstrate the antioxidant activity of carotenoids. Dietary supplementation with lycopene-rich foods for 14 days resulted in marked protection of human lymphocytes against the reactive species $NO^{\bullet}_2$ and $^1O_2$ (Böhm et al., 2001). With the consumption of 25 g tomato puree for 14 days, an inverse relationship was found between plasma and lymphocyte lycopene concentrations and oxidative DNA damage (Porrini and Riso, 2000). Ingestion of a beverage called Lyc-o-Mato, which contained natural tomato extract, significantly reduced DNA damage in lymphocytes subjected to oxidative stress (Porrini et al., 2005). Patients with localized prostate adenocarcinoma who consumed tomato sauce–based pasta for 3 weeks before their scheduled radical prostatectomy had significant uptake of lycopene into prostate tissue and a reduction of DNA damage in both leukocyte and prostate tissue (L. Chen et al., 2001; Bowen et al., 2002).

Dietary supplementation with practical amounts of tomato products decreased LDL oxidizability, suggesting a protective in vivo role of carotenoids and other tomato components against lipid peroxidation, a risk factor of atherosclerosis/cardiovascular disease (Visioli et al., 2003). Consumption of processed tomato soup or juice for 15 days significantly enhanced the protection of lipoproteins to ex vivo oxidative stress (Hadley et al., 2003). Daily intake of tomato juice for 2 weeks (Bub et al., 2000) and of 160 g of a high-lycopene tomato sauce (Abete et al., 2013) reduced LDL oxidation. Dietary lycopene provided by tomato juice, spaghetti sauce, and tomato oleoresin for a period of 1 week each, significantly decreased lipid peroxidation and LDL oxidation (Agarwal and Rao, 1998). In 60 postmenopausal women (aged 50–60 years), lycopene supplementation (capsule or juice) for 4 months resulted in significantly increased total antioxidant capacity, as well as decreased lipid peroxidation, protein oxidation, and N-telopeptide (Mackinnon et al., 2011). The results suggest that lycopene reduced oxidative stress and bone resorption markers and might lower the risk of osteoporosis.

Supplementation with lutein increased plasma lutein concentration and antioxidant capacity, and reduced plasma lipid peroxidation and C-reactive protein in healthy nonsmokers (M.-X. Wang et al., 2013).

Of 20 supplementation studies (17 with tomato and tomato products) reviewed by Basu and Imrhan (2007), only two observed no effect on LDL oxidation and lipid peroxidation. The others found a decrease in biomarkers of oxidative stress (decrease in LDL oxidizability and in protein and lipid oxidation, increase in LDL lag time, decreased DNA damage).

In other studies, however, no or limited antioxidant effects were observed. A single dose of tomato sauce increased plasma lycopene level but had limited antioxidant effect (C.-Y.J. Lee et al., 2009). Plasma carotenoids were significantly lower in the obese compared to control subjects (Markovitz et al., 2009). After 4 weeks of lycopene supplementation (tomato-derived Lyc-O-Mato) (30 mg daily), a significant elevation of plasma carotenoids, specifically lycopene, occurred in the treatment vs. the placebo group. However, markers of inflammation and oxidation products were not altered. Consumption of a fruit and vegetable soup caused an increase of serum β-carotene and lycopene by more than 100% after 3 and 4 weeks. Oxidative markers did not show any variation except for glutathione peroxidase (Martinez-Tomas et al., 2012). Similarly, Paterson et al. (2006) found that supplementation with fruit and vegetable soups and beverages for 4 weeks increased plasma carotenoid concentrations but did not affect markers of oxidative stress or cardiovascular risk factors. Supplementation with tomato or carrot juice for 2 weeks did not affect lipid peroxidation in the plasma and feces (Briviba et al., 2004).

On the other hand, nonantioxidant mechanisms have been increasingly reported for carotenoids such as retinoid-dependent signaling, modulation of carcinogen metabolism, regulation of cell growth, inhibition of cell proliferation and/or apoptosis induction, enhancement of cell differentiation, stimulation of intercellular gap junctional communication, gene and transcription regulation, modulation of DNA repair mechanisms, induction of detoxifying enzymes, hormonal and immune system modulation, redox activity, modulation of cytokine expression, inhibition of inflammation, hypocholesterolemic effect, and filtering of blue light (Astorg, 1997; Bertram, 1999; Rao and Agarwal, 1999; Olson, 1999; Stahl et al., 2000b, 2002; Heber and Lu, 2002; Sharoni et al., 2002, 2004; Chew and Park, 2004; Tapiero et al., 2004; Krinsky and Johnson, 2005; Rao and Rao, 2007; Pan et al., 2009; Palozza et al., 2011).

11.4 PROTECTION AGAINST CANCER

Historically, β-carotene was the first carotenoid to draw researchers' attention to possible health-promoting roles of carotenoids other than the provitamin A activity. In the 1980s to early 1990s, numerous epidemiological studies, supported by in vitro and animal studies, strongly and consistently showed that β-carotene had protective effect against cancer, especially lung cancer. Prospective (cohort) and retrospective studies in different countries showed an inverse relation between the incidence of cancer, especially lung cancer, and the consumption of fruits and vegetables rich in β-carotene or the serum level of β-carotene. Intervention studies were being awaited and expected to confirm this important role in human health.

A randomized, double-blind, placebo controlled trial, the α-Tocopherol, β-Carotene Cancer Prevention Study (ATBC, 1994) was undertaken in Finland. Male smokers (29,133), 50 to 69 years old, were randomly assigned into four groups, supplemented with (a) 20 mg β-carotene, (b) 50 mg α-tocopherol, (c) 20 mg β-carotene + 50 mg α-tocopherol, or (d) placebo. Supplementation was administered daily for 5–8 years. Unexpectedly, instead of reducing the incidence of lung cancer, there was an 18% increase in the groups that received β-carotene. There was no negative or positive effect of the supplementation with α-tocopherol.

This troubling finding was corroborated by a U.S. study, the CARET study (β-Carotene and Retinol Efficiency Trial) (Omenn et al., 1996). Men and women (18,314 smokers, former smokers, or workers exposed to asbestos) were divided into two groups: (a) supplemented daily with 30 mg of β-carotene and 25,000 IU of vitamin A and (b) placebo. The intervention was stopped 21 months earlier than planned because the supplemented group had 28% higher incidence of lung cancer than the placebo group. In this and the previous intervention study, supplementation with β-carotene did not affect the incidence of other types of cancer.

In order to explain the results of these intervention trials, a comparison of the fundamental differences between epidemiological and intervention should be done (Olson, 1999). Epidemiological studies focus on food, which is a multicomponent system, while intervention studies involve individual compounds. Additionally, the compound of interest in epidemiological studies is consumed in a much lower amount than that utilized in intervention studies.

The Carotenoid Research Interactive Group (CARIG, 1996) pointed out that the applied doses of β-carotene in the intervention studies were too high: 20 mg per day in the ATBC study and 30 mg per day plus 25,000 IU vitamin A in the CARET study. In the epidemiological studies in which β-carotene intakes were inversely associated with decreased risk of cancer, the daily intake of β-carotene was about 4 mg. Moreover, the diets in the epidemiological studies had other carotenoids or other food constituents that could act jointly with β-carotene; in the intervention trial, β-carotene was administered mostly alone or with vitamin A or α-tocopherol. Additionally, the intervention trials' participants were high-risk smokers or workers exposed to asbestos; oxidative stress or the cancer process might have reached a point at which carotenoids could no longer be effective.

In Linxian, China, one of the regions with the highest incidence of gastric and stomach cancer in the world and where ingestion of micronutrients is insufficient, 29,584 residents were supplemented with eight different combinations of retinol, zinc, riboflavin, niacin, vitamin C, molybdenum, β-carotene, vitamin E, and selenium (Blot et al., 1993). There was a 21% reduction of deaths due to gastric cancer in the group supplemented with β-carotene, vitamin E, and selenium. Since a mixture was administered, it was not possible to affirm which component was responsible for the decrease. On the other hand, the result of this study could be taken as among the first indications that a number of components, rather than individual compounds, are responsible for lowering the risk of chronic diseases.

Mayne and others (Mayne, 1996; Mayne et al., 1996) and X.-D. Wang and Russell (1999) also offered explanations for what appeared to be a prooxidant behavior of beta-carotene. These included the generation of relatively high amounts of deleterious oxidation products (typically epoxides) brought about by exposure to the reactive oxygen species (ROS) found in tobacco smoke (or produced as a consequence of asbestosis or by metabolic processes via increased retinoic acid catabolism or interference with retinoid signal transduction).

After these intervention trials, which had a dramatic impact on consumers and the scientific community, investigations on the possible effects of carotenoids on cancer continued but were extended to other carotenoids. In a study of 587 incident primary lung cancer cases and 624 controls, the results indicated that consumption of a wide variety of vegetables had greater bearing on lung cancer risk in a population of smoking and nonsmoking women than intake of a specific carotenoid or total carotenoids (Wright et al., 2003). Other phytochemicals or interactions among phytochemicals, including carotenoids, might be more important in lung cancer prevention.

Lycopene's role in human health has drawn considerable interest (Clinton, 1998; Giovannucci, 1999; Rao and Agarwal, 1999; Agarwal and Rao, 2000; Khachik et al., 2002; Rao and Rao, 2004; J.K. Collins and Perkins-Veazie, 2006; Singh and Goyal, 2008; X.-D. Wang, 2012), especially in relation to prostate cancer (Giovannucci, 2002a; Hadley et al., 2002; Miller et al., 2002; Campbell et al., 2004; Wertz et al., 2004; Stacewicz-Sapuntzakis and Bowen, 2005; Holzapfel et al., 2013).

The majority of epidemiological studies concluded that tomato and tomato products were associated with a reduced risk of prostate cancer, a conclusion highly supported by numerous in vitro and animal studies. Several clinical trials have also suggested that supplementation with tomato or tomato products decreases prostate cancer risk. This finding has been largely attributed to lycopene, but the possibility that other components, perhaps in combination with lycopene, may be responsible for the health effect is increasingly acknowledged.

The huge and comprehensive U.S. Health Professionals Follow-up Study investigated the relation between intake of various carotenoids, retinol, fruits, and vegetables and reduced risk of prostate cancer (Giovannucci et al., 1995). A cohort of 47,894 male subjects, who completed a 131-item food frequency questionnaire, was followed from 1986 to 1992. It was concluded that the consumption of fresh tomatoes, tomato sauce, and pizza, which accounted for 82% of the total intake, was significantly associated with a lower incidence of prostate cancer. Subsequently, results from 1992 through 1998 confirmed the previous finding of an inverse relation between frequent tomato or lycopene intake and risk of prostate cancer (Giovannucci et al., 2002). For the entire period (1986–1998), lycopene intake was associated with reduced risk of prostate cancer, but intake of tomato sauce, the main source of bioavailable lycopene, was associated with greater reduction in prostate cancer risk, especially for extraprostatic cancer.

In a meta-analysis of 72 epidemiological studies, 57 reported an inverse relation between lycopene intake or serum lycopene level and the risk of cancer at a defined anatomic site (Giovannucci, 1999). Thirty-five of these inverse associations were statistically significant. No study indicated that higher consumption of tomato or blood lycopene level significantly increased the risk of cancer at any of the sites investigated. The evidence for a benefit was strongest for cancers of the prostate, lung, and stomach.

In a review, Giovannucci (2002a) cited five studies that supported a 30% to 40% reduction in the risk of prostate cancer associated with high tomato or lycopene consumption, three studies that were consistent with a 30% reduction but the results were not statistically significant, and seven studies that were not supportive of an association. The largest dietary study found that consumption of two to four servings of tomato sauce per week was associated with about 35% risk reduction of total prostate and 50% reduction of advanced prostate cancer. In the largest plasma-based study, very similar risk reductions were observed for total and advanced prostate cancer. The author attributed inconsistencies of some results to insufficient sample size, low intake of lycopene, failure to account for bioavailability, reliance on a single dietary assessment, and heterogeneity of prostate cancer (Giovannucci, 2002b).

In a meta-analysis, after a systematic search of the literature, 21 studies (11 case-control and 10 cohort studies or nested case-control studies) that met inclusion criteria were chosen (Etminan et al., 2004). The results showed that tomato products might play a role in the prevention of prostate cancer, but this effect was modest, restricted to high amounts of tomato intake. The preventive effect was slightly stronger for high intakes of cooked tomato products than for high intakes of raw tomatoes.

Supplementation with 15 mg of lycopene daily for 3 weeks decreased the levels of PSA (prostate specific antigen) as well as the growth of prostate cancer in newly diagnosed prostate cancer patients prior to radical prostatectomy (Kucuk and Wood, 2002; Kucuk et al., 2001). In another study (L. Chen et al., 2001), tomato sauce–based pasta (30 mg lycopene/day) was administered for the 3 weeks preceding prostatectomy in men diagnosed with prostate cancer. Serum and prostate lycopene levels were elevated significantly, serum PSA level declined significantly (20%), and oxidative damage of DNA was reduced.

Supplementation studies indicate that lycopene may be involved in the prevention and treatment of the disease. A recent review (Holzapfel et al., 2013), however, affirms that there is still no clearly proven clinical evidence supporting the use of lycopene in the prevention and treatment of prostate cancer, due to the limited number of published randomized clinical trials and the varying quality of existing studies.

In recent years, the question has been raised as to whether the effect of lycopene on human health is mediated by direct action of lycopene itself or of its derivatives (X.-D. Wang, 2012), formed either by enzymatic or nonenzymatic oxidation (Sharoni et al., 2012).

Lycopene has also been associated with lung (Ito et al., 2003), pancreatic (Nkondjock et al., 2005), colorectal (Erhardt et al., 2003) and digestive-tract cancers (Franceshi et al., 1994).

Palozza et al. (2011) reviewed both experimental and human studies on tomato lycopene and lung cancer prevention. Experimental studies demonstrated that lycopene may inhibit the growth of several cultured lung cancer cells and prevent lung tumorigenesis in animal models. Various potential mechanisms have been proposed: redox activity, inhibition of cell proliferation and/or apoptosis induction, interference with growth factor signaling, modulation of cytokine expression, induction of phase II enzymes, enhancement of gap junctional communication, regulation of transcription, hypocholesterolemic effects, and inhibition of invasion and metastasis. However, the authors found it difficult to relate available experimental data to human pathology and called for more well-controlled human studies, taking into consideration subject selection, specific markers of analysis, the levels of carotenoids to be tested, metabolism and isomerization of lycopene, and interaction with other bioactive food components.

In a cohort study in Singapore of 63,257 Chinese men and women, ages 45–74 years, from 1993 to 1998, high levels of dietary β-cryptoxanthin were associated with reduced risk of lung cancer (Yuan et al., 2003). α-Carotene, β-carotene, lycopene, lutein/zeaxanthin, vitamins A and E, and folate were not associated significantly with lung cancer risk after adjustment for cigarette smoking.

In a case-control study in Nebraska involving 124 esophageal adenocarcinoma cases, 124 distal stomach cancer cases, and 449 controls, significant inverse associations were observed with risk of esophageal adenocarcinoma for dietary intakes of vitamin A, β-cryptoxanthin, riboflavin, folate, zinc, dietary fiber, protein, and carbohydrate (H.L. Chen et al., 2002). For distal stomach cancer, only vitamin C, dietary fiber, and carbohydrate were inversely associated with risk. In a case-control Italian study (198 cases, 594 controls), carotenoids (notably α-carotene and β-carotene) were inversely related to nasopharyngeal carcinoma risk (Polesel et al., 2012).

In the European Prospective Investigation into Cancer and Nutrition (330 gastric cancer cases among 520,000 men and women), a protective role for citrus fruit consumption was observed for gastric cardia cancer (Gonzalez et al., 2006). In the Netherlands Cohort Study on vegetables and fruits consumption, citrus fruits, including mandarin, orange, and fresh orange juice, were inversely associated with esophageal adenocarcinoma and gastric cardia adenocarcinoma risks (Steevens et al., 2011).

From data collected from 1,993 case subjects with first primary incident adenocarcinoma of the colon and 2,410 population-based control subjects, dietary lutein was inversely associated with colon cancer in both men and women (Slattery et al., 2000). Associations with other carotenoids (α-carotene, β-carotene, lycopene, zeaxanthin, and β-cryptoxanthin) were unremarkable.

11.5 PROTECTION AGAINST CARDIOVASCULAR DISEASE

A cross-sectional analysis of data from the U.S. National Health and Nutrition Examination Survey III (NHANES III), on a representative population-based sample of 11,327 men and women (aged 35 to over 90 years), showed serum concentrations of α-carotene, β-carotene, and β-cryptoxanthin to be significantly associated with decreased risk for angina pectoris (Ford and Giles, 2000). There was no significant association between serum vitamins A, C, E, and B_{12}; serum and red blood cell folate; and angina pectoris, indicating no protective effect against ischemic heart disease, even after multiple factors were adjusted. In female nurses (73,286) followed for 12 years, a modest but significant inverse association between the highest quintiles of β-carotene and α-carotene intakes and the risk of coronary artery disease was observed (Osganian et al., 2003). There was no significant relation with intakes of lutein/zeaxanthin, lycopene, or β-cryptoxanthin.

The association between carotenoids and the risk of congestive heart failure, a leading cause of cardiovascular death and morbidity in the Western world, was examined by Karppi et al. (2013b). Men with the lowest quartile of β-carotene had an almost three-fold increased risk of congestive heart failure; serum concentrations of lycopene and α-carotene were not related to this risk. Karppi et al. (2013c) investigated the relation between serum concentration of carotenoids and the risk of sudden cardiac death in a study population of 1,031 Finnish men aged 45–65 years. While lycopene and α-carotene showed no relation, men in the lowest tertile of serum β-carotene had a two-fold increased risk of sudden cardiac death, compared to those in the highest tertile. In addition, low serum concentrations of β-carotene were associated with an increased risk of cardiovascular disease and total mortality.

In a study comprising 468 elderly men and women living in the United Kingdom, the men with higher plasma concentrations of vitamin E, vitamin C, and β-carotene had thinner artery walls and little or no plaque in their carotid arteries (Gale et al., 2001b). There was no significant trend between plasma concentrations of the antioxidant vitamins and either measure of carotid atherosclerosis in the women.

In a Japanese cross-sectional study of 390 men and 666 women, after adjusting for possible confounders, higher serum levels of α-carotene were associated with lower risk of elevated serum N-terminal pro-brain-type natriuretic peptide (NT-proBNP) in both men and women, suggesting that diets rich in this carotenoid could help prevent cardiac overload in the Japanese population (Suzuki et al., 2013). NT-pro BNP was significantly associated with serum canthaxanthin and β-cryptoxanthin only in women.

In an epidemiological study involving 304 men and 269 women (aged 40 to 60 years), an inverse association between lutein and the progression of intima-media thickness of the common carotid arteries over 18 months suggested that intake of lutein-rich foods had a protective effect on progression of early atherosclerosis (Dwyer et al., 2001). Serum concentrations of lutein and zeaxanthin in 40 early atherosclerosis patients aged 45–68 years were lower than those of control subjects (Xu et al., 2012). Serum carotenoids were associated with reduced risk of atherosclerosis. Connor et al. (2004) surveyed the diet in 19 countries and coronary mortality in 16 countries. They concluded that a diet low in foods containing folate and carotenoids (β-carotene and lutein/zeaxanthin) might be a major contributing factor to increased coronary risk observed in the countries of central and eastern Europe.

In a study population of 1,847 Finnish subjects (620 women and and 1,227 men) aged 61–82 years, from the Kuopio Ischaemic Heart Disease Risk Factor study cohort, low plasma concentrations of lutein and zeaxanthin were associated with an increased risk of atrial fibrillation, a common arrhythmia in elderly population (Karppi et al., 2013a). Lycopene, β-cryptoxanthin, α-carotene, and total carotenoids were not associated with the risk of atrial fibrillation. β-carotene had borderline significance.

A randomized, double-blind, placebo-controlled trial of lutein supplementation in 117 healthy nonsmokers, randomly assigned to receive 10 to 20 mg/day of lutein or placebo, was conducted for 12 weeks (M.-X. Wang et al., 2013). There was a significant reduction in malondialdehyde in the 20 mg lutein group, and C-reactive protein decreased in a dose-dependent manner. Serum C-reactive protein was directly related to the change in plasma lutein and total antioxidant capacity for both supplemented groups. Lutein supplemention therefore significantly reduced biomarkers of cardiovascular diseases via lipid peroxidation and inflammatory response.

The possible role of lycopene in the prevention of cardiovascular diseases has been widely investigated, but the results are markedly inconsistent (Riccioni, 2009). Mordente et al. (2011) comprehensively and critically reviewed epidemiological and interventional studies on the association between lycopene or tomato products and cardiovascular diseases. Out of 61 epidemiological studies, 35 (including 3 reports with significant relation only for women) found a significant inverse association between plasma or tissue lycopene levels and the incidence of cardiovascular diseases or risk factors. Twenty-six epidemiological studies did not observe such relationships. Fifty-four clinical trials, in which supplementation was done with tomato and tomato products except for two studies with lycopene capsules, were also examined. The outcomes were in terms of LDL and protein oxidation, lipid peroxidation, DNA oxidative damage, blood pressure, platelet activation, antioxidant enzymes, and inflammatory markers. The number of subjects varied from 12 to 100, the dose from 4 to 80 mg/day, and the duration from 1 to 60 days. The authors considered the picture emerging from these intervention trials as unclear and complex, with several studies reporting conflicting results. Further studies and long-term intervention trials were considered necessary.

Sesso et al. (2003) determined whether the intake of lycopene or tomato-based foods was associated with the risk of cardiovascular diseases in a prospective cohort of 39,876 middle-aged and older women initially free of this disease and cancer, followed during 7.2 y. Dietary lycopene was not strongly associated with the risk of cardiovascular diseases. However, possible inverse associations were noted for higher levels of tomato-based products, particularly tomato sauce and pizza, with cardiovascular diseases, suggesting that dietary lycopene or other phytochemicals consumed as oil-based tomato products confer cardiovascular benefits.

Not being a regular component of the diet, astaxanthin has not been the subject of epidemiological studies, but even intervention studies have been limited. Twelve weeks of supplementation with astaxanthin significantly lowered LDL cholesterol and apolipoprotein B in overweight subjects (Choi et al., 2011). Oxidative stress biomarkers including malondialdehyde, isoprostane, superoxide dismutase, and total antioxidant capacity were improved by astaxanthin in moderately hyperlipidemic subjects (Hiroshi et al., 2010).

Randomized, placebo-controlled administration of astaxanthin at 6, 12, and 18 mg/day for 12 weeks on 61 nonobese healthy subjects (41 men and 20 women), aged 25–60 y, did not affect LDL-cholesterol but decreased triacylglycerols and increased HDL-cholesterol and adiponectin significantly (Yoshida et al., 2010).

11.6 PROTECTION AGAINST CATARACT AND MACULAR DEGENERATION

Lutein (3R,3′R,6′R), zeaxanthin (3R,3′R), and meso-zeaxanthin (3R,3′S) selectively accumulate in the macula of the human retina (Bone et al., 1997, 2000; Landrum and Bone, 2001) and are collectively called the macular pigment. Zeaxanthin is dominant in the macula lutea while lutein predominates in the peripheral retina (Bone et al., 1997; Whitehead et al., 2006). Unlike lutein and zeaxanthin, which are supplied by the diet, meso-zeaxanthin is a metabolite of lutein (Bone et al., 1993, 1997). This conversion only requires the migration of the 4′,5′-double bond in lutein to the 5′,6′-position in meso-zeaxanthin (Bone et al., 1997).

Ingestion of lutein and zeaxanthin in food or supplemental form increased serum concentrations and macular pigment density (Bone et al., 1997; Landrum et al., 1997, 2001; Berendschot et al., 2000; Richer et al., 2004; Carpentier et al., 2009) and could improve visual function in patients suffering from age-related macular degeneration and cataract (Olmedilla et al., 2001, 2003). Among subjects with early macular degeneration, supplementation with lutein and zeaxanthin (10 mg/day each) improved macular pigment and visual function (Ma et al., 2012).

Although some studies found no significant association of lutein and zeaxanthin and age-related macular degeneration (Cho et al., 2008; Mares-Perlman et al., 2001), most epidemiological studies showed that dietary intake or serum level of lutein and zeaxanthin was associated with reduced risk of macular degeneration (EDCC, 1993; Seddon et al., 1994; Snodderly, 1995; Vanden Langenberg, 1998; Bone et al., 2000, 2001; Gale et al., 2003; van Leeuwen et al., 2005; Delcourt et al., 2006; Moeller, et al., 2006; Basu et al., 2007; Tan et al., 2008; Carpentier et al., 2009). Similarly, for cataract, some studies reported no significant relation (Mares-Perlman et al., 1995; Lyle et al., 1999b), but most studies observed association of lutein and zeaxanthin with decreased risk of cataract development (Brown et al., 1999; Chasan-Taber et al., 1999; Lyle et al., 1999a; Moeller et al., 2000; Gale et al., 2001a; Jacques et al., 2001; Taylor et al., 2002; Delcourt et al., 2006; Dherani et al., 2008;). Reviewing observational studies, Moeller et al. (2000) noted that generous intake of lutein and zeaxanthin, particularly from certain xanthophyll-rich foods like spinach, broccoli, and eggs, is associated with a significant reduction of cataract (up to 20%) and age-related macular degeneration (up to 40%).

Lutein and zeaxanthin may act in two ways: (a) as filters of damaging blue light, and (b) as antioxidants quenching excited triplet state sensitizers or singlet oxygen and scavenging harmful reactive oxygen species like lipid peroxides or the superoxide radical anion (Krinsky et al., 2003). Supplementation with lutein for 140 days was estimated to produce a 30% to 40% reduction in blue light reaching the macular photoreceptors (Landrum et al., 1997).

A systematic review yielded only six longitudinal cohort studies, considered of fair to good quality, involving 1,709 to 71,494 participants (Ma et al., 2012a). A meta-analysis of these studies showed that dietary intake of lutein and zeaxanthin was significantly related with reduced risk of late macular degeneration, and had a statistically significant inverse association with neovascular age-related macular degeneration risk. However, dietary lutein and zeaxanthin were not significantly associated with decreased risk of early macular degeneration.

Although noting that supplementation trials are limited by several factors, including small number of subjects and inadequate masking, preventing definitive conclusions to be drawn, Sabour-Pickett et al. (2012) concluded that there is biologically plausible rationale whereby the macular pigment protects against development and progression of age-related macular degeneration. It was further stated that the literature demonstrates that supplementation with the macular carotenoids is probably the best means of fortifying the antioxidant defenses of the macula, thus putatively reducing the risk of macular degeneration and/or its progression.

11.7 PROTECTION OF COGNITIVE FUNCTIONS

Lutein and zeaxanthin also accumulate preferentially in the human brain (Johnson, 2012) and may influence neural function in the elderly. A significant relationship was found between serum levels of lutein and zeaxanthin and cognitive function in a population-based study that looked at biological, psychological, and social factors that play a role in longevity and survival of centenarians (Johnson et al., 2011). Postmortem lutein levels in brain tissue were also found to be significantly related to antemortem measures of global cognitive function, executive function, and dementia severity after adjusting for age, gender, education, hypertension, and diabetes.

As part of the Irish Longitudinal Study on Aging, the relation between macular pigment optical density and cognitive function was investigated in 4,453 adults aged ≥50 years (Feeney et al., 2013). Lower macular pigment optical density was associated with poorer performance on the mini-mental state examination and on the Montreal cognitive assessment. Individuals with lower macular pigment optical density also had poorer prospective memory, took longer time to complete a trail-making task, and had slower and more variable reaction times on a choice reaction time task. However, there was no significant association between macular pigment optical density and verbal fluency, word recall, visual reasoning, or picture memory.

In a 4-month double-blind, placebo-controlled trial, older women were supplemented with lutein (12 mg/day), alone or in combination with docosahexaenoic acid (DHA) (Johnson et al., 2008). Verbal fluency scores improved significantly in the DHA, lutein, and combined treatment groups. Memory scores and rate of learning improved significantly in the combined treatment group that also displayed a trend toward more efficient learning.

In the Nurses' Health Study, higher lycopene intake was related to slower cognitive decline while greater carotenoid intake was strongly associated with better overall cognition (Devore et al., 2013).

11.8 OTHER HEALTH BENEFITS

β-cryptoxanthin was shown by epidemiological studies to be associated with reduced risk of inflammatory disorders. In a prospective cohort study of 29,368 women (aged 55 to 69 years at baseline) carried out from 1986 through 1997, only β-cryptoxanthin and zinc intake had statistically significant inverse association with risk of rheumatoid arthritis (Cerhan et al., 2003). There was no association with total carotenoid, α- or β-carotene, lycopene, or lutein/zeaxanthin. The European Prospective Investigation of Cancer Incidence Norfolk Study, a population-based prospective study of >25,000 subjects, also found that β-cryptoxanthin was significantly associated with a reduced risk of inflammatory polyarthritis after adjustments were made for total energy and protein intakes and for cigarette smoking (Pattison et al., 2005). The results of this study indicate that a modest increase in β-cryptoxanthin intake, equivalent to one glass of freshly squeezed orange juice per day, is associated with a reduced risk of inflammatory disorders such as rheumatoid arthritis.

Cross-sectional data from the U.S. National Health and Nutrition Examination Surveys (2005–2006) on adults aged 25–85 years were analyzed, the final sample consisting of 1,798 adults with complete data (Beydoun et al., 2013). Total carotenoid (mainly β-carotene and lutein + zeaxanthin) in the serum was significantly associated with reduced levels of depressive symptoms. None of the other serum antioxidants (retinol, retinyl esters, vitamin C, and vitamin E) had a significant association with depressive symptoms.

A tomato-rich diet has also been recently inversely related to depressive symptoms. In a cross-sectional survey consisting of 986 elderly Japanese individuals aged 70 years or older, a tomato-rich diet was independently related to lower prevalence of depressive symptoms (Niu et al., 2013).

A systematic review and meta-analysis of observational studies published between 1996 and March 2005 identified eight studies (six case-control, one cohort, and one cross-sectional) about the effect of vitamin C, vitamin E, and β-carotene intake on the risk of Parkinson's disease (Etminan et al., 2005). It was concluded that dietary vitamin E might have a neuroprotective effect attenuating the risk of Parkinson's disease, but the studies did not suggest any protective effects associated with vitamin C or β-carotene.

In the Framingham Osteoporosis Study, cross-sectional and longitudinal analyses were carried out in 334 men and 540 women (Sahni et al., 2009). Few cross-sectional associations were observed with carotenoid intake. Significant associations were found between lycopene intake and 4-year change in lumbar spine bone mineral density in women, and between intakes of total carotenoids, β-carotene, lycopene and lutein + zeaxanthin, and 4-year change in trochanter bone mineral density in men. No significant associations were observed at other bone sites. The results, although not consistent across all bone mineral density sites, were considered supportive of a protective role of carotenoids for bone mineral density in older men and women.

In an intervention study, 33 female and 20 male subjects (aged 63–86 y) consumed 330 mL/d (47.1 mg/d lycopene) tomato juice or mineral water for 8 wk (Watzl et al., 2000). Prolonged tomato juice consumption increased plasma lycopene concentrations but did not significantly affect cell-mediated immunity in well-nourished elderly subjects.

According to Sies and Stahl (2004) and Köpcke and Krutmann (2008), in a review and a meta-analysis, respectively, human intervention studies show moderate UV protective effects of β-carotene in the skin. Ultraviolet light-induced erythema on the dorsal skin (back) was significantly diminished after 8 weeks of supplementation, the suppression being greater with a combination of carotenoids and vitamin E than with the carotenoids alone (Stahl et al., 2000a). Photoprotection through individual dietary carotenoids such as β-carotene or lycopene is considerably lower in terms of sun protection factor than that provided by topical sunscreens (Stahl and Sies, 2012). However, an optimal supply of antioxidant micronutrients in the skin increases basal dermal defense against UV irradiation, gives longer-term protection, and contributes to maintenance of skin health and appearance.

β-carotene, used as oral sun protectant for the prevention of sunburn, was shown to be effective either alone or in combination with other carotenoids or antioxidant vitamins (Stahl and Sies, 2005). Ingestion of tomato paste, corresponding to 16 mg lycopene/day, for 10 weeks led to increases in serum levels of lycopene and total carotenoids in the skin (Stahl et al., 2001). Erythema formation was lower in the group that consumed tomato paste, compared to the control. In a double-blind placebo-controlled human study, volunteers' diets were supplemented with a kale extract, resulting in slow but significant and effective uptake of carotenoids in the skin (Meinke et al., 2013). This significantly increased the radical scavenging activity and protection against stress-induced radical formation.

11.9 CONCLUDING REMARKS

Although numerous studies report the protective effect of carotenoids against chronic diseases, there are some inconsistent or inconclusive results. The consensus, however, is that there is ample evidence to support and recommend increased consumption of carotenoid-rich foods. However, caution and more investigations are recommended to evaluate the benefits and risks of supplements.

References

Abete I, Perez-Cornago A, Navas-Carretero S, Bondia-Pons I, Zulet MA, Martinez JA. 2013. A regular lycopene enriched tomato sauce consumption influences antioxidant status of healthy young subjects: a crossover study. *J Funct Foods* 5:28–35.

Agarwal M, Parameswari RP, Vasanthi HR, Das DK. 2012. Dynamic action of carotenoids in cardioprotection and maintenance of cardiac health. *Molecules* 17:4755–69.

Agarwal S, Rao AV. 1998. Tomato lycopene and low density lipoprotein oxidation: a human dietary intervention study. *Lipids* 33:981–4.

Agarwal S, Rao AV. 2000. Tomato lycopene and its role in human health and chronic diseases. *Can Med Assoc J* 163:739–44.

Ashwell M. 2002. *Concepts of functional foods. ILSI Europe Concise Monograph Series*. Brussels: International Life Sciences Institute Europe.

Astley SB, Hughes DA, Wright AJA, Elliot RM, Southon S. 2004a. DNA damage and susceptibility to oxidative damage in lymphocytes: effects of carotenoids in vitro and in vivo. *Brit J Nutr* 91:53–61.

Astley SB, Elliot RM, Archer DB, Southon, S. 2004b. Evidence that dietary supplementation with carotenoids and carotenoid-rich foods modulates the DNA damage: repair balance in human lymphocytes. *Brit J Nutr* 91:63–72.

Astorg P. 1997. Food carotenoids and cancer prevention: an overview of current research. *Trends Food Sci Technol* 8:406–13.

ATBC (Alpha-Tocopherol, Beta-Carotene Cancer Prevention Study Group). 1994. The effect of vitamin E and beta carotene on the incidence of lung cancer and other cancers in male smokers. *New Engl J Med* 330:1029–35.

Basu A, Imrhan V. 2007. Tomatoes versus lycopene in oxidative stress and carcinogenesis: conclusions from clinical trials. *Eur J Clin Nutr* 61:295–303.

Bazzano LA, He J, Ogden LG, Loria CM, Vupputuri S, Myers L, Wheldon PK. 2002. Fruit and vegetable intake and the risk of cardiovascular disease in US adults: the first National Health and Nutrition Examination Survey Epidemiologic Follow-up Study. *Am J Clin Nutr* 76:93–9.

Berendschot TTJM, Goldbohm RA, Klöpping WAA, van de Kraats J, van Norel J, van Norren D. 2000. Influence of lutein supplementation on macular pigment, assessed with two techniques. *Invest Ophthalmol Vis Sci* 41:3322–6.

Bertram JS. 1999. Carotenoids and gene regulation. *Nutr Rev* 57:182–91.

Beydoun MA, Beydoun HA, Boueiz A, Shroff MR, Zonderman AB. 2013. Antioxidant status and its association with elevated depressive symptoms among US adults: National Health and Nutrition Examination Surveys 2005–6. *Brit J Nutr* 109:1714–29.

Blot WJ, Li J-Y, Taylor PR, Guo W, Dawsey S, Wang G-Q, Yang CS, Zheng S-F, Gail M, Li G-Y, Yu Y, Liu B-Q, Tangrea J, Sun Y-H, Liu F, Fraumeni JF, Zhang Y-H Jr, Li B. 1993. Nutrition intervention trials in Linxian, China: supplementation with specific vitamin/mineral combinations, cancer incidence, and disease specific mortality in the general population. *J Natl Cancer Inst* 85:1483–92.

Boffetta P, Couto E, Wichmann J, Ferrari P, Trichopoulas D, Bueno-de-Mesquita HB, van Duijnhoven FJB, Büchner FL, Key T, Boeing H and others. 2010. Fruit and vegetable intake and overall cancer risk in the European Prospective Investigation into Cancer and Nutrition (EPIC). *J Natl Cancer Inst* 102:529–37.

Böhm F, Edge R, Burke M, Truscott TG. 2001. Dietary uptake of lycopene protects human cells from singlet oxygen and nitrogen dioxide: ROS components from cigarette smoke. *J Photochem Photobiol B: Biol* 64:176–8.

Bone RA, Landrum JT, Dixon Z, Chen Y, Llerena CM. 2000. Lutein and zeaxanthin in the eyes, serum and diet of human subjects. *Exp Eye Res* 71:239–45.
Bone RA, Landrum JT, Friedes LM, Gomez CM, Kilburn MD, Menendez E, Vidal I, Wang W. 1997. Distribution of lutein and zeaxanthin stereoisomers in the human retina. *Exp Eye Res* 64:211–8.
Bone RA, Landrum JT, Hime GW, Cains A, Zamor J. 1993. Stereochemistry of the human macular carotenoids. *Invest Ophthalmol Vis Sci* 34:2033–40.
Bone RA, Landrum JT, Mayne ST, Gomez CM, Tibor SE, Twaroska EE. 2001. Macular pigment in donor eyes with and without AMD: a case-control study. *Invest Ophthalmol Vis Sci* 42:235–40.
Borel P. 2012. Genetic variations involved in interindividual variability in carotenoid status. *Mol Nutr Food Res* 56:228–40.
Bowen P, Chen L, Stacewicz-Sapuntzakis M, Duncan C, Sharifi R, Ghosh L, Kim H-S, Christov-Tzelkov K, van Breemen R. 2002. Tomato sauce supplementation and prostate cancer: lycopene accumulation and modulation of biomarkers of carcinogenesis. *Exp Biol Med* 227:886–93.
Britton G. 1995. Structure and properties of carotenoids in relation to functions. *FASEB J* 9:1551–8.
Briviba K, Schnäbele K, Rechkemmer G, Bub A. 2004. Supplementation of a diet low in carotenoids with tomato or orange juice does not affect lipid peroxidation in plasma and feces of healthy men. *J Nutr* 134:1081–3.
Brown L, Rimm EB, Seddon JM, Giovannucci EL, Chasan-Tauber L, Spiegelman D, Willett WC, Hankinson SE. 1999. A prospective study of carotenoid intake and risk of cataract extraction in US men. *Am J Clin Nutr* 70:517–24.
Bub A, Watzl B, Abrahamse L, Delincée H, Adam S, Wever J, Müller H, Rechkemmer G. 2000. Moderate intervention with carotenoid-rich vegetable products reduces lipid peroxidation in men. *J Nutr* 130:2200–6.
Campbell JK, Canene-Adams K, Lindshield BL, Boileau TW-M, Clinton SK, Erdman JW Jr. 2004. Tomato phytochemicals and prostate cancer risk. *J Nutr* 134:S3486–92.
CARIG (Carotenoid Research Interactive Group). 1996. Beta-carotene and the carotenoids: beyond the intervention trials. *Nutr Rev* 54:185–8.
Carpentier S, Knaus M, Suh M. 2009. Associations between lutein, zeaxanthin, and age-related macular degeneration. *Crit Rev Food Sci Nutr* 49:313–26.
Cerhan JR, Saag KG, Merlino LA, Mikuls TR, Criswell LA. 2003. Antioxidant micronutrients and risk of rheumatoid arthritis in a cohort of older women. *Am J Epidemiol* 157:345–54.
Chan JM, Wang F, Holly EA. 2005. Vegetable and fruit intake and pancreatic cancer in a population-based case-control study in the San Francisco Bay Area. *Cancer Epidemiol Biomarkers Prev* 14:2093–7.
Chasan-Taber L, Willett WC, Seddon JM, Stampfer MJ, Rosner B, Colditz GA, Speizer FE, Hankinson SE. 1999. A prospective study of carotenoid and vitamin A intakes and the risk of cataract extraction in US women. *Am J Clin Nutr* 70:509–16.
Chen HL, Tucker KL, Graubard BI, Heineman EF, Markin RS, Potischman NA, Russell RM, Weisenburger DD, Ward MH. 2002. Nutrient intakes and adenocarcinoma of the esophagus and distal stomach. *Nutr Cancer Int J* 42:33–40.
Chen L, Stacewicz-Sapuntzakis M, Duncan C, Sharifi R, Ghosh L, van Breemen R, Ashton D, Bowen PE. 2001. Oxidative DNA damage in prostate cancer patients consuming tomato sauce-based entrees as whole-food intervention. *J Natl Cancer Inst* 93:1872–9.
Chew BP, Park JS. 2004. Carotenoid action on the immune response. *J Nutr* 134:S257–61.
Cho E, Hankinson SE, Rosner B, Willet WC, Colditz GA. 2008. Prospective study of lutein/zeaxanthin intake and risk of age-related macular degeneration. *Am J Clin Nutr* 87:1837–43.
Choi HD, Youn YK, Shin WG. 2011. Positive effects of astaxanthin on lipid profiles and oxidative stress in overweight subjects. *Plant Foods Hum Nutr* 66:363–9.
Chong EWT, Wong TY, Kreis AJ, Simpson JA, Guymer RH. 2007. Dietary antioxidants and primary prevention of age related macular degeneration: systematic review and meta-analysis. *Brit Med J* 335:755–62.
Clinton SK. 1998. Lycopene: chemistry, biology, and implications for human health and disease. *Nutr Rev* 56:35–51.
Cohen JH, Kristal AR, Stanford JL. 2000. Fruit and vegetable intakes and prostate cancer risk. *J Natl Cancer Inst* 92:61–8.
Collins AR. 2001. Carotenoids and genomic stability. *Mutation Res* 475:21–8.
Collins JK, Perkins-Veazie P. 2006. Lycopene: from plants to humans. *Hortsci* 41:1101–366.
Connor SL, Ojeda LS, Sexton G, Weidner G, Connor WE. 2004. Diets lower in folic acid and carotenoids are associated with coronary disease epidemic in central and eastern Europe. *J Am Diet Assoc* 104:1793–9.

Dauchet L, Amouyel P, Dallongeville J. 2005. Fruit and vegetable consumption and risk of stroke: a meta-analysis of cohort studies. *Neurology* 65:1193–7.

Dauchet L, Amouyel P, Hercberg S, Dallongeville J. 2006. Fruit and vegetable consumption and risk of coronary heart disease: a meta-analysis of cohort studies. *J Nutr* 136:2588–93.

Dauchet L, Kesse-Guyot E, Czernichow S, Bertais S, Estaquio C, Péneau, S, Vergnaud A-C, Chat-Yung S, Castetbon K, Deschamps, V, Brindel, P, Hercberg S. 2007. Dietary patterns and blood pressure change over 5-y follow-up in the SU.VI.MAX cohort. *Am J Clin Nutr* 85:1650–6.

Delcourt C, Carriere I, Delage M, Barbenger-Gateau P, Schalch W. 2006. Plasma lutein and zeaxanthin and other carotenoids as modifiable risk factors for age-related maculopathy and cataract; the POLA Study. *Invest Opthalmol Vis Sci* 47:2329–35.

Devore EE, Kang JH, Stampfer MJ, Grodstein F. 2013. The association of antioxidants and cognition in the Nurses' Health Study. *Am J Epidemiol* 177:33–41.

Dherani M, Murthy GVS, Gupta SK, Young IS, Maraini G, Camparini M, Price GM, John N, Chakravarthy U, Fletcher AE. 2008. Blood levels of vitamin C, carotenoids and retinol are inversely associated with cataract in a North Indian population. *Invest Ophthalmol Vis Sci* 49:3328–35.

Dwyer JH, Navab M, Dwyer KM, Hassan K, Sun P, Shircore A, Hama-Levy S, Hough G, Wang X, Drake T, Merz CNB, Fogelman AM. 2001. Oxygenated carotenoid lutein and progression of early atherosclerosis: the Los Angeles Atherosclerosis study. *Circulation* 103:2922–7.

EDCC (Eye Disease Case-Control) Study Group (1993). Antioxidant status and neovascular age-related macular degeneration. *Arch Ophthalmol* 111:104–9.

Edge R, McGarvey DJ, Truscott TG. 1997. The carotenoids as anti-oxidants: a review. *J Photochem Photobiol* 41:189–200.

Erhardt JG, Meisner C, Bode JC, Bode C. 2003. Lycopene, β-carotene, and colorectal adenomas. *Am J Clin Nutr* 78:1219–24.

Etminan M, Gill SS, Samii A. 2005. Intake of vitamin E, vitamin C, and carotenoids and the risk of Parkinson's disease: a meta-analysis. *Lancet Neurol* 4:362–5.

Etminan M, Takkouche B, Caamaño-Isorna F. 2004. The role of tomato products and lycopene in the prevention of prostate cancer: a meta-analysis of observational studies. *Cancer Epidemiol Biomarkers Prev* 13:340–5.

Feeney J, Finucane C, Savva GM, Cronin H, Beatty S, Nolan JM, Kenny RA. 2013. Low macular pigment optical density is associated with lower cognitive performance in a large population-based sample of older adults. *Neurobiol Aging* 34:2449–56.

Ford ES, Giles WH. 2000. Serum vitamins, carotenoids, and angina pectoris: findings from the National Health and Nutrition Examination Survey III. *Ann Epidemiol* 10:106–16.

Franceschi S, Bidioli E, La Vecchia C, Talamini R, D'Avanzo B, Negri E. 1994. Tomatoes and risk of digestive-tract cancers. *Int J Cancer* 59:181–4.

Freedman ND, Park Y, Subar AF, Hollenbeck AR, Leitzmann MF, Schatzkin A, Abnet CC. 2008. Fruit and vegetable intake and head and neck cancer risk in a large United States prospective cohort study. *Int J Cancer* 122:2330–6.

Fung TT, Willett WC, Stampfer MJ, Manson JE, Hu FB. 2001. Dietary patterns and the risk of coronary heart disease in women. *Arch Inter Med* 161:1857–62.

Gale CR, Hall NF, Phillips DIW, Martyn CN. 2001a. Plasma antioxidant vitamins and carotenoids and age-related cataract. *Ophthalmology* 108:1992–8.

Gale CR, Ashurst HE, Powers HJ, Martyn CN. 2001b. Antioxidant vitamin status and carotid atherosclerosis in the elderly. *Am J Clin Nutr* 74:402–8.

Gale CR, Hall NF, Phillips DIW, Martyn CN. 2003. Lutein and zeaxanthin status and risk of age-related macular degeneration. *Invest Opthalmol Vis Sci* 44:2461–5.

Genkinger JM, Platz EA, Hoffman SC, Comstock GW, Helzlsouer KJ. 2004. Fruit, vegetable, and antioxidant intake and all-cause, cancer, and cardiovascular disease mortality in a community-dwelling population in Washington County, Maryland. *Am J Epidemiol* 160:1223–33.

Giovannucci E. 1999. Tomatoes, tomato-based products, lycopene, and cancer: review of the epidemiologic literature. *J Natl Cancer Inst* 91:317–31.

Giovannucci E. 2002a. A review of epidemiologic studies of tomatoes, lycopene and prostate cancer. *Exp Bio Med* 227:852–9.

Giovannucci E. 2002b. Lycopene and prostate cancer risk: methodological considerations in the epidemiologic literature. *Pure Appl Chem* 74:1427–34.

Giovannucci E, Ascherio A, Rimm EB, Stampfer MJ, Colditz GA, Willett WC. 1995. Intake of carotenoids and retinol in relation to risk of prostate cancer. *J Natl Cancer Inst* 87:1767–76.

Giovannucci E, Rimm EB, Liu Y, Stampfer MJ, Willett WC. 2002. A prospective study of tomato products, lycopene, and prostate cancer risk. *J Natl Cancer Inst* 94:391–8.

Gonzalez CA, Pera G, Agudo A, Bueno de Mesquita HB, Ceroti M, Boieng H, et al. 2006. Fruit and vegetable intake and the risk of stomach and oesophagus adenocarcinoma in the European Prospective Investigation into Cancer and Nutrition (EPIC-EURGAST). *Int J Cancer* 118:2559–66.

Hadley CW, Clinton SK, Schwartz SJ. 2003. The consumption of processed tomato products enhances plasma lycopene concentrations in association with a reduced lipoprotein sensitivity to oxidative damage. *J Nutr* 133:727–32.

Hadley CW, Miller EC, Schwartz SJ, Clinton SK. 2002. Tomatoes, lycopene, and prostate cancer: progress and promise. *Exp Biol Med* 227:869–80.

He FJ, Nowson CA, Lucas M, MacGregor GA. 2007. Increased consumption of fruit and vegetable is related to a reduced risk of coronary heart disease: meta-analysis of cohort studies. *J Hum Hypertens* 21:717–28.

He FJ, Nowson CA, MacGregor GA. 2006. Fruit and vegetable consumption and stroke: meta-analysis of cohort studies. *Lancet* 367:320–6.

Heber D, Lu Q-Y. 2002. Overview of mechanisms of action of lycopene. *Exp Biol Med* 227:920–3.

Heidermann C, Schulze MB, Franco OH, van Dam RM, Mantzoros CS, Hu FB. 2008. Dietary patterns and risk of mortality from cardiovascular disease, cancer, and all-causes in a prospective cohort of women. *Circulation* 118:230–7.

Hiroshi Y, Hidekatsu Y, Kumie I, Yoshiharu T, Takashi K, Hiroki T, Norio T. 2010. Administration of natural astaxanthin increases serum HDL-cholesterol and adiponectin in subjects with mild hyperlipidemia. *Atherosclerosis* 209:520–3.

Holzapfel NP, Holzapfel BM, Champ S, Feldthusen J, Clements J, Hutmacher DW. 2013. The potential role of lycopene for the prevention and therapy of prostate cancer: from molecular mechanisms to clinical evidence. *Int J Mol Sci* 14:14620–46.

Hung HC, Joshipura KJ, Jiang R, Hu FB, Hunter D, Smith-Warner SA, Colditz GA, Rosner B, Spidelman D, Willet WC. 2004. Fruit and vegetable intake and the risk of major chronic disease. *J Nat'l Cancer Inst* 96:1577–84.

Ito Y, Wakai K, Suzuki K, Tamakoshi A, Seki N, Ando M, Nishino Y, Kondo T, Watanabe Y, Ozasa K, Ohno Y for the JACC Study Group. 2003. Serum carotenoids and mortality from lung cancer: a case-control study nested in the Japan Collaborative Cohort (JACC) Study. *Cancer Sci* 94:57–63.

Jacques PF, Chylack LT Jr, Hankinson SE, Khu PM, Gail Rogers G, Judith Friend J, Tung W, Wolfe JK, Padhye N, Willett WC, Taylor A. 2001. Long-term nutrient intake and early age-related nuclear lens opacities. *Arch Ophthalmol* 119:1009–19.

Johnson EJ. 2012. A possible role for lutein and zeaxanthin in cognitive function in the elderly. *Am J Clin Nutr* 96:S1161–5.

Johnson EJ, McDonald K, Caldarella SM, Chung HY, Troen AM, Snodderly DM. 2008. Cognitive findings of an exploratory trial of docosahexaenoic acid and lutein supplementation in older women. *Nutr Neurosc* 11:75–83.

Johnson EJ, Vishwanathan R, Schalch W, Poon L, Wittwer J, Johnson MA, Hausman D, Davey A, Green R, Gearing M, Woodard J, Nelson P, Miller LS, Scott TM. 2011. Brain levels of lutein (L) and zeaxanthin (Z) are related to cognitive function in centenarians. *FASEB J* 25:975.21.

Joshipura KJ, Hu FB, Manson JE, Stampfer MJ, Rimm EB, Speizer FE, Colditz G, Ascherio A, Rosner B, Spiegelman D, Willett WC. 2001. The effect of fruit and vegetable intake on risk for coronary heart disease. *Ann Inter Med* 134:1106–14.

Kaliora AC, Dedoussis GVZ, Schmidt H. 2006. Dietary antioxidants in preventing atherogenesis. *Atherosclerosis* 187:1–17.

Karppi J, Kurl S, Mäkikallio TH, Ronkainen K, Laukkanen JA. 2013a. Low levels of plasma carotenoids are associated with an increased risk of atrial fibrillation. *Eur J Epidemiol* 28:45–53.

Karppi J, Kurl S, Mäkikallioi TH, Ronkainen K, Laukkanen JA. 2013b. Serum β-carotene concentrations and the risk of congestive heart failure in men: a population-based study. *Int J Cardiol* 168:1841–6.

Karppi J, Laukkanen JA, Mäkikallio TH, Ronkainen K, Kurl S. 2013c. Serum β-carotene and the risk of sudden cardiac death in men: a population-based follow-up study. *Atherosclerosis* 226:172–7.

Kaur C, Kapoor HC. 2001. Antioxidants in fruits and vegetables: the millennium's health. *Int J Food Sci Technol* 36:703–7.

Khachik F, Carvalho L, Bernstein PS, Muir GJ, Zhao D-Y, Katz NB. 2002. Chemistry, distribution, and metabolism of tomato carotenoids and their impact on human health. *Exp. Biol. Med* 227:845–51.
Kiokias S, Gordon MH. 2004. Antioxidant properties of carotenoids in vitro and in vivo. *Food Rev Int* 20:99–121.
Köpcke W, Krutmann J. 2008. Protection from sunburn with β-carotene: a meta-analysis. *Photochem Photobiol* 84:284–8.
Krinsky NI. 1989. Antioxidant functions of carotenoids. *Free Radic Biol Med* 7:617–35.
Krinsky NI. 2001. Carotenoids as antioxidants. *Nutr* 17:815–7.
Krinsky NI, Johnson EJ. 2005. Carotenoid actions and their relation to health and disease. *Mol Aspects Med* 26:459–516.
Krinsky NI, Landrum JT, Bone RA. 2003. Biologic mechanisms of the protective role of lutein and zeaxanthin in the eye. *Annu Rev Nut* 23:171–201.
Kucuk O, Sarkar FH, Sakr W, Djuric Z, Pollak MN, Khachik F, Li Y-W, Banerjee M, Grignon D, Bertram JS, Crissman JD, Pontes EJ, Wood DP Jr. 2001. Phase II randomized clinical trial of lycopene supplementation before radical prostatectomy. *Cancer Epidemiol Biomark Prev* 10:861–8.
Kucuk O, Wood DP Jr. 2002. Response of hormone rerfractory prostate cancer to lycopene. *J Urol* 167:651.
Landrum JT, Bone RA. 2001. Lutein, zeaxanthin, and the macular pigment. *Arch Biochem Biophys* 385:28–40.
Landrum JT, Bone RA, Joa H, Kilburn MD, Moore LL, Sprague KE. 1997. A one year study of the macular pigment: the effect of 140 days of a lutein supplement. *Exp Eye Res* 65:57–62.
Lee C-YJ, Isaac HB, Huang SH, Long LH, Wang H, Gruber J, Ong CN, Kelly RP. 2009. Limited antioxidant effect after consumption of a single dose of tomato sauce by young males, despite a rise in plasma lycopene. *Free Radic Res* 43:622–8.
Lee L, Kang SA, Lee HO, Lee B-H, Park JS, Kim J-H, Jung IK, Park YJ, Lee JE. 2001. Relationships between dietary intake and cognitive function level in Korean elderly people. *Public Health* 115:133–8.
Liu S, Lee, I-M, Ajani U, Cole SR, Buring JE, Manson JE. 2001. Intake of vegetables rich in carotenoids and risk of coronary heart disease in men: the Physicians' Health Study. *Int J Epidemiol* 30:130–5.
Liu S, Manson JE, Lee I-M, Cole SR, Hennekens CH, Willet WC, Buring JE. 2000. Fruit and vegetable intake and the risk of cardiovascular disease: the Women's Health Study. *Am J Clin Nutr* 72:922–8.
Lyle BJ, Mares-Perlman JA, Klein BEK, Klein R, Greger JL. 1999a. Antioxidant intake and risk of incident age-related nuclear cataracts in the Beaver Dam Eye Study. *Am J Epidemiol* 149:801–9.
Lyle BJ, Mares-Perlman JA, Klein BEK, Klein R, Palta M, Bowen PE, Greger JL. 1999b. Serum carotenoids and tocopherols and incidence of age-related nuclear cataract. *Am J Clin Nutr* 69:272–7.
Ma L, Dou H-L, Wu Y-Q, Huang Y-M, Huang Y-B, Xu X-R, Zou Z-Y, Lin X-M. 2012. Lutein and zeaxanthin intake and the risk of age-related macular degeneration: a systematic review and meta-analysis. *Br J Nutr* 107:350–9.
Mackinnon ES, Rao AV, Josse RG, Rao LG. 2011. Supplementation with the antioxidant lycopene significantly decreases oxidative stress parameters and the bone resorption marker N-telopeptide of type I collagen in postmenopausal women. *Osteoporos Int* 22:1091–101.
Mares-Perlman A, Brady WE, Klein BE, Klein R, Palta M, Bowen P, Stacewicz-Sapuntzakis M. 1995. Serum carotenoids and tocopherols and severity of nuclear and cortical opacities. *Invest Opthalmol Vis Sci* 36:276–88.
Mares-Perlman JA, Fisher AI, Klein R, Palta M, Block G, Millen AE, Wright JD. 2001. Lutein and zeaxanthin in the diet and serum and their relation to age-related maculopathy in the Third National Health and Nutrition Examination Survey. *Am J Epidemiol* 153:424–32.
Markovits N, Ben Amotz A, Levy Y. 2009. The effect of tomato-derived lycopene on low carotenoids and enhanced systemic inflammation and oxidation in severe obesity. *Israel Med Assoc J* 11:598–601.
Martinez-Tomás R, Larqué E, González-Silvera D, Sánchez-Campillo M, Burgos MI, Wellner A, Parra S, Bialek L, Alminger M, Pérez-Llamas F. 2012. Effect of the consumption of a fruit and vegetable soup with high in vitro carotenoid bioaccessibility on serum carotenoid concentrations and markers of oxidative stress in young men. *Eur J Nutr* 51:231–9.
Mayne ST. 1996. Beta-carotene, carotenoids, and disease prevention. *FASEB J* 10:690–701.
Mayne ST, Handelman GJ, Beecher G. 1996. β-carotene and lung cancer promotion in heavy smokers—a plausible relationship? *J Natl Cancer Inst* 88:1513–5.
Meinke MC, Friedrich A, Tscherch K, Haag SF, Darvin ME, Vollert H, Groth N, Lademann J, Rohn S. 2013. Influence of dietary carotenoids on radical scavenging capacity of the skin and skin lipids. *Eur J Pharm Biopharm* 84:365–73.

Michels KB, Giovannucci E, Chan AT, Singhania R, Fuchs CS, Willett WC. 2006. Fruit and vegetable consumption and colorectal adenomas in the Nurses' Health Study. *Cancer Res* 66:3942–53.

Miller EC, Giovannucci E, Erdman JW Jr, Bahnson R, Schwartz SJ, Clinton S. 2002. Tomato products, lycopene and prostate cancer risk. *Urol Clin N Am* 29:83–93.

Moeller SM, Jacques PF, Blumberg JB. 2000. The potential role of dietary xanthophylls in cataract and age-related macular degeneration. *J Am Coll Nutr* 19:S522–7.

Moeller SM, Parekh N, Tinker L, Ritrenbaugh C, Blodi B, Wallace RB, Mares JA. 2006. Associations between intermediate age-related macular degeneration and lutein and zeaxanthin in the Carotenoids in Age-related Eye Disease Study (CAREDS): Ancillary study of the Women's Health Initiative. *Arch Opthalmol* 124:1151–62.

Mordente A, Guantario B, Meucci E, Silvestrini A, Lombardi E, Martorana GE, Giardina B, Böhm V. 2011. Lycopene and cardiovascular diseases: an update. *Curr Med Chem* 18:1146–63.

Morris MC, Evans DA, Tangney CC, Bienias JL, Wilson RS. 2006. Associations of vegetable and fruit consumption with age-related cognitive change. *Neurology* 67:1370–6.

Niu K, Guo H, Kakizaki M, Cui Y, Ohmori-Matsuda K, Guan L, Hozawa A, Kuriyama S, Tsuboya T, Ohrui T, Furukawa K, Arai H, Tsuji I, Nagatomi R. 2013. A tomato-rich diet is related to depressive symptoms among an elderly population aged 70 years and over: a population-based, cross-sectional analysis. *J Affect Disord* 144:165–70.

Nkondjock A, Ghadirian P, Johnson KC, Krewski D, the Canadian Cancer Registries Epidemiology Research Group. 2005. Dietary intake of lycopene is associated with reduced pancreatic cancer risk. *J Nutr* 135:592–7.

Nöthlings U, Schulze MB, Weikert C, Boeing H, van der Schouw YT Christina Bamia C, Benetou V, Lagiou P, Krogh V, Beulens JWJ, Peeters PHM et al. 2008. Intake of vegetables, legumes, and fruit, and risk for all-cause, cardiovascular, and cancer mortality in a European diabetic population. *J Nutr* 138:775–81.

Olmedilla B, Granado F, Blanco I, Vaquero M. 2003. Lutein, but not alpha-tocopherol, supplementation improves visual function in patients with age-related cataracts: a 2-year double-blind, placebo-controlled pilot study. *Nutrition* 19:21–4.

Olmedilla B, Granado F, Blanco I, Vaquero M, Cajigal C. 2001. Lutein in patients with cataracts and age-related macular degeneration: a long-term supplementation study. *J Sci Food Agric* 81:904–9.

Olson JA. 1999. Carotenoids and human health. *Arch Latinoamer Nutr* 49:7S–11S.

Omenn GS, Goodman GE, Thornquist MD, Balmes J, Cullen MR, Glass A, Keogh JP, Meyskens FL Jr, Valanis B, Williams JH Jr, Barnhart S, Hammar S. 1996. Effects of a combination of beta carotene and vitamin A on lung cancer and cardiovascular disease. *New Eng J Med* 334:1150–5.

Ortega RM, Requejo AM, Andrés P, Lopez-Sobaler AM, Quintas ME, Redondo MR, Navia B, Rivas T. 1997. Dietay intake and cognitive function in a group of elderly people. *Am J Clin Nutr* 66:803–9.

Osganian, SK, Stampfer MJ, Rimm E, Spiegelman D, Manson JE, Willet WC. 2003. Dietary carotenoids and risk of coronary artery disease in women. *Am J Clin Nutr* 77:1390–99.

Palace VP, Khaper N, Qin Q, Singal PK. 1999. Antioxidant potentials of vitamin A and carotenoids and their relevance to heart disease. *Free Radic Biol Med* 26:746–61.

Palozza P, Krinsky NI. 1992. Antioxidant effects of carotenoids in vivo and in vitro: an overview. *Methods Enzymol* 213:403–20.

Palozza P, Simone RE, Catalano A, Mele MC. 2011. Tomato lycopene and lung cancer prevention: from experimental to human studies. *Cancers* 3:2333–57.

Pan M-H, Lai C-S, Dushenkov S, Ho C-T. 2009. Modulation of inflammatory genes by natural dietary bioactive compounds. *J Agric Food Chem* 57:4467–77.

Paterson E, Gordon MH, Niwat C, George TW, Parr L, Waroonphan S, Lovegrove JA. 2006. Supplementation with fruit and vegetable soups and beverages increases plasma carotenoid concentrations but does not alter markers of oxidative stress or cardiovascular risk factors. *J Nutr* 136:2849–55.

Pattison DJ, Symmons DPM, Lunt M, Welch A, Bingham SA, Day NE, Silman AJ 2005. Dietary β-cryptoxanthin and inflammatory polyarthritis: results from a population-based prospective study. *Am J Clin Nutr* 82:451–5.

Polesel J, Negri E, Serraino D, Parpinel M, Barzan L, Libra M, Bosetti C, Garavello W, Montella M, La Vecchia A, Franceschi S, Talamini R. 2012. Dietary intakes of carotenoids and other nutrients in the risk of nasopharyngeal carcinoma: a case-control study in Italy. *Brit J Cancer* 107:1580–3.

Pomerleau J, Lock K, McKee M. 2006. The burden of cardiovascular disease and cancer attributable to low fruit and vegetable intake in the European Union: differences between old and new member states. *Public Health Nutr* 9:575–83.

Porrini M, Riso P. 2000. Lymphocyte lycopene concentration and DNA protection from oxidative damage is increased in women after a short period of tomato consumption. *J Nutr* 130:189–92.
Porrini M, Riso P, Brusamolino A, Berti C, Guarnieri S, Visioli F. 2005. Daily intake of a formulated tomato drink affects carotenoid plasma and lymphocyte concentrations and improved cellular antioxidant protection. *Br J Nutr* 93:93–9.
Rao AV, Agarwal S. 1999. Role of lycopene as antioxidant carotenoid in the prevention of chronic diseases: a review. *Nutr Res* 19:305–23.
Rao AV, Rao LG. 2004. Lycopene and human health. *Curr Top Nutr Res* 2:127–36.
Rao AV, Rao LG. 2007. Carotenoids and human health. *Pharmacol Res* 55:207–16.
Riccioni G. 2009. Carotenoids and cardiovascular disease. *Curr. Atherosclerosis Rep.* 11:434–9.
Richer S, Stiles W, Statkute L, Pulido J, Frankowski J, Rudy D, Pei K, Tsipursky M, Nyland J. 2004. Double-masked, placebo-controlled, randomized trial of lutein and antioxidant supplementation in the intervention of atrophic age-related macular degeneration: the Veteran's LAST study (Lutein Antioxidant Supplementation Trial). *Optometry* 75, 216–230.
Sabour-Pickett S, Nolan JM, Loughman J, Beatty S. 2012. A review of the evidence germane to the putative protective role of the macular carotenoids for age-related macular degeneration. *Mol Nutr Food Res* 56:270–86.
Sahni S, Hannan, MT, Blumberg J, Cupples LA, Kiel DP, Tucker KL. 2009. Inverse association of carotenoid intakes with 4-y change in bone mineral density in elderly men and women: the Framingham Osteoporosis Study. *Am J Clin Nutr* 89:416–24.
Seddon JM, Ajani UA, Sperduto RD, Hiller R, Blair N, Burton TC, Farber MD, Gragoudas ES, Haller J, Miller DT, Lawrence A, Yannuzzi LA, Willet W. 1994. Dietary carotenoids, vitamins A, C, and E, and advanced age-related macular degeneration: Eye Disease Case-Control Study Group. *JAMA* 272:1413–20.
Sesso HD, Liu S, Gaziano JM, Buring JE. 2003. Dietary lycopene, tomato-based food products and cardiovascular disease in women. *J Nutr* 133:2336–41.
Sharoni Y, Danilenko M, Dubi N, Ben-Dor A, Levy J. 2004. Carotenoids and transcription. *Arch Biochem Biophys* 430:89–96.
Sharoni Y, Danilenko M, Walfish S, Amir, H, Nahum, A, Ben-Dor, A, Hirsch K, Khanin M, Steiner M, Agemy L, Zango G, Levy J. 2002. Role of gene regulation in the anticancer activity of carotenoids. *Pure Appl Chem* 764:1469–77.
Sharoni Y, Linnewiel-Hermoni K, Zango G, Khanin M, Salman H, Veprik A, Danilenko M, Levy J. 2012. The role of lycopene and its derivatives in the regulation of transcription systems: implications for cancer prevention. *Am J Clin Nutr* 96:S1173–8.
Sies H, Stahl W. 2004. Nutritional protection against skin damage from sunlight. *Annu Rev Nutr* 24:173–200.
Singh P, Goyal GK. 2008. Dietary lycopene: its properties and anticarcinogenic effects. *Comp Rev Food Sci Food Safety* 7:255–70.
Slattery ML, Benson J, Curtin K, Ma K-N, Schaeffer D, Potter JD. 2000. Carotenoids and colon cancer. *Am J Clin Nutr* 71:575–82.
Snodderly DM. 1995. Evidence for protection against age-related macular degeneration by carotenoids and antioxidant vitamins. *Am J Clin Nutr* 62:S1448–61.
Stacewicz-Sapuntzakis M, Bowen PE. 2005. Role of lycopene and tomato products in prostate health. *Biochim Biophys Acta* 1740:202–5.
Stahl W, Ale-Agha N, Polidori MC. 2002. Non-antioxidant properties of carotenoids. *Biol Chem* 383:553–8.
Stahl W, Heinrich U, Jungmann H, Sies H, Tronnier H. 2000a. Carotenoids and carotenoids plus vitamin E protect against ultraviolet light-induced erythema in humans. *Am J Clin Nutr* 71:795–8.
Stahl W, Heinrich U, Wiseman S, Eichler O, Sies H, Tronnier H. 2001. Dietary tomato paste protects against ultraviolet light-induced erythema in humans. *J Nutr* 131:1449–51.
Stahl W, Sies H. 2003. Antioxidant activity of carotenoids. *Mol Aspects Med* 24:345–51.
Stahl W, Sies H. 2005. Bioactivity and protective effects of natural carotenoids. *Biochim Biophys* 1740:101–7.
Stahl W, Sies H. 2012. β-carotene and other carotenoids in protection from sunlight. *Am J Clin Nutr* 96:S1179–84.
Stahl W, von Laer J, Martin HD, Emmerich T, Sies H. 2000b. Stimulation of gap junctional communication: comparison of acyclo-retinoic acid and lycopene. *Arch Biochem Biophys* 373:271–4.

Stanner SA, Hughes J, Kelly CNM, Buttriss J. 2003. A review of the epidemiological evidence for the 'antioxidant hypothesis.' *Publ Health Nutr* 7:407–22.

Steevens J, Schouten LJ, Goldbohm RA, van den Brandt PA. 2011. Vegetables and fruits consumption and risk of esophageal and gastric cancer subtypes in the Netherland Cohort Study. *Inter J Cancer* 129:2681–93.

Steinmetz KA, Potter JD. 1996. Vegetables, fruit, and cancer prevention: a review. *J Am Diet Assoc* 96:1027–39.

Suzuki K, Ishii J, Kitagawa F, Kuno A, Kusuhara Y, Ochiai J, Ichino N, Osakabe K, Sugimoto K, Yamada H, Ito Y, Hamajima N, Inoue T. 2013. Association of serum carotenoid levels with N-terminal pro-brain-type natriuretic peptide: a cross-sectional study in Japan. *J Epidemiol* 232:163–8.

Tan JSL, Wang JJ, Flood V, Rochtchina E, Smith W, Mitchell P. 2008. Dietary antioxidants and the long-term incidence of age-related macular degeneration: the Blue Mountain Eye Study. *Opthalmology* 115:334–41.

Tanaka T, Shnimizu M, Moriwaki H. 2012. Cancer chemoprevention by carotenoids. *Molecules* 17:3202–42.

Tapiero H, Townsend DM, Tew KD. 2004. The role of carotenoids in the prevention of human pathologies. *Biomed Pharmacother* 58:100–10.

Taylor A, Jacques PF, Chylack LT Jr, Hankinson SE, Khu PM, Rogers G, Friend J, Tung W, Wolfe JK, Padhye N, Willett WC. 2002. Long-term intake of vitamins and carotenoids and odds of early age-related cortical and posterior subcapsular lens opacities. *Am J Clin Nutr* 75:540–9.

Temple NJ. 2000. Antioxidants and disease: more questions than answers. *Nutr Res* 20:449–59.

Trichopoulou A, Costacou T, Bamia C, Trichopoulos D. 2003. Adherence to a Mediterranean diet and survival in a Greek population. *N Eng J Med* 348:2599–608.

USFDA. 2005. *Qualified health claims: letter of partial denial—tomatoes and prostate cancer (lycopene health claim coalition).* College Park MD: Center for Food Safety and Applied Nutrition.

Vanden Langenberg GM, Mares-Perlman JA, Klein R, Klein BEK, Brady WE, Palta M. 1998. Associations between antioxidant and zinc intake and the 5-year incidence of early age-related maculopathy in the Beaver Dam Eye Study. *Am J Epidemiol* 148:204–14.

van Leeuwen R, Boekhoorn S, Vingerling JR, 2005. Dietary intake of antioxidants and risk of age-related macular degeneration. *JAMA* 294:3101–7.

van't Veer P, Jansen MCJF, Klerk M, Kok FJ. 2000. Fruits and vegetables in the prevention of cancer and cardiovascular disease. *Public Health Nutr* 3:103–7.

Visioli F, Riso P, Grande S, Galli C, Porrini M. 2003. Protective activity of tomato products on *in vivo* markers of lipid oxidation. *Eur J Nutr* 42:201–6.

Voorrips LE, Goldbohm RA, van Poppel G, Sturmans F, Hermus RJJ, van den Brandt PA. 2000. Vegetable and fruit consumption and risks of colon and rectal cancer in a prospective cohort study. The Netherlands Cohort Study on Diet and Cancer. *Am J Epidemiol* 152:1081–92.

Voutilainen S, Nurmi T, Mursu J, Rissanen TH. 2006. Carotenoids and cardiovascular health. *Am J Clin Nutr* 83:1265–71.

Wang M-X, Jiao J-H, Li Z-Y, Liu R-R, Shi Q, Ma L. 2013. Lutein supplementation reduces lipid peroxidation and C-reactive protein in healthy nonsmokers. *Atherosclerosis* 227:380–5.

Wang S, Melnyk JP, Tsao R, Marcone MF. 2011. How natural dietary antioxidants in fruits, vegetables and legumes promote vascular health. *Food Res Int* 44:14–22.

Wang X-D. 2012. Lycopene metabolism and its biological significance. *Am J Clin Nutr* 96:S1214–22.

Wang X-D, Russell RM. 1999. Procarcinogenic and anticarcinogenic effects of β-carotene. *Nutr Rev* 57:263–72.

Watzl B, Bub A, Blockhaus M, Herbert BM, Lührmann PM, Neuhäuser-Berthold M, Rechkemmer G. 2000. Prolonged tomato juice consumption has no effect on cell-mediated immunity of well-nourished elderly men and women. *J Nutr* 130:1719–23.

Wertz K, Siler U, Goralczyk R. 2004. Lycopene: modes of action to promote prostate health. *Arch Biochem Biophys* 430:127–34.

Whitehead AJ, Mares JA, Danis RP. 2006. Macular pigment: a review of current knowledge. *Arch Opthalmol* 124:1038–45.

Willcox JK, Ash SL, Catignani GL. (2004). Antioxidants and prevention of chronic disease. *Crit Rev Food Sci Nutr* 44:275–95.

World Cancer Research Fund (WCRF)/American Institute for Cancer Research (AICR). 2007. *Food, nutrition, and the prevention of cancer: a global perspective.* Washington DC: AICRF.

Wright ME, Mayne ST, Swanson CA, Sinha R, Alavanja MCR. 2003. Dietary carotenoids, vegetables, and lung cancer risk in women: the Missouri Women's Health Study (United States). *Cancer Causes Control* 14:85–96.

Xu X-R, Zou Z-Y, Huang Y-M, Xiao X, Ma L, Lin X-M. 2012. Serum carotenoids in relation to risk factors for the development of atherosclerosis. *Clin Biochem* 45:1357–61.

Yoshida H, Yanai H, Ito K, Toomo Y, Koikeda T, Tsukahara H, Tada N. 2010. Administration of natural astaxanthin increases serum HDL-cholesterol and adinopectin in subjects with mild hyperlipidemia. *Atherosclerosis* 209:520–3.

Young AJ, Lowe GM. 2001. Antioxidant and prooxidant properties of carotenoids. *Arch Biochem Biophys* 385:20–7.

Yuan J-M, Stram DO, Arakawa K, Lee H-P, Yu MC. 2003. Dietary cryptoxanthin and reduced risk of lung cancer: the Singapore Chinese Health Study. *Cancer Epidemiol Biomarkers Prev* 12:890–8.

Index

Food Carotenoids: Chemistry, Biology, and Technology, First Edition. Delia B. Rodriguez-Amaya.